BSAVA Manual of Canine and Feline Endocrinology
fifth edition

Editors:

Carmel T. Mooney
MVB MPhil PhD DipECVIM-CA MRCVS
Small Animal Clinical Studies, School of Veterinary Medicine,
University College Dublin, Stillorgan Road, Belfield, Dublin 4, Ireland

Mark E. Peterson
DVM DipACVIM
Animal Endocrine Clinic,
21 W 100th Street, New York, NY 10025, USA

Robert E. Shiel
MVB ProfDipUTL PhD DipECVIM-CA
School of Veterinary Medicine, Murdoch University,
Loneragan Building, Murdoch WA 6150, Australia

Published by:

British Small Animal Veterinary Association
Woodrow House, 1 Telford Way, Waterwells Business Park,
Quedgeley, Gloucester GL2 2AB

A Company Limited by Guarantee in England
Registered Company No. 2837793
Registered as a Charity

Save 15% off the digital version of this manual. By purchasing this print edition we are pleased to offer you a reduced price on online access at www.bsavalibrary.com • Enter offer code 15END508 on checkout

Please note the discount only applies to a purchase of the full online version of the *BSAVA Manual of Canine and Feline Endocrinology, 5th edition* via **www.bsavalibrary.com**. The discount will be taken off the BSAVA member price or full price, depending on your member status. The discount code is for a single purchase of the online version and is for your personal use only. If you do not already have a login for the BSAVA website you will need to register in order to make a purchase.

Printed in the UK by Cambrian Printers Ltd, Dowlais CF48 3TD.

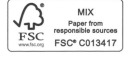

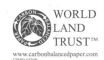

WORLD LAND TRUST™
www.carbonbalancedpaper.com
CBP019708

Carbon Balancing is delivered by World Land Trust, an international conservation charity, who protects the world's most biologically important and threatened habitats acre by acre. Their Carbon Balanced Programme offsets emissions through the purchase and preservation of high conservation value forests.

Titles in the BSAVA Manuals series

For further information on these and all BSAVA publications, please visit our website: **www.bsava.com**

Contents

Contributors

Ellen Behrend
VMD PhD DipACVIM(SAIM)
Department of Clinical Sciences,
College of Veterinary Medicine,
Auburn University, USA

Ghita Benchekroun
DMV PhD DipECVIM-CA
Ecole Nationale Vétérinaire d'Alfort,
CHUVA, Unité de médecine interne,
Maisons Alfort, F-94700, France

Alisdair Boag
BSc BVetMed PhD DipECVIM-CA MRCVS
Royal (Dick) School of Veterinary Studies,
The University of Edinburgh, Easter Bush Campus,
Midlothian EH25 9RG

Amanda K. Boag
MA VetMB DipECVECC DipACVECC DipACVIM FHEA FRCVS
IVC Evidensia,
The Chocolate Factory, Keynsham,
Bristol BS31 2AU

Miguel Campos
DVM PhD DipECVIM

Rosario Cerundolo
DVM CertVD DipECVD FRCVS
Dick White Referrals,
Veterinary Specialist Centre, Station Farm,
London Road, Six Mile Bottom,
Cambridgeshire CB8 0UH

Sylvie Daminet
DVM PhD DipACVIM DipECVIM-CA
Companion Animal Clinic,
University of Ghent, Salisburylane 133,
9820, Belgium

Lucy J. Davison
MA VetMB PhD DSAM DipECVIM-CA MRCVS
Department of Clinical Science and Services,
Royal Veterinary College, London

Luca Ferasin
DVM PhD CertVC PGCert(HE) DipECVIM-CA(Cardiology)
GPCert(B&PS) FRCVS
Specialist Veterinary Cardiology Consultancy,
Four Marks, Hampshire

Samuel Fowlie
BSc(Hons) BVSc(Hons) MVM DipECVIM-CA MRCVS
Southfields Veterinary Specialists,
Cranes Point, Gardiners Lane South,
Basildon SS14 3AP

Federico Fracassi
DVM PhD DipECVIM-CA
Department of Veterinary Medical Sciences,
University of Bologna,
Ozzano dell'Emilia, Italy

Sara Galac
DVM PhD
Department of Clinical Sciences,
Faculty of Veterinary Medicine,
Utrecht University, Heidelberglaan 8
3584 CS Utrecht, The Netherlands

Susan Gottlieb
BVSc BSc BAppSc MANZCVS
The Cat Clinic,
Brisbane, Queensland, Australia

Peter A. Graham
BVMS PhD CertVR SFHEA DipECVCP MRCVS
School of Veterinary Medicine and Science,
The University of Nottingham, College Road,
Stanford, Sutton Bonington, Loughborough LE12 5RD

Eilidh Gunn
BVMS DVMS DipECVIM-CA MRCVS
North Downs Specialist Referrals,
Brewerstreet Dairy Business Park, Brewer Street,
Bletchingley RH1 4QP

Michael E. Herrtage
MA BVSc DVSc DVetMed(h.c.) DVR DVD DSAM DipECVIM-CA
DipECVDI FRCVS
Department of Veterinary Medicine,
University of Cambridge, Madingley Road,
Cambridge CB3 0ES

Hans S. Kooistra
DVM PhD DipECVIM-CA
Department of Clinical Sciences,
Faculty of Veterinary Medicine, Utrecht University,
Heidelberglaan 8, 3584 CS Utrecht,
The Netherlands

Patty Lathan
VMD MS DipACVIM
College of Veterinary Medicine,
Mississippi State University,
MS 39762, USA

Carlos Melián
DVM PhD Acre. AVEPA Internal Medicine
Veterinary Teaching Hospital,
School of Veterinary Medicine,
University Las Palmas de Gran Canaria,
Trasmontaña, Arucas, Spain

Richard Mellanby
BSc BVMS PhD DSAM DipECVIM-CA FRSE FRCVS
Royal (Dick) School of Veterinary Studies,
The University of Edinburgh, Easter Bush Campus,
Midlothian EH25 9RG

Carmel T. Mooney
MVB MPhil PhD DipECVIM-CA MRCVS
Small Animal Clinical Studies,
School of Veterinary Medicine, University College Dublin,
Stillorgan Road, Belfield, Dublin 4, Ireland

Kevin Murtagh
MVB CertSAM DipECVIM-CA MRCVS
School of Veterinary Medicine,
University College Dublin, Stillorgan Road,
Belfield, Dublin 4, Ireland

Stijn Niessen
DVM PhD DipECVIM PGCert VetEd FHEA MRCVS
Royal Veterinary College,
University of London,
North Mymms AL9 7TA

Laura Pérez-López
DVM MSc PhD
Biomedical and Health Research Institute,
University Las Palmas de Gran Canaria,
Las Palmas de Gran Canaria, Spain

Mark E. Peterson
DVM DipACVIM
Animal Endocrine Clinic,
21 W 100th Street, New York, NY 10025, USA

Ian K. Ramsey
BVSc PhD DSAM DipECVIM FHEA FRCVS
Small Animal Hospital,
University of Glasgow, 464 Bearsden Road,
Bearsden, Glasgow G61 1QH

Jacquie Rand
BVSc DVSc MANZCVS DipACVIM
School of Veterinary Science,
The University of Queensland, Gatton 4343,
Queensland, Australia

Johan P. Schoeman
BVSc MMedVet PhD DSAM DipECVIM-CA FRCVS
Department of Companion Animal Clinical Studies,
Faculty of Veterinary Science, University of Pretoria,
M35, Onderstepoort, Pretoria, 0110, South Africa

Robert E. Shiel
MVB ProfDipUTL PhD DipECVIM-CA
School of Veterinary Medicine,
Murdoch University, Loneragan Building,
Murdoch WA 6150, Australia

Barbara J. Skelly
MA VetMB PhD CertSAM DipACVIM DipECVIM-CA AFHEA MRCVS
Queen's Veterinary School Hospital,
Department of Veterinary Medicine, University of
Cambridge, Madingley Road, Cambridge CB3 0ES

Annemarie M.W.Y. Voorbij
DVM PhD DipECVIM-CA
Department of Clinical Sciences,
Faculty of Veterinary Medicine,
Utrecht University, Heidelberglaan 8
3584 CS Utrecht, The Netherlands

Brett Wasik
DVM DipACVIM(SAIM)
Canine Internal Medicine, Endocrinology,
Veterinary Information Network, 777 W. Covell Blvd.,
Davis, CA 95616, USA

Tim Williams
MA VetMB PhD AFHEA FRCPath DipECVCP MRCVS
Department of Veterinary Medicine,
University of Cambridge, Madingley Road,
Cambridge CB3 0ES

Panagiotis G. Xenoulis
DVM DrMedVet PhD
Clinic of Medicine,
Faculty of Veterinary Medicine, University of Thessaly,
Trikalon, 224, 43100 Karditsa, Greece

Foreword

I was honoured to be asked to write this foreword for this newest edition of the *BSAVA Manual of Canine and Feline Endocrinology*.

Endocrinology is endlessly fascinating, sitting as it does at the interface of physiology and clinical medicine. Excessive or inadequate secretion of a single hormone can cause multisystemic clinical signs resulting in a complex clinical picture that needs to be unravelled by the discerning clinician. That complexity, however, can be off-putting for the busy small animal clinician in general practice, given the time pressures that they are often working under. This book helps to address this by being both comprehensive and accessible. The level of detail given, and the consistency in the layout of the chapters, makes it easy to find information when researching an individual case quickly between consults. As a complete text though it can also be studied more completely and would be invaluable to those studying for certificate exams as well as highly performing veterinary students.

The editors, Carmel Mooney, Mark Peterson and Robert Shiel, as well as contributing their own expertise to write key chapters, have assembled an acclaimed group of authors from around the globe. They are commended for managing to harness the detailed knowledge of each of the contributors without swamping the reader with excessive levels of detail. The book is laid out in a logical fashion with initial chapters on the principles of hormone synthesis, action and endocrine testing. There is also a new chapter on the genetics of endocrine disease, an emerging field in veterinary endocrinology. Chapters on the systemic effects of endocrine disease are next, followed by individual endocrine diseases or clinical presentations.

This book belongs in every small animal veterinary practice. I am sure that I will refer to my copy often.

Harriet Syme
BSc BVetMed PhD FHEA DipACVIM DipECVIM MRCVS
Professor of Small Animal Internal Medicine
The Royal Veterinary College, London

Preface

This is the fifth edition of the *BSAVA Manual of Canine and Feline Endocrinology*. It is over 10 years since the last edition was published and the advances in our knowledge of endocrine diseases continue unabated. As with so many projects, the COVID-19 pandemic intervened and delayed our progress to completion. Even during the final production of the Manual, new discoveries were made and, while we may have limited in-depth knowledge of some of them, we were able to introduce their inherent concepts – who would have thought of an oral drug enhancing renal excretion of glucose for diabetic cats or the possibility of a once-weekly insulin injection for dogs?

We have modified the structure of the Manual to enhance its suitability for clinical practice. The first section provides the reader with information on the aetiology of endocrine diseases and principles for interpreting endocrine test results. This section covers sample handling, providing easy access to relevant advice. It is followed by several chapters dedicated to how endocrine diseases affect other organ systems such as the cardiovascular and renal systems, lipid metabolism and the skin. Testament to the growing importance of this field, there is a chapter dedicated to the genetics of endocrine disease. The next 26 chapters focus on individual endocrine glands and their inherent diseases. Where applicable there are separate chapters on the dog or cat. If relevant to an endocrine gland, chapters are included on solving associated problems (e.g. polyuria/polydipsia, hypo- and hypercalcaemia, hypo- and hyperglycaemia and unstable diabetes). Finally, the remaining chapters are dedicated to investigating whether multiple endocrine neoplasia or autoimmune polyglandular syndromes exist in dogs or cats, and erythropoietin excess and gastrointestinal endocrine tumours.

The Manual has only been possible with the support of the 34 contributing authors who emanate from Europe, Australia and the USA. They have each been a pleasure to work with and we are grateful for their invaluable input. Their varied areas of expertise and geographical location contribute to the international appeal of the Manual.

The new edition of the *BSAVA Manual of Canine and Feline Endocrinology* provides the reader with the most up to date information available. Like other Manuals in this series, it provides a valuable resource not just to those with a general interest in small animal internal medicine but also to those with a specific interest in endocrinology, be they veterinary practitioners, veterinary nurses, technicians or undergraduate students. We hope that you find it a modern addition to your library.

Carmel T. Mooney, Mark E. Peterson and Robert E. Shiel
June 2023

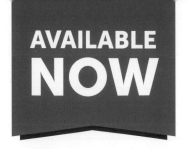
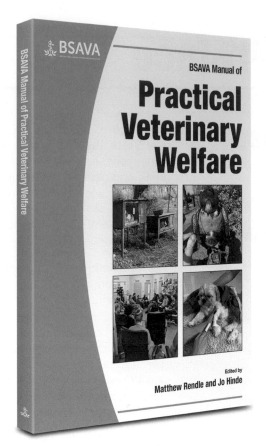

Chapter 1

Principles of endocrine disease

Hans S. Kooistra

Introduction

The classical or traditional subject of endocrinology deals with glands that produce hormones. The term 'hormone' is derived from the Greek word *ormao*, which is the verb for 'excite' or 'arouse'. Indeed, hormones are agents that stimulate activity in different parts of the body after they have been released into the bloodstream by an endocrine cell. The word 'endocrine' contrasts the actions of substances secreted internally into the bloodstream with those secreted externally (exocrine) into ducts such as the lumen of the gastrointestinal tract.

Endocrinology is part of what is often referred to as intercellular communication. Classical or traditional endocrinology deals with the endocrine glands, which produce hormones that are released into the systemic circulation and interact with target cells expressing specific receptors for these hormones (Figure 1.1). However, the capacity to form hormones is not limited to endocrine glands. The traditional view of the endocrine system's glandular nature has broadened to include production of hormones in specialized endocrine cells scattered in organs whose primary function is not endocrine, such as the stomach, the small intestine, the heart, the kidneys and adipose tissue.

Modern endocrinology now includes hormones that are not primarily released into the systemic circulation. Examples include hormones that circulate primarily in restricted compartments, such as the releasing and inhibiting factors in the hypothalamic–pituitary portal system. Modern endocrinology also deals with hormones that are secreted into the interstitial fluid to act on adjacent cells (paracrine effect) or on the cell of origin (autocrine effect) (Figure 1.2). Hormones may even have an effect within the cell of origin (intracrine effect). Many hormones, of which insulin is an example, have both paracrine actions in the tissues in which they are formed and classical endocrine actions at peripheral sites. Other forms of intercellular communication studied by endocrinologists include exocrine secretion (e.g. in milk and semen) and the release of pheromones (in air or water).

There are strong similarities in signalling mechanisms between the endocrine and nervous systems. The same molecule can act as both a hormone and a neurotransmitter. For example, catecholamines are hormones when released by the adrenal medulla and neurotransmitters when released by nerve terminals.

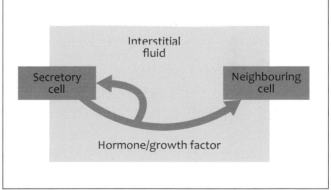

1.2 Schematic illustration of paracrine and autocrine effects. Endocrine cells produce hormones that are secreted into the interstitial fluid to act on neighbouring cells (paracrine effect) or on the cell of origin (autocrine effect).

Hormone groups

Hormones can be divided into two major groups: hydrophilic and lipophilic. The hydrophilic hormones contain amino acids and include proteins (including glycoproteins), peptides or peptide derivatives (e.g. arginine vasopressin), and amino acid analogues (e.g. adrenaline (epinephrine) and noradrenaline (norepinephrine)). Polypeptide hormones are direct translation products of specific messenger RNA (mRNA) sequences, cleavage products of larger precursor proteins or modified peptides. They can be as small as thyrotropin-releasing hormone (three amino acids) or as

1.1 Schematic illustration of the endocrine system. The endocrine glands produce hormones that are released into the systemic circulation and interact with target cells expressing specific receptors for these hormones.

large and complex as growth hormone and follicle-stimulating hormone, which each contain approximately 200 amino acid residues.

The lipophilic hormones are mainly derived from cholesterol or fatty acids. The thyroid hormones, derived from the amino acid tyrosine, are an exception to this rule, because of the lipophilic character of tyrosine. Hormones derived from cholesterol may have an intact steroid nucleus, as in the steroid hormones from the gonads and the adrenal cortex, or a steroid nucleus with an open B ring, as in vitamin D and its metabolites. Retinoids, prostaglandins, leucotrienes and thromboxanes are derived from fatty acids (Figure 1.3).

Hormone signalling and action

The majority of hydrophilic hormones are transported in blood without binding to specific proteins. This explains the plasma half-life of only a few minutes for most of the non-glycosylated peptide hormones. The more insoluble a hormone is in water, the more important the role of its transport protein. Thyroid and steroid hormones are largely transported in the circulation bound to proteins, which partly explains their relatively long half-life compared with the hydrophilic hormones. Protein-bound hormones cannot enter cells *per se* but serve as a reservoir from which free hormone is liberated for cellular uptake. The distribution

Amines

Noradrenaline

Tripeptides

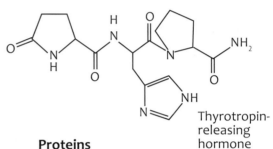

Thyrotropin-releasing hormone

Polypeptides

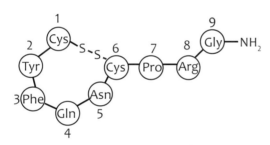

Vasopressin

Proteins

H_2N

COOH

Growth hormone

Steroids

Cortisol

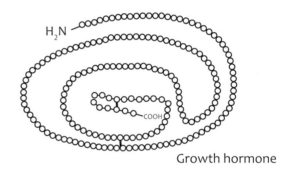

1,25-dihydroxycholecalciferol

Retinoids

Vitamin A$_1$ (retinol)

Prostaglandins

Prostaglandin F$_{2\alpha}$ (PGF$_{2\alpha}$)

1.3 Examples of different types of hormones.
(Reproduced from Rijnberk and Kooistra (2010) with permission)

between bound and free hormone in plasma is determined by the concentration of the hormone and the concentration, affinity and capacity of the proteins that bind it. The free hormone enters and interacts with its specific receptor in target cells and participates in the regulatory feedback mechanisms. Hence, changes in the concentration of transport proteins can cause considerable changes in the total hormone concentration in plasma without producing signs of hormone deficiency or excess. If the regulatory feedback mechanisms that control hormone synthesis are intact, they maintain the concentration of free hormone within a fixed (normal) range.

Hormones exert their effects by binding to specific receptors, which can be in the cell membrane or intracellular. Hydrophilic hormones operate via receptors located in the cell membrane. Activated cell-surface receptors often activate second messengers, which amplify and pass on the molecular information. Alternatively, activated cell-surface receptors may change the function of ion channels in the cell membrane. Many hydrophilic hormones ultimately signal via regulation of protein phosphorylation. This allows hydrophilic hormones to rapidly change the conformation and thus the function of existing cell enzymes (i.e. enzyme activation or inactivation).

Lipophilic hormones act via intracellular receptors. Small amounts of (free) lipophilic hormones are transported into the cytosol and bind to specific receptor proteins to form a hormone–receptor complex. This complex can bind to (positive and negative) response elements in promoter regions of genes in chromosomal DNA, thereby acting as a regulator of gene transcription. As a result, the formation of mRNA is increased or decreased and thus the synthesis and secretion of proteins (enzymes, hormones) is enhanced or suppressed. Consequently, the effect of lipophilic hormones is usually slower but longer lasting than that of hydrophilic hormones. However, apart from this classical genomic mechanism of lipophilic hormone action, lipophilic hormones can also mediate rapid effects by non-genomic mechanisms, for example, by interaction with a membrane-bound receptor.

Endocrine disorders

Endocrine disorders can be divided into the following broad categories, most of which can be further subdivided:

- **Primary hypofunction** – if the endocrine glands are injured or destroyed by autoimmune disorders, neoplasia, infection or haemorrhage, the resulting hypofunction is said to be primary. Primary hypofunction may also be due to agenesis of an endocrine gland, or it may be iatrogenic (e.g. gonadal hypofunction resulting from castration)
- **Dyshormonogenesis** – this is a special form of primary hypofunction. Genetic defects, for example, resulting in an enzyme defect, can cause abnormalities in hormone synthesis. Occasionally, this leads to both hormone deficiency and manifestations of a compensatory adaptation, such as goitre resulting from defective thyroid hormone synthesis and ensuing hypersecretion of thyrotropin (thyroid-stimulating hormone (TSH)). Another example of dyshormonogenesis is iodine deficiency resulting in primary hypothyroidism and goitre
- **Secondary hypofunction** – endocrine hypofunction can also be due to inadequate stimulation of the endocrine gland and is then said to be secondary. An example is secondary hypothyroidism resulting from a deficiency of TSH as a consequence of a pituitary disorder

- **Primary hyperfunction** – if the endocrine glands autonomously secrete excessive amounts of hormones, often because of neoplasia, the resulting hyperfunction is said to be primary (Figure 1.4a). An example is primary hyperaldosteronism as a result of an adrenocortical tumour

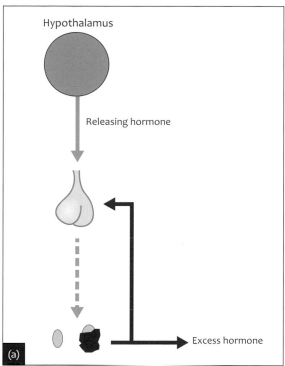

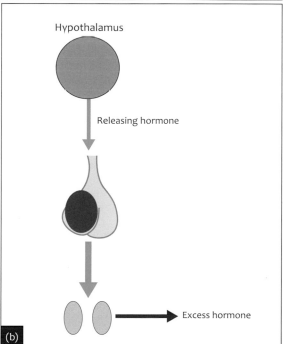

1.4 Generalized hypothalamic–pituitary system and related endocrine glands. (a) Primary hyperfunction. The neoplastic endocrine gland secretes excess hormone into the systemic circulation (red arrows), resulting in clinical signs. In addition, the high plasma hormone concentration provides negative feedback on the hypothalamic–pituitary system, resulting in low tropic hormone secretion by the pituitary (dashed green arrow) and subsequent atrophy of the non-neoplastic endocrine gland. (b) Secondary hyperfunction. The neoplastic pituitary gland secretes excess tropic hormone into the systemic circulation. Consequently, the related endocrine glands secrete excess hormone into the systemic circulation, resulting in clinical signs and, eventually, hyperplastic glands.

- **Secondary hyperfunction** – endocrine hyperfunction can also be due to hyperstimulation of the endocrine gland and is then said to be secondary (Figure 1.4b). An example is secondary hypercortisolism due to excessive secretion of adrenocorticotropic hormone (ACTH) by a corticotropic adenoma in the pituitary gland
- **Paraneoplastic endocrine hyperfunction** – excessive hormone production may also be traced to cells that are not normally the primary source of circulating hormone. An example is hypercalcaemia due to secretion of parathyroid hormone-related peptide into the systemic circulation by an adenocarcinoma of the anal sac
- **Ectopic receptors** – expression of receptors in an endocrine gland that does not normally harbour receptors of this type may also result in endocrine hyperfunction. A similar outcome can result from altered activity of eutopic receptors. For example, the adrenal cortex may express aberrant receptors such as gastric inhibitory polypeptide receptors, which may result in food-dependent hypercortisolism in dogs
- **Iatrogenic disease** – when hormones are used to treat non-endocrine diseases or when hormone replacement for an endocrine deficiency is excessive, the resulting syndrome of hormone excess is said to be iatrogenic. An example is secondary hypercortisolism as a consequence of treatment of an immune-mediated disorder with pharmacological dosages of prednisolone. Similarly, excessive treatment of endocrine hyperfunction with an inhibitor may result in iatrogenic hypofunction. For example, treatment of cats with hyperthyroidism with too high a dosage of thiamazole may result in iatrogenic hypothyroidism
- **Resistance to hormone action** – hormone resistance is defined as a defect in the capacity of normal target tissues to respond to a hormone. It may be an inherited disorder involving one or more molecular deviations, including abnormalities in receptors or post-receptor mechanisms. Hormone resistance may also be acquired, as is insulin resistance in some forms of diabetes mellitus. A common feature of hormone resistance is an increased concentration of the hormone in the circulation in the presence of diminished or absent hormone action
- **Abnormalities that do not impair function** – these include tumours, cysts and infiltrative diseases that do not lead to significant impairment of hormone secretion.

Recognition of endocrine disorders in the clinical setting

Recognition or diagnosis requires several pieces of evidence taken concurrently. The primary indication for pursuing a diagnosis of an endocrine disorder is the presence of one or more clinical signs; a thorough history and physical examination are crucial. Failure to identify multiple indicators for an endocrine disorder does not rule out endocrine disease. However, the more abnormalities identified, the stronger the indication to pursue testing.

Historical and clinical features

When an endocrine disorder is suspected, the diagnostic process is hampered by the inaccessibility for physical examination of all of the endocrine glands except the thyroid and parathyroid glands and testes. However,

deranged hormone secretion has consequences for the function of other organ systems, usually leading to multiple abnormalities that often result in characteristic features. The diagnosis of an endocrine disease thus often begins with the recognition of these features in the medical history and physical examination (Rijnberk and Kooistra, 2009).

Many syndromes of hormone excess or deficiency lead to manifestations that are readily apparent at the time of the initial presentation of the animal. Especially now that a definitive diagnosis can often be secured by laboratory data, veterinary surgeons (veterinarians) have learned to recognize the physical characteristics of endocrine disorders. Nevertheless, in some cases the changes are subtle and it is necessary to rely on laboratory testing and diagnostic imaging. This is especially true when an endocrine disease is being considered in the differential diagnosis of non-specific presenting problems such as polyuria and polydipsia, weakness, lethargy, and weight loss or gain.

Basal hormone concentrations

Increased or decreased basal hormone concentrations are theoretically synonymous with endocrine hyper- and hypofunction, respectively. However, often basal plasma hormone concentrations do not accurately reflect the true functional status of an endocrine organ. There are several reasons for caution in assessing isolated measurements of circulating hormone concentration:

- Several hormones are secreted in a pulsatile manner (Figure 1.5) and/or their circulating concentrations may exhibit a circadian or diurnal rhythm
- Some hormones are secreted in restricted compartments, such as the hypothalamic–pituitary portal system, and do not reach the systemic circulation in appreciable quantities
- Steroid and thyroid hormones are transported in plasma largely bound to proteins. The small percentage of unbound hormone exerts the biological effect, but often the total plasma hormone concentration is determined. The total plasma hormone concentration reflects the concentration of free hormone only if the concentration and the affinity of the binding protein remain constant or fluctuate within narrow limits

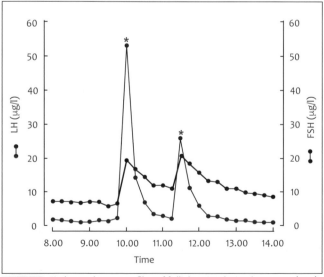

1.5 Six-hour plasma profiles of follicle-stimulating hormone (FSH) and luteinizing hormone (LH) in a 3-year-old Beagle bitch. Asterisks indicate significant pulses of both FSH and LH.

- Hormones may be activated outside the endocrine organs, e.g. by proteolytic cleavage of protein prohormones in the vascular bed or inside the target cell. Consequently, determination of the plasma concentration of an inactive prohormone, such as angiotensin I in the renin–angiotensin–aldosterone system, may not provide relevant information regarding the endocrine system
- The range of reference values for most hormones is fairly broad. Thus, it is possible for the concentration in an individual animal to double or to decrease by half and yet still be in the reference interval. For this reason it is often useful to measure the concentrations of a related pair of hormones simultaneously (e.g. thyroxine and TSH)
- Reference intervals are usually determined for the general animal population and do not necessarily consider the effects of age, breed, sex, nutritional status, concurrent illnesses, sexual cycle or pregnancy (see Chapter 4)
- Paracrine, autocrine and intracrine effects of hormones are usually not reflected by circulating hormone concentrations
- Exocrine secretion of hormones and the release of pheromones cannot be determined by measuring the hormone concentration in plasma/serum.

Dynamic endocrine tests

Dynamic testing may be very helpful in the diagnostic process if the basal hormone concentration does not truly reflect the functional status of an endocrine organ. Dynamic testing involves either stimulation or suppression of endogenous hormone production. Stimulation tests are utilized most often when hypofunction of an endocrine organ is suspected. In the most commonly employed stimulation tests, a tropic hormone is administered to test the capacity of a target gland to increase hormone production. The tropic hormone can be a hypothalamic releasing hormone such as corticotropin-releasing hormone (CRH), in which case the target gland is the pituitary and the measured response is the increment in the plasma ACTH concentration, or a pituitary hormone such as ACTH, with the adrenal cortex as the target gland being assessed by measurement of the increment in the circulating cortisol concentration. Suppression tests are utilized when endocrine hyperfunction is suspected; they are designed to determine whether negative feedback control is intact. A hormone or other regulatory substance is administered, and the inhibition of endogenous hormone secretion is assessed. An example is the dexamethasone suppression test used when hypercortisolism is suspected.

Diagnostic imaging

The inaccessibility of most of the endocrine glands for direct physical examination has been progressively overcome over the past decades through the use of diagnostic imaging techniques such as ultrasonography, scintigraphy, computed tomography and magnetic resonance imaging. The first technique is relatively inexpensive but requires extensive operator experience, whereas the latter three may be easier to perform but require expensive equipment as well as immobilization of the patient, which necessitates sedation or anaesthesia.

References and further reading

Rijnberk A and Kooistra HS (2009) Endocrine glands. In: *Medical History and Physical Examination in Companion Animals, 2nd edn*, ed. A Rijnberk and FJ van Sluijs, pp. 207–212. Elsevier, Oxford

Rijnberk A and Kooistra HS (2010) Introduction. In: *Clinical Endocrinology of Dogs and Cats, 2nd edn*. Ed. A Rijnberk and HS Kooistra, pp. 3–12. Schlütersche Verlagsgesellschaft mbH & Co, Hanover

Chapter 2

The genetics of endocrine disease

Lucy Davison

Glossary

Alleles: Alternative versions of a DNA sequence at a particular locus.

Codon: A sequence of three nucleotides that codes for a specific amino acid or indicates the start or stop of translation.

Exon: A region of a gene that is transcribed into messenger RNA, some of which encodes the amino acid sequence.

Genetic variant: A change in the DNA sequence (e.g. single nucleotide polymorphism, insertion, deletion or copy number variant) that is permanent. Variation can occur within genes but also in intergenic regions.

Genotype: The alleles carried by an individual – either at a particular locus or across the whole genome.

Haplotype: A set of DNA variations that is inherited together, often because of close proximity on the same chromosome.

Intron: A region within a gene that lies in between two exons, which may have a regulatory function.

Locus: The specific fixed position on a chromosome where a particular genetic marker is located.

Nucleotides: The base units that make up the building blocks of DNA, comprising adenine (A), thymine (T), guanine (G) and cytosine (C).

Phenotype: The observable physical or behavioural properties of an organism, tissue or cell, determined by a combination of genotype and environment.

Single nucleotide polymorphism (SNP): The most common form of genetic variation resulting from a change in the nucleotide code at a single site. May be found in exons, introns or intergenic regions.

Introduction

Every individual is the product of their genes and their environment. This chapter reviews the ways in which genetic variation can contribute to the risk of endocrine disease, the tools available to identify risk-associated genes and variants, and the endocrine conditions in dogs and cats for which some aspects of the genetic basis of risk are already understood.

Determination of the genetic basis of endocrine disease

Investigation of the genetic basis of a disease usually begins with the observation that the disease occurs more commonly in related individuals. These individuals may be as closely related as members of the same litter, may be from the same breed or may share a common ancestor. There are many known susceptibilities to endocrine disorders in specific dog breeds, and a small number of similar observations have been made in cats.

From a genetic research perspective, it is also important to study breeds from the same species in which a specific disease is present at a particularly low prevalence, as these breeds may hold important information about genetic protection from the condition.

Examples of high- and low-risk breeds for a range of endocrine conditions are presented in Figure 2.1.

Condition	High-risk breed examples	Low-risk breed examples
Diabetes mellitus	Samoyed, Tibetan Terrier	Boxer, German Shepherd Dog, Golden Retriever
Hypercortisolism	Bichon Frise, Standard Dachshund, Yorkshire Terrier	Labrador Retriever, German Shepherd Dog
Hyperparathyroidism	Keeshond, Beagle	
Hypoadrenocorticism	Bearded Collie, Labradoodle, Standard Poodle	
Hypothyroidism	Purebred dogs, Boxer, Labrador Retriever, Giant Schnauzer	Crossbreed dogs
Pituitary dwarfism	German Shepherd Dog	
Insulinoma	Boxer, West Highland White Terrier, German Shepherd Dog	

2.1 Examples of high- and low-risk breeds for endocrine conditions in dogs.

BSAVA Manual of Canine and Feline Endocrinology, fifth edition. Edited by Carmel T. Mooney, Mark E. Peterson and Robert E. Shiel. ©BSAVA 2023

The importance of investigating the genetics of endocrine disease

A deeper understanding of the genetic elements of endocrine disease can inform clinical decisions and improve outcomes.

- **Precision screening and preventive healthcare** – identifying the genes and pathways involved in disease susceptibility improves understanding of pathogenesis. This could lead to the discovery of novel treatment or preventive targets for endocrine disorders. Understanding risk factors enables targeted screening for early identification of disease and helps stratify populations by underlying risk when analysing clinical trials.
- **Breeding** – although the impact of genetic variants on disease risk varies, genetic testing for informed breeding is very effective in preventing diseases caused by a monogenic disease-causing variant.
- **Precision medicine** – advanced genetic testing has facilitated more precisely targeted and effective treatment of conditions such as neonatal diabetes mellitus, thyroid cancer and phaeochromocytoma in humans. Similar studies of endocrine genetics might also be transformational for the treatment of endocrine disease in veterinary species.

As well as the delivery of benefits for veterinary species, findings that could be translated to human health may arise from the study of veterinary endocrine genetics. This includes highlighting the importance of novel pathways in pathogenesis and identification of genes of unknown function for further study.

Mechanisms by which genes may affect disease risk

Monogenic *versus* complex disease

In monogenic diseases, a variation or mutation in a single gene results in the condition developing, typically in a dominant or recessive fashion. Every chromosome carries one copy of each gene, and one copy of each chromosome is inherited from each parent. If the variant has a dominant effect, then one copy, from one parent, is enough to cause the disease. If a recessive variant is associated with disease, an individual must inherit two copies of the variant – one from each parent – to be affected with the disease. In such a recessive model, heterozygous 'carriers' are clinically unaffected.

The majority of endocrine diseases with a genetic basis are described as 'complex' because the genetic risk results from multiple variants of small effect, combined with an unknown number of environmental influences. The role of the environment in human autoimmune endocrine diseases such as type 1 diabetes mellitus is demonstrated by the disease concordance in genetically identical twins being less than 100%, as well as by a range of studies evaluating environmental factors. The role of environmental triggers in canine and feline endocrine disorders is less well explored, apart from the clear relationship between obesity and diabetes mellitus in cats.

Types of variation and their impact

The genome of an individual is unique and contains millions of small variations, some of which may have a direct or indirect functional impact on the protein they encode. The precise impact of a variation on the function of a gene depends on a number of factors, including the nature of the variation and its location within or outside the protein-coding region of a gene.

Endocrine disorders are typically divided into hyperfunctional and hypofunctional states and can arise through a variety of mechanisms, including congenital abnormalities of organ development, hyperplasia, neoplasia, impaired hormone production, impaired transport or signalling, autoimmunity, and other mechanisms of endocrine tissue damage or necrosis. Genetic variations can contribute to all of these mechanisms.

Genetic variants are usually inherited from parents but can also be acquired (somatic mutations), for example, during neoplastic processes. Sometimes, important variations for endocrine disease risk are found in genes proximal to the endocrine system itself (e.g. thyroid-stimulating hormone receptor mutations) but they can also be present in genes involved in pathways relevant to specific disease development (e.g. the immune system in autoimmune disorders).

Single nucleotide polymorphism

Single nucleotide polymorphisms are among the most common forms of variation in the genome, with millions already catalogued. If an SNP falls in an exon, and changes the amino acid sequence of a protein, it is known as a non-synonymous SNP (nsSNP); if it does not change the amino acid sequence, it is a known as a synonymous SNP (sSNP). Non-synonymous SNPs may impact on disease risk because the amino acid change can alter the function of a protein. However, SNPs may also have an important effect on disease risk by changing the function of a regulatory region. The regulatory effect of SNPs may be apparent only in certain tissues or at certain times in development, so may be very challenging to identify. Many SNPs in the dog and cat genome have now been described, and knowledge of SNP maps has been crucial in understanding normal variation within species.

Insertion/deletion

Insertion/deletion (INDEL) variations are insertions or deletions in the genome and can be difficult to discover by some commonly used genomic analysis techniques. The consequences of INDELs depend on their size and location, but they can generally impact on gene function in a similar way to SNPs.

Structural variant

Structural variants include copy number variants (CNVs) and variations in the length of repetitive sequences known as short and long interspersed retrotransposable elements (SINEs and LINEs). Similar to some types of INDEL, these can be challenging to identify and can impact on the function or transcription of nearby genes, depending on where they are located. Larger rearrangements of whole sections of chromosome are also possible (e.g. inversions).

Epigenetics and imprinting

Epigenetic changes refer to external modifications of DNA as a result of environmental influences that may impact gene expression or function without alteration of the genetic sequence itself. These heritable changes depend on a range of factors including gestational and neonatal environment, ageing, and exposure to toxins and micro-organisms. Epigenetic changes include methylation of DNA as well as modification of the proteins (histones) around which DNA is wrapped, both of which prevent gene transcription. Non-coding RNA sequences are also encoded within the genomic DNA; whilst not translated into protein, these can influence gene expression, for example, by attaching to protein-encoding RNA sequences. Most epigenetic changes are not detected by standard DNA sequencing techniques.

In a small number of regions of the genome, only genes from one parent are expressed – a process known as genomic imprinting. For some genes, only the paternal copy is expressed and for others, only the maternal copy. In humans, imprinted genes can affect the risk of endo-crinopathies, but this has not yet been investigated in veterinary species.

Tools

It is important for clinicians to understand the strengths and limitations of different tools for studying the genetic basis of endocrine disease.

- **Linkage studies** – these use genetic data from affected and unaffected individuals related within the same family pedigree to identify the locus of a disease-associated gene. Such studies are only effective for monogenic disorders.
- **Candidate gene studies** – these use polymerase chain reaction (PCR)-based 'Sanger' sequencing to determine the DNA sequence of a particular gene that is hypothesized to be associated with disease risk.
- **Genome-wide association studies (GWASs)** – these involve analysing thousands of SNPs across the genome in many cases and controls, using 'SNP chips' to determine whether a particular allele of any SNP is present at a higher frequency in the diseased or control population. This technique associates a region of the genome with a disease but a lot more work is needed to 'fine-map' the signal and determine which gene in the region is responsible, and it does not allow 'new' variants to be discovered.
- **Whole-genome and whole-exome sequencing** – high-throughput sequencing technologies can sequence a whole genome in a few days to weeks and an exome (all the exons) even more rapidly, but the amount of data generated requires time-consuming specialist bioinformatics analysis and follow-up study. This also requires high-performance cluster computing capacity; however, this is becoming more rapid, efficient and cost-effective every year.
- **Functional studies** – once a region, gene or variant has been identified, further studies are usually required to confirm association with disease and to investigate causality. It can take many years to prove causality of a candidate variant at a functional level and this can be very costly.

Challenges

There are a number of challenges in the study of the genetics of endocrine disease in dogs and cats.

- **Phenocopies** – phenocopies are cases that share clinical presentations but have different underlying causes, with a different pathogenesis and potential genetic basis (e.g. diabetes mellitus related to hypercortisolism, dioestrus or pancreatitis in dogs). Careful phenotyping and grouping of clinical cases for genetic study is required, especially if multiple mechanisms may result in the same clinical diagnosis.
- **Statistical power** – most genetic studies require a large number of case and control samples, so proactive sample archiving and a collaborative approach are essential. The control population must not contain phenocopies, unrecognized or undiagnosed cases, or animals that are too young for clinical signs to appear (e.g. cats <10 years of age when studying feline hyperthyroidism).
- **Population structure** – as a result of domestication and breed formation, dogs and cats have a unique population structure characterized by high genetic variability between breeds and limited genetic variability within breeds, as well as geographical differences. Cases and controls must always be carefully selected to avoid false-positive results due to, for example, geographical differences.
- **'Fixed risk' within breeds** – where a whole breed is known to be at increased risk of a disease, this risk may affect the entire breed equally, with mainly environmental factors deciding whether an animal acquires a disease; cases and controls of a single breed may exhibit no genetic differences. To identify variants associated with a fixed high risk in a particular breed, comparisons with low-risk breeds must be made.
- **Environmental influences** – cases and controls may be genetically similar but differ in the environmental factors to which they have been exposed, which can reduce the power of genetic studies. Genetic studies need to take into account suitable covariates (e.g. body condition score) and consider that some individuals might carry a high genetic potential for a disease, yet never develop it because they do not encounter sufficient environmental triggers.
- **Normal variation** – any genetic variations discovered in a diseased individual must be considered in the context of known variations in the species. Canine and feline SNP maps are not yet complete and are not as detailed as those for humans, so it can be difficult to determine which variations in a particular animal are most signifi-cant. Collaborative approaches such as the Dog 10K genomes project and the 99 Lives Cat Genome Sequencing Initiative are working to bridge this gap.
- **Complex diseases** – the large number of variants with small but additive effects in complex diseases makes analysis very challenging. Variants can be associated with disease one by one, using statistical analysis, but it is possible that variant interactions exist such that certain haplotypes, when combined, lead to an even greater risk of disease. Examples exist of dominant protective variants that limit disease risk regardless of risk alleles of other genes. In addition, some variants that contribute to autoimmune endocrine disease risk become relevant only in certain circumstances. 'Genetic risk scores' present a potential solution in human medicine and may be an important area for further study in veterinary species.

The major histocompatibility complex

The genes encoding the major histocompatibility complex (MHC) are of particular significance to the risk of auto-immune endocrine diseases in dogs. Genes encoded within the MHC play critical roles in the regulation of the adaptive immune response. This includes involvement in immune tolerance, allowing distinction of 'self' antigens from 'non-self' antigens, and influencing the level and nature of the immune response that develops to particular antigens.

In the dog, there are four functional MHC class II genes – DLA-DRA1, -DRB1, -DQA1 and -DQB1 – known as the dog leucocyte antigen (DLA) genes. These encode cell-surface heterodimers which bind antigenic peptides in a peptide-binding groove and present them to T cells. There is potential for extreme diversity in the MHC regions because three of the canine MHC class II genes are highly polymorphic. This means that there are many different alleles and haplotypes present in the canine population, similar to human leucocyte antigen (HLA) haplotypes in humans. Notably, within some breeds, there is limited DLA diversity as a result of selective breeding, despite the wide variety of haplotypes seen across breeds. In humans, certain HLA polymorphisms are highly associated with the development of auto-immune endocrine conditions, including type 1 diabetes mellitus and hypoadrenocorticism. Particular alleles are often inherited together (in a haplotype), so the three-locus DLA haplotype terminology, describing the variation at DLA-DRB1, -DQA1 and -DQB1, is usually used to describe DLA associations with disease in dogs. An association with MHC genes implicates the adaptive immune response in the pathogenesis of a disease.

The genetic basis of specific canine and feline endocrine disorders

Canine primary hyperparathyroidism

One of the earliest genetic endocrine diseases in a single breed to receive specific attention was primary hyper-parathyroidism in the Keeshond. Here, a candidate gene approach was employed, as well as studies of segregation of the disease in certain families. Initial work ruled out certain mutations commonly associated with the disease in humans and documented autosomal dominant inheritance with age-related expression (also known as penetrance) of the disease phenotype. This work, followed by further mapping studies, eventually led to the discovery of a positional candidate for the disease, from which a commercially available genetic test was developed (Goldstein et al., 2007).

Canine pituitary dwarfism

Early reports of proportionate dwarfism in German Shepherd Dogs and pedigree analysis suggested a simple autosomal recessive monogenic inheritance (Andresen and Willeberg, 1976). More recently, this condition has been mapped by linkage analysis to a deletion in intron 5 of the LHX3 gene, leading to aberrant gene splicing and abnormal pituitary development (Voorbij et al., 2011). Subsequently, LHX3 gene mutations have been reported in association with pituitary dwarfism in additional breeds, including the Saarloos Wolfdog, Czechoslovakian Wolfdog and Tibetan Terrier (Voorbij et al., 2014; Thaiwong et al., 2021), and a genetic test is now available. More recently, a further intronic mutation in a gene called POU1F1 has been associated with pituitary dwarfism in the Karelian Bear Dog (Kyöstilä et al., 2021). Additionally, a 6-month-old Chihuahua bitch has been described with pituitary dwarfism and a deletion of six base pairs in exon five of the growth hormone gene, GH1 (Iio et al., 2020; see Chapter 12).

Canine hypothyroidism

The first genetic mutation associated with canine hypo-thyroidism was found in TPO, the gene encoding thyroid peroxidase, in a candidate gene study of congenital hypo-thyroidism of Tenterfield and Toy Fox Terriers (Fyfe et al., 2003). Since then, TPO mutations have been identified in congenital hypothyroidism in a French Bulldog (Major et al., 2015) and a Rat Terrier (Pettigrew et al., 2007). A family of Shih Tzus with congenital hypothyroidism and goitre were found to have a mutation in a different gene associated with thyroid hormone synthesis. In affected dogs, a homozygous mutation of the splice acceptor site in intron 9 of the SLC5A5 gene, encoding the sodium/iodide symporter, was identified (Arias et al., 2018).

Despite these interesting monogenic findings, most cases of canine hypothyroidism are characterized by a complex inheritance made more complicated by the heterogeneity of disease. Some dogs demonstrate lymphocytic thyroid infiltrates and autoantibodies, and others thyroid atrophy. This makes the condition challenging to study due to the potential presence of phenocopies.

Despite these challenges, phenotyping tools such as autoantibody measurements have assisted in ensuring a shared pathogenesis amongst cases undergoing genetic investigation. Unsurprisingly, the first genetic region associated with disease risk was the DLA (Kennedy et al., 2006a), where haplotypes containing the DQA1*00101 allele were found to be associated with hypothyroidism in certain breeds. The same allele was also identified in a haplotype associated with autoimmune lymphocytic thyroiditis in the Giant Schnauzer (Wilbe et al., 2010). The alleles DQB1*00201 and DQA1*00101 were subsequently associated with hypothyroidism in Gordon and English Setters, respectively (Ziener et al., 2015). More recently, another hypothyroidism-associated region on canine chromosome 12, outside the DLA gene cluster, was identified in a GWAS of the Gordon Setter, Hovawart and Rhodesian Ridgeback (Bianchi et al., 2015). These findings support an immune-mediated pathogenesis for hypothyroidism in these breeds.

Whole-genome sequencing has also been employed in the study of canine hypothyroidism in the Giant Schnauzer (Bianchi et al., 2020). A deletion falling between two predicted interferon (IFN)-alpha genes was associated with protection from hypothyroidism, although the functional impact of this variant is unclear.

Feline hyperthyroidism

The publication of the feline genome sequence has enabled tremendous advances in the study of feline genetics, although the availability of data regarding normal feline variation is still limited. Although feline hyperthyroidism is a very common disease, any underlying genetic cause remains elusive. Some breeds, such as the Burmese, Persian and Siamese, appear relatively protected from hyperthyroidism compared with non-purebred Domestic

Shorthaired cats, implying that there may be protective genetic variants fixed within certain breeds. Several candidate gene studies have attempted to examine mutations of thyroid-related genes in feline thyroid adenomas, with limited success. In some thyroid nodules, missense mutations in the *TSHR* gene and/or the Gs alpha gene have been reported, but none can explain the disease completely (Watson *et al.*, 2005). A recent feline GWAS identified an SNP on chromosome B2 that was significantly associated with hyperthyroidism in Domestic Shorthaired cats, although further work is required to fine-map this association to a causal gene (Hernandez *et al.*, 2022).

Canine hypoadrenocorticism

Early heritability work on canine hypoadrenocorticism in the Standard Poodle suggested an autosomal recessive inheritance (Famula *et al.*, 2003); however, this is now thought to be less likely. Early candidate gene studies in canine hypoadrenocorticism focused on genes associated with this condition in humans, with functions mainly in the adaptive immune system. Of the four candidate genes studied in the Nova Scotia Duck Tolling Retriever (*AIRE*, *CD28*, *CTLA4* and *PTPN22*), one – *CTLA4* – showed a weak association with disease (Hughes *et al.*, 2011). This gene was also associated with hypoadrenocorticism in a separate candidate gene study of the Cocker Spaniel, Labrador Retriever and Springer Spaniel, as were *COL4A4*, *PTPN22*, *OSBPL9* and *STXBP5* (Short *et al.*, 2013). More recently, a promoter polymorphism in *CTLA4* has been associated with hypoadrenocorticism in Springer and Cocker Spaniels (Boag *et al.*, 2020).

Further evidence for the role of the immune system in the pathogenesis of canine hypoadrenocorticism has been provided by DLA studies. The first study demonstrated that the haplotype *DRB1*01502/DQA*00601/DQB1*02301* was significantly more prevalent in affected Nova Scotia Duck Tolling Retrievers. A further study identified a hypoadrenocorticism-associated DLA haplotype in Cocker Spaniels, known as *DRB1*015:01/DQA1*006:01/DQB1*023:01* (Massey *et al.*, 2013). In the same study, hypoadrenocorticism in Cocker Spaniels and Bearded Collies was also associated with the *DRB1*009:01/DQA1*001:01/DQB1*008* haplotype, whilst the *DRB1*001:01/DQA1*001:01/DQB1*002:01* haplotype was found to be associated with hypoadrenocorticism in the Labrador Retriever and the West Highland White Terrier. Notably, in the Standard Poodle, two haplotypes (*DRB1*015:01/DQA1*006:01/DQB1*023:01* in males and *DRB1*009:01/DQA1*001:01/DQB1*008:01:1* in females) have been found to affect risk of hypoadrenocorticism in a sex-specific manner (Treeful *et al.*, 2019).

Single nucleotide polymorphism array genotyping and whole-genome sequencing have also been employed to study the genetics of hypoadrenocorticism in the Standard Poodle. However, no significant variants were identified when comparing cases and controls within the breed, which may be related to a fixed breed risk (Friedenberg *et al.*, 2017). Similarly, GWASs within the Bearded Collie found only suggestive associations, with a potential additive risk, and did not account for the potential fixed risk within the breed (Gershony *et al.*, 2020). Ongoing studies comparing high- and low-risk breeds are likely to find further susceptibility genes.

Other adrenal disorders

The genetic basis of another adrenal disorder, congenital adrenal hyperplasia-like syndrome in Pomeranians, has

also been investigated using a candidate gene approach based on the genetics of a similar condition in humans. However, no mutations of the canine 21-hydroxylase enzyme were identified (Takada *et al.*, 2002).

Studies have also been undertaken to evaluate the role of a potentially activating mutation in *CRHR1*, the gene encoding corticotropin-releasing hormone receptor 1, in hypercortisolism in Poodles. This mutation was identified in only one dog out of 50 cases and 50 control dogs studied (De-Marco *et al.*, 2017), making it an unlikely contributor to the risk of hypercortisolism in this breed. Similarly, studies to investigate somatic (acquired) mutations in corticotropic adenomas of dogs with pituitary-dependent hypercortisolism have not revealed any candidate causal variants in genes encoding signal transduction proteins (Van Wijk *et al.*, 1997). Familial pituitary-dependent hypercortisolism in Wire Haired Dachshunds has also been reported, but no associated genetic mutation has been identified (Stritzel *et al.*, 2008).

Feline diabetes mellitus and hypersomatotropism

Based on the wide variety of treatment options utilized in human type 1, type 2 and monogenic diabetes, canine and feline diabetes mellitus hold particular promise for precision veterinary medicine. Evidence for a genetic basis for feline diabetes mellitus includes the increased prevalence of the disease in the UK and Australian Burmese cat population compared with Domestic Shorthaired cats (Samaha *et al.*, 2019). Notably, healthy Burmese cats also have a different metabolic profile compared with other breeds, which implies that there might be an underlying genetic difference in energy homeostasis in this breed (Öhlund *et al.*, 2021).

Feline diabetes mellitus is challenging to study because of the role of obesity in diabetes risk, and hence the possibility that a genetically high-risk cat may never become diabetic if it is kept at a healthy bodyweight and body condition score. In addition, there are likely to be genetic factors driving appetite and obesity that may be independent of diabetes risk. Another complicating feature of feline diabetes mellitus is the heterogeneity of mechanisms by which a cat might become diabetic, and therefore the high likelihood of phenocopies. This includes the fact that a proportion of diabetic cats have hypersomatotropism as the underlying cause of their insulin resistance and diabetes. If cases are not screened for this condition, meaning that hypersomatotropic and non-hypersomatotropic cats are considered as 'diabetic cases' together, statistical power will be reduced if the genetic basis for the two subgroups of diabetes is different. Similarly, it is not clear whether pancreatitis, another risk factor for feline diabetes mellitus, has a genetic basis in the cat. Therefore, a different prevalence of pancreatitis in cases and controls might also impact on statistical power in genetic studies of diabetes mellitus.

The first genetic variation to be associated with diabetes mellitus in the overweight Domestic Shorthaired cat was a polymorphism in the melanocortin 4 receptor gene (*MC4R*), identified in a candidate gene study (Forcada *et al.*, 2014). This was selected as a candidate gene because of its relationship with obesity in humans. A GWAS combined with whole-genome sequencing in Australian Burmese cats identified diabetes-associated haplotypes across the Burmese breed on chromosomes A3, B1 and E1, with B1 being a particular focus as this appeared to be relatively fixed in the Burmese population, using a technique called selective sweep analysis. Promising candidate genes in this region include *ANK1*, *EPHX2* and *LOXL2*, which are implicated in diabetes mellitus and lipid dysregulation (Balmer *et al.*, 2020). A second GWAS in Australian Burmese cats, with follow-up genotyping, identified SNPs in six genetic regions of interest associated with diabetes risk. The nearest genes to these SNPs were *SLC8A1*, *E2F6*, *TRA2B*, *CHCHD4*, *IGF2BP2* and *SENP2*, although functional and causality studies are yet to be undertaken (Balmer *et al.*, 2020). A recent feline GWAS also identified an SNP on chromosome D4 that was significantly associated with diabetes mellitus in Domestic Shorthaired and Maine Coon cats, although the study did not specifically screen for hypersomatotropism within the diabetic population (Hernandez *et al.*, 2022). Ongoing work utilizing GWAS and whole-genome sequencing is likely to reveal many more diabetes-associated variants in both Burmese and non-Burmese cats, which may offer novel preventive or therapeutic targets in the future.

Canine diabetes mellitus

As with feline diabetes mellitus, the challenge of phenocopies is critically important in canine diabetes mellitus, where many mechanisms can result in the familiar clinical signs of hyperglycaemia, glucosuria, polyuria, polydipsia, and weight loss. The relationship between obesity and diabetes mellitus risk is less clear in dogs than in cats; however, a deletion in the pro-opiomelanocortin gene (*POMC*) has been associated with increased appetite and obesity in Labrador Retrievers (Raffan *et al.*, 2016).

Although progress is being made using technologies such as whole-genome sequencing by consortia such as the Canine Diabetes Genetics Partnership, to date most published work on genetic susceptibility to canine diabetes mellitus relates to candidate genes.

The earliest report of a potential genetic basis to canine diabetes mellitus was a form of insulin-dependent juvenile-onset diabetes in the Keeshond (Kramer *et al.*, 1980). Although the genetic basis was not determined, histological studies revealed an absence of pancreatic beta cells. Isolated cases of juvenile diabetes have since been reported in a number of breeds, for example, in combination with exocrine pancreatic insufficiency in a German Shepherd Dog, in a Dogue de Bordeaux with lymphocytic insulitis (Jouvion *et al.*, 2006) and in a small number of Labrador Retrievers (Catchpole *et al.*, 2005). However, to date, no single gene defects have been identified to account for these cases. Familial diabetes has also been reported in the Samoyed (Kimmel *et al.*, 2002) and recent analyses of heritability in the Australian Terrier and American Eskimo Dog suggested polygenic inheritance in these breeds (Mui *et al.*, 2020).

Similar to canine hypothyroidism, the first gene region to be associated more broadly with canine diabetes mellitus risk was the DLA (Kennedy *et al.*, 2006b), and this work has more recently been expanded to examine breed-specific DLA haplotypes (Denyer *et al.*, 2020). Breeds in which the DLA genes appear to be important include the Cocker Spaniel, Cavalier King Charles Spaniel, Border Terrier, Labrador Retriever and West Highland White Terrier. Some diabetes risk haplotypes, such as *DRB1*001:01/DQA1*001:01/DQB1*002:01* in the Labrador Retriever, have been associated with different endocrinopathies such as hypoadrenocorticism and hypothyroidism. Notably, no MHC association has been identified in some breeds at high risk of diabetes, including the Samoyed, Tibetan Terrier and Cairn Terrier, which may be due to the fixed nature of the genetic risk in these breeds.

Alternatively, this might be because the adaptive immune response does not play a critical role in diabetes risk in these breeds. A separate DLA study of canine diabetes identified four new *DQB1* alleles restricted to diabetic dogs and highlighted the high level of linkage disequilibrium (LD) in the region. Linkage disequilibrium refers to the non-random inheritance of alleles that are close together on a chromosome, inherited together as a 'block'. This means that diabetes associations found with variants in the MHC region might also reflect diabetes associations with variants in genes outside the DLA region that are in high LD with the DLA genes (Seddon *et al.*, 2010).

Using SNP discovery and a candidate gene approach, polymorphisms in several cytokine and immune-response genes have also been associated with risk of diabetes mellitus in certain breeds. The implicated genes include those encoding IFN-gamma, interleukin (IL)-10, IL-12-beta, IL-6, IL-4, PTPN22 and tumour necrosis factor-alpha, and associations were most common in terriers and spaniels (Short *et al.*, 2007, 2009). In addition, similar to canine hypoadrenocorticism, variations in the immune response gene *CTLA4* have been associated with diabetes risk in the Samoyed, Miniature Schnauzer, West Highland White Terrier, Border Terrier and Labrador Retriever (Short *et al.*, 2010). In these immune-response candidate gene studies, many alleles were associated with protection or susceptibility in only a single breed (e.g. *IL10* polymorphisms in the Cavalier King Charles Spaniel) and, interestingly, some SNPs were monomorphic (existed in only one form) within breeds. The potential role of the immune system in canine diabetes is also highlighted by GWASs and whole-genome sequencing studies suggesting that a region containing the immunoglobulin heavy chain gene cluster is associated with diabetes in high-risk breeds (Sanz *et al.*, 2021).

Another approach has been to study the genes associated with type 1, type 2 and monogenic forms of diabetes in humans (Catchpole *et al.*, 2013; Short *et al.*, 2014). Six canine allelic associations to genes that are causative for human monogenic forms of diabetes were identified. Single nucleotide polymorphisms associated with canine diabetes mellitus were identified in the Bichon Frise (*ZFP57* gene), Samoyed (*ZFP57* gene), Miniature Dachshund (*HNF4A* gene) and Cocker Spaniel (*MTTL1*, *PAX4* and *INS* genes), although none of the associated SNPs changed the amino acid sequence of the protein or fully explained diabetes risk in any given breed. The insulin gene, which has been associated with type 1 diabetes in humans, has also been the subject of investigations in the Samoyed and the Australian Terrier. Single nucleotide polymorphism array analysis of variants in the region of the insulin gene in cases and controls suggested that variation in or near this region might also contribute to diabetes risk in these breeds.

Future developments

Understanding of the genetics of endocrine disease in veterinary species is still in its infancy. However, the advent of precision veterinary medicine, in which personalized veterinary care is informed by a range of factors specific to an individual, is driving a need for improved understanding of canine and feline genetics. The next decade promises to be a very exciting and informative phase for the study of the genetics of endocrine disease in dogs and cats.

References and further reading

Andresen E and Willeberg P (1976) Pituitary dwarfism in German shepherd dogs: additional evidence of simple, autosomal recessive inheritance. *Nordisk Veterinaermedicin* **28**, 481–486

Arias ES, Castillo V, Garcia J and Fyfe J (2018) Congenital dyshormonogenic hypothyroidism with goiter caused by a sodium/iodide symporter (SLC5A5) mutation in a family of Shih-Tzu dogs. *Domestic Animal Endocrinology* **65**, 1–8

Balmer L, O'Leary CA, Menotti-Raymond M *et al.* (2020) Mapping of diabetes susceptibility loci in a domestic cat breed with an unusually high incidence of diabetes mellitus. *Genes* **11**, 1369

Bianchi M, Dahlgren S, Massey J *et al.* (2015) A multi-breed genome-wide association analysis for canine hypothyroidism identifies a shared major risk locus on CFA12. *PLoS One* **10**, e0134720

Bianchi M, Rafati N, Karlsson Å *et al.* (2020) Whole-genome genotyping and resequencing reveal the association of a deletion in the complex interferon alpha gene cluster with hypothyroidism in dogs. *BMC Genomics* **21**, 307

Boag AM, Short A, Kennedy LJ *et al.* (2020) Polymorphisms in the *CTLA4* promoter sequence are associated with canine hypoadrenocorticism. *Canine Medicine and Genetics* **7**, 2

Catchpole B, Adams JP, Holder AL *et al.* (2013) Genetics of canine diabetes mellitus: are the diabetes susceptibility genes identified in humans involved in breed susceptibility to diabetes mellitus in dogs? *The Veterinary Journal* **195**, 139–147

Catchpole B, Ristic J, Fleeman L and Davison L (2005) Canine diabetes mellitus: can old dogs teach us new tricks? *Diabetologia* **48**, 1948–1956

De-Marco V, Carvalho LR, Guzzo MF *et al.* (2017) An activating mutation in the *CRHR1* gene is rarely associated with pituitary-dependent hyperadrenocorticism in poodles. *Clinics (Sao Paulo)* **72**, 575–581

Denyer AL, Massey JP, Davison LJ *et al.* (2020) Dog leucocyte antigen (DLA) class II haplotypes and risk of canine diabetes mellitus in specific dog breeds. *Canine Medicine and Genetics* **7**, 15

Famula T, Belanger J and Oberbauer A (2003) Heritability and complex segregation analysis of hypoadrenocorticism in the standard poodle. *Journal of Small Animal Practice* **44**, 8–12

Forcada Y, Holder A, Church D and Catchpole B (2014) A polymorphism in the melanocortin 4 receptor gene (*MC4R:c.92C>T*) is associated with diabetes mellitus in overweight domestic shorthaired cats. *Journal of Veterinary Internal Medicine* **28**, 458–464

Friedenberg SG, Lunn KF and Meurs KM (2017) Evaluation of the genetic basis of primary hypoadrenocorticism in Standard Poodles using SNP array genotyping and whole-genome sequencing. *Mammalian Genome* **28**, 56–65

Fyfe JC, Kampschmidt K, Dang V *et al.* (2003) Congenital hypothyroidism with goiter in toy fox terriers. *Journal of Veterinary Internal Medicine* **17**, 50–57

Gershony LC, Belanger JM, Hytönen MK *et al.* (2020) Genetic characterization of Addison's disease in Bearded Collies. *BMC Genomics* **21**, 833

Goldstein RE, Atwater DZ, Cazolli DM *et al.* (2007) Inheritance, mode of inheritance, and candidate genes for primary hyperparathyroidism in Keeshonden. *Journal of Veterinary Internal Medicine* **21**, 199–203

Hernandez I, Hayward JJ, Brockman JA *et al.* (2022) Complex feline disease mapping using a dense genotyping array. *Frontiers in Veterinary Science* **9**, 862414

Hughes AM, Bannasch DL, Kellett K and Oberbauer AM (2011) Examination of candidate genes for hypoadrenocorticism in Nova Scotia Duck Tolling Retrievers. *The Veterinary Journal* **187**, 212–216

Iio A, Maeda S, Yonezawa T, Momoi Y and Motegi T (2020) Isolated growth hormone deficiency in a Chihuahua with a *GH1* mutation. *Journal of Veterinary Diagnostic Investigation* **32**, 733–736

Jouvion G, Abadie J, Bach J-M *et al.* (2006) Lymphocytic insulitis in a juvenile dog with diabetes mellitus. *Endocrine Pathology* **17**, 283–290

Kennedy L, Quarmby S, Happ G *et al.* (2006a) Association of canine hypothyroidism with a common major histocompatibility complex DLA class II allele. *Tissue Antigens* **68**, 82–86

Kennedy LJ, Davison LJ, Barnes A *et al.* (2006b) Identification of susceptibility and protective major histocompatibility complex haplotypes in canine diabetes mellitus. *Tissue Antigens* **68**, 467–476

Kimmel SE, Ward CR, Henthorn PS and Hess RS (2002) Familial insulin-dependent diabetes mellitus in Samoyed dogs. *Journal of the American Animal Hospital Association* **38**, 235–238

Kramer JW, Nottingham S, Robinette J *et al.* (1980) Inherited, early onset, insulin-requiring diabetes mellitus of Keeshond dogs. *Diabetes* **29**, 558–565

Kyöstilä K, Niskanen JE, Arumilli M *et al.* (2021) Intronic variant in *POU1F1* associated with canine pituitary dwarfism. *Human Genetics* **140**, 1553–1562

Major S, Pettigrew R and Fyfe J (2015) Molecular genetic characterization of thyroid dyshormonogenesis in a French bulldog. *Journal of Veterinary Internal Medicine* **29**, 1534–1540

Massey J, Boag A, Short AD *et al.* (2013) MHC class II association study in eight breeds of dog with hypoadrenocorticism. *Immunogenetics* **65**, 291–297

Mui ML, Famula TR, Henthorn PS and Hess RS (2020) Heritability and complex segregation analysis of naturally-occurring diabetes in Australian Terrier Dogs. *PLoS One* **15**, e0239542

Öhlund M, Müllner E, Moazzami A *et al.* (2021) Differences in metabolic profiles between the Burmese, the Maine coon and the Birman cat – Three breeds with varying risk for diabetes mellitus. *PLoS One* **16**, e0249322

Pettigrew R, Fyfe J, Gregory B *et al.* (2007) CNS hypomyelination in Rat Terrier dogs with congenital goiter and a mutation in the thyroid peroxidase gene. *Veterinary Pathology* **44**, 50–56

Raffan E, Dennis RJ, O'Donovan CJ *et al.* (2016) A deletion in the canine *POMC* gene is associated with weight and appetite in obesity-prone Labrador retriever dogs. *Cell Metabolism* **23**, 893–900

Samaha G, Beatty J, Wade C and Haase B (2019) The Burmese cat as a genetic model of type 2 diabetes in humans. *Animal Genetics* **50**, 319–325

Sanz C, Sevane N, Pérez-Alenza M, Valero-Lorenzo M and Dunner S (2021) Polymorphisms in canine immunoglobulin heavy chain gene cluster: a double-edged sword for diabetes mellitus in the dog. *Animal Genetics* **52**, 333–341

Seddon J, Berggren K and Fleeman L (2010) Evolutionary history of DLA class II haplotypes in canine diabetes mellitus through single nucleotide polymorphism genotyping. *Tissue Antigens* **75**, 218–226

Short AD, Boag A, Catchpole B *et al.* (2013) A candidate gene analysis of canine hypoadrenocorticism in 3 dog breeds. *Journal of Heredity* **104**, 807–820

Short AD, Catchpole B, Kennedy LJ *et al.* (2007) Analysis of candidate susceptibility genes in canine diabetes. *Journal of Heredity* **98**, 518–525

Short AD, Catchpole B, Kennedy LJ *et al.* (2009) T cell cytokine gene polymorphisms in canine diabetes mellitus. *Veterinary Immunology and Immunopathology* **128**, 137–146

Short AD, Holder A, Rothwell S *et al.* (2014) Searching for "monogenic diabetes" in dogs using a candidate gene approach. *Canine Genetics and Epidemiology* **1**, 8

Short AD, Saleh N, Catchpole B *et al.* (2010) *CTLA4* promoter polymorphisms are associated with canine diabetes mellitus. *Tissue Antigens* **75**, 242–252

Stritzel S, Mischke R, Philipp U *et al.* (2008) Familiäres Auftreten des kaninen hypophysären Hyperadrenokortizismus beim Rauhaardackel [Familial canine pituitary-dependent hyperadrenocorticism in wirehaired Dachshunds]. *Berliner und Münchener Tierärztliche Wochenschrift* **121**, 349–358

Takada K, Kitamura H, Takiguchi M, Saito M and Hashimoto A (2002) Cloning of canine 21-hydroxylase gene and its polymorphic analysis as a candidate gene for congenital adrenal hyperplasia-like syndrome in Pomeranians. *Research in Veterinary Science* **73**, 159–163

Thaiwong T, Corner S, Forge SL and Kiupel M (2021) Dwarfism in Tibetan Terrier dogs with an *LHX3* mutation. *Journal of Veterinary Diagnostic Investigation* **33**, 740–743

Treeful AE, Rendahl AK and Friedenberg SG (2019) DLA class II haplotypes show sex-specific associations with primary hypoadrenocorticism in Standard Poodle dogs. *Immunogenetics* **71**, 373–382

Van Wijk P, Rijnberk A, Croughs R *et al.* (1997) Molecular screening for somatic mutations in corticotrope adenomas of dogs with pituitary-dependent hyperadrenocorticism. *Journal of Endocrinological Investigation* **20**, 1–7

Voorbij AMWY, Leegwater P and Kooistra H (2014) Pituitary dwarfism in Saarloos and Czechoslovakian wolfdogs is associated with a mutation in *LHX3*. *Journal of Veterinary Internal Medicine* **28**, 1770–1774

Voorbij AMWY, Van Steenbeek FG, Vos-Loohuis M *et al.* (2011) A contracted DNA repeat in *LHX3* intron 5 is associated with aberrant splicing and pituitary dwarfism in German shepherd dogs. *PLoS ONE* **6**, e27940

Watson S, Radford A, Kipar A, Ibarrola P and Blackwood L (2005) Somatic mutations of the thyroid-stimulating hormone receptor gene in feline hyperthyroidism: parallels with human hyperthyroidism. *Journal of Endocrinology* **186**, 523–537

Wilbe M, Sundberg K, Hansen I *et al.* (2010) Increased genetic risk or protection for canine autoimmune lymphocytic thyroiditis in Giant Schnauzers depends on DLA class II genotype. *Tissue Antigens* **75**, 712–719

Ziener ML, Dahlgren S, Thoresen SI and Lingaas F (2015) Genetics and epidemiology of hypothyroidism and symmetrical onychomadesis in the Gordon setter and the English setter. *Canine Genetics and Epidemiology* **2**, 12

Chapter 3

Hormone assays, quality control and sample collection

Peter A. Graham

Hormone assay methods

Almost all routine hormone measurement methods are immunoassays relying on antibodies interacting with the hormone of interest in order to estimate its concentration. A few veterinary laboratories and specialist human reference laboratories have recently implemented alternative technologies, such as mass spectrometry, but these are not yet widely available.

Immunoassay types

An immunoassay system can take one of many forms. However, all have antibodies and a 'tracer', that is, either a hormone or a labelled antibody that can be detected by a suitable detection system. Most will have a mechanism of separating hormone that is bound to antibodies from that which is not. Calibrators of known and diagnostically useful hormone concentration are required so that the detected signal can be compared to a standard curve and converted to a concentration.

The antibodies used can be polyclonal (limited supply raised in a hormone-inoculated animal) or monoclonal (unlimited supply produced in a laboratory using cultured hybridomas of lymphocytes extracted from inoculated mice). Some assays will use a single antibody and others may use more than one directed at different parts of the hormone molecule. The exact molecule the antibody reacts or cross-reacts with is an important determinant of assay performance.

The separation system could be as simple as the 'capture' antibody being bound to a reaction vessel wall, cellulose membrane or magnetic bead, or antibody-bound hormone being precipitated and centrifuged prior to decanting and washing steps. Alternatively, unbound hormone could be separated from antibody-bound hormone by charcoal absorption.

In a classical competitive radioimmunoassay (RIA), the hormone in the sample competes with a radiolabelled version of the hormone for binding sites on antibodies that are bound to something solid (vessel wall, bead) and, after a washing step, the bound radioactivity is detected and compared against a calibration or standard curve (Figure 3.1a). An alternative format is to have a labelled antibody that binds to hormone already captured by another antibody bound to a solid surface, a so-called immunoradiometric assay (IRMA) (Figure 3.1b).

Most other immunoassays follow one of these two formats but with a detection system that does not rely on

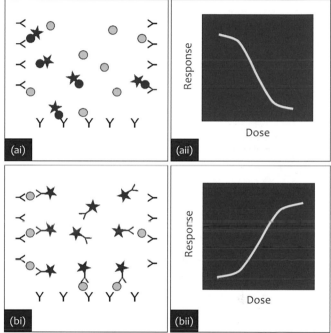

3.1 Classical immunoassays. (ai–ii) Radioimmunoassay: the amount of labelled hormone bound to the antibody is inversely proportional to the concentration of unlabelled hormone in the sample. (bi–ii) Immunoradiometric assay: the amount of labelled antibody remaining after washing is directly proportional to the concentration of hormone in the sample. In these examples the assay antibody binding sites are bound to the reaction vessel wall, but these could also be bound to a bead or a membrane. A wash step removes all unbound components prior to the detection stage. ✶ = radiolabelled antibody (could be labelled with an enzyme in non-isotopic method); ● = sample hormone; ✶ = radiolabelled assay hormone.

radioisotopes. Hormones or antibodies can be labelled with enzymes in enzyme immunoassays (EIAs). Such enzymes allow detection by inducing a colour change (e.g. enzyme-linked immunosorbent assay (ELISA), lateral flow), light emission (e.g. chemiluminescent immunoassay, capillary electrophoresis immunoassay) or fluorescence (e.g. fluorescent immunoassay, enzyme-linked fluorescence assay (ELFA), fluorescent EIA).

To avoid the usual necessity of wash steps and therefore simplify the mechanics of the analytical process, techniques such as 'homogeneous enzyme immunoassay' and 'surface plasmon-enhanced fluorescence' have been developed in which there is no separation and wash step. A homogeneous EIA (DRI Thyroxine Assay, Thermo/Microgenics) has become a popular method to measure total thyroxine (T4) in commercial reference laboratories because it can be implemented on a clinical chemistry analyser, rather than a specialist immunoassay analyser. This reduces the costly logistical inconvenience of separating samples for use in two different analysers to complete a panel of results that includes total T4. This method utilizes an enzyme, glucose-6-phosphate dehydrogenase (G6PDH), bound to T4 that competes with sample T4 for binding sites on liquid-phase anti-T4 antibodies (Figure 3.2). At low sample concentrations, antibodies bind to the G6PDH-T4 conjugate, preventing the enzyme from catalysing the conversion of nicotinamide adenine dinucleotide (NAD) to its reduced form (NADH) and an associated colour change. At high sample total T4 concentrations, fewer antibodies are free to interact with the conjugate and the colour-change reaction can proceed. The same reaction principle is also used in an in-clinic format (VetScan T4/Cholesterol Panel, Zoetis). Surface plasmon-enhanced fluorescence (AU10V, Fujifilm) avoids the need for separation by only detecting fluorescence close to the vessel wall (attached to antibodies) rather than throughout the whole reaction chamber.

(a)

(b)

3.2 Glucose-6-phosphate dehydrogenase (G6PDH) homogeneous immunoassay for total thyroxine (T4). The conversion of nicotinamide adenine dinucleotide (NAD) to its reduced form (NADH) is monitored by ultraviolet light absorbance at 340 nm and compared with a calibration curve.
(a) At low hormone concentrations, G6PDH cannot convert NAD to NADH because the enzymatic site is blocked by antibody interacting with enzyme-bound hormone.
(b) At high hormone concentrations, G6PDH can convert NAD to NADH because the enzymatic site is not blocked by antibody, which is instead interacting with sample hormone.

Reference laboratories most often use RIA (believed by many to still be the 'gold standard') and chemiluminescence (or DRI Thyroxine Assay, Thermo/Microgenics), whereas technologies designed for in-clinic use employ variants of colour-change EIA or fluorescence.

Reference laboratory *versus* point of care

Measurement of hormones including total T4, thyrotropin (thyroid-stimulating hormone (TSH)), cortisol and progesterone is possible using in-clinic technology. Technologies include: ELISA in lateral flow format (SNAP, IDEXX); dry multi-layered slide (Catalyst, IDEXX); homogeneous EIA (Vetscan, Zoetis); surface plasmon-enhanced fluorescence (AU10V, Fujifilm) and, in larger hospital environments, fluorescence EIA (Tosoh AIA and VIDAS (ELFA)). The analytical performance of some but not all of these technologies has been independently evaluated or compared with reference laboratory methods. If in-clinic hormone analysis is used for clinical decision-making, clinicians should first be assured of the suitability of their local method through independent verification and understanding the requirement for continued quality control (QC) and quality assurance (QA). In-clinic analysis offers the advantage of speed but the disadvantage that the clinic carries the responsibility for verifying the method's clinical suitability, maintenance and the management of QC that can effectively spot clinically impactful errors. The quality of in-clinic analysis varies by method, manufacturer and analyte such that only a local verification will determine whether it performs well enough. The speed of a quick-turnaround in-clinic result is no advantage to the animal if it is incorrect and causes an inappropriate clinical decision. The advantages of commercial laboratory analyses are that validation, maintenance, QC and QA are taken care of, and the analytical performance is usually higher. The disadvantage is turnaround time but, for many of the chronic conditions diagnosed or monitored by hormone tests, waiting a day or two has limited clinical impact.

Variation between methods

Some hormones, such as steroids and thyroid hormones, are structurally identical (conserved) across species. Others, particularly peptides, are more likely to have species-dependent structure (non-conserved). In the case of non-conserved hormones, variation between methods is expected as different antibodies from different assay manufacturers will have different degrees of cross-reactivity against veterinary species of interest. Many commercial assays used in veterinary endocrinology employ antibodies that have been raised against the human version of the molecule. If the calibrators are also the human version of the molecule then the estimated hormone concentration is technically 'equivalent immunoreactivity'; for example, it cannot be assumed that the sample actually has 35 µIU/ml of insulin, only that the insulin that is there is reacting equivalently to a human sample with 35 µIU/ml of insulin. This would have limited clinical impact if all laboratories used the same methods and they were never altered. However, a change in method or a result from a different method at a different laboratory will have a different cross-reactivity, result and reference interval. This is one reason that laboratories occasionally change their immunoassay reference intervals. It also makes it difficult to apply thresholds from textbooks that have derived cut-offs from a different method (e.g. insulin:glucose will vary from method to method).

The nature of the calibrators being used may need to be confirmed in detail from method specifications. For example, calibrators may be described as 'canine calibrators' when they are actually a human (or other species) version of the hormone added to canine serum.

It is easily understood that different laboratories are likely to have different reference intervals and diagnostic cut-off values for non-conserved hormones. However, the conserved hormones can also be subject to similar variability between methods as a result of differences in antibody, antibody cross-reaction with similar biological molecules and calibration (Figure 3.3).

When an assay based on polyclonal antibody exhausts the original antibody pool, manufacturers may replace the antibody with one that works equivalently for their target market (human samples) but that changes the results or stops the assay working completely for animals. They may not communicate that change to veterinary laboratories. Such a change might only be detected by a laboratory using species-relevant QC material (see 'Quality control', below). In this circumstance, and when assays are discontinued and replaced, laboratories may have to adjust their reference intervals accordingly – making it important to rely on communication with the laboratory, rather than textbooks or other publications, for interpretative guidance.

Even when hormone structure is conserved across species, an assay that works well in one species may not work well in another, because of either so-called 'matrix effects' or differences in typical concentrations. For example, the circulating concentration of total T4 in dogs and cats is generally lower than in humans, so the assays used in veterinary laboratories need to be more sensitive (have a lower limit of detection). This concept may even extend to breeds; sighthounds would need an even more sensitive assay for total T4 than other canine breeds. Matrix effects include observable differences in assay function between species that cannot be explained by hormone structure or antibody specificity. It is not usually established what these differences are specifically, but when observed they suggest that there is something different about the serum in a more general sense (e.g. differences in protein structure or distribution of proteins and how they interact with assay components).

Other methods

Hormone molecules can be separated by chromatographic methods. Liquid chromatography elutes different molecules at different rates from a separation column and each molecular fraction is detected by light, electrochemistry, mass spectrometry or fluorescence. An example application is high-performance liquid chromatography for catecholamines.

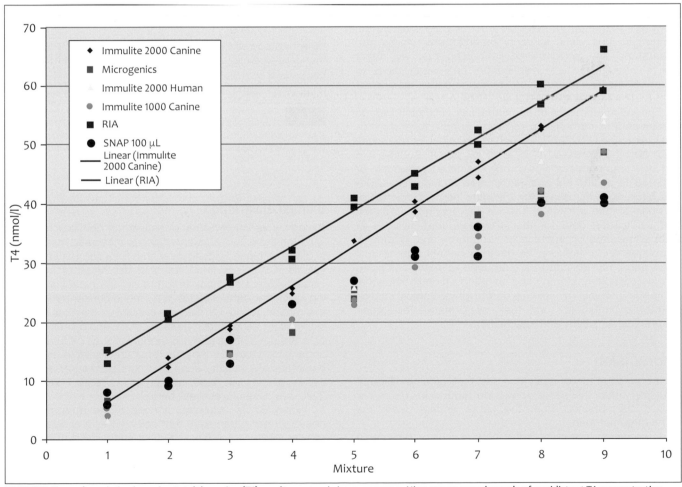

3.3 Example variation in canine total thyroxine (T4) results across six immunoassays. Nine serum sample pools of equidistant T4 concentration were measured in duplicate on each immunoassay. Concentrations reported for the highest values ranged from 40 to >60 nmol/l and those around the lower canine reference limit ranged from 10 to 20 nmol/l depending on the method used. Using pools of equidistant concentration also allows visualization of how well individual methods agree with themselves. A method with good linearity and precision should generate results through which a single straight line can be drawn. RIA = radioimmunoassay.
(Reproduced from Graham (2010))

In mass spectrometry, molecules are fragmented, separated and then measured based on the mass:charge of the fragments. In recent years, the combination of liquid chromatography and two mass analysers in tandem (liquid chromatography–tandem mass spectrometry (LC–MS/MS)) has been applied to hormone measurement. Such an approach mitigates the disadvantages of relying on antibodies and their various affinities and cross-reactivities and represents a new 'gold standard'. There is still variability between laboratories, suggesting that LC–MS/MS does not always offer a guaranteed 'true' result, although results from this technology would be more likely to enable harmonization across laboratories.

Hormone assay validation

The techniques chosen for hormone measurement should be fit for the intended clinical or research purpose. There are physiological factors that can complicate the interpretation of hormone results (see Chapter 4), a task that can only be made easier with high confidence in the analytical quality of results. Adding diagnostic uncertainty on top of analytical uncertainty increases the chances of error in clinical decision-making.

Laboratories that bring in new methods of analysis, often adapting assays for human samples, must fully *validate* their assay to ensure that it is fit for purpose in the intended veterinary species. Clinics that acquire in-clinic analysers marketed for veterinary use should evaluate the method in their clinic to verify manufacturer claims and understand any performance limitations that will affect clinical use. The term *verification* has been used to describe this less onerous 'performance check' as distinct from a full validation (Arnold *et al.*, 2019).

The initial elements of immunoassay validation include assessment of imprecision, accuracy, specificity and sensitivity (Arnold *et al.*, 2019). Potential analytical interferences must also be assessed (Arnold *et al.*, 2019). Studies that use new immunoassays (e.g. not evaluated previously or targeted to a different species) should include full validation. Studies using assays for the same intended species or purpose should include a citation for previous validation and verification data for the laboratory that includes at least some data on imprecision, accuracy and sensitivity. Subsequently, to achieve the greatest benefit from clinical application, further studies are required to derive optimized sample collection, storage and shipping recommendations, reference intervals (by species and/or physiological status), diagnostic thresholds and their performance evaluation (diagnostic sensitivity and specificity).

Imprecision

As a consequence of analytical and biological variation, it is unlikely that the same endocrine laboratory result will always be obtained from the same animal under the same circumstance.

Imprecision is a measure of how similar or repeatable the results are when the same sample is analysed multiple times. It is assessed in the short term within-assay or within-day (depending on whether the analytical method operates as a batch or continuously) and in the long term between-assay or between-day. Imprecision is expressed as a coefficient of variation (CV), which is the ratio of standard deviation (SD) to mean of a set of more than 20 replicate results, given as a percentage (Arnold *et al.*,

2019). Imprecision varies across the analytical range of an immunoassay and so it is important that it is evaluated at more than one concentration and helpful if the chosen evaluation concentration is close to a clinical decision limit (Figure 3.4). A lower number of replicates would be appropriate for verification of an in-clinic analyser to check against manufacturer claims.

Compared with other types of serum chemistry analyses that can achieve CVs less than 2%, immunoassays are generally less precise, with typical CVs in the range of 5–10% and occasionally higher. Consequently, it is somewhat misleading to see numerical results such as 100.5 nmol/l from assays with CVs of 5% and there is an argument that results should be rounded to the nearest whole number that represents the relevant imprecision (e.g. 95, 100 or 105 nmol/l) or reported with the imprecision noted (e.g. 100 ± 10 nmol/l). This is not done in practice but would reduce the temptation to make clinical judgements based on small changes in results that the analytical method cannot truly discern.

Imprecision should be low enough that extremes of possible results would not cause different clinical decisions.

Method	Very low canine serum pool	Low canine serum pool	High feline serum pool
Mean (nmol/l)	7.2	12.6	60
Radioimmunoassay	5.8%	6.2%	2.8%
Immulite 2000 Canine Total T4	9.1%	4.6%	4.1%
Immulite 1000 Canine T4	11.6%	4.3%	3.5%
Thermo Microgenics DRI T4	18.8%	7.4%	5.1%
Immulite 2000 Human Total T4	30.5%	13.6%	7.1%
IDEXX SNAP T4*		18.2%	

3.4 Coefficient of variation for a 10-replicate study of three diagnostically relevant thyroxine (T4) concentration pools on six analytical methods. * = using SNAP T4 Test method and 100 μl protocol with Snapshot DX – a newer version of this assay is now available (SNAP Total T4 Test).
(Data from Graham (2010))

Biological variation

Biological variation (BV) is a measure of how much natural variation there is in concentrations of measured substances in blood within individuals over time (CV_I) and between individuals (CV_G). It is important that the noise of analytical variation is not so great as to prevent the detection of biologically important changes in hormone concentrations. For this reason, where BV data are available, analytical imprecision should be less than 25–50% of BV. Biological variation data are not available for all hormones or all circumstances under which they are measured but are available for thyroid parameters in healthy dogs and cats (Jensen *et al.*, 1993; Jensen and Høier, 1996; Iversen *et al.*, 1999; Prieto *et al.*, 2020; see 'Useful websites', below).

When BV is available, it creates the opportunity to derive further parameters that can help with assessing the clinical suitability of the analytical method (total allowable error (TEa); see below) and determining whether two numerically distinct concentrations represent a biologically relevant difference (reference change value (RCV) and critical difference), which assists with clinical interpretation, particularly around thresholds and diagnostic cut-off values. The availability of TEa derived from BV also informs the choice of QC strategy through 'sigma metrics' (see 'Quality control', below).

Assessing biologically relevant change

RCV% for a unidirectional change in a normally distributed analyte at $p < 0.05 = 2.33 \times (CV_A^2 + CV_I^2)^{0.5}$

RCV% for a unidirectional change in a normally distributed analyte at $p < 0.01 = 3.29 \times (CV_A^2 + CV_I^2)^{0.5}$

CV_A = Analytical coefficient of variation (%) at a concentration close to the interpretative threshold

CV_I = Within individual biological coefficient of variation (%)

RCV% multiplied by the first obtained result gives the RCV in analytical units.

More complicated log transformed approaches are required for calculating RCV for non-normally distributed analytes. Prieto *et al.* (2020) calculated that from an initial feline TSH concentration of 0.1 ng/ml, the second result would have to be below 0.04 ng/ml or above 0.29 ng/ml to represent a biologically relevant change when using the Siemens Immulite 2000 Canine TSH method.

Rearrangement of the RCV formula can provide a Z-score as an indication of the probability that there has been a biologically relevant change:

Z = %difference / $[2^{0.5} \times (CV_A^2 + CV_I^2)^{0.5}]$

$Z > 1.65$ indicates probability $p < 0.05$; $Z > 2.33$ indicates $p < 0.01$ (Fraser and Sandberg, 2018).

Accuracy

Accuracy is a measure of how closely the results generated match the 'true' concentration, and the term *bias* is commonly used to describe any difference observed. It is best measured at a concentration that has clinical relevance (close to a diagnostic threshold). There are two main ways of assessing method bias in the laboratory: a method comparison study and spike/recovery experiments. In the longer term, data can be used from participation in external quality assessment (EQA) schemes (see below).

A method comparison study generally requires a minimum of 40 independent samples measured in both a reference assay and the method being evaluated across a range of diagnostically relevant concentrations. Guidelines for determining bias and the acceptability of method comparisons are widely available (Jensen and Kjelgaard-Hansen, 2006). The terms *systematic* (or *constant*) and *proportional* bias are used to describe whether the bias can be best summarized as results that are generally different by a measurement unit amount (e.g. cortisol results that are generally 20 nmol/l higher than true values) or different by a proportion (e.g. results that are generally 20% higher than true values), respectively, across a range of concentrations.

A spike/recovery study involves the addition of a purified and accurately measured concentration of the hormone of interest to a relevant species matrix and checking whether the results agree with what was known to have been added. This approach is problematic when species-specific purified hormone is not available. However, for example, structurally identical and available porcine insulin could be used to assess an insulin assay for dogs. By participating in an EQA scheme, a laboratory can discover how its results compare to those produced by other laboratories and can calculate bias as the difference from EQA target values.

To determine whether an assay is measuring the intended hormone, an inference can be made by assessing whether or not the assay generates physiologically expected results: for example, is the hormone concentration increased in the serum of animals when predicted (e.g. high erythropoietin concentrations in regenerative anaemia samples) and expectedly low in the right conditions (e.g. low erythropoietin concentrations in chronic kidney disease cases)?

Once the potential errors from imprecision and bias are known for a diagnostically relevant concentration, they can be summarized by a combined single value of 'total error' (TE), which can be calculated using measurement units ($TE_{units} = Bias_{units} + 2 \times SD$) or percentages ($TE\% = Bias\% + 2 \times CV\%$) (Harr *et al.*, 2013). For example, a method with a bias of 10% and a CV of 6% would have an observed TE of ±22%. Recommendations for how much error can be tolerated from a method without it adversely affecting clinical decisions (TEa) are published from time to time based on expert opinion or biological variation studies (Harr *et al.*, 2013; see 'Useful websites', below). Few TEa recommendations and BV data exist presently for veterinary hormones and, when they are not available, laboratories rely on human recommendations (Figure 3.5).

Analyte	Species	TEa based on biological variation			Human CLIA proposal 2019
		Optimal TEa	*Desirable TEa*	*Minimum TEa*	
Total T4	Dog	9.9	19.8	28.5	20 (or 13 nmol/l)
Free T4	Dog	12.3	24.6	35.3	15 (or 3.9 pmol/l)
TSH	Dog	11.3	22.6	31.7	20
Total T4	Cat	7.6	15.2	21.6	20 (or 13 nmol/l)
Total T4	Cat	6.1	12.2	17.5	20 (or 13 nmol/l)
Free T4	Cat	6.4	12.8	18.4	15 (or 3.9 pmol/l)
Insulin	Cat	32.3	64.7	93.6	
TSH	Cat	25.8	51.6	73.3	20
IGF-1	Cat	11.1	22.2	30.1	
Cortisol					20

3.5 Examples of total allowable error (TEa) based on biological variation in endocrinology. Values are ±% from true or target value. Minimum TEa refers to the TEa that provides minimally acceptable performance. Biological variation studies listed were performed in healthy animals. Further information is available from VetBiologicalVariation.org. CLIA = Clinical Laboratory Improvement Amendments. IGF-1 = insulin-like growth factor-1, T4 = thyroxine, TSH = thyroid-stimulating hormone.
(Data from Jensen *et al.*, 1993; Jensen and Høier, 1996; Iversen *et al.*, 1999; Strage, 2015; Strage *et al.*, 2015; Falkenö *et al.*, 2016; Department of Health and Human Services, 2019; Prieto *et al.*, 2020)

Specificity

Specificity is a measure of whether the assay results could be influenced by the presence of related molecules or if truly only the hormone of interest is being measured. The choice of assay antibody has the greatest influence on this. Specificity is assessed by adding known quantities of suspected related molecules to samples to see if it changes the measured concentration of the hormone of interest. For example, prednisolone will interact with most cortisol immunoassays, causing falsely high results, and some adrenocorticotropic hormone (ACTH) methods are influenced by corticotropin-like intermediate peptide (CLIP), causing higher results than attributable to true ACTH alone (Knowles et al., 2018). Manufacturers often provide data on assay specificity for a range of substances chemically similar to the hormone of interest.

Specificity can also be assessed by parallelism studies, and this may be the only measure of specificity when purified related compounds are difficult to obtain. A parallelism study is conducted by progressively diluting a sample with high expected hormone concentration with serum or other matrix from which the hormone is absent and checking that the resulting decrease parallels the calibration or standard curve. If related molecules or other components of the serum matrix influence the result, the line of measured concentrations will diverge from the line of the standard curve.

A quick and simple experiment that captures aspects of imprecision and specificity can be performed by mixing exactly 50:50 volumes of samples containing expected high and low concentrations to create samples that should generate a result exactly between the results of the high and low samples. This can be further extended by mixing the middle sample 50:50 with the low and high samples to create a series of five (or nine, with one more mixing step) equidistant concentrations. Results from these sample mixtures should lie exactly on a straight line plotted equidistantly on the x-axis with concentration on the y-axis. An exact fit suggests that precision and specificity are likely to be high. Deviations from the straight line suggest one or more issues with the assay (see Figure 3.3).

Sensitivity

The definition of analytical sensitivity in immunoassays varies but the most practical measures to quote are the lowest detectable concentration (limit of detection (LoD)) and lowest quantifiable concentration (limit of quantification (LoQ)). The LoD can be assessed by replicate measurement of a sample that does not contain the hormone of interest. The mean + 2SD of these values estimates the lowest concentration that is 'different' from zero. The LoQ takes a more applied view and is the lowest concentration that can be reported with acceptable imprecision. In some assay set-ups that utilize a log-transformed calibration curve, the lowest reportable value is the assigned concentration of the lowest non-zero calibrator (e.g. 27.59 nmol/l for cortisol). Methods with a LoQ that is not low enough to document endocrine hypofunction will not be useful; for example, some human total T4 methods have a LoQ near the lower reference limit for dogs.

The upper reporting limit can be determined by progressively diluting a sample with an extremely high hormone concentration to discover the highest point at which the results follow a linear relationship with the dilution factor. Alternatively, the highest reportable value may be assigned to the highest calibrator used and results above this are simply reported as 'greater than'.

Analytical interference

Analytical interference studies again look for things that can cause an undesirable influence on the measured result. Common things that are tested include haemolysis, lipaemia and icterus, anticoagulants and serum separator gel.

Some physiological interferences become apparent only after initial clinical application because not all molecules can be tested for all assays in advance. Example interferences in free T4 by dialysis methods include free fatty acids and furosemide, which both increase the free fraction of T4 potentially resulting in a hypothyroid concentration appearing euthyroid (Stockigt and Lim, 2009). As immunoassays rely on the interaction of assay antibodies with hormone molecules, the presence of antibodies in the sample that interact with the molecule (e.g. T4 autoantibody) or the assay monoclonal antibody (anti-mouse antibodies) will generate false results (Bergman et al., 2019a,b).

Quality assurance

Once a method is validated or verified, its performance should be managed and monitored to ensure it remains fit for purpose at each use. These processes are QA and QC. Quality assurance in this context most often means the overall system that is in place to ensure quality results, including standard operating procedures, operator manuals, staff training, staff proficiency checks, cleaning and maintenance schedules and environmental controls, as well as QC and EQA.

Quality control

Quality control is a process that runs contemporaneously with sample analysis. It informs the laboratory technician as to whether the analysis has worked correctly and the sample results are safe to release for clinical decision-making. It involves running one or more samples of quality control material (QCM) in the same way as the other samples and verifying that the QCM result(s) is consistent with what is expected from that material by checking whether it meets (pass) or does not meet (fail, reject) certain acceptance rules.

Efficient QC design depends on using acceptance rules based on the clinical purpose of the measurement and TEa guidelines where available. Stable (low imprecision), accurate (low bias), low TE methods may need less stringent QC rules than less reliable methods because it would take a significant shift in performance to exceed the allowable error and have a clinical impact. How resistant a method is against potential clinically significant error can be represented by the sigma metric (σ = (TEa% − Bias%) / CV%), which is a single scale of analytical performance related to clinical impact that can be applied across many analytical methods (Arnold et al., 2019). The least stringent QC approach can be taken with methods whose sigma metric exceeds a value of 6, such as a simple QC rule on a single level QCM. For example, using only the Westgard 1_{3s} rule, there is no concern about clinically impactful malfunction in the assay unless the QC sample result is more than 3 SDs away from its historic mean. More complicated and sensitive combinations of QC acceptance rules are required for lower sigma metric assays.

Quality control material can be obtained from commercial suppliers or created locally from in-house pools of surplus samples. Commercial QCMs containing veterinary species hormones are not easily obtained and there is, therefore, an advantage to using local species-specific serum pools. For example, if an assay modification happens that does not affect the target human market, commercial QCM may not detect an impact on veterinary analysis that a veterinary species QCM would. Where commercial QCM is used, it is better to derive mean and historical SD values locally rather than accept the usually overly broad and insensitive limits provided by the manufacturer. These should normally be derived from around 20 local replicates of each independent lot number of QCM.

In analyses that are performed by RIA in a batch, the QCM and sample result experience the same process and results for both become available at the same time. The operator then knows if that whole batch passed or failed and whether results can be safely released. However, in automated systems, the equipment may be used as required (occasionally, continuously) rather than in sample batches. In commercial laboratories that are generating tens or hundreds of automated sample results a day, QC will be performed frequently (at the beginning and end of the day and sometimes even more than once in between) because the laboratory needs to know at the earliest opportunity if there is a problem with their methods. When a QC fails, all results since the last passed QC are questionable and potentially require re-analysis once the malfunction has been addressed. In a high-volume laboratory, it is in the operator's interest to keep the number of questionable results to a manageable minimum. When deciding on appropriate in-clinic QC frequency, the same approach is relevant; that is, how many samples is the clinic comfortable having to review or how many samples will they re-analyse at their cost when there is a QC failure.

With regard to in-clinic hormone measurement, the responsibility for QA falls on the veterinary clinic, not the manufacturer, and the QA and QC approach of reference laboratories should be replicated in the in-clinic environment if the clinician is to be confident that their clinical decisions are not being impacted by analytical

error. If in-clinic QC limits are not derived locally and manufacturers' limits are used, they should at least be reviewed from a clinical application standpoint – would it be clinically reasonable for results from one sample to match the upper and lower control limits? For example, if a manufacturer provided acceptance limits for a cortisol QCM of 100–250 nmol/l, would that fit with clinicians' expectations of acceptable performance – that a single sample could generate a result as low as 100 nmol/l or as high as 250 nmol/l if the system was working properly?

Some analysers perform internal electronic checks on their systems, including incubation temperature, light source and detector performance checks. Whilst these provide some reassurance against serious mechanical malfunction, they do not replace the value of a QCM-based QC system.

External quality assessment

Laboratories and clinics should participate in an EQA programme for the hormones they measure. External quality assessment informs how results compare with others and may detect shifts in performance that are not detected by local QC. It is infrequent, retrospective and does not immediately inform the decision whether it is safe to release sample results. Ideally, the selected EQA scheme participants should not only be other users of identical equipment. Specific veterinary endocrine EQA schemes have been set up by the Society for Comparative Endocrinology and European Society of Veterinary Endocrinology (see 'Useful websites', below). However, common analyses such as total T4 may be included in general chemistry EQA schemes provided commercially. The review of variation in results obtained by different laboratories from the same sample evident in EQA reports can inform clinicians about the degree of caution required when utilizing textbook or literature-based decision thresholds (Figure 3.6).

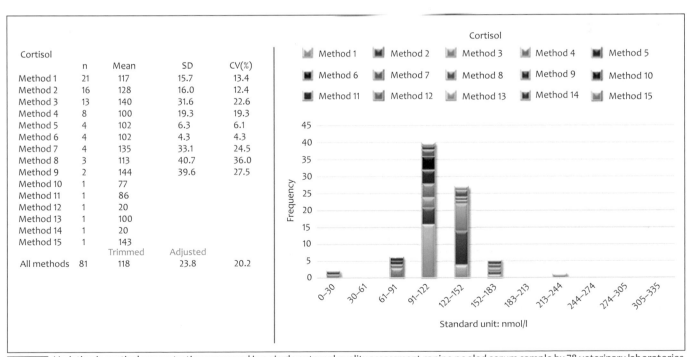

Cortisol	n	Mean	SD	CV(%)
Method 1	21	117	15.7	13.4
Method 2	16	128	16.0	12.4
Method 3	13	140	31.6	22.6
Method 4	8	100	19.3	19.3
Method 5	4	102	6.3	6.1
Method 6	4	102	4.3	4.3
Method 7	4	135	33.1	24.5
Method 8	3	113	40.7	36.0
Method 9	2	144	39.6	27.5
Method 10	1	77		
Method 11	1	86		
Method 12	1	20		
Method 13	1	100		
Method 14	1	20		
Method 15	1	143		
		Trimmed	Adjusted	
All methods	81	118	23.8	20.2

3.6 Variation in cortisol concentration measured in a single external quality assessment canine pooled serum sample by 78 veterinary laboratories using 15 different analytical methods in 20 countries. Results range from 20 to 223 nmol/l (trimmed mean = 118 nmol/l, coefficient of variation = 20%). Although Method 14 yielded a low result compared with the consensus, it was reported against a lower reference interval than most other laboratories. Methods 8 and 11 were in-clinic analysers. CV = coefficient of variation
(Data from European Society of Veterinary Endocrinology, 2020)

Sample collection and handling

Guidance on sample collection, handling and shipping depend on the analyses of interest and also to a lesser extent on the laboratory method being used.

There are sample handling studies available in the literature, but laboratories may conduct their own shipping and storage experiments and devise their own recommendations, meaning that sample submission requirements may vary between laboratories. The suitability of environmental shipping temperatures will also vary by regional climate. The laboratory is the best source of information on sample collection and shipping.

In broad terms, steroids and total thyroid hormones are more stable in transit than peptides that could be subject to protease activity. Some peptides are particularly labile and will need cold handling or protease inhibitors (EDTA, aprotinin) to mitigate losses during shipping.

Free T4 is an example where cold shipping does not stop the hormone itself from being degraded but instead preserves the relationship between the hormone and its binding proteins.

Sample tube selection can be important not just for anti-protease activity. The gel in serum separator tubes may bind a proportion of the analyte of interest (particularly relevant if low concentrations are important, e.g. pre-ovulatory canine progesterone) or the anticoagulant may interfere in the analytical method. For example, EDTA is not recommended for Immulite total T4 or cortisol assays, perhaps because unwashed residue chelates the ions required for the alkaline phosphatase activity that generates luminescence (Schechter et al., 2020).

Figure 3.7 compiles example sample type and sample handling recommendations from two veterinary endocrinology laboratories: Michigan State University Veterinary Diagnostic Laboratory (USA) and NationWide Specialist Laboratories (UK).

Test	Sample required	Special shipping and handling
Adrenocorticotropic hormone	EDTA plasma	• Freeze; ship on ice or frozen via overnight courier • Must arrive below 16°C
Aldosterone	EDTA or heparin plasma or serum	• Refrigerate or freeze; ship on ice. Should arrive either overnight or next day • Separate EDTA plasma samples within 30 minutes of collection • No special sample handling
Anti-Müllerian hormone	Serum or heparin plasma	• No special sample handling
Cortisol	Serum or heparin plasma	• Refrigerate or freeze; ship on ice. Should arrive either overnight or next day • Separate samples within 30 minutes of collection • No special sample handling
Erythropoeitin	Serum	• No special sample handling
Gastrin	Serum	• Refrigerate or freeze; ship on ice during hot months
17-alpha-hydroxyprogesterone	Serum or heparin plasma	• No special sample handling
Insulin	Serum	• Refrigerate or freeze; ship on ice • Animal should be fasted before collection • No special sample handling
Insulin-like growth factor-1	Serum or heparin plasma	• Refrigerate or freeze; ship on ice • No special sample handling
Insulin antibodies	Serum	• No special sample handling
Metanephrines (blood)	EDTA plasma	• Freeze; ship on dry ice
Metanephrines (urine)	Urine	• Acidified • Plain • Freeze; ship on ice
Oestradiol	Serum or heparin plasma	• No special sample handling
Parathyroid hormone	Serum or EDTA plasma	• Refrigerate or freeze; ship on ice or frozen via overnight courier • Must arrive below 16°C • Avoid lipaemia and haemolysis
Parathyroid hormone-related protein	EDTA plasma	• Freeze; ship on ice or frozen via overnight courier • Must arrive below 16°C • Avoid lipaemia and haemolysis • Do not send an EDTA tube without separating the plasma
Progesterone	Serum or heparin plasma No gel tubes	• Refrigerate or freeze; ship on ice. Should arrive either overnight or next day • No special sample handling
Relaxin	Heparin plasma	• No special sample handling
Renin	EDTA plasma	• Freeze; ship frozen by overnight courier
Testosterone	Serum or heparin plasma	• Refrigerate or freeze; ship on ice • No special sample handling
Thyroglobulin and thyroid hormone autoantibodies	Serum or heparin plasma	• Avoid haemolysis and lipaemia • No special sample handling

3.7 Sample type and handling recommendations for veterinary hormone measurement. The handling recommendations are generally compiled from Michigan State University – Veterinary Diagnostic Laboratory (USA) and NationWide Laboratories (UK) guidance. Note the variation in sample handling requirements for individual hormones. This emphasizes the need to refer to the individual laboratory being used. (continues) ▶

Test	Sample required	Special shipping and handling
Thyrotropin (thyroid-stimulating hormone) (canine)	Serum or heparin plasma	• Avoid haemolysis and lipaemia • No special sample handling
Thyroxine (total)	Serum or heparin plasma	• Avoid haemolysis and lipaemia • No special sample handling
Thyroxine (free by analogue assay)	Serum or heparin plasma	• Avoid haemolysis and lipaemia • No special sample handling
Thyroxine (free by equilibrium dialysis)	Serum or heparin plasma	• Refrigerate or freeze; ship on ice. Should arrive either overnight or next day • Avoid haemolysis and lipaemia • No special sample handling
Urinary cortisol:creatinine	Urine	• Refrigerate or freeze; ship on ice. Should arrive either overnight or next day • No special sample handling
Vitamin D: 25-hydroxycholecalciferol and 1,25-dihydroxycholecalciferol (calcitriol, active vitamin D)	Serum	• Animal should be fasted overnight before collection • Centrifuge within 1 hour • Refrigerate or freeze; ship on ice via overnight courier • Avoid exposure to sunlight • No special sample handling

3.7 (continued) Sample type and handling recommendations for veterinary hormone measurement. The handling recommendations are generally compiled from Michigan State University Veterinary Diagnostic Laboratory (USA) and NationWide Laboratories (UK) guidance. Note the variation in sample handling requirements for individual hormones. This emphasizes the need to refer to the individual laboratory being used.

References and further reading

Arnold JE, Camus MS, Freeman KP et al. (2019) ASVCP Guidelines: Principles of Quality Assurance and Standards for Veterinary Clinical Pathology (version 3.0). Veterinary Clinical Pathology 48, 542–618

Bergman D, Larsson A, Hansson-Hamlin H, Åhlén E and Holst BS (2019a) Characterization of canine anti-mouse antibodies highlights that multiple strategies are needed to combat immunoassay interference. Scientific Reports 9, 14521

Bergman D, Larsson A, Hansson-Hamlin H and Holst BS (2019b) Investigation of interference from canine anti-mouse antibodies in hormone immunoassays. Veterinary Clinical Pathology 48 Suppl 1, 59–69

Department of Health and Human Services (2019) Clinical Laboratory Improvement Amendments of 1988 (CLIA) Proficiency Testing Regulations Related to Analytes and Acceptable Performance: Proposed Rule. Federal Register 84, 1536–1567

European Society of Veterinary Endocrinology (2020) European Veterinary Endocrine Quality Assurance Scheme (EVF-QAS). Available from: www.esve.org/esve/eve-qas

Falkenö U, Hillström A, von Brömssen C and Strage EM (2016) Biological variation of 20 analytes measured in serum from clinically healthy domestic cats. Journal of Veterinary Diagnostic Investigation 28, 699–704

Fraser CG and Sandberg S (2018) Biological variation. In: Tietz Textbook of Clinical Chemistry and Molecular Diagnostics, 6th edn, ed. N Rifai, AR Horvath and C Wittwer, pp. 157–169. Elsevier, St. Louis

Graham PA (2010) Impact of Analytical Method on Endocrine Diagnosis. Presented at ECVIM 2010

Harr KE, Flatland B, Nabity M and Freeman KP (2013) ASVCP guidelines: allowable total error guidelines for biochemistry. Veterinary Clinical Pathology 42, 424–436

Iversen L, Jensen AL, Høier R and Aaes H (1999) Biological variation of canine serum thyrotropin (TSH) concentration. Veterinary Clinical Pathology 28, 16–19

Jensen AL and Høier R (1996) Evaluation of thyroid function in dogs by hormone analysis: effects of data on biological variation. Veterinary Clinical Pathology 25, 130–134

Jensen AL, Høier R and Pedersen HD (1993) Evaluation of an enzyme linked immunosorbent assay for the determination of free thyroxine in canine plasma samples assisted by data on biological variation. Zentralblatt für Veterinärmedizin A 40, 539–545

Jensen AL and Kjelgaard-Hansen M (2006) Method comparison in the clinical laboratory. Veterinary Clinical Pathology 35, 276–286

Knowles EJ, Moreton-Clack MC, Shaw S et al. (2018) Plasma adrenocorticotropic hormone (ACTH) concentrations in ponies measured by two different assays suggests seasonal cross-reactivity or interference. Equine Veterinary Journal 50, 672–677

Prieto JM, Carney PC, Miller ML et al. (2020) Short-term biological variation of serum thyroid hormones concentrations in clinically healthy cats. Domestic Animal Endocrinology 71, 106389

Schechter DA, Lee HP, Kemppainen RJ and Behrend EN (2020) Effect of EDTA on measurement of cortisol and thyroxine by chemiluminescent enzyme immunoassay in dogs. Journal of Veterinary Diagnostic Investigation 32, 363–368

Stockigt JR and Lim CF (2009) Medications that distort in vitro tests of thyroid function, with particular reference to estimates of serum free thyroxine. Best Practice & Research: Clinical Endocrinology & Metabolism 23, 753–767

Strage E (2015) Biological variation of serum insulin concentrations in healthy cats. Acta Veterinaria Scandinavica 57 Suppl 1, O14

Strage EM, Theodorsson E, Holst BS, Lilliehöök I and Lewitt MS (2015) Insulin-like growth factor I in cats: validation of an enzyme-linked immunosorbent assay and determination of biologic variation. Veterinary Clinical Pathology 44, 542–551

Useful websites

European Society of Veterinary Endocrinology
www.esve.org

Society for Comparative Endocrinology
www.veterinaryendocrinology.org

Vet Biological Variation – curated database of biological variation in veterinary species
www.vetbiologicalvariation.org

Chapter 4

Principles of interpreting endocrine test results

Peter A. Graham

General guidelines

The interpretation of endocrine laboratory test results can be more complicated than that of other types of clinical chemistry. The interrelatedness of endocrine systems with other physiological systems and their responsiveness to environmental factors makes them subject to a number of influences other than simply the presence or absence of pathology. Endocrine systems are dynamic and responsive, meaning that changes in hormone test results will occur physiologically as well as pathologically, and in many cases there is a fine and ill-defined line distinguishing the two. In practice, this means that a clear-cut laboratory diagnosis cannot always be made.

However, not all endocrine results are ambiguous and, with an understanding of endocrine physiology, the impact of non-endocrine factors and the limitations of the diagnostic tests employed, it is possible to confidently confirm the presence or absence of endocrine disease.

For many endocrine disorders, diagnosis is often a judgement taking the above factors and clinical presentation into account. Knowing in which of those judgements to be confident and which should remain open to re-evaluation is the basis of successful endocrine interpretation.

For other clinical chemistry results, it is common to rely on reference intervals and make diagnostic decisions based on whether results are within or outside those intervals. However, the responsive nature of the endocrine system means that in many endocrine disorders a particular test result may remain within its reference interval but still provide strong evidence for the presence or classification of disease. The key to interpreting results in these circumstances is recollection of, and reliance upon, the concept of negative feedback. With this approach, the focus shifts from 'is it normal?' to 'is it appropriate?' Incorporating negative feedback into the interpretive process makes it possible to, for example:

- Interpret reference interval parathyroid hormone (PTH) results as primary hyperparathyroidism in canine hypercalcaemia
- Classify adrenocorticotropic hormone (ACTH)-dependent hypercortisolism with reference interval endogenous ACTH concentrations
- Diagnose insulinoma with reference interval insulin concentrations
- Understand why a low-dose dexamethasone suppression (LDDS) test can be immediately followed by an ACTH response test, but not *vice versa*.

Diagnostic test performance

There can be considerable overlap in endocrine test results between physiological and pathological responses. As a consequence, many of the hormone concentrations measured for investigating endocrine disease provide less than perfect diagnostic performance. For example, the hypothalamic–pituitary–adrenal response to stress and other illnesses is frequently associated with test results expected in canine hypercortisolism, resulting in poor diagnostic specificity (many false-positives). Similarly, the total thyroxine (T4) response to non-thyroidal illness (NTI) makes this measurement poorly specific for canine hypothyroidism.

Diagnostic sensitivity and specificity

Once the analytical performance of a laboratory test has been established (see Chapter 3), the next step is to determine its diagnostic performance. This provides information on how well the test distinguishes the presence of a given disease from its absence.

To assess diagnostic performance, dichotomized outcomes are generally used (i.e. the test result is either positive or negative, and the pathological condition or disease is either present or absent). However, while this is the best understood and most commonly used approach, it is a system of two extremes (not diseased or diseased). It does not allow for grey area or equivocal results, nor does it take into account the different aetiologies and the varying degrees of pathology that can be a feature of endocrine disorders, particularly those that take time to develop.

Diagnostic sensitivity

The diagnostic sensitivity (not to be confused with analytical sensitivity; see Chapter 3) is the proportion of individuals with the disease that are correctly identified by the test. The derivation of this proportion requires a diseased population of reasonable size that has been well characterized as having the disorder, usually by an independent and gold-standard diagnostic method or technique.

> Dixon and Mooney (1999) derived the diagnostic sensitivity of free T4 by equilibrium dialysis (fT4d) by measuring it in 30 dogs confirmed as hypothyroid using thyrotropin (thyroid-stimulating hormone (TSH)) response test results. Of these 30 dogs, 24 yielded fT4d results below a diagnostic cut-off of 5.42 pmol/l. ▶

> Diagnostic sensitivity – 24/30 = 0.80 (80%)
>
> Gold *et al.* (2016) derived the diagnostic sensitivity of a basal cortisol concentration cut-off of 22 nmol/l for hypoadrenocorticism. Of 163 dogs with hypoadrenocorticism based on results of an ACTH response test, 158 had results below the cut-off.
>
> Diagnostic sensitivity = 158/163 = 0.969 (96.9%)

Because this attribute is a proportion based on a sample, confidence intervals for the population proportion can be estimated as ± 1.96 x the estimated standard error of the proportion.

95% confidence limits for sensitivity =
sensitivity ± 1.96 x $\sqrt{}$ [sensitivity x (1 – sensitivity) / n]

Consequently, the larger the size of the diseased study group, the narrower the confidence intervals will be and, therefore, the more reliable the estimated sensitivity. Diagnostic sensitivity studies based on a small number of animals will generate wide confidence intervals, meaning that they are a less reliable source of sensitivity than studies based on larger numbers. In the above fT4d example, the 95% confidence interval ranged from 61% to 92%, and in the larger basal cortisol study example the interval was narrower (93–99%).

Diagnostic sensitivity is synonymous with the true-positive rate. As sensitivity is derived from only within the diseased population, the higher the sensitivity, the lower the false-negative rate must be. Greater confidence can be placed on negative results being true because false-negatives are rare. Therefore, tests of high diagnostic sensitivity are particularly useful for ruling out disease (Figure 4.1).

Test result	Diseased animals
Positive	True-positives
Negative	False-negatives
Example 1	
Positive	80
Negative	20
Total	100
Example 2	
Positive	99
Negative	1
Total	100

4.1 The derivation of diagnostic sensitivity. In example 1, diagnostic sensitivity is 80% and the false-negative rate is 20%. In example 2, diagnostic sensitivity is 99% and the false-negative rate is 1%.

> A commonly used memory aid is 'SnOut' (sensitivity is good for ruling out disease).

The derived diagnostic sensitivity can be swayed, to some extent, by the selection of the diseased group. Often the diseased group contains cases that are easily categorized and, consequently, may have 'severe' or 'obvious' disease. 'Mild' or 'early' cases that are more difficult to categorize may be omitted. As a consequence, sensitivity may be overestimated in studies that do not include a representative range of severities of presentation. If a high diagnostic sensitivity is quoted for a new test, it is prudent to check whether the diseased group really represented the complete range or continuum of presentations appropriately.

Diagnostic specificity

The diagnostic specificity (not to be confused with analytical specificity; see Chapter 3) is the proportion of individuals without the disease that are correctly identified by the test. The derivation of this proportion requires a well characterized population that is known not to have the pathology in question. Ideally, this should not simply be a healthy group, but instead should include animals of a similar signalment that have some attribute or clinical sign suggestive of the disease in question. Specificity is calculated in the same manner as sensitivity except in the non-diseased group.

> Dixon and Mooney (1999) derived the diagnostic specificity of fT4d by measuring it in 77 dogs confirmed as euthyroid (i.e. not hypothyroid) using TSH response test results. Of these 77 dogs, 72 yielded results greater than or equal to the diagnostic cut-off of 5.42 pmol/l.
>
> Diagnostic specificity = 72/77 = 0.935 (93.5%)
>
> Gold *et al.* (2016) derived the diagnostic specificity of a basal cortisol concentration cut-off of 22 nmol/l for hypoadrenocorticism. Of 351 dogs that did not have hypoadrenocorticism based on the results of an ACTH response test, 336 had results above the cut-off.
>
> Diagnostic specificity = 336/351 = 0.957 (95.7%)

Confidence intervals for diagnostic specificity are derived in an identical manner to those for sensitivity. In the above fT4d example, the 95% confidence interval ranged from 85% to 98% and, again, in the larger basal cortisol study example the interval was narrower (93.0–97.6%).

Diagnostic specificity is synonymous with the true-negative rate. As specificity is derived from within the non-diseased population, the higher the specificity, the lower the false-positive rate. Greater confidence can be placed on positive results being true because false-positives are rare. Therefore, tests of high diagnostic specificity are particularly useful for ruling in disease (Figure 4.2).

Test result	Non-diseased animals
Positive	False-positives
Negative	True-negatives
Example 1	
Positive	7
Negative	93
Total	100
Example 2	
Positive	1
Negative	99
Total	100

4.2 The derivation of diagnostic specificity. In example 1, diagnostic specificity is 93% and the false-positive rate is 7%. In example 2, diagnostic specificity is 99% and the false-positive rate is 1%.

> A commonly used memory aid is 'SpIn' (specificity is good for ruling in disease).

Estimates of diagnostic specificity can be swayed by the choice of subjects in the non-diseased population. As already mentioned, it is important that the chosen subjects are appropriately under investigation for the disorder in question. For example, a study on the specificity of a test for canine hypercortisolism using very young animals with no compatible clinical or presenting signs is likely to over-estimate diagnostic specificity significantly. If a high diagnostic specificity is quoted for a new test, it is prudent to check whether the non-diseased group is representative of the signalment and various presentations appropriate to the disease in question.

Ideally, the choice of diagnostic test should give the best available diagnostic sensitivity when the main aim is to rule out or exclude disease and the best specificity when the aim is to rule in or confirm disease. That may not necessarily require a different test but could be the same test using a different interpretive cut-off value, for example, a urinary cortisol:creatinine threshold of 26.5 for ruling out and 161.2 for ruling in hypercortisolism (Zeugswetter et al., 2010), or a basal cortisol of 5.5 nmol/l to rule in and 55 nmol/l to rule out hypoadrenocorticism (Gold et al., 2016).

Assessment of diagnostic performance

The combination of a test's diagnostic sensitivity and specificity across a range of possible cut-off values represented graphically is termed a receiver operating characteristic (ROC) curve. The overall usefulness of a test is conveyed by the area under such a curve. This approach allows comparison between diagnostic methods independent of the cut-off values that different clinical researchers may assign. The ROC curve and related data such as differential positive rate (DPR) can be used to determine the most suitable diagnostic cut-off values with the most appropriate combination of sensitivity and specificity.

Positive and negative predictive value and the effect of prevalence

The diagnostic sensitivity and specificity provide useful information on how a test performs in populations of well defined disease status created by researchers developing or assessing a new test. However, when clinically applied, users will want to know the likelihood of a positive test result being a true- or a false-positive – in other words, how much confidence they can have in positive or negative results. The probability of positive or negative test results correctly classifying the disease status is called a *predictive value*; positive predictive value (PPV) and negative predictive value (NPV), respectively. The PPV and NPV are derived from sensitivity and specificity combined with prevalence (Figure 4.3).

The true prevalence of the condition within the clinical population of animals under test is usually unknown. However, understanding the behaviour of the test in different circumstances of prevalence can alter the weight placed on the result, and can influence the type of animals upon which the test is performed.

Another way to consider prevalence is the probability that the disease is present before the test is performed (pre-test probability). Pre-test probability can be significantly improved by performing the test only on animals that already have a high likelihood of having the disease (appropriate age, breed or sex, compatible clinical signs and routine clinicopathological abnormalities, other differential diagnoses ruled out, etc).

As illustrated in Figure 4.4, prevalence (pre-test probability) has a dramatic effect on predictive values, particularly when the diagnostic sensitivity or specificity is relatively poor, as is often the case for tests for endocrine diseases.

- Tests of low diagnostic sensitivity have a poor NPV in high-prevalence (high pre-test probability) situations, such as those where there are appropriate supporting data for the disorder in question.
- Tests of low diagnostic specificity have a poor PPV in low-prevalence (low pre-test probability) situations when there is limited supporting clinical data for the diagnosis. Such a low prevalence is not uncommon when screening large populations for a relatively uncommon disease.

The effect of prevalence on PPV can be dramatic. When prevalence (pre-test probability) is as low as 5%, the PPV of the LDDS test for diagnosing canine hypercortisolism falls to an unacceptable 15% (Figure 4.4). Faced with a positive LDDS test result, and despite the result being 'positive', it is far more likely (85%) that the animal does not, in fact, have hypercortisolism. It is for this reason that the LDDS test is not suitable for 'screening' dogs for hypercortisolism, unless there is strong supporting evidence of such (high prevalence or pre-test probability).

Tests of low diagnostic specificity are common in veterinary endocrinology, hence the advice to increase pre-test probability (prevalence) before using total T4 for canine hypothyroidism or the LDDS test for canine hypercortisolism. In the case of total T4 for canine hypothyroidism, it is also important to avoid testing dogs in situations that are known to increase the risk of false-positive results (e.g. NTI, certain drug therapies). Alternatively, confidence in the diagnosis of hypothyroidism can be improved by using a combination of thyroid function tests with better specificity, rather than relying on total T4 alone.

For diagnosing feline hyperthyroidism, total T4 has high specificity but lower sensitivity. It is therefore a good test for screening older cats as there is confidence in diagnosing hyperthyroidism with a positive test result. However, when prevalence (pre-test probability) is high, the NPV decreases and hyperthyroidism cannot be definitively ruled out with a reference interval total T4 value. An appropriate course of action is re-testing or combining with a higher-sensitivity test, such as fT4d.

Test result	Diseased animals	Non-diseased animals	Total	Predictive values and prevalence
Positive	True-positives (TP)	False-positives (FP)	TP + FP	PPV = TP / (TP + FP)
Negative	False-negatives (FN)	True-negatives (TN)	FN + TN	NPV = TN / (FN + TN)
Total	TP + FN	FP + TN		Prevalence = (TP + FN) / (TP + FN + FP + TN)
	Sensitivity = TP / (TP + FN)	Specificity = TN / (FP + TN)		

4.3 The derivation of positive predictive value (PPV) and negative predictive value (NPV).

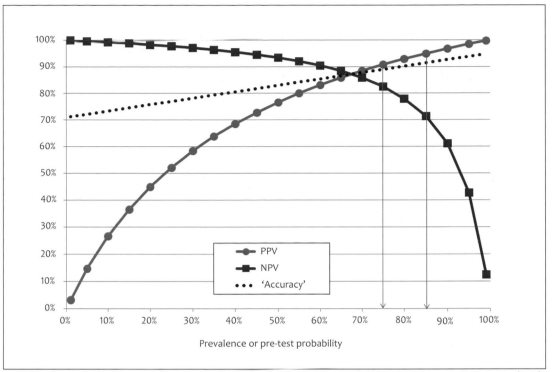

4.4 Effect of pre-test probability (prevalence) on positive predictive value (PPV) and negative predictive value (NPV) and diagnostic accuracy using the low-dose dexamethasone suppression test for diagnosing canine hypercortisolism. The NPV and PPV are calculated from the 95% sensitivity and 71% specificity reported by Van Liew *et al.* (1997). At low prevalence, PPV is low (5% prevalence is associated with 15% PPV). To have 90% confidence in a positive test result being true requires a pre-test probability of 75%, and a PPV >95% requires a pre-test probability of 85% (purple arrows). However, at such high pre-test probabilities, the confidence in negative results falls. Confidence in a negative test result is >90% at all pre-test probabilities below 60%.

Published predictive values do not apply universally. As demonstrated in Figure 4.4, they are entirely dependent on prevalence (pre-test probability) within the studied population and, as a consequence, predictive values should be mistrusted unless prevalence is also stated. For application to the clinical setting, the cited prevalence must be similar to the clinician's expectations.

Some studies quote test accuracy (all correct results as proportion of all tests). This measure of performance is affected by prevalence in the same way as predictive values (Figure 4.4) and therefore should be critically evaluated in a similar manner.

Sensitivity and specificity data can also be combined to generate *likelihood ratios* (LRs) of positive (LR+) or negative (LR–) results. An LR+ conveys the likelihood of a given result in an animal with the condition compared with the likelihood of that same result in one without the condition. The more the LR+ exceeds 1, the more likely the disease is present. An LR– can be used similarly with regard to negative results. The more the LR– is less than 1, the more likely the disease is absent. Likelihood ratios can be created for multiple hormone concentrations. An added advantage of LRs is that they can be combined with known or assumed pre-test odds to generate post-test odds for the presence of disease.

LR+ = sensitivity / (1 – specificity)
LR– = (1 – sensitivity) / specificity
Pre-test odds = pre-test probability /
                (1 – pre-test probability)
Post-test odds = pre-test odds x LR
Post-test probability = post-test odds /
                        (post-test odds + 1)

Interpretive caution near reference limits and cut-off values

Chapter 3 highlights assay imprecision as a source of variation when comparing results to the laboratory-derived cut-offs and reference limits. Laboratory total error (TE) (bias combined with imprecision) is relevant when comparing results to limits derived outside that laboratory. Laboratories and in-clinic equipment providers should provide imprecision and TE values for analyte concentrations close to interpretive limits, which can be used to inform the clinician how much grey zone surrounds a cut-off value. This information alone provides a minimum estimate of grey zone without the addition of potential variation due to biological variation (see Chapter 3).

For example, at an interpretive cut-off of 140 nmol/l for cortisol and an intra-assay imprecision coefficient of variation (CV) of 5%, samples analysed at that laboratory that truly have a concentration of 140 nmol/l could yield results anywhere between 126 and 154 nmol/l. If the CV imprecision between laboratories taken from an external quality assessment (EQA) report was 15%, and a clinician wanted to use any laboratory and compare their result to a published cut-off of 140 nmol/l, in the absence of a specific TE value from the chosen laboratory, they might have to consider a wider grey zone of 98–182 nmol/l. Both of these examples do not take into account the additional potential impact of biological variation. Considering CV is often worst at low concentrations, the grey zone surrounding an 8-hour LDDS cut-off of 40 nmol/l could be between 32 and 48 nmol/l at a CV of 10% and between 24 and 56 nmol/l at a CV of 20%.

When trying to determine whether two results from the same animal using the same laboratory method represent a genuine change (e.g. worsening pathology, therapeutic response), a *reference change value* (RCV) (or *critical difference*) can be helpful and can be calculated if both analytical and biological variation are known (see Chapter 3). If only analytical imprecision is known, it can be expressed as a minimum estimate.

Another concern when comparing results to an upper or lower reference interval is the convention that reference intervals typically encompass 95% of the healthy population. Results that are close to but outside the reference limits may be representative of the 5% of the healthy population outside the interval or could be abnormal. For analytes that have a normal distribution, the limit beyond which a result is likely to represent abnormality can be crudely estimated by dividing the reference interval by four and extending the reference interval by that result and, in so doing, estimating a three-standard-deviation limit.

There are other reasons for being cautious in interpreting close-to-limit results. Endocrine reference intervals are not always well constructed or may not appropriately represent the population of animals under investigation.

Discordant results

When a laboratory result does not fit the clinical expectation, and particularly when obtaining a replacement blood sample would be inconvenient, there are three main approaches to result checking:

- Repeat the measurement with the same sample on the same analytical method. The two results can be considered similar if they are within approximately three standard deviations of each other
  - Analytically acceptable difference in duplicate analysis = mean of results x analytical coefficient of variation (CV_A) x 2.77
- Repeat analysis of the sample diluted 1 in 2, 1 in 4, and so on. All results should multiply back up to the original value if there is no interferent present
- Use an alternative analytical methodology but be mindful that a different reference interval is likely to apply.

Effects of non-endocrine factors

In some instances, non-endocrine factors can significantly affect the interpretation of endocrine test results and can influence the tests chosen. They may even dictate whether a test is performed at all. Specific effects of non-endocrine factors on individual endocrine system test results are discussed in the relevant chapters.

For many situations, the effects of non-endocrine factors are subtle. A change in test results due to a physiological factor may be seen in an individual animal or between the results of groups of animals. However, such a change is often not sufficient to cause a significant change in diagnostic category. In these situations, even when a physiological factor has 'pushed' a result over a diagnostic threshold, it is likely that the result would be 'borderline' and viewed with an appropriately low level of diagnostic confidence, rather than the animal being con-

fidently misclassified as diseased or healthy. However, there are some particular situations in which non-endocrine factors can result in significant and frequent misclassification of health *versus* disease.

Breed

The physical characteristics of dogs vary greatly, and so the risk of diagnostic misclassification when using general all-breed reference intervals is unsurprising; breed-specific reference intervals may be considered more appropriate. Since wide breed variability is less of an issue in cats, this problem is of greater concern in dogs.

The necessity for breed-specific reference intervals is dependent on studies of large numbers of healthy individuals within each breed of interest. So far, only a limited number of studies have been completed and, from those, a strong case for breed-specific intervals has been made in only a few specific circumstances (Hegstad-Davies *et al.*, 2015).

It is now widely accepted that dolichocephalic sighthound breeds have a much lower reference interval for total T4 and, in some instances, free T4. In these dogs, the lower end of their reference interval may be below the limit of detection of most commercially available assays. Outside this group, and despite insistence by some breed societies, there is little evidence that the general all-breed reference interval is inappropriate.

Circulating concentrations of insulin-like growth factor-1 (IGF-1), produced by the liver under the influence of growth hormone (GH), are measured for suspected hypersomatotropism and pituitary dwarfism, and to determine nutritional status. These are strongly affected by the size (and age, see below) of the dog. Smaller breeds have naturally lower IGF-1 concentrations than larger breeds and this needs to be taken into account when interpreting results.

Where a breed-specific reference interval is unavailable, it may be helpful to submit a 'control' sample from an age- and breed-matched healthy dog.

Age

Very young and growing animals may have significantly different circulating hormone concentrations from their adult counterparts. For example, in the first few weeks of life, thyroid hormone concentrations are likely to be high, and in growing animals, IGF-1 concentrations are much higher than in adults.

There may be more subtle changes in hormone concentration as adult animals age; for example, total T4 appears to decline slowly with age, while TSH increases. However, in general, these changes are not sufficient to result in significant diagnostic misclassification when using an all-age reference interval.

Sex

For most of the common hormone measurements used to document endocrine pathology, the differences in results due to sex are unlikely to cause diagnostic misclassifications. However, there are some examples of sex-specific reference intervals, such as for the interpretation of adrenal steroid precursors (adrenal sex hormones). Clearly, the interpretation of gonadal steroid concentrations will depend on sex and neuter status, and these may be used to investigate, for example, neuter status and remnant or retained gonadal tissue.

Time of day

Although there may be a strong circadian or diurnal pattern for circulating concentrations of commonly measured hormones in humans and other mammals, this may be of limited or no relevance in dogs and cats, despite being frequently cited in textbooks. It has been shown that cortisol in the dog has a cyclic and pulsatile pattern of secretion, but a diurnal pattern has not been demonstrated. Consequently, advice that investigation of canine adrenal function be carried out at a particular time of day is unfounded and unnecessary.

Some hormones are released into the circulation in a pulsatile manner and the measured concentration will depend on when the sample was obtained in relation to the timing of the associated peaks and troughs. Such pulsatile patterns of secretion can create wide reference intervals that are sometimes so wide that they mask biologically relevant changes in concentration. Examples include the inability to diagnose ACTH-dependent hypercortisolism with endogenous ACTH concentrations alone, or hypersomatotropism in cats based on a single GH measurement.

The time of day (or, more correctly, time since last medication) is of greater importance when using tests for therapeutic monitoring, such as thyroid hormone supplementation in the treatment of canine hypothyroidism or trilostane in the treatment of canine hypercortisolism.

Drugs

There is a long list of commonly used veterinary drugs that have been investigated for their potential to alter endocrine test results. By far the majority of such investigations discover only subtle or minimal effects, such that diagnostic misclassification is unlikely. However, there are some drugs that can exert a diagnostically significant effect. Common examples include:

- Sulphonamides, which can cause primary but reversible hypothyroidism
- Barbiturates, which suppress total T4 and, through induction of metabolic enzymes, could result in false-positive ACTH response and LDDS test results
- Glucocorticoids, which suppress thyroid hormone concentrations and exert negative feedback on the pituitary–adrenal axis, influencing adrenal function tests.

Ideally, endocrine investigations should not be performed when these drug therapies are being used. If barbiturates or glucocorticoids cannot be avoided, specialist laboratory approaches (e.g. fT4d) or other diagnostic techniques should be considered.

Non-endocrine illness

Non-endocrine illness poses the greatest challenge and risk of misclassification. Non-endocrine illnesses significantly influence the results of the two most commonly investigated endocrine systems in companion animals: the thyroid and adrenal.

As discussed above, the diagnostic specificity of tests such as total T4 for hypothyroidism and the LDDS test for hypercortisolism, and the diagnostic sensitivity of total T4 for feline hyperthyroidism, are far from perfect. The most important reason for this is the effect of NTI or non-adrenal illness.

- Any significant NTI, either acute or chronic, has the potential to suppress total T4 concentrations below the reference interval. Thyroid testing should therefore be postponed in dogs with a known NTI until it has abated or been stabilized with treatment. Alternatively, as the effect of NTI is less dramatic on fT4d results, measuring this parameter improves the chances of correctly diagnosing hypothyroidism.
- The effect of NTI presents a similar difficulty in the investigation of feline hyperthyroidism, whereby cats need to be re-tested after recovery from NTI or with the additional measurement of fT4d for correct diagnosis.
- Any illness that might be described as 'metabolically stressful' has the potential to result in false-positive results on hypercortisolism testing. The simplistic explanation is that the physiological demand for glucocorticoids in stressful illness increases the production capacity, and this can be misinterpreted by dynamic endocrine testing (e.g. ACTH response and LDDS tests) as evidence for pathological excess (hypercortisolism).

Effects of endocrine disease

Concurrent endocrinopathy

The pre-existence of one endocrinopathy may affect the ability to reliably confirm or exclude the presence of another. For example, the routine clinicopathological abnormalities expected in a poorly controlled diabetic dog are similar to those expected in a dog with hypercortisolism. In this scenario, the significance of increased liver enzyme activities and cholesterol concentration in supporting a diagnosis of hypercortisolism must be discounted. Similarly, a dog with hypercortisolism is likely to have a low circulating total T4 concentration, even when truly euthyroid.

Hyperlipidaemia

Several endocrine diseases can result in hyperlipidaemia. Lipaemia is capable of interfering with the test results of some analytes, using certain methods of analysis. The degree of this effect is generally known by commercial laboratories for each particular analyte measured using their technology. When there is interference, it is often because the lipid present alters the equipment's ability to detect light or a colour change in a sample. Antibody interactions with the analyte and the separation of antibody-bound hormone from free hormone are less commonly affected. In general, radioimmunoassays are free from the effects of this type of interference, because light or a colour change is not integral to these assays. However, for fT4d, an increased concentration of free fatty acids in the sample will, by displacement from binding proteins, result in an increased free hormone fraction.

Endogenous antibodies

As discussed in Chapter 3, immunoassays are almost exclusively used for the measurement of hormones. The principle of an immunoassay relies on an antibody directed against the hormone under investigation. By using a uniform amount of anti-hormone antibody in both samples and assay standards, the interaction is controlled and a reliable estimate of the hormone concentration in the sample can be made. However, if antibodies that can cross-react with the hormone under test are already present in the sample or interfere with the assay antibody directly, control over the hormone–antibody interaction is lost. As a consequence, a reliable estimate of hormone concentration can no longer be made and false results are generated.

Anti-thyroglobulin autoantibodies

A common scenario in which false results are generated relates to the presence of anti-thyroglobulin autoantibodies (TgAAs) that cross-react with triiodothyronine (T3) and T4 (T3AAs and T4AAs). These occur in up to approximately 30% and 10% of hypothyroid dogs, respectively. Whether TGAAs cause a false high or false low value depends on the intricacies of the immunoassay design. However, false highs (not necessarily above but often close to the upper end of the reference interval) are a common consequence in traditional radioimmunoassays; with other measurement approaches, false low values are more common. These autoantibodies have no physiological consequence for the animal in terms of the availability of thyroid hormones, but their effect on correctly measuring the hormones is great.

Anti-insulin antibodies

False high results due to anti-insulin antibody interference may also be seen when measuring insulin, either before treatment or, more commonly, following treatment with insulin that is antigenically distinct from the endogenous insulin (Davison et al., 2011).

Anti-mouse antibodies

Assays that depend on monoclonal antibodies (mAbs) derived from murine hybridomas (such as the commonly available canine TSH assay) are at risk from circulating anti-mouse antibodies. This is seen in human patients occupationally exposed to mice or mouse serum products or those treated with mAb therapeutic products. This phenomenon has been recognized recently in dogs but reports on its effect on different immunoassays are limited (Bergman et al., 2019a,b).

Endocrine therapy

Although the design of immunoassays for measuring hormones should be as specific as possible for the hormone in question, in some assays the antibody used will cross-react with related compounds. For example, prednisolone will cause falsely increased cortisol results but dexamethasone will not, and the steroid precursors accumulating during trilostane therapy will contribute to a more marked increase in 17-alpha-hydroxyprogesterone concentrations than expected.

If 'empirical' treatment is undertaken without confirmation of the underlying condition, accurate interpretation can be hindered. The treatment of calcium disorders without identifying the underlying condition can be problematic. If the treatment normalizes circulating calcium concentration, the interpretation of PTH results is compromised. Similarly, the treatment of suspected hypoadrenocorticism prior to confirmatory endocrine testing may compromise the investigation if it is later conducted after glucocorticoid administration. In such circumstances, aldosterone measurement may be more helpful.

Exogenous glucocorticoid, including topical eye, ear and skin medications, will often result in suppressed ACTH response test results that should not be interpreted as evidence of adrenal deficiency.

References and further reading

Bergman D, Larsson A, Hansson-Hamlin H, Åhlén E and Holst BS (2019a) Characterization of canine anti-mouse antibodies highlights that multiple strategies are needed to combat immunoassay interference. *Scientific Reports* **9**, 14521

Bergman D, Larsson A, Hansson-Hamlin H and Holst BS (2019b) Investigation of interference from canine anti-mouse antibodies in hormone immunoassays. *Veterinary Clinical Pathology* **48** Suppl 1, 59–69

Davison LJ, Herrtage ME and Catchpole B (2011) Autoantibodies to recombinant canine proinsulin in canine diabetic patients. *Research in Veterinary Science* **91**, 58–63

Dixon RM and Mooney CT (1999) Evaluation of serum free thyroxine and thyrotropin concentrations in the diagnosis of canine hypothyroidism. *Journal of Small Animal Practice* **40**, 72–78

Fraser CG and Sandberg S (2018) Biological variation. In: *Tietz Textbook of Clinical Chemistry and Molecular Diagnostics, 6th edn*, ed. N Rifai, AR Horvath and C Wittwer, pp. 157–169. Elsevier, St. Louis

Gold AJ, Langlois DK and Refsal KR (2016) Evaluation of basal serum or plasma cortisol concentrations for the diagnosis of hypoadrenocorticism in dogs. *Journal of Veterinary Internal Medicine* **30**, 1798–1805

Hegstad-Davies RL, Torres SM, Sharkey LC et al. (2015) Breed-specific reference intervals for assessing thyroid function in seven dog breeds. *Journal of Veterinary Diagnostic Investigation* **27**, 716–727

Iversen L, Jensen AL, Høier R and Aaes H (1999) Biological variation of canine serum thyrotropin (TSH) concentration. *Veterinary Clinical Pathology* **28**, 16–19

Jensen AL and Høier R (1996) Evaluation of thyroid function in dogs by hormone analysis: effects of data on biological variation. *Veterinary Clinical Pathology* **25**, 130–134

Jensen AL, Høier R and Pedersen HD (1993) Evaluation of an enzyme linked immunosorbent assay for the determination of free thyroxine in canine plasma samples assisted by data on biological variation. *Zentralblatt für Veterinärmedizin A* **40**, 539–545

Prieto JM, Carney PC, Miller ML et al. (2020) Short-term biological variation of serum thyroid hormones concentrations in clinically healthy cats. *Domestic Animal Endocrinology* **71**, 106389

Van Liew CH, Greco DS and Salman MD (1997) Comparison of results of adrenocorticotropic hormone stimulation and low-dose dexamethasone suppression tests with necropsy findings in dogs: 81 cases (1985–1995). *Journal of the American Veterinary Medical Association* **211**, 322–325

Zeugswetter F, Bydzovsky N, Kampner D and Schwendenwein I (2010) Tailored reference limits for urine corticoid:creatinine ratio in dogs to answer distinct clinical questions. *Veterinary Record* **167**, 997–1001

Chapter 5

The effect of endocrine disease on the cardiovascular system

Luca Ferasin

Introduction

Several clinical manifestations of cardiovascular disease can arise from either excess or deficiency of hormone production. This chapter reviews the spectrum of cardiac abnormalities that may result from changes in specific endocrine gland function, which can affect autonomous cardiovascular modulation, cardiomyocyte function, vascular smooth muscle cells, and other target cells and tissues.

Thyroid gland disorders

The heart and thyroid gland have a close physiological relationship, which is confirmed by predictable changes in cardiovascular function in dogs and cats with hyperthyroidism and hypothyroidism. Indeed, many of the most characteristic clinical signs of thyroid disease result from the effects of thyroid hormones on the cardiovascular system (Klein and Danzi, 2016).

Cellular mechanisms of thyroid hormones

Thyroid function influences every structure of the heart and its specialized conducting system. Moreover, thyroid hormones have indirect effects mediated through the autonomic nervous system, the renin–angiotensin–aldosterone system (RAAS), vascular compliance, vasoreactivity and kidney function.

The thyroid gland primarily secretes thyroxine (T4). However, the heart relies mainly on circulating triiodothyronine (T3) because there is no significant cardiomyocyte intracellular deiodinase activity, and it appears that only T3, and not T4, is transported into cardiac muscle cells. Thyroid hormones alter the expression of key structural and regulatory genes within cardiomyocytes (Klein and Danzi, 2007). Triiodothyronine exerts its cellular actions by binding to thyroid hormone nuclear receptors, thereby inducing transcription of positively regulated genes, such as those encoding alpha-myosin heavy chain and sarco/endoplasmic reticulum calcium ATPase. Conversely, transcription of negatively regulated cardiac genes, such as those encoding beta-myosin heavy chain and phospholamban, is induced in the absence of T3 and suppressed in its presence. Triiodothyronine also induces non-genomic effects on the cardiovascular system, through various membrane ion channels (i.e. sodium, potassium and calcium) and a variety of intracellular signalling pathways in the heart and vascular smooth muscle cells.

Effects of thyroid hormones

The efffects of thyroid hormones on the heart and peripheral vasculature are summarized in Figure 5.1 and include:

- Decreased systemic vascular resistance (SVR)
- Increased resting heart rate (Graham et al., 2007)
- Increased ventricular contractility
- Increased blood volume.

Decreased systemic vascular resistance

Thyroid hormones can increase production of nitric oxide in endothelial cells, which subsequently acts on adjacent cells to induce vascular relaxation. Furthermore, T3 increases the serum concentration of adrenomedullin, another potent vasodilator. Vasodilation ultimately causes a decrease in arterial blood pressure and increased RAAS activation, leading to increases in renal sodium resorption and plasma volume. This combination of reduced SVR, and increased venous return and preload contributes to the increased cardiac output in hyperthyroid animals. Indeed, cardiac output may double in hyperthyroidism and, conversely, may decrease by as much as 30–40% in hypothyroidism.

Increased resting heart rate

Thyroid hormones induce a positive chronotropic effect (increased heart rate). The resultant resting sinus tachycardia is probably the most consistent cardiovascular sign in feline hyperthyroidism. The precise mechanism of increased heart rate is not completely clear, but it may be caused by unbalanced sympathovagal tone due to a relative adrenergic overdrive and direct effects on the sinoatrial node (San José et al., 2020), increasing its rate of both depolarization and repolarization. Furthermore, beta-1 adrenergic receptors are positively regulated by thyroid hormones and this may contribute to the increased heart rate (Osuna et al., 2017).

Increased ventricular contractility

Increased myocardial function is primarily caused by direct genomic and non-genomic effects on the myocardial components. Beta-adrenergic receptor density is also increased, resulting in increased tissue sensitivity to catecholamines. An increase in left ventricular fractional shortening has been shown in hyperthyroid cats (Connolly et al., 2005). Administration of beta-blockers (e.g. propranolol) to hyperthyroid humans slows the heart rate

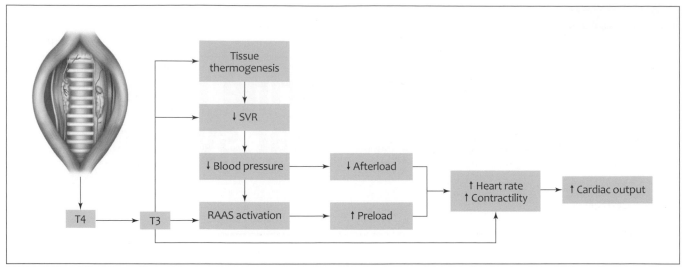

5.1 Thyroid hormone effects on the heart and peripheral vasculature. RAAS = renin–angiotensin–aldosterone system; SVR = systemic vascular resistance; T3 = triiodothyronine; T4 = thyroxine.
(Redrawn after Klein and Danzi, 2007)

but does not affect systolic or diastolic performance, confirming that T3 acts directly on the cardiac muscle. Therefore, beta-blocker treatment should reduce heart rate without affecting the direct inotropic effects of T3.

Increased blood volume

The activation of the RAAS mentioned above increases sodium resorption and blood volume. In turn, this leads to increased preload and ultimately a significant increase in stroke volume. In addition, there is evidence that T3 directly stimulates the synthesis of renin substrate in the liver. Triiodothyronine also increases erythropoietin concentrations, leading to a further increase in blood volume and a rise in cardiac preload.

Hyperthyroidism

Clinical hyperthyroidism is characterized by an exacerbation of the cardiovascular effects of thyroid hormones described above. Therefore, a hyperthyroid animal often presents with tachycardia, exercise intolerance, occasional structural and functional myocardial changes and, in severe cases, congestive heart failure (CHF).

Persistent tachycardia can deteriorate cardiac performance (tachycardia-induced cardiomyopathy) and result in high-output CHF, which can be responsible for exercise intolerance. Exercise intolerance may also result from the inability of the body to further increase heart rate and contractility or lower SVR as normally observed during exercise in healthy individuals. Humans with hyperthyroidism can develop angina and electrocardiographic changes suggestive of cardiac ischaemia secondary to coronary vasospasm. Successful treatment of the hyperthyroidism has been associated with a reversal of these symptoms.

Myocardial ischaemia is also considered an important cause of the myocardial changes observed in hyperthyroid cats. Concentric left ventricular myocardial hypertrophy (LVH), mimicking hypertrophic cardiomyopathy (HCM), is often reported as an expected myocardial change in cats with hyperthyroidism. However, in analogy to humans, echocardiographic examination of hyperthyroid cats rarely reveals concentric LVH, while non-specific myocardial changes are more commonly observed, especially in hyperthyroid cats presenting with signs of CHF (Figure 5.2). Concentrations of cardiac troponin-I and NT-proBNP can also be increased in hyperthyroid cats in response to myocardial damage and myocardial stretch, respectively (Connolly et al., 2005; Menaut et al., 2012). In affected cats, CHF can develop in response to LVH, tachycardiomyopathy, coronary ischaemia, loss of sinoatrial node modulation and plasma expansion leading to volume overload.

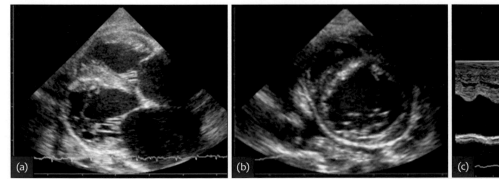

5.2 Echocardiographic images obtained from a cat with overt hyperthyroidism and acute signs of congestive heart failure. (a) Right parasternal four-chamber long-axis view. (b) Right parasternal short-axis view at the level of the chordae tendineae. Both images show severe myocardial damage characterized by four-chamber dilatation, thinning of the left ventricular free wall, bridging scar in the mid-left ventricular cavity and mild pleural effusion. (c) M-mode image of the left ventricle in right parasternal short-axis view at the level of the chordae tendineae showing a thin left ventricular free wall, which also displayed increased echogenicity and regional hypokinesis suggestive of replacement fibrosis secondary to myocardial ischaemia.

Hypertension is traditionally reported as a common finding in feline hyperthyroidism, although based on the reduced SVR, a reduction in arterial blood pressure would be expected instead. Indeed, systemic hypertension is not a common finding in humans with hyperthyroidism because the reduction of SVR causes mild hypotension; a small increase in blood pressure can still be observed, mostly associated with atherosclerotic changes (Berta *et al.*, 2019). Historically, mild systemic hypertension has been reported in hyperthyroid cats (87% of cases) based on a small case series of 39 cats (Kobayashi *et al.*, 1990). However, more recent studies indicated a much lower prevalence of hypertension (22%) in cats with increased circulating thyroid hormone concentrations (Williams *et al.*, 2013). Interestingly, 23% of normotensive hyperthyroid cats develop hypertension after treatment for hyperthyroidism and restoration of euthyroid status (Morrow *et al.*, 2009), and although RAAS activation occurs in hyperthyroid cats, this does not seem to be associated with the development of hypertension (Williams *et al.*, 2013). These findings are supported by the expected physiological response of the vascular smooth muscle to excessive circulating thyroid hormone, suggesting that, if present, hypertension may not be directly related to hyperthyroidism. Hypertension after treatment of hyperthyroidism can develop without concurrent pre-existing or unmasked kidney disease, suggesting that its development may be secondary to the decreased vasodilatory effect due to the reduction of circulating thyroid hormone concentrations.

Heart murmurs are commonly detected in hyperthyroid cats and this is attributable to the high output states that can cause or exacerbate dynamic right and/or left outflow tract obstruction.

Hyperthyroid cats should be handled with particular care because additional stress can easily exacerbate underlying cardiovascular changes, in particular tachycardia and increased contractility, leading to a rapid development of signs of CHF. This should not be confused with the onset of 'thyroid storm' described in humans, which is characterized by hyperthermia, neurological signs, agitation, delirium, stupor, obtundation and even coma and is caused by a rapid increase in serum thyroid hormone concentrations. Thyroid storm has also been reported in cats, but it has not been convincingly confirmed. It is a controversial topic in feline endocrinology (Peterson, 2016).

Treatment of hyperthyroid cats with concomitant signs of heart disease is not always straightforward, especially when the cardiac investigation reveals sustained tachycardia and advanced myocardial remodelling. Clinicians should prioritize stabilization of the case before considering treatment of hyperthyroidism because some cats with severe underlying cardiac disease largely depend on their increased cardiac output. Signs of pulmonary oedema should be controlled with diuretics, while significant cavitary effusion, in particular pleural effusion, should be drained accordingly. Beta-blockers (e.g. atenolol) can be considered for a satisfactory control of rapid sustained sinus tachycardia, although this intervention should only be reserved for cats that do not have overt or incipient signs of CHF.

Hypothyroidism

The most common cardiovascular signs of hypothyroidism are diametrically opposed to those described for hyperthyroidism and may include bradycardia, cold intolerance and fatigue. Bradycardia with low QRS voltage is the most consistent finding in dogs with hypothyroidism and it is often characterized by a regular rhythm rather than the more typical slow sinus arrhythmia frequently observed in healthy dogs (Figure 5.3).

Mild diastolic hypertension can also be observed due to increased SVR with subsequent narrowed pulse pressure (pulse pressure = systolic pressure – diastolic pressure), although this is not commonly recognized in dogs.

The lack of thyroid hormone activity can result in decreased serum erythropoietin concentration, explaining the normochromic normocytic anaemia found in some dogs with hypothyroidism. This also contributes to plasma volume contraction and reduced stroke volume, which, in combination with a reduced heart rate, lead to reduced cardiac output. These factors contribute to the development of lethargy and exercise intolerance.

In the past, canine hypothyroidism was also reported as a cause of systolic dysfunction and ventricular dilatation, mimicking echocardiographic signs of idiopathic dilated cardiomyopathy (DCM) (Dukes-McEwan *et al.*, 2003). However, if this were the case, systolic function and time intervals would be expected to improve with thyroid hormone supplementation, but this is rarely observed. Diagnosis of DCM in dogs is challenging *per se*, and the suppressive effect of non-thyroidal illness (including heart failure) on thyroid hormone concentrations makes this association even weaker. More recent studies have discredited a cause–effect relationship between canine hypothyroidism and DCM, indicating that a lack of T4 does not play any role in the aetiology and pathophysiology of DCM (Beier *et al.*, 2015; Guglielmini *et al.*, 2019), although a degree of left ventricular dilatation in diastole might be expected due to the increased preload associated with underlying bradycardia.

Atherosclerosis is a common complication of the hypercholesterolaemia and lipid abnormalities induced by hypothyroidism in humans. It has also been reported as a rare but serious complication of hypothyroidism in dogs since atherosclerosis can also affect the coronary arteries, resulting in myocardial ischaemia, impaired cardiac function and heart failure (Liu *et al.*, 1986; Zeiss and Waddle, 1995).

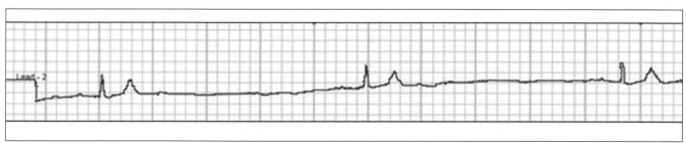

5.3 Electrocardiographic recording from a dog with hypothyroidism. The trace shows profound sinus bradycardia at approximately 25 bpm with low-voltage QRS complexes (50 mm/s, 10 mm/mV, lead II).

Pituitary gland disorders

The somatotropic cells of the anterior pituitary gland secrete growth hormone (GH) and direct effects of this hormone can be seen in numerous tissue types and organs, including the cardiovascular system. Many actions of GH are mediated by insulin-like growth factor-1 (IGF-1), which is synthesized in the liver, kidneys and many other tissues. Tissue growth is promoted by IGF-1 acting in concert with GH, and they both play an important role in cardiac development as well as modulation of myocardial structure and function in the adult heart (Meyers and Cuneo, 2003).

Hypersomatotropism

In humans with hypersomatotropism, an excess of GH can affect the cardiovascular system causing cardiomegaly, hypertension and a specific acromegalic cardiomyopathy within which LVH is the hallmark cardiac lesion. This form of cardiomyopathy is also characterized by progressive interstitial fibrosis that impairs both systolic and diastolic function of the heart.

Most cats with hypersomatotropism have evidence of structural or functional cardiac disease, most commonly characterized by LVH, left atrial enlargement, abnormal diastolic function and, eventually, heart failure, often mimicking severe HCM (HCM-phenotype) (Figure 5.4). Interestingly, these echocardiographic changes can be reversible after hypophysectomy and normalization of the IGF-1 concentration (Myers *et al.*, 2014; Borgeat *et al.*, 2018). Aortic aneurysm and significant aortic regurgitation are additional echocardiographic abnormalities observed in humans with hypersomatotropism (van der Klaauw *et al.*, 2008) and similar changes have also been observed in affected cats, with complete reverse remodelling following hypophysectomy (Figure 5.5). These findings indicate that in cats with hypersomatotropism, an extension of the cardiac evaluation to the aortic root offers a more in-depth assessment of the state of the individual acromegalic cardiomyopathy.

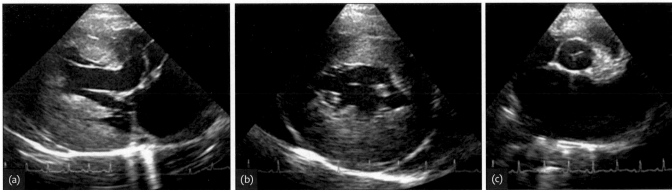

5.4 Echocardiographic images of a diabetic cat with hypersomatotropism and congestive heart failure. (a) Right parasternal four-chamber long-axis view. (b) Right parasternal short-axis view at the level of the chordae tendineae. Both images show significant left ventricular myocardial thickening. (c) Right parasternal short-axis view at the level of the heart base showing significant left atrial enlargement.

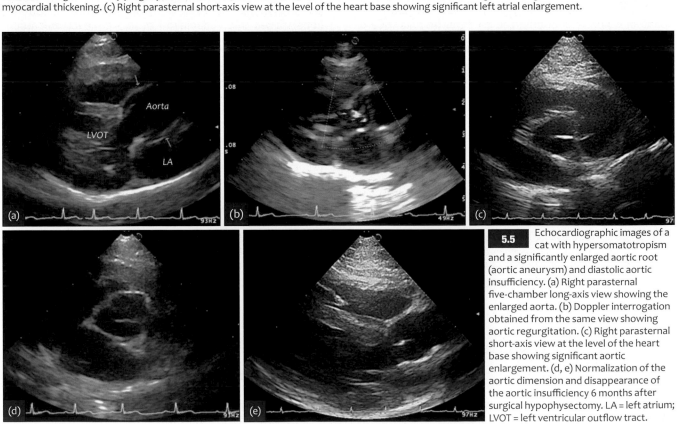

5.5 Echocardiographic images of a cat with hypersomatotropism and a significantly enlarged aortic root (aortic aneurysm) and diastolic aortic insufficiency. (a) Right parasternal five-chamber long-axis view showing the enlarged aorta. (b) Doppler interrogation obtained from the same view showing aortic regurgitation. (c) Right parasternal short-axis view at the level of the heart base showing significant aortic enlargement. (d, e) Normalization of the aortic dimension and disappearance of the aortic insufficiency 6 months after surgical hypophysectomy. LA = left atrium; LVOT = left ventricular outflow tract.

Interestingly, increased IGF-1 concentrations, similar to values found in confirmed hypersomatotropism, have been demonstrated in a small proportion (<10%) of non-diabetic cats with HCM (Steele *et al.*, 2021). It is unclear whether these high concentrations represent hypersomatotropism and associated HCM or are the result of other unknown factors.

Dogs with hypersomatotropism commonly present with respiratory stridor, mostly due to the increased soft tissue mass in the orolingual, oropharyngeal and orolaryngeal region (Eigenmann, 1984). Cardiovascular abnormalities have not yet been documented in affected dogs.

Growth hormone deficiency

Mortality in humans with GH deficiency (hyposomatotropism or pituitary dwarfism) is more than doubled due to cardiovascular disease associated with atherosclerosis and endothelial dysfunction. Furthermore, decreased left ventricular wall thickness, decreased contractility and reduced cardiac output, accompanied by exercise intolerance and cardiovascular abnormalities, which improve following GH replacement therapy have been described (Meyers and Cuneo, 2003). Hyposomatotropism is rare in dogs and cats, and cardiovascular abnormalities associated with growth hormone deficiency have not been reported to date.

Adrenal gland disorders

Cardiovascular effects can be associated with deficiency or excess of glucocorticoids or mineralocorticoids, or excess of catecholamines.

Hypercortisolism

Cardiovascular effects of hypercortisolism are due to the action of excess glucocorticoids on the heart and vessels. Systemic hypertension is the most common cardiovascular abnormality in humans with hypercortisolism, arising through a variety of mechanisms including alterations in peripheral and renovascular resistance and vascular remodelling. Activation of the RAAS via enhanced hepatic production of angiotensinogen has also been described. However, low renin concentrations are observed in humans with hypercortisolaemia due to the negative feedback produced by cortisol's inherent mineralocorticoid activity, suggesting that there are other activation mechanisms. Increased concentrations of endothelin-1, a potent vasoconstrictor, are observed in hypercortisolism, and play an important role in the development of cortisol-induced hypertension. In addition, glucocorticoids inhibit the expression of nitric oxide synthase, which is essential for adequate peripheral vasodilation, and this may also contribute to hypertension. Finally, cortisol can also bind to mineralocorticoid receptors, mimicking aldosterone action, when its concentration exceeds the capacity of the body to inactivate cortisol to cortisone, resulting in higher sodium uptake and potassium excretion at the renal level. The blood volume expansion that follows suppresses endogenous renin secretion (Barbot *et al.*, 2019).

Systemic hypertension is observed in most dogs with hypercortisolism, and blood pressure does not always normalize after treatment with trilostane (Smets *et al.*, 2012; San José *et al.*, 2020). Hypercortisolism can also cause significant LVH in dogs but this is rarely associated with systemic hypertension, suggesting alternative mechanisms for myocardial hypertrophy, such as a direct effect of cortisol on myocardial tissue (Takano *et al.*, 2015). Feline hypercortisolism is a rare endocrine disorder and cardiovascular signs are rarely reported.

Hyperaldosteronism

The main cardiovascular effect of primary hyperaldosteronism (Conn's syndrome) is hypertension due to sodium and water retention. Sustained hypertension will ultimately damage target tissues such as the retina, kidney, brain and heart. Within the heart, sustained hypertension leads to concentric LVH and fibrosis. In addition, proliferation of vascular endothelium and smooth muscle occurs, which, in turn, contributes to development of refractory hypertension. Myocardial hypertrophy can potentially lead to cardiac ischaemia, arrhythmias and heart failure. Furthermore, increased aldosterone concentrations can cause hypokalaemia, which can lead to the cardiac arrhythmias (mostly ventricular) frequently observed in cats with hyperaldosteronism (Kooistra *et al.*, 2009; Djajadiningrat-Laanen *et al.*, 2011; Abad-Cardiel *et al.*, 2013). Primary hyperaldosteronism is extremely rare in dogs, but hypertension has been reported in those affected.

Hypoadrenocorticism

In humans, there have been multiple reports of cardiomyopathy as the initial presentation in both adults and children with untreated adrenal insufficiency (Schumaecker *et al.*, 2016). However, in dogs and cats, the primary cardiovascular manifestations of hypoadrenocorticism are associated with electrocardiographic abnormalities and haemodynamic disturbances (Figure 5.6). Most electrocardiographic changes are secondary to hyperkalaemia, although they do not occur in proportion to the increase in potassium concentration, likely due to concomitant metabolic acidosis as well as other electrolyte imbalances, such as hyponatraemia, hypercalcaemia, hypermagnesaemia and hypochloridaemia. Hypoadrenocorticism can induce profound sinus bradycardia (with associated prolongation of the PQ interval), atrial standstill, atrial fibrillation, decreased R-wave and increased T-wave amplitude, widened QRS complex and even cardiac arrest from asystole (Riesen and Lombard, 2006; Van Lanen and Sande, 2014).

Haemodynamic changes are caused by severe hypovolaemia, which ultimately results in reduced cardiac output, regardless of ventricular intrinsic contractile state, and secondary exercise intolerance, lethargy and hypotension. Hypovolaemia is also the cause of the typical changes on thoracic radiographs: reduced size of the heart (microcardia), pulmonary vessels and venae cavae. Hypovolaemia can also induce pseudo-hypertrophy (thickened myocardial wall, reduced left ventricular diameters and reduced left atrial size) demonstrable by echocardiography. In animals with electrocardiographic abnormalities and hypotension, emergency treatment should target both hyperkalaemia and hypovolaemia, as detailed in Chapters 28 and 31.

Phaeochromocytoma

Phaeochromocytomas are relatively frequently identified as the cause of adrenal masses in dogs, while an antemortem diagnosis of phaeochromocytoma is very rare in cats. Clinical signs are caused by the direct presence of a space-occupying mass or by excess catecholamine secretion,

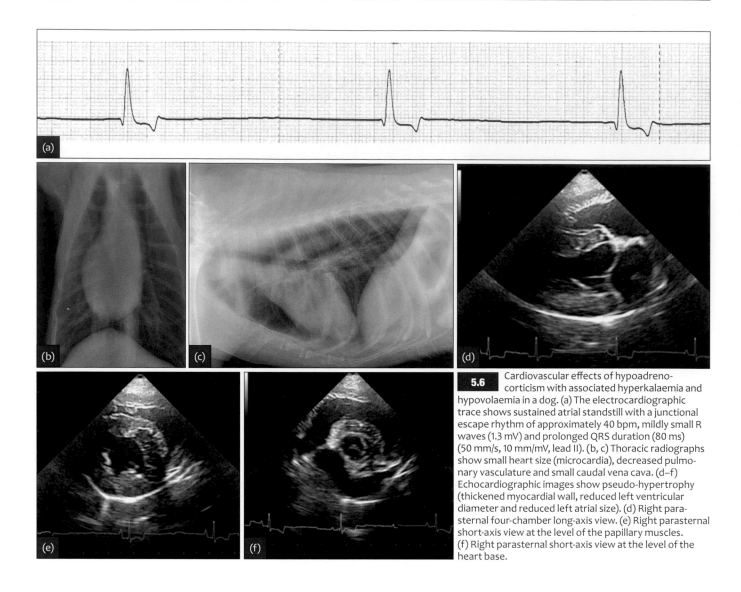

5.6 Cardiovascular effects of hypoadreno-corticism with associated hyperkalaemia and hypovolaemia in a dog. (a) The electrocardiographic trace shows sustained atrial standstill with a junctional escape rhythm of approximately 40 bpm, mildly small R waves (1.3 mV) and prolonged QRS duration (80 ms) (50 mm/s, 10 mm/mV, lead II). (b, c) Thoracic radiographs show small heart size (microcardia), decreased pulmonary vasculature and small caudal vena cava. (d–f) Echocardiographic images show pseudo-hypertrophy (thickened myocardial wall, reduced left ventricular diameter and reduced left atrial size). (d) Right parasternal four-chamber long-axis view. (e) Right parasternal short-axis view at the level of the papillary muscles. (f) Right parasternal short-axis view at the level of the heart base.

which can evoke cardiovascular signs such as systemic hypertension and cardiac arrhythmias. However, both of these abnormalities can potentially be missed due to the paroxysmal release of catecholamines. Ambulatory electro-cardiogram (Holter) recording can significantly increase the diagnostic yield of intermittent arrhythmias, mainly represented by ventricular and atrial ectopic beats, as well as episodes of paroxysmal sinus tachycardia (Figure 5.7).

Pancreatic disorders

Insulin and associated glucose derangements may affect cardiovascular function.

Diabetes mellitus

In diabetes mellitus, the lack of insulin production and associated hyperglycaemia can cause cardiovascular abnormalities. The association between diabetes mellitus and cardiovascular disease is widely documented in humans (Petrie *et al.*, 2018). However, only a few studies have evaluated the cardiovascular consequences in small animals. Two independent studies reported a compelling association between diabetes mellitus and the development of heart failure in cats, with a relative risk 10 times higher than in non-diabetic cats (Laluha *et al.*, 2004; Little and Gettinby, 2008). A more recent study revealed diastolic cardiac dysfunction in cats with diabetes mellitus prior to instituting antidiabetic therapy, resembling the 'diabetic cardiomyopathy' observed in humans. Furthermore, this dysfunction appeared to progress rather than normalize after 6 months, despite insulin therapy (Pereira *et al.*, 2017). Diastolic dysfunction has also been reported in diabetic dogs, although progression to heart failure appears to be uncommon in this species (Vichit *et al.*, 2018).

Systemic hypertension is common in humans with diabetes mellitus due to upregulation of the RAAS, oxidative stress, inflammation and activation of the immune system (Petrie *et al.*, 2018). However, the incidence of hypertension in diabetic dogs and cats appears negligible (Sennello *et al.*, 2003; Herring *et al.*, 2014).

Insulinoma

Hypoglycaemia can be associated with tachycardia as a result of increased adrenergic tone, although in rare cases bradycardia has been demonstrated. However, given the episodic nature of hypoglycaemia and its other potential effects in animals with insulinoma, cardiovascular signs are rarely specifically recognized.

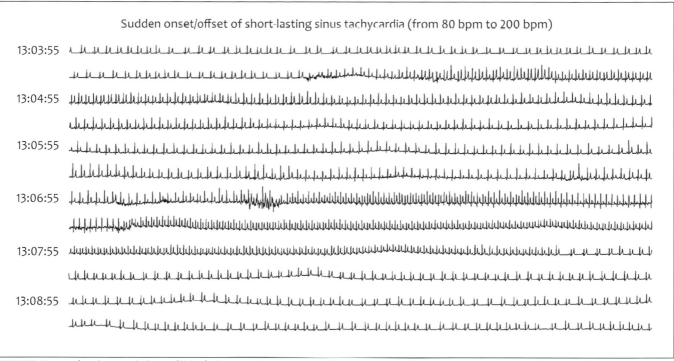

Sudden onset/offset of short-lasting sinus tachycardia (from 80 bpm to 200 bpm)

13:03:55

13:04:55

13:05:55

13:06:55

13:07:55

13:08:55

5.7 Twenty-four hour ambulatory (Holter) electrocardiography recording from a dog with phaeochromocytoma and hypertension. The trace shows approximately 3 minutes of inappropriate (during resting) sinus tachycardia, approaching 200 bpm and characterized by abrupt onset and cessation.

References and further reading

Abad-Cardiel M, Alvarez-Alvarez B, Luque-Fernandez L et al. (2013) Hypertension caused by primary hyperaldosteronism: increased heart damage and cardiovascular risk. Revista Española de Cardiología (English Edition) **66**, 47–52

Barbot M, Ceccato F and Scaroni C (2019) The pathophysiology and treatment of hypertension in patients with Cushing's syndrome. Frontiers in Endocrinology **10**, 321

Beier P, Reese S, Holler PJ et al. (2015) The role of hypothyroidism in the etiology and progression of dilated cardiomyopathy in Doberman Pinschers. Journal of Veterinary Internal Medicine **29**, 141–149

Berta E, Lengyel I, Halmi S et al. (2019) Hypertension in thyroid disorders. Frontiers in Endocrinology **10**, 482

Borgeat K, Niessen SJM, Wilkie L et al. (2018) Time spent with cats is never wasted: lessons learned from feline acromegalic cardiomyopathy, a naturally occurring animal model of the human disease. PLoS ONE **13**, e0194342

Connolly DJ, Guitian J, Boswood A and Neiger R (2005) Serum troponin I levels in hyperthyroid cats before and after treatment with radioactive iodine. Journal of Feline Medicine and Surgery **7**, 289–300

Djajadiningrat-Laanen S, Galac S and Kooistra H (2011) Primary hyperaldosteronism: expanding the diagnostic net. Journal of Feline Medicine and Surgery **13**, 641–650

Dukes-McEwan J, Borgarelli M, Tidholm A et al. (2003) Proposed guidelines for the diagnosis of canine idiopathic dilated cardiomyopathy. Journal of Veterinary Cardiology **5**, 7–19

Eigenmann JE (1984) Acromegaly in the dog. Veterinary Clinics of North America: Small Animal Practice **14**, 827–836

Graham PA, Refsal KR and Nachreiner RF (2007) Etiopathologic findings of canine hypothyroidism. Veterinary Clinics of North America: Small Animal Practice **37**, 617–631

Guglielmini C, Berlanda M, Fracassi F et al. (2019) Electrocardiographic and echocardiographic evaluation in dogs with hypothyroidism before and after levothyroxine supplementation: a prospective controlled study. Journal of Veterinary Internal Medicine **33**, 1935–1942

Herring IP, Panciera DL and Werre SR (2014) Longitudinal prevalence of hypertension, proteinuria, and retinopathy in dogs with spontaneous diabetes mellitus. Journal of Veterinary Internal Medicine **28**, 488–495

Klein I and Danzi S (2007) Thyroid disease and the heart. Circulation **116**, 1725–1735

Klein I and Danzi S (2016) Thyroid disease and the heart. Current Problems in Cardiology **41**, 65–92

Kobayashi DL, Peterson ME, Graves TK, Lesser M and Nichols CE (1990) Hypertension in cats with chronic renal failure or hyperthyroidism. Journal of Veterinary Internal Medicine **4**, 58–62

Kooistra HS, Galac S, Buijtels JJ and Meij BP (2009) Endocrine diseases in animals. Hormone Research **71** Suppl 1, 144–147

Laluha P, Gerber B, Laluhova D, Boretti FS and Reusch CE (2004) Stress hyperglycemia in sick cats: a retrospective study over 4 years. Schweizer Archiv für Tierheilkunde **146**, 375–383

Little CJ and Gettinby G (2008) Heart failure is common in diabetic cats: findings from a retrospective case-controlled study in first-opinion practice. Journal of Small Animal Practice **49**, 17–25

Liu SK, Tilley LP, Tappe JP and Fox PR (1986) Clinical and pathologic findings in dogs with atherosclerosis: 21 cases (1970-1983). Journal of the American Veterinary Medical Association **189**, 227–232

Menaut P, Connolly DJ, Volk A et al. (2012) Circulating natriuretic peptide concentrations in hyperthyroid cats. Journal of Small Animal Practice **53**, 673–678

Meyers DE and Cuneo RC (2003) Controversies regarding the effects of growth hormone on the heart. Mayo Clinic Proceedings **78**, 1521–1526

Morrow LD, Adams VJ, Elliott J et al. (2009) Hypertension in hyperthyroid cats: prevalence, incidence and predictors of its development. Proceedings of the 2009 ACVIM Forum & Canadian Veterinary Medical Association Convention, Montreal, Canada, 3–6 June 2009, 699

Myers JA, Lunn KF and Bright JM (2014) Echocardiographic findings in 11 cats with acromegaly. Journal of Veterinary Internal Medicine **28**, 1235–1238

Osuna PM, Udovcic M and Sharma MD (2017) Hyperthyroidism and the heart. Methodist DeBakey Cardiovascular Journal **13**, 60–63

Pereira NJ, Novo Matos J, Baron Toaldo M et al. (2017) Cats with diabetes mellitus have diastolic dysfunction in the absence of structural heart disease. The Veterinary Journal **225**, 50–55

Peterson ME (2016) Thyroid storm: does this syndrome really exist in cats? Journal of Feline Medicine and Surgery **18**, 936–937

Petrie JR, Guzik TJ and Touyz RM (2018) Diabetes, hypertension, and cardiovascular disease: clinical insights and vascular mechanisms. Canadian Journal of Cardiology **34**, 575–584

Riesen SC and Lombard CW (2006) ECG of the Month. Atrial fibrillation secondary to hypoadrenocorticism. Journal of the American Veterinary Medical Association **229**, 1890–1892

San José PG, Arenas Bermejo C, Clares Moral I, Cuesta Alvaro P and Alenza MDP (2020) Prevalence and risk factors associated with systemic hypertension in dogs with spontaneous hyperadrenocorticism. Journal of Veterinary Internal Medicine **34**, 1768–1778

Schumaecker MM, Larsen TR and Sane DC (2016) Cardiac manifestations of adrenal insufficiency. Reviews in Cardiovascular Medicine **17**, 131–136

Sennello KA, Schulman RL, Prosek R and Siegel AM (2003) Systolic blood pressure in cats with diabetes mellitus. Journal of the American Veterinary Medical Association **223**, 198–201

Smets PM, Lefebvre HP, Meij BP *et al.* (2012) Long-term follow-up of renal function in dogs after treatment for ACTH-dependent hyperadrenocorticism. *Journal of Veterinary Internal Medicine* **26**, 565–574

Steele MME, Borgeat K, Payne JR *et al.* (2021) Increased insulin-like growth factor 1 concentrations in a retrospective population of non-diabetic cats diagnosed with hypertrophic cardiomyopathy. *Journal of Feline Medicine and Surgery* **23**, 952–958

Takano H, Kokubu A, Sugimoto K *et al.* (2015) Left ventricular structural and functional abnormalities in dogs with hyperadrenocorticism. *Journal of Veterinary Cardiology* **17**, 173–181

van der Klaauw AA, Bax JJ, Smit JW *et al.* (2008) Increased aortic root diameters in patients with acromegaly. *European Journal of Endocrinology* **159**, 97–103

Van Lanen K and Sande A (2014) Canine hypoadrenocorticism: pathogenesis, diagnosis, and treatment. *Topics in Companion Animal Medicine* **29**, 88–95

Vichit P, Rungsipipat A and Surachetpong SD (2018) Changes of cardiac function in diabetic dogs. *Journal of Veterinary Cardiology* **20**, 438–450

Williams TL, Elliott J and Syme HM (2013) Renin-angiotensin-aldosterone system activity in hyperthyroid cats with and without concurrent hypertension. *Journal of Veterinary Internal Medicine* **27**, 522–529

Zeiss CJ and Waddle G (1995) Hypothyroidism and atherosclerosis in dogs. *Compendium on Continuing Education for the Practicing Veterinarian* **17**, 1117–1129

Chapter 6

The effect of endocrine disease on the renal system

Tim Williams

Introduction

The effect of endocrine disease on the renal system is clinically relevant because some endocrine diseases might cause or exacerbate renal damage and complicate the diagnosis of concurrent kidney disease (Figure 6.1). In addition, kidney disease itself may affect the endocrine system and make the diagnosis of some endocrinopathies more problematic.

Endocrine disease (in order of importance)	Effects on renal function
Hyperthyroidism	↑ GFR*, reduced urine-concentrating ability*, proteinuria*
Hypothyroidism (primary and iatrogenic)	↓ GFR*
Hypercortisolism	↑ GFR*, reduced urine-concentrating ability*, proteinuria*
Diabetes mellitus	Variable effects on GFR, proteinuria*
Hypoadrenocorticism	↓ GFR, altered tubular handling of sodium and potassium*
Primary hyperaldosteronism	Altered tubular handling of sodium and potassium
Primary hyperparathyroidism	Dystrophic calcification and tubular injury
Hypersomatotropism	↑ GFR
Hyposomatotropism	↓ GFR, retarded renal development

6.1 List of endocrine diseases that affect renal function (glomerular and/or tubular functions). * = has been observed in dogs and/or cats; GFR = glomerular filtration rate.

Interplay between thyroid and renal function

Both hyperthyroidism and hypothyroidism have well recognized effects on glomerular filtration rate (GFR), such that hyperthyroidism can 'mask' biochemical evidence of concurrent kidney disease, and hypothyroidism can exaggerate biochemical evidence of renal dysfunction. This means that accurate assessment of renal function in animals with thyroid dysfunction is difficult and cannot be fully attained until thyroid disease is successfully managed.

Effect of thyroid disease on renal function

Assessment of GFR is regarded as the gold standard measure of functional renal mass, with a low GFR generally attributed to kidney disease. However, thyroid hormones also directly influence GFR, with hyperthyroidism increasing GFR and hypothyroidism decreasing GFR. The changes in GFR associated with thyroid dysfunction (Figure 6.2) are hypothesized to be secondary to any or a combination of:

- Altered cardiac output
- Altered systemic vascular resistance
- Activation of the renin–angiotensin–aldosterone system (RAAS)
- Altered tubuloglomerular feedback within the kidney.

Therefore, the GFR in animals with thyroid dysfunction may not be an accurate reflection of the true functional renal mass in that animal.

In addition to its effects on renal glomerular function, thyroid disease also affects renal tubular function (Figure 6.2). In humans with hyperthyroidism, altered sensitivity of the distal renal tubule to arginine vasopressin is observed, which can reduce urine-concentrating ability. However, reduced urine-concentrating ability in hyperthyroidism could also occur secondary to reduced medullary sodium concentration (consequent to increased renal blood flow and medullary washout) or osmotic diuresis associated with increased filtered solute. In human and animal models of hypothyroidism, impaired water excretion is also observed, associated with changes in renal water handling that are both dependent on and independent of increased arginine vasopressin secretion. Increased renal phosphate resorption also occurs in hyperthyroid rats, leading to hyperphosphataemia, and this is hypothesized to also occur in cats as many hyperthyroid cats without concurrent chronic kidney disease (CKD) are hyperphosphataemic. Renal protein excretion is increased in feline hyperthyroidism, such that proteinuria (urine protein:creatinine (UPCR) >0.4) is common, although the vast majority of hyperthyroid cats are only mildly proteinuric (UPCR <1). Studies to date have indicated increased urinary excretion of albumin, N-acetyl-beta-D-glucosaminidase (NAG), retinol-binding protein (RBP) and vascular endothelial growth factor in hyperthyroid cats, which suggests that the pathogenesis of proteinuria is a combination of reduced tubular resorption and increased tubular excretion of proteins.

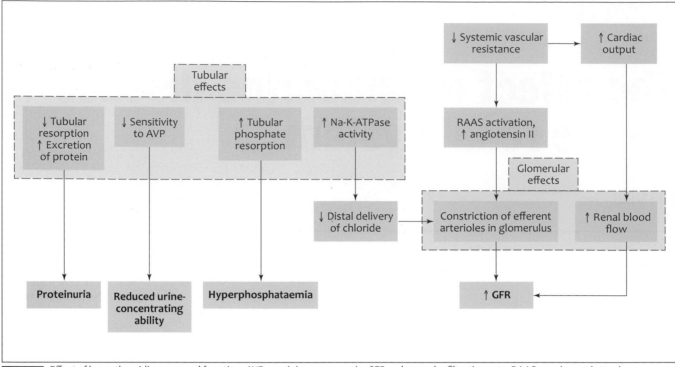

6.2 Effect of hyperthyroidism on renal function. AVP = arginine vasopressin; GFR = glomerular filtration rate; RAAS = renin–angiotensin–aldosterone system.

Is thyroid disease damaging to the kidney?

Hyperthyroidism

Hyperthyroidism and CKD are both common morbidities of senior and geriatric cats, and it is not uncommon for them to occur in the same cat concurrently. Early studies suggested that the overall prevalence of azotaemic CKD in hyperthyroid cats, calculated by totaling those cats with azotaemia prior to treatment (20–23%) and those that developed azotaemia following treatment (up to 49%), was higher than the reported prevalence of CKD in the general feline senior and geriatric population. For this reason, it has been postulated that hyperthyroidism causes damage to the kidney, which contributes to the increased prevalence of CKD in the hyperthyroid population.

There are a number of clinicopathological changes that occur in hyperthyroidism that could be damaging to the kidney. These include the induction of proteinuria, activation of the RAAS and derangements in calcium and phosphate homeostasis; however, hyperthyroid cats with proteinuria, hyperphosphataemia and hyperparathyroidism are not more likely to develop azotaemia following treatment, which suggests that these changes are not damaging to the kidney *per se*.

The increased prevalence of azotaemic CKD in the hyperthyroid population, which led to the hypothesis that hyperthyroidism might be damaging to the kidney, may in fact reflect the reduction in GFR that occurs secondary to iatrogenic hypothyroidism, as this was not accounted for in previous studies. It is possible that approximately 50% of cats with iatrogenic hypothyroidism have reversible azotaemia, which may have led to an overestimation of the prevalence of azotaemia in hyperthyroid cats following treatment. More recent data from hyperthyroid cats treated in first-opinion practice using antithyroid medication alone or in combination with thyroidectomy suggest that the prevalence of azotaemic CKD in hyperthyroid cats is lower than previously thought, with 10% of hyperthyroid cats having azotaemia prior to treatment and approximately 25% of well controlled hyperthyroid cats developing azotaemic CKD following treatment (Williams *et al.*, 2010b). As a result, the prevalence of azotaemic CKD in hyperthyroid cats overall would be approximately 35%, which is consistent with the prevalence of azotaemic CKD in a senior and geriatric feline population of this age (up to 31%). Therefore, at present, there is no evidence to support the premise that hyperthyroidism itself is damaging to the kidney in cats.

Hypothyroidism

Hypothyroid dogs have reduced GFR, which increases following thyroid supplementation, although in one study approximately half of hypothyroid dogs maintained a decreased GFR (<2 ml/min/kg) even after euthyroidism had been restored (Gommeren *et al.*, 2009). This could indicate some ongoing renal dysfunction, perhaps secondary to previous hypothyroidism. However, concurrent CKD in hypothyroid dogs is an uncommon finding, perhaps suggesting that the subnormal GFR observed in the hypothyroid dogs before and after treatment is not clinically relevant.

Unlike dogs with naturally occurring disease, cats with iatrogenic hypothyroidism have a higher prevalence of post-treatment azotaemic CKD compared with euthyroid cats, and hypothyroid cats with concurrent azotaemia also have reduced survival times compared with hypothyroid cats without azotaemia (Williams *et al.*, 2010a), although the cause of reduced survival in this group of cats is unclear. It could be speculated that hypothyroidism causes more rapid progression of existing CKD, but further studies are required to investigate if hypothyroidism can cause or exacerbate existing renal injury in dogs and cats.

Effect of thyroid dysfunction on diagnosis of kidney disease

Although whether thyroid disease could cause damage to the kidney is still an open question, there is no doubt that thyroid dysfunction does have a profound effect on the diagnosis of concurrent CKD (Figure 6.3). Consequently, full biochemical assessment of renal function cannot be made until thyroid disease has been successfully treated.

Hyperthyroidism	Hypothyroidism
Serum creatinine ↓ Serum SDMA ↓ Serum urea ↑ or ↓ Serum phosphate ↑ Serum total and ionized calcium ↓ Urine specific gravity ↓ Urine protein:creatinine ↑	Serum creatinine ↑ Serum SDMA ↑ or ↓

6.3 Biochemical parameters of renal function affected by thyroid dysfunction. SDMA = symmetric dimethylarginine.

Serum creatinine and urea concentrations in thyroid disease

As GFR is inversely proportional to serum creatinine concentration, hyperthyroid cats (with increased GFR) have reduced serum creatinine concentrations, and hypothyroid dogs and cats (with decreased GFR) have increased serum creatinine concentrations. Serum creatinine concentrations are also influenced by muscle mass, which is reduced in hyperthyroid cats secondary to increased protein breakdown and catabolism, and by alterations in endogenous creatinine production, which is reduced in hypothyroid dogs (Panciera and Lefebvre, 2009). The composite effects of thyroid-hormone-mediated changes in GFR, muscle mass and endogenous creatinine production mean that the use of serum creatinine concentrations as a biomarker of renal function is confounded in animals with thyroid dysfunction. Therefore, approximately two thirds of hyperthyroid cats with concurrent CKD have serum creatinine concentrations within the reference interval at presentation. Subsequently, creatinine concentrations increase above the reference interval once the hyperthyroidism has been treated and GFR decreases to 'normal' for that cat. However, it is important for clinicians to realize that the development of mild to moderate azotaemia after starting treatment of hyperthyroidism does not adversely affect the survival of that cat, provided that iatrogenic hypothyroidism is avoided (Williams et al., 2010a). Clinicians should aim for a serum total thyroxine (T4) concentration in the lower half of the laboratory reference interval together with a reference interval thyrotropin (thyroid-stimulating hormone (TSH)) concentration, thus avoiding both biochemical and subclinical hypothyroidism.

Hypothyroidism (both iatrogenic and naturally occurring) can increase the prevalence of azotaemia (due to reductions in GFR) that may not reflect 'true' renal dysfunction. Renal function should be rechecked after euthyroidism is restored (by thyroid supplementation or adjustments to the dosage of antithyroid medications). However, despite the limitations associated with the interpretation of serum creatinine concentrations in thyroid disease, the detection of an increased serum creatinine concentration (in conjunction with urine specific gravity (SG) <1.035) in an uncontrolled hyperthyroid cat indicates concurrent CKD, and a hypothyroid dog or cat without concurrent azotaemia is unlikely to have concurrent CKD.

Serum urea concentrations are also unreliable markers of GFR in hyperthyroid cats because of the divergent effects of polyphagia and increased protein catabolism (which will increase serum urea concentrations), and thyroid-hormone-mediated increases in GFR (which will decrease serum urea concentrations).

Serum symmetric dimethylarginine concentrations in thyroid disease

Symmetric dimethylarginine (SDMA) might be advantageous as a biomarker of renal dysfunction in thyroid disease, particularly hyperthyroidism, because SDMA is less influenced by changes in body muscle mass. Recent studies have documented that increased serum SDMA concentrations might be a useful, albeit poorly sensitive, marker of concurrent CKD (based on post-treatment renal status) in hyperthyroid cats compared with serum creatinine concentrations (Peterson et al., 2018), although other studies have observed that some hyperthyroid cats have increased serum SDMA concentrations despite no other biochemical evidence of CKD (Buresova et al., 2019; Yu et al., 2020). This could indicate that the metabolic derangements associated with the hyperthyroid state can also influence SDMA metabolism, decreasing its diagnostic specificity for CKD.

In hypothyroid dogs, serum SDMA concentrations are increased in approximately 50% of untreated cases, likely reflecting the reduction in GFR; however, serum SDMA concentrations normalized in the majority of cases after at least 2 weeks of thyroid hormone supplementation (Di Paola et al., 2021).

Urinary biomarkers in thyroid disease

The interpretation of urinary biomarkers of kidney disease is also confounded in hyperthyroidism, with urine-concentrating ability compromised and urine protein excretion increased regardless of the presence or absence of concurrent CKD (Williams et al., 2010b).

Effect of kidney disease on thyroid physiology and diagnosis of thyroid disease

Not only can thyroid disease influence renal function, but renal dysfunction can also have effects on thyroid physiology, which can complicate the diagnosis of concurrent thyroid disease. For instance, the diagnosis of hyperthyroidism and hypothyroidism is complicated in animals with non-thyroidal illnesses (NTIs), such as CKD, because NTIs can cause suppression of serum total T4 concentrations, thus decreasing its diagnostic sensitivity and specificity for hyperthyroidism and hypothyroidism, respectively. Evaluation of serum TSH concentrations may be useful to distinguish between low total T4 values associated with hypothyroidism and NTI. Non-thyroidal illness can also increase free T4 concentrations in some euthyroid cats, which could lead to a false-positive diagnosis of hyperthyroidism; therefore, free T4 concentrations should not be used as a stand-alone test for hyperthyroidism. Conversely, severe NTIs can also suppress free T4 concentrations; therefore, both total T4 and free T4 concentrations should be interpreted with caution in animals with CKD.

Interplay between adrenal and renal function

The adrenal glands produce both glucocorticoids (predominantly cortisol) and mineralocorticoids (predominantly aldosterone), both of which can independently impact renal function. Excess glucocorticoids (hypercortisolism) and mineralocorticoids (hyperaldosteronism) might also have detrimental effects on the kidney, although evidence to support this in dogs and cats is currently weak.

Effect of adrenal disease on renal function

Dogs with hypercortisolism have increased GFR (and thus low or low-normal serum creatinine concentrations) and GFR decreases (and serum creatinine increases) after treatment. The increase in GFR observed in hypercortisolism (Figure 6.4) may reflect any or all of a combination of:

- Mineralocorticoid activity of glucocorticoids (that enhances sodium and water retention, thus causing volume expansion)
- Direct and indirect vasodilatory and vasoconstrictive effects of glucocorticoids on the afferent and efferent arterioles in the glomerulus
- Decreased renal vascular resistance
- Increased protein catabolism that leads to an increase in circulating amino acids, which in turn directly stimulates an increase in GFR.

Conversely, hypoadrenocorticism (usually a combination of hypocortisolism and hypoaldosteronism) is associated with a reduction in GFR due to volume depletion associated with increased renal sodium and water excretion and the lack of other actions of glucocorticoids that help to maintain GFR.

Proteinuria is a relatively common feature in dogs with hypercortisolism (44–75% of cases), and is caused by increased excretion of albumin, high-molecular-weight proteins (such as immunoglobulin G (IgG)) and low-molecular-weight proteins (such as RBP and NAG) (Smets *et al.*, 2012a). These data suggest that a combination of both increased glomerular protein permeability and decreased renal tubular protein resorption is occurring in these cases.

Polyuria is also a common feature in canine hypercortisolism, caused by a reduction in renal tubular concentrating ability that may be secondary to disturbed osmoregulation and arginine vasopressin secretion, inhibition of responsiveness of the renal tubules to arginine vasopressin or lower interstitial osmolality (due to a glucocorticoid-mediated reduction in expression of urea transporters) that impairs urine-concentrating ability.

Hypoadrenocorticism can occasionally be associated with the production of poorly concentrated urine (SG <1.015), which may reflect a failure of sodium and chloride delivery to the loop of Henle (due to a whole body sodium and chloride deficit), thus limiting the ability of the kidney to maintain medullary hypertonicity. Hyponatraemia could also reduce the osmotic stimulus for arginine vasopressin secretion, thereby promoting renal water excretion.

When cortisol is in excess, it is able to activate mineralocorticoid receptors and increase expression of the renal epithelial sodium channel and the basolateral Na-K-ATPase, thus increasing sodium and water resorption and potassium excretion. However, alterations in serum sodium or potassium concentrations are not commonly observed in dogs with hypercortisolism or, when present, are mild and unlikely to be of clinical significance. In contrast, cats with hyperaldosteronism frequently demonstrate marked hypokalaemia, with high-normal to occasionally mildly increased serum sodium concentrations. Cortisol-mediated changes in sodium resorption secondarily cause a reduction in renal calcium resorption, leading to hypercalciuria and an increased prevalence of calcium-containing urolithiasis in dogs with hypercortisolism.

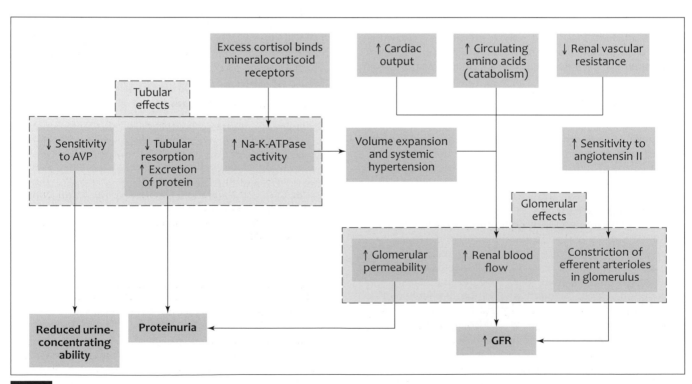

6.4 Effect of hypercortisolism on renal function. AVP = arginine vasopressin; GFR = glomerular filtration rate.

Is adrenal disease damaging to the kidney?

Hypercortisolism

Hypercortisolism is associated with systemic hypertension in dogs (37–86% of cases), which could cause glomerular injury and proteinuria. Furthermore, proteinuria itself might directly cause tubular injury. However, a combination of hypercortisolism and kidney disease is relatively rare in humans, although a possible association between hypercortisolism and nephrotic syndrome has been suggested based on the resolution of nephrotic syndrome after treatment of hypercortisolism, which implies a possible causal association.

Concurrent hypercortisolism and clinically appreciable kidney disease is also uncommon in dogs; however, in one study, approximately one-third of dogs treated for hypercortisolism had subnormal GFR (<2 ml/min/kg) and approximately half of the dogs were mildly proteinuric (UPCR <1) 12 months after treatment, which could reflect permanent renal dysfunction. The same study also identified histological evidence of glomerular and tubulo-interstitial lesions in two of these dogs (Smets et al., 2012b). However, whether this reflects a causal association between hypercortisolism and kidney disease or the identification of two unrelated comorbidities requires additional investigation.

Primary hyperaldosteronism

It has been postulated that primary hyperaldosteronism could contribute to renal injury, because aldosterone can cause podocyte injury and promote interstitial inflammation and renal fibrosis. Serum urea and creatinine concentrations increased over time in a single observational study of cats with primary hyperaldosteronism; however, since a control group was not included, this finding could reflect declining renal function with age that is independent of the effects of aldosterone.

Effect of adrenal disease on diagnosis of kidney disease

Figure 6.5 outlines the biochemical parameters of renal function that are affected by adrenal dysfunction.

Hypercortisolism	Hypoadrenocorticism
Serum creatinine ↓ Urine specific gravity ↓ Urine protein:creatinine ↑	Serum creatinine ↑ Urine specific gravity ↓

6.5 Biochemical parameters of renal function affected by adrenal dysfunction.

Hypercortisolism

Glucocorticoids stimulate an increase in GFR and consequently a decrease in serum creatinine concentrations, which may also be exacerbated by muscle atrophy. These factors mean that biochemical evidence of concurrent CKD could be 'masked' in animals with hypercortisolism, although the coexistence of hypercortisolism and CKD in dogs is low. Following treatment, GFR will decrease and serum creatinine concentrations will increase (Smets et al., 2012b), although the subsequent development of azotaemia is uncommon.

The effects of hypercortisolism on urine-concentrating ability and protein excretion will also complicate the diagnosis of concurrent CKD, particularly as mild proteinuria can persist after treatment in approximately 50% of dogs (Smets et al., 2012b). However, normal urine-concentrating ability should recover following successful medical treatment of hypercortisolism. Animals treated by hypophysectomy may not recover normal urine-concentrating ability because of impaired secretion of arginine vasopressin.

Hypoadrenocorticism

Hypoadrenocorticism can be associated with azotaemia that is usually prerenal in origin (secondary to dehydration and hypovolaemia), although the biochemical and clinical features of hypoadrenocorticism mimic those of acute kidney injury (AKI). Prerenal azotaemia and electrolyte abnormalities associated with hypoaldosteronism are usually rapidly corrected after appropriate fluid and hormone therapy, whereas AKI will often be associated with persistent azotaemia, thus aiding in their differentation.

Effect of kidney disease on adrenal physiology and the diagnosis of adrenal disease

Hypercortisolism

Although it is relatively rare for dogs with hypercortisolism to have concurrent CKD, renal dysfunction could potentially have clinically relevant effects on the diagnostic tests for hypercortisolism. In humans with CKD, assessment of cortisol concentrations is confounded because of reduced binding of cortisol to albumin (which can cause spuriously increased cortisol concentrations), and a reduction in renal excretion of cortisol and cortisol metabolites, leading to a prolonged serum half-life of cortisol and accumulation of metabolites that can interfere with cortisol assays.

All of the commonly used diagnostic tests for hypercortisolism in dogs can yield false-positive results in animals with non-adrenal illnesses, including CKD, either due to either adrenal hyperplasia that is consequent to chronic illness or the previously described effects of non-adrenal illnesses on cortisol metabolism.

Primary hyperaldosteronism

Chronic kidney disease, which is a frequent comorbidity in feline primary hyperaldosteronism, can itself be associated with RAAS activation (secondary hyperaldosteronism), which could confound the diagnosis of primary hyperaldosteronism. Differentiation between primary hyperaldosteronism and secondary hyperaldosteronism can be achieved by evaluation of the plasma renin:aldosterone, although measurement of plasma renin activity is not widely available.

Interplay between diabetes mellitus and renal function

Diabetic nephropathy is a common comorbidity and cause of mortality in human diabetic patients; however, relatively little is known about the influence of diabetes mellitus on renal function in dogs and cats with naturally occurring disease.

Effect of diabetes mellitus on renal function

In humans, the prediabetic and early diabetic phases are associated with an increased GFR secondary to the effects of hyperglycaemia, abnormal insulin concentrations and obesity. These factors cause nephron hypertrophy through the actions of various cytokines and growth factors, leading to glomerular hyperfiltration and increased GFR. However, in the later phases of diabetic disease, structural lesions in the kidney, such as thickening of the basement membrane and mesangial expansion, lead to a progressive reduction in GFR.

Relatively little is known about the GFR of diabetic dogs and cats. Glomerular filtration rate is increased in dogs with experimentally induced diabetes mellitus; however, increased GFR was not observed in a small cohort of dogs with naturally occurring disease (Marynissen et al., 2016). Glomerular filtration rate was also not significantly different between healthy cats and cats with diabetes mellitus in one study, although most cats included were already receiving insulin therapy, which may have confounded the analysis (Paepe et al., 2014).

Diabetes mellitus is also associated with proteinuria in dogs and cats (28–44% of dogs, 39–70% of cats), which is likely to reflect increased renal excretion of albumin and other proteins (including IgG, RBP and NAG) (Paepe et al., 2014; Marynissen et al., 2016). Thus, increased proteinuria in diabetes mellitus probably reflects a combination of increased glomerular permeability and decreased tubular resorption of protein.

Is diabetes mellitus damaging to the kidney?

Hyperglycaemia, oxidative stress, inflammatory cytokines, profibrotic growth factors and microvascular changes in diabetes mellitus may all cause renal injury. In humans, diabetes mellitus is known to be associated with structural changes in the kidney, including accumulation of extracellular matrix, which leads to thickening of the basement membrane, mesangial expansion, podocyte injury and, eventually, tubulointerstitial expansion and injury.

In dogs with experimentally induced diabetes mellitus, morphological lesions similar to those observed in human diabetic nephropathy have been observed. However, few studies have investigated renal morphology in naturally occurring diabetes mellitus in dogs and cats. In one small cohort of diabetic dogs, some histological changes consistent with human diabetic nephropathy were observed (Jeraj et al., 1984). Differences in renal histological lesions were not identified between diabetic cats and age-matched control cats (Zini et al., 2014).

Observational studies do not generally support an association between diabetes mellitus and significant CKD in dogs, as no change in serum creatinine (or GFR) or biochemical evidence of CKD was observed during a 12–24-month follow-up period (Herring et al., 2014; Marynissen et al., 2016), and azotaemic CKD is not typically identified as a comorbidity in diabetic dogs. In cats, there is some discordance in the literature, as one study has identified diabetic cats with a higher prevalence of concurrent CKD compared with the general adult cat population (Pérez-López et al., 2019), whereas another larger study identified a lower prevalence of diabetes mellitus in cats with CKD compared with an age-matched control population (Greene et al., 2014). Therefore, it remains unclear whether diabetes mellitus is a true risk factor for CKD in cats.

Taken together, there is currently no or limited evidence to support an association between diabetes mellitus and kidney disease in dogs and cats. It may be the case that the limited lifespan of dogs and cats means that there is insufficient time for renal lesions to develop in diabetic individuals, unlike in humans, who may be diabetic for many decades.

Effect of diabetes mellitus on diagnosis of kidney disease

Diabetic animals can demonstrate some clinicopathological features of kidney disease, which could complicate the diagnosis of concurrent CKD. As mentioned previously, a significant proportion of diabetic dogs and cats are proteinuric. In dogs, proteinuria can be persistent even after attainment of good glycaemic control (Herring et al., 2014), which could suggest ongoing or underlying comorbid renal dysfunction and disease.

Diabetic animals with glucosuria may be hypovolaemic secondary to osmotic diuresis, which may lead to prerenal azotaemia. However, the osmotic diuresis associated with glucosuria can also decrease urine SG, which could lead to the conclusion that there is tubular dysfunction in azotaemic animals. Therefore, reassessment of renal biochemical parameters and urinalysis is recommended once glucosuria has resolved.

Diabetes mellitus may also influence some of the biochemical markers of renal function, and perhaps biochemically 'mask' concurrent CKD. In one study of 17 cats with CKD, 17 cats with diabetes mellitus and 20 healthy controls, serum SDMA and creatinine concentrations were significantly lower in cats with diabetes mellitus than in healthy controls, which could lead to reference interval SDMA concentrations in diabetic cats with concurrent CKD (Langhorn et al., 2018). An inverse association between fructosamine and serum SDMA concentrations in cats has also been observed (Pérez-López et al., 2020). The reduced serum creatinine concentrations may reflect reduced muscle mass or perhaps increased GFR in diabetic cats. Symmetric dimethylarginine should be influenced less by changes in muscle mass; therefore, reduced SDMA concentrations in diabetes mellitus could reflect changes in arginine metabolism, altered cellular uptake, increased hepatic metabolism or increased GFR. Studies in diabetic dogs have not identified reduced serum creatinine concentrations, and no studies have yet evaluated serum SDMA concentrations in this group.

Effect of kidney disease on diagnosis of diabetes mellitus

In general, kidney disease will not affect interpretation of the commonly used tests for diabetes mellitus (blood glucose concentrations, fructosamine concentration), although some normoglycaemic animals with AKI or severe end-stage CKD can be glucosuric secondary to renal tubular injury and reduced tubular resorption of glucose.

Glucosuria is also expected in animals with congenital or acquired defects in renal tubular glucose handling (Fanconi syndrome, primary renal glucosuria). In addition, one study reported that 20% of non-diabetic cats with CKD had increased serum beta-hydroxybutyrate concentrations (Gorman et al., 2016); therefore, increased serum beta-hydroxybutyrate concentrations are not specific for diabetes mellitus.

Interplay between other endocrine disorders and renal function

Other less common endocrinopathies have also been associated with kidney disease, although the rarity of these disorders means that only a small number of cases of kidney disease in animals with these endocrinopathies have been reported; hence, it is difficult to extrapolate a cause–effect relationship.

Growth hormone (GH) and insulin-like growth factors (IGFs) are involved in pre- and postnatal development of the kidney, and IGFs also influence GFR and tubular handling of phosphate. Growth hormone deficiency is also associated with reduced GFR; therefore, GH deficiency would be expected to result in kidney disease and dysfunction. In human patients, GH replacement therapy will at least partially normalize the GFR, and this would also be expected to support postnatal renal development. In contrast, GH excess results in kidney hypertrophy as well as sodium retention, leading to volume expansion and hypertension. Growth hormone excess (hypersomatotropism) will also lead to insulin resistance and the development of diabetes mellitus, which in itself may have detrimental effects on renal function (see above). There is sparse literature reporting renal function in animals with GH disorders, although one 3-month-old cat with hyposomatotropism did become azotaemic within 1 year of diagnosis, which could reflect the renal consequences of GH deficiency. In addition, one study reported that 7 of 14 cats with hypersomatotropism developed azotaemia during a 3-year follow up period; however, the kidneys were normal to large in size, and histopathological findings in one cat indicated glomerulonephropathy with lesions resembling those observed in human diabetic nephropathy.

Disorders of calcium and phosphate homeostasis may also be detrimental to renal function, since dystrophic calcification of the kidney may lead to kidney injury. Primary hyperparathyroidism causes hypercalcaemia, and one study reported that the degree of hypercalcaemia correlated with the presence of kidney disease, thus suggesting that hypercalcaemia and/or hyperparathyroidism are detrimental to renal function. However, the reported prevalence of kidney disease in canine primary hyperparathyroidism is variable, with one study observing renal azotaemia in 24% of dogs (Gear *et al.*, 2005), whereas another larger study reported azotaemia in only 3–4% of dogs (Feldman *et al.*, 2005). Additional studies would be useful to clarify the prevalence of CKD in canine primary hyperparathyroidism.

Hyperparathyroidism can also be observed secondary to CKD (secondary renal hyperparathyroidism). However, the role of this in the onset and progression of CKD is controversial. Feeding of phosphate-restricted diets to cats with CKD does reduce plasma parathyroid hormone (PTH) concentrations and is associated with improved survival times. However, more recent data in cats suggest that circulating concentrations of the phosphaturic hormone fibroblast growth factor 23 (FGF-23), rather than PTH, are associated with the progression of CKD – perhaps indicating that secondary hyperparathyroidism itself is not a mechanism for renal injury.

References and further reading

Buresova E, Stock E, Paepe D *et al.* (2019) Assessment of symmetric dimethylarginine as a biomarker of renal function in hyperthyroid cats treated with radioiodine. *Journal of Veterinary Internal Medicine* **33**, 516–522

Di Paola A, Carotenuto G, Dondi F *et al.* (2021) Symmetric dimethylarginine concentrations in dogs with hypothyroidism before and after treatement with levothyroxine. *Journal of Small Animal Practice* **62**, 89–96

Feldman EC, Hoar B, Pollard R and Nelson RW (2005) Pretreatment clinical and laboratory findings in dogs with primary hyperparathyroidism: 210 cases (1987–2004). *Journal of the American Veterinary Medical Association* **227**, 756–761

Gear RNA, Neiger R, Skelly BJS and Herrtage ME (2005) Primary hyperparathyroidism in 29 dogs: diagnosis, treatment, outcome and associated renal failure. *Journal of Small Animal Practice* **46**, 10–16

Gommeren K, van Hoek I, Lefebvre HP *et al.* (2009) Effect of thyroxine supplementation on glomerular filtration rate in hypothyroid dogs. *Journal of Veterinary Internal Medicine* **23**, 844–849

Gorman L, Sharkey LC, Armstrong PJ, Little K and Rendahl A (2016) Serum beta hydroxybutyrate concentrations in cats with chronic kidney disease, hyperthyroidism, or hepatic lipidosis. *Journal of Veterinary Internal Medicine* **30**, 611–616

Greene JP, Lefebvre SL, Wang M *et al.* (2014) Risk factors associated with the development of chronic kidney disease in cats evaluated at primary care veterinary hospitals. *Journal of the American Veterinary Medical Association* **244**, 320–327

Herring IP, Panciera DL and Werre SR (2014) Longitudinal prevalence of hypertension, proteinuria, and retinopathy in dogs with spontaneous diabetes mellitus. *Journal of Veterinary Internal Medicine* **28**, 488–495

Jeraj K, Basgen J, Hardy RM, Osborne CA and Michael AF (1984) Immunofluorescence studies of renal basement membranes in dogs with spontaneous diabetes. *American Journal of Veterinary Research* **45**, 1162–1165

Langhorn R, Kieler IN, Koch J, Christiansen LB and Jessen LR (2018) Symmetric dimethylarginine in cats with hypertrophic cardiomyopathy and diabetes mellitus. *Journal of Veterinary Internal Medicine* **32**, 57–63

Marynissen SJJ, Smets PMY, Ghys LFE *et al.* (2016) Long-term follow-up of renal function assessing serum cystatin C in dogs with diabetes mellitus or hyperadrenocorticism. *Veterinary Clinical Pathology* **45**, 320–329

Paepe D, Ghys LFE, Smets PMY *et al.* (2014) Routine kidney variables, glomerular filtration rate and urinary cystatin C in cats with diabetes mellitus, cats with chronic kidney disease and healthy cats. *Journal of Feline Medicine and Surgery* **17**, 880–888

Panciera DL and Lefebvre HP (2009) Effect of experimental hypothyroidism on glomerular filtration rate and plasma creatinine concentration in dogs. *Journal of Veterinary Internal Medicine* **23**, 1045–1050

Peterson ME, Varela FV, Rishniw M and Polzin DJ (2018) Evaluation of serum symmetric dimethylarginine concentration as a marker for masked chronic kidney disease in cats with hyperthyroidism. *Journal of Veterinary Internal Medicine* **32**, 295–304

Pérez-López L, Boronat M, Melián C, Brito-Casillas Y and Wägner AM (2020) Kidney function and glucose metabolism in overweight and obese cats. *Veterinary Quarterly* **40**, 132–139

Pérez-López L, Boronat M, Melián C *et al.* (2019) Assessment of the association between diabetes mellitus and chronic kidney disease in adult cats. *Journal of Veterinary Internal Medicine* **33**, 1913–1925

Smets PMY, Lefebvre HP, Kooistra HS *et al.* (2012a) Hypercortisolism affects glomerular and tubular function in dogs. *Veterinary Journal* **192**, 532–534

Smets PMY, Lefebvre HP, Meij BP *et al.* (2012b) Long-term follow-up of renal function in dogs after treatment for ACTH-dependent hyperadrenocorticism. *Journal of Veterinary Internal Medicine* **26**, 565–574

Williams TL, Elliott J and Syme HM (2010a) Association of iatrogenic hypothyroidism with azotemia and reduced survival time in cats treated for hyperthyroidism. *Journal of Veterinary Internal Medicine* **24**, 1086–1092

Williams TL, Peak KJ, Brodbelt D, Elliott J and Syme HM (2010b) Survival and the development of azotemia after treatment of hyperthyroid cats. *Journal of Veterinary Internal Medicine* **24**, 863–869

Yu L, Lacorcia L, Finch S and Johnstone T (2020) Assessment of serum symmetric dimethylarginine and creatinine concentrations in hyperthyroid cats before and after a fixed dose of orally administered radioiodine. *Journal of Veterinary Internal Medicine* **34**, 1423–1431

Zini E, Benali S, Coppola L *et al.* (2014) Renal morphology in cats with diabetes mellitus. *Veterinary Pathology* **51**, 1143–1150

Chapter 7

The effect of endocrine disease on lipid metabolism

Panagiotis G. Xenoulis

Introduction

Disorders of lipid metabolism have received limited attention in canine and feline medicine. In contrast to humans, hyperlipidaemia has been traditionally considered a relatively benign condition in cats and dogs, and clinical experience with and research into hyperlipidaemia have been limited in these species. In the past decade, several studies in both humans and dogs have associated specific forms of hyperlipidaemia with a much wider range of diseases than previously thought. Therefore, canine hyperlipidaemia is emerging as an important clinical condition that requires a systematic diagnostic approach and appropriate treatment. In cats, disorders of lipid metabolism are considered less common than in dogs and the related bibliography is sparse. The clinical importance of hyperlipidaemia is largely unknown in this species, as is its diagnosis and treatment.

Many endocrine diseases are known to affect lipoprotein metabolism in various ways. This chapter aims to provide a concise approach to hyperlipidaemia in dogs and cats with emphasis on the relationship between hyperlipidaemia and endocrine disease.

The basics of lipoprotein metabolism

Lipids

Lipids are water-insoluble organic compounds that are essential for many normal functions of living organisms: lipids are important components of cell membranes, are used to store energy, and play a significant role as enzyme cofactors, hormones and intracellular messengers. Of the many groups of lipids, three are most important from a clinical perspective:

- **Fatty acids** – these are relatively simple lipids and are also important components of many other more complex lipids
- **Sterols** – cholesterol is the main sterol in animal tissues. Dietary intake is the major source of cholesterol, but it can also be synthesized endogenously by the liver and other tissues. It plays a fundamental role in central metabolic pathways, such as bile acid metabolism and steroid hormone and vitamin D synthesis

- **Acylglycerols** – the acylglycerols are esters of glycerol and fatty acids, and can be classified as triglycerides, diglycerides and monoglycerides. Triglycerides are the most common and efficient form of stored energy in mammals. They can be derived from both dietary sources and endogenous (hepatic) production.

Lipoproteins and apolipoproteins

As lipids are water-insoluble molecules, they cannot be transported in aqueous solutions, such as plasma. For that reason, lipids are transported in plasma as macromolecular complexes known as lipoproteins. Lipoproteins are spherical structures that consist of a hydrophobic core containing lipids (i.e. triglycerides and/or cholesterol esters) and an amphiphilic (i.e. both hydrophobic and hydrophilic) outer layer of phospholipids, free cholesterol and proteins that forms a protective envelope surrounding the lipid core.

Plasma lipoproteins differ in their physical and chemical characteristics such as size, density and composition, as well as in function. Lipoproteins can be divided based on their hydrated density into four major classes:

- Chylomicrons
- Very-low-density lipoproteins (VLDLs)
- Low-density lipoproteins (LDLs)
- High-density lipoproteins (HDLs), which can be further subdivided into HDL_1 (unique to dogs), HDL_2 and HDL_3.

The protein components of lipoproteins are known as apolipoproteins (or apoproteins). Lipoproteins can contain one or a variety of apolipoproteins. In general, apolipoproteins are involved in regulation of the physiological functions of lipoproteins, including facilitation of lipid transport, maintenance of structural integrity and activation of certain enzymes that play key roles in lipid metabolism.

Serum lipid enzymes

Lipoprotein lipase is an enzyme that is located on the luminal surface of capillary endothelial cells. The enzyme hydrolyses blood triglycerides within lipoproteins into free fatty acids, monoglycerides, diglycerides and glycerol for transport into the cell. Apolipoprotein C2 (apo C2) is an important cofactor of lipoprotein lipase. The activity of lipoprotein lipase is affected by several hormones, the most important being insulin (stimulating effect), thyroxine (T4) (stimulating effect), cortisol (inhibitive effect) and growth hormone (inhibitive effect).

Hormone-sensitive lipase is responsible for the hydrolysis of triglycerides in adipose tissue. The products of this reaction enter the circulation for subsequent use as an energy source. The activity of hormone-sensitive lipase is regulated by several hormones that have the opposite function on this enzyme compared with lipoprotein lipase; insulin and T4 inhibit, and cortisol and growth hormone stimulate, hormone-sensitive lipase.

Hepatic triglyceride lipase, also known as hepatic lipase, is located on endothelial cells of hepatic sinusoids and several extrahepatic tissues, and is involved in hepatic uptake of triglycerides and phospholipids from chylomicrons and VLDL remnants, the conversion of VLDLs to LDLs, and the conversion of HDL_2 to HDL_3.

Lecithin–cholesterol acyltransferase (LCAT) circulates in the blood mainly bound to HDL. Lecithin–cholesterol acyltransferase acts on HDL molecules to convert cholesterol into cholesteryl esters and plays a crucial role in a pathway known as reverse cholesterol transport.

In humans, an additional enzyme, cholesteryl ester transfer protein (CETP), is involved in lipid metabolism. The role of this enzyme is to transport triglycerides from VLDLs and chylomicrons to HDL_2, and cholesteryl esters from HDL_2 to VLDLs and LDLs. Cholesteryl ester transfer protein activity has not been documented in cats or dogs.

Lipoprotein metabolism

The basic principles of lipoprotein metabolism are illustrated in Figure 7.1. Lipid metabolism occurs via one of two basic pathways: the exogenous pathway, which is associated with the metabolism of exogenous (dietary) lipids, and the endogenous pathway, which is associated with the metabolism of endogenously produced lipids.

Exogenous pathway

The first step of dietary lipid metabolism is digestion. Dietary lipids that reach the duodenum undergo emulsification and are then hydrolysed by the pancreatic and intestinal lipases. Hydrolysis products are transferred to the microvilli of the intestinal epithelial cell brush border in the form of micelles, where they diffuse through the epithelial cell membranes into the enteric mucosal cells. In the intestinal mucosal cells, free fatty acids and monoglycerides reassemble to form new triglycerides, which then combine with phospholipids, free and esterified cholesterol, and the apo B48 protein to form chylomicrons.

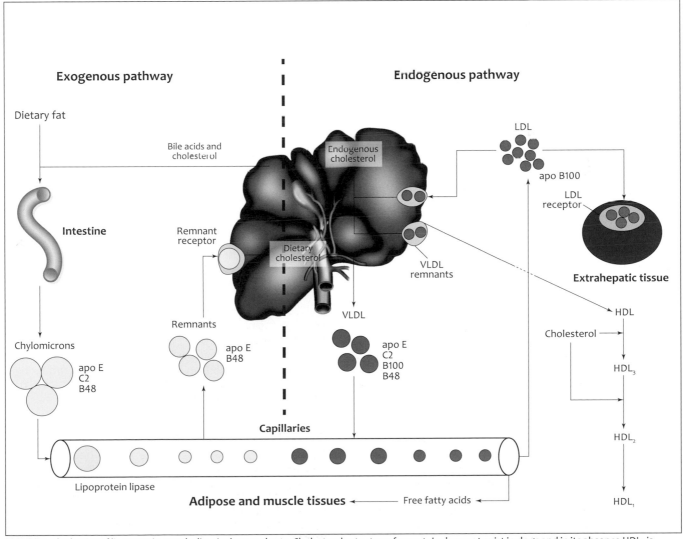

7.1 The basics of lipoprotein metabolism in dogs and cats. Cholesteryl ester transfer protein does not exist in dogs and in its absence HDL_2 is transformed into HDL_1. apo = apolipoprotein; HDL = high-density lipoprotein; LDL = low-density lipoprotein; VLDL = very-low-density lipoprotein.

Chylomicrons are the lipoprotein class responsible for transfer of dietary lipids. After formation in the enterocytes, chylomicrons, which mainly contain triglycerides, are secreted into the lacteals and enter first the lymphatic and later the blood circulation, where they acquire apolipoproteins C and E from circulating HDL molecules. Apolipoprotein C2, which is exposed on the chylomicron surface, activates the lipoprotein lipase attached to the capillary beds in adipose and muscle tissues, which in turn hydrolyses triglycerides into free fatty acids and glycerol. Free fatty acids enter the muscle cells (where they are used for energy production) or adipocytes (for storage). The remaining cholesteryl ester-rich particles (chylomicron remnants) return their apo C2 molecules to HDLs and are recognized by specific hepatic apo E receptors that rapidly remove them from the circulation by endocytosis. The cholesterol found in chylomicron remnants can be used for VLDL or bile acid formation or stored as cholesteryl esters.

Endogenous pathway

While chylomicrons are responsible for the transport of dietary lipids, VLDLs, LDLs and HDLs are mainly involved in the metabolism of endogenously produced lipids. Endogenously synthesized triglycerides and cholesterol (and cholesteryl esters) combine with phospholipids, apo B100 and apo B48 to form VLDLs. After VLDL molecules reach the vasculature, they acquire apolipoproteins C and E from HDL. Very-low-density lipoprotein apo C2 activates lipoprotein lipase located in the capillary beds, which in turn leads to hydrolysis of triglycerides and the production of free fatty acids and glycerol. The VLDL molecules remaining after hydrolysis of VLDL triglycerides (VLDL remnants) are either removed from the circulation by the liver or undergo further transformation by lipoprotein lipase and/or hepatic lipase to form LDLs.

Low-density lipoproteins, which contain mainly cholesteryl esters, circulate in the blood and bind to specific receptors that are widely distributed throughout tissues. Their main function is to deliver cholesterol, which can be used for the synthesis of steroid hormones and cell membranes and for hepatic metabolism. One of the main organs expressing LDL receptors that plays an important role in LDL metabolism is the liver.

High-density lipoproteins, which are synthesized primarily in the liver, act as donors and acceptors of apolipoproteins C and E and various lipids from other lipoproteins in the circulation. They play a fundamental role in the reverse cholesterol transport pathway, through which cholesterol is transferred from peripheral tissues to the small circulating discoid HDL molecules, thus converting them to nascent HDL_3 molecules. Cholesterol is then esterified by the action of LCAT, after which the cholesteryl esters move to the core of the HDL molecule, thus allowing more free cholesterol to be absorbed into their surface. Continued absorption of free cholesterol, and subsequent esterification by LCAT, leads to the formation of the larger, cholesteryl-ester-rich HDL_2. In dogs, due to the absence of the enzyme CETP (which is present in humans), HDL_2 molecules continuously acquire cholesteryl esters, resulting in the formation of HDL_1 molecules. Cholesteryl esters within HDL_1 molecules are transferred from tissues to the liver for disposal or reuse, unlike those within LDL or VLDL molecules, which transfer cholesterol to peripheral tissues. Thus, it is this function of HDL_1 that accounts for the lower incidence of atherosclerotic disorders in dogs compared with humans. The existence of HDL_1 has not been confirmed in cats.

Definitions and measurement of serum lipid concentrations

The term *hyperlipidaemia* refers to an increased concentration of lipids (i.e. triglycerides, cholesterol or both) in the blood (serum or plasma). Specifically, an increased blood concentration of triglycerides is referred to as *hypertriglyceridaemia*, while an increased blood concentration of cholesterol is referred to as *hypercholesterolaemia*. Because both triglycerides and cholesterol are transported in the blood combined with apolipoproteins (the lipid–protein complex is referred to as lipoprotein), the term *hyperlipoproteinaemia* is often used interchangeably with the term hyperlipidaemia. The term *lipaemia* is used to describe a grossly visible turbid or lactescent appearance of serum or plasma (Figure 7.2). Lipaemia is a result of moderate and severe hypertriglyceridaemia (typically >2.26–3.39 mmol/l), but not hypercholesterolaemia or mild hypertriglyceridaemia. Finally, the term *dyslipidaemia* is a more general term, the use of which is not limited to describing increases in blood lipid concentrations, but rather any kind of disturbance in the quality and/or quantity of blood lipids and/or lipoproteins.

Determination of serum lipid concentrations is routinely done after a fast of at least 12 hours. Fasting should be ensured because an increase in serum lipid concentrations is expected after a meal and is normal in most cases. Although there is strong evidence that measurement of lipid concentrations during the postprandial state is a more sensitive way to detect lipid abnormalities than during the fasting state, there are currently no established guidelines or reference intervals for interpretation of these values in dogs or cats. The existing reference intervals for most laboratories are for the fasting state and cannot be used to evaluate postprandial serum lipid concentrations. As a result, postprandial serum lipid measurements are not suitable for routine use at the time of writing.

The most basic laboratory procedures for the detection and evaluation of lipid disorders are determinations of serum triglyceride and total cholesterol concentrations, typically measured with spectrophotometric or enzymatic methods. Other tests that have occasionally been used to further characterize or investigate the cause of hyperlipidaemia (mainly primary hyperlipidaemia) include the following:

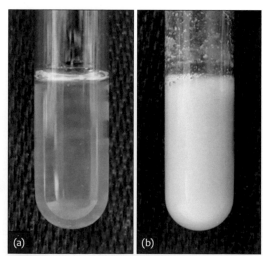

(a) (b)

7.2 Lipaemia. (a) Serum samples with reference interval triglyceride concentrations are clear. (b) Lactescent serum indicates severely increased serum triglyceride concentrations.

- **The chylomicron test** – this is a simple test to determine whether lipaemia is due to the presence of chylomicrons, VLDLs or both. Lipaemic serum samples are left for 12 hours undisturbed at 4°C. Due to their lower density, chylomicrons (if present) float to the top of the sample and form a cream layer. Therefore, the presence of a cream layer at the top of the sample indicates the presence of chylomicrons. The absence of a cream layer indicates the absence of chylomicrons in the sample. The remaining serum (below the cream layer) can be clear or turbid. In the first case, the hyperlipidaemia is due to increased chylomicrons alone; in the latter case, an excess of VLDLs is also indicated. If no chylomicrons are present, there is no cream layer and the serum remains turbid, indicating an excess of VLDLs
- **Indirect measurement of plasma lipoprotein lipase activity** – for this test, serum triglyceride concentrations are measured before and, usually, 10 minutes after intravenous administration of 40–90 IU/kg heparin. Heparin stimulates the release of lipoprotein lipase from the capillary endothelium, leading to a transient increase in the hydrolysis of chylomicrons and VLDLs. If there is an obvious decrease in plasma triglyceride concentrations after the administration of heparin, lipoprotein lipase is functional. A lack of change is an indirect indicator of decreased or absent lipoprotein lipase activity
- **Further characterization by lipoprotein electrophoresis, ultracentrifugation or measurement of specific apolipoproteins** – the availability of these tests is limited; therefore, they are not used routinely in clinical cases.

Consequences of hyperlipidaemia in dogs and cats

Hyperlipidaemia *per se* does not appear to lead to any clinical signs. However, many animals develop diseases as a result of hyperlipidaemia and clinical signs develop as a result of those diseases.

Pancreatitis

Hyperlipidaemia, and more specifically hypertriglyceridaemia, has long been suspected as a risk factor for canine pancreatitis. Two recent clinical studies provided evidence that hypertriglyceridaemia, especially severe hypertriglyceridaemia, is a risk factor for pancreatitis in Miniature Schnauzers (Xenoulis and Steiner, 2010; Xenoulis *et al.*, 2011a). In one of those studies, Miniature Schnauzers with a history of pancreatitis were five times more likely to have hypertriglyceridaemia than age- and breed-matched controls (Xenoulis *et al.*, 2011a).

Insulin resistance

Serum triglyceride concentrations are considered to be one of the major determinants of insulin resistance in both human and animal models. Evidence of insulin resistance has been documented in Miniature Schnauzers with primary hypertriglyceridaemia (Xenoulis *et al.*, 2011b). The association between hyperlipidaemia, insulin resistance and type 2 diabetes is not clear in cats.

Hepatobiliary disease

Clinical studies and anecdotal observations suggest that two hepatic disorders are associated with hypertriglyceridaemia in dogs: diffuse vacuolar hepatopathy and gallbladder mucocoele. In one study, primary hypertriglyceridaemia was found to be associated with increased serum hepatic enzyme activities in clinically healthy Miniature Schnauzers, presumably due to hyperlipidaemia-associated vacuolar hepatopathy (Xenoulis *et al.*, 2008). Gallbladder mucocoeles have been commonly reported in dog breeds that are predisposed to primary hyperlipidaemia (e.g. Miniature Schnauzers and Shetland Sheepdogs).

Atherosclerosis

Although dogs appear to be resistant to atherosclerosis due to their lipoprotein composition and metabolism, they have been reported to develop atherosclerosis in both experimental and clinical studies. Spontaneous atherosclerosis has been reported in dogs mainly in association with secondary hypercholesterolaemia due to endocrinopathies. Cats appear to be resistant to atherosclerosis.

Ocular disease

Several ocular manifestations of hyperlipidaemia, such as lipaemia retinalis, lipaemic aqueous and lipid keratopathy, have been described in dogs and cats.

Xanthomatosis

Xanthomas are benign granulomatous lesions that are believed to result from disrupted lipid metabolism and transport. Formation of single or, more commonly, multiple xanthomas has been reported most frequently in the skin and internal organs (e.g. liver, spleen, kidneys, adrenal glands, intestine, mesentery) of cats with primary hyperchylomicronaemia and may also be seen in cats with uncontrolled severe secondary hyperlipidaemia.

Proteinuria and glomerular lipidosis

Hypertriglyceridaemia in Miniature Schnauzers has been associated with proteinuria, glomerular lipidosis and glomerular lipid thromboembolism. The clinical importance and long-term consequences of such findings are unknown and warrant further investigation.

Neurological disease

Seizures, ischaemic strokes and other neurological signs have been reported to potentially occur as a result of severe hyperlipidaemia in dogs and may also be seen in cats. Cats with severe primary hyperchylomicronaemia have been reported to develop peripheral neuropathy, most commonly encountered as hindlimb paralysis.

Clinical syndrome of transient hyperlipidaemia in kittens

Several cases of transient hyperlipidaemia have been described in young kittens. Affected kittens are usually between 3 and 8 weeks of age and they appear heathy prior to the development of clinical signs. Affected kittens become lethargic, weak, anorexic and dyspnoeic, and typically collapse and die within 48 hours if left untreated.

Non-endocrine causes of hyperlipidaemia

Postprandial hyperlipidaemia is physiological and typically resolves within 7–12 hours after a meal. Persistent fasting hyperlipidaemia can be either primary (typically due to an inborn inherited error in lipid metabolism) or secondary to other diseases or drug administration.

Secondary hyperlipidaemia is the most common form of hyperlipidaemia in dogs and cats and is most commonly the result of an endocrine disorder. However, other causes are possible. Hyperlipidaemia (hypertriglyceridaemia and/or hypercholesterolaemia) has also been associated with naturally occurring pancreatitis in dogs. Results of a recent study in dogs with naturally occurring pancreatitis indicate that when concurrent diseases (e.g. diabetes mellitus, hypothyroidism) and use of certain drugs that can cause hyperlipidaemia are excluded, hypertriglyceridaemia and hypercholesterolaemia occur infrequently (18% and 24%, respectively) as a possible result of pancreatitis and are typically mild (Xenoulis et al., 2020). The mechanism by which pancreatitis causes hyperlipidaemia is unclear but could potentially involve cholestasis. Assigning cause or effect is complicated given that hyperlipidaemia is a known risk factor for pancreatitis. No such association between hyperlipidaemia and pancreatitis has been confidently identified in cats.

Other possible causes of hyperlipidaemia in dogs and/or cats include obesity, protein-losing nephropathy (nephrotic syndrome), cholestasis, high-fat diets (dogs), hepatic lipidosis (cats) and possibly other conditions (e.g. infections, inflammation, neoplasia, congestive heart failure). Administration of certain drugs, mainly glucocorticoids and oestrogens (e.g. megoestrol acetate), can induce marked hyperlipidaemia. Other drugs reported to cause hyperlipidaemia in dogs, such as phenobarbital, potassium bromide and progestins, may also cause hyperlipidaemia in cats.

Primary lipid abnormalities in dogs are usually, but not always, associated with certain breeds. Depending on the breed, the prevalence of a primary lipid abnormality can vary widely. Primary hyperlipidaemia is very common in Miniature Schnauzers in the USA. This disorder is typically characterized by hypertriglyceridaemia resulting from an abnormal accumulation of VLDLs or a combination of VLDLs and chylomicrons. Although hypercholesterolaemia may also be present, it is not found in all affected dogs and is always present in association with hypertriglyceridaemia. Primary hyperlipidaemia (mainly hypercholesterolaemia but in some cases with concurrent hypertriglyceridaemia) has also been reported in Shetland Sheepdogs. Primary hyperlipidaemia with hypercholesterolaemia and hypertriglyceridaemia has been reported in Beagles. Primary hypercholesterol-aemia without hypertriglyceridaemia has been described in Briards and a family of Rough Collies from the UK. In addition, primary hypercholesterolaemia has been reported anecdotally in Dobermanns and Rottweilers.

Primary lipid abnormalities are uncommon in cats. Sporadic case reports since the early 1980s have documented several individual cats or families of cats with hyperlipidaemia. Burmese cats have been reported to commonly have a familial lipoprotein metabolism disorder. Although some of these cats can have mild to moderate fasting hypertriglyceridaemia, many cats have normal fasting serum triglyceride concentrations, and their lipid disorder is identified only after a fatty meal challenge producing marked postprandial hypertriglyceridaemia and delayed clearance of serum triglycerides.

Lipid abnormalities in endocrine disease

Secondary hyperlipidaemia is a common clinicopathological abnormality in several endocrine diseases in both dogs and cats, most commonly hypothyroidism, hypercortisolism and diabetes mellitus. The presence of hyperlipidaemia in association with compatible clinical signs should raise suspicion for endocrine disease.

Hypothyroidism

Hypothyroidism has long been associated with increases in serum cholesterol and, to a lesser degree, triglyceride concentrations in humans. Hypothyroidism typically leads to increased concentrations of total and LDL cholesterol in the blood. Other subclasses of lipoproteins are also affected but to a lesser degree. Serum triglyceride concentrations are either not affected or only mildly affected. Restoration of thyroid function in humans with hypothyroidism typically results in correction of lipid abnormalities.

Thyroid hormones regulate the expression and activity of several key enzymes and receptors involved in lipoprotein metabolism. Thyroid hormone deficiency leads to decreased lipoprotein lipase and increased hormone-sensitive lipase activity, contributing to hypercholesterolaemia and hypertriglyceridaemia. Thyroid hormones also stimulate the expression of LDL receptors in the liver by increasing sterol regulatory element-binding protein (SREBP)-2 and by direct effects on the LDL receptor promoter. Decreased concentrations of thyroid hormones lead to a decrease in hepatic LDL receptors, resulting in reduced clearance of circulating LDL. This leads to increased serum LDL and total cholesterol concentrations. In addition, evidence from experimental animal models suggests that thyroid hormones increase the conversion of cholesterol into bile acids and increase biliary secretion of bile acids and cholesterol. Finally, because thyroid hormones reduce intestinal absorption of dietary cholesterol, hypothyroidism might lead to increased cholesterol absorption from the intestine. Several other pathways involved in lipoprotein metabolism have been shown to be affected in experimental animals.

Hypercholesterolaemia and hypertriglyceridaemia are common clinicopathological features in dogs with hypothyroidism and are seen in approximately 75% of cases. Studies have shown an increase in VLDL, LDL and HDL fractions as well as an increase in the cholesterol content of those lipoproteins. Hypothyroidism may also cause hypercholesterolaemia and possibly hypertriglyceridaemia in cats, albeit less consistently and much less commonly than in dogs.

Hypercortisolism

Increased serum cholesterol and triglyceride concentrations are commonly seen in humans with hypercortisolism. These are typically the result of increases in serum LDL and VLDL concentrations, respectively. Hyperlipidaemia typically improves with correction of increased cortisol concentrations, although complete normalization of serum lipid and lipoprotein concentrations is often not achieved.

Glucocorticoids affect several pathways and key enzymes involved in lipoprotein metabolism in different ways. Glucocorticoids, and potentially other hormones secreted by the adrenal glands, decrease hepatic LDL receptor expression, potentially contributing to delayed clearance of serum LDL and hypercholesterolaemia. Glucocorticoids also stimulate fatty acid synthesis in the liver (by increasing the activity of acetyl coenzyme A (CoA)) and increase the formation and secretion of VLDL. The increased concentration of VLDL released in the blood, leads to hypertriglyceridaemia and might potentially con-tribute to hypercholesterolaemia. Finally, glucocorticoids increase the expression of hormone-sensitive lipase in adipose tissue, resulting in triglyceride hydrolysis and the release of free fatty acids in the blood, which are then utilized by the liver to produce VLDL molecules. Glucocorticoids also have effects on the production of several lipoproteins and on hepatic lipase and LCAT activity.

The majority of dogs with hypercortisolism have hypercholesterolaemia (73–90%) and/or hypertriglyceridaemia (67%). Both hypercholesterolaemia and hypertriglyceridaemia can range from mild to marked. Hypertriglyceridaemia is mainly due to an increase in serum VLDL concentration, while hypercholesterolaemia is due to increased LDL, HDL and VLDL concentrations. Alterations of lipid content within lipoprotein fractions are also evident. Hyperlipidaemia typically resolves or dramatically improves with adequate control of the primary disorder.

Hypercortisolism is much less common in cats than in dogs. In addition, many cats with hypercortisolism have concurrent diabetes mellitus and, therefore, lipid abnormalities may be due to the latter or a combination of the two diseases. In one study, 38% of cats with hypercortisolism had hypercholesterolaemia and 71% had hypertriglyceridaemia, but 90% had concurrent diabetes mellitus (Valentin et al., 2014).

Diabetes mellitus

Hypertriglyceridaemia and hypercholesterolaemia are both common in humans with diabetes mellitus. These are due to increased concentrations of VLDL and LDL in the blood. Uncontrolled or poorly controlled diabetes mellitus is associated with major lipid abnormalities. Good glycaemic control in humans with type 1 diabetes mellitus leads to correction of lipid abnormalities, while in type 2 diabetes, even with good glycaemic control, lipid abnormalities persist in up to 60% of cases.

Insulin increases the activity of lipoprotein lipase and decreases the activity of hormone-sensitive lipase. Decreased insulin concentration or insulin resistance leads to increased activity of hormone-sensitive lipase, which leads to increased hydrolysis of triglycerides in adipose tissue and increased release of free fatty acids into the circulation. Free fatty acids are taken up by the liver to synthesize triglycerides that are packed and released in the blood within VLDL molecules. This leads to hypertriglyceridaemia. Decreased insulin concentration or insulin resistance leads to decreased activity of lipoprotein lipase, which leads to decreased clearance of serum triglycerides, contributing to hypertriglyceridaemia. Insulin also increases de novo synthesis of fatty acids in the liver (by stimulating the activity of SREBP-1c, a transcription factor that increases the expression of the enzymes required for the synthesis of fatty acids), resulting in increased VLDL synthesis and secretion.

Both hypercholesterolaemia and hypertriglyceridaemia are common in dogs with diabetes mellitus, and both can range from mild to marked. In these dogs, most lipoprotein fractions are increased, including VLDL, LDL and HDL. The lipid content of those lipoproteins is also altered; for example, most lipoprotein fractions have increased cholesterol content compared with controls. Due to their significant lipoprotein abnormalities, dogs with diabetes mellitus are at increased risk of atherosclerosis compared with dogs without diabetes mellitus. Approximately 30–50% of cats with diabetes mellitus have hyperlipidaemia (hypertriglyceridaemia and/or hypercholesterolaemia), which is usually mild to moderate (up to three times the upper limit of their respective reference intervals). Hyperlipidaemia typically resolves or at least improves with successful management of diabetes mellitus.

Serum triglyceride concentrations are considered to be one of the major determinants of insulin resistance in both human and animal models. Evidence of insulin resistance has also been documented in Miniature Schnauzers with primary hypertriglyceridaemia (Xenoulis et al., 2011b). In that study, the percentage of dogs with increased serum insulin concentrations was significantly greater in the hypertriglyceridaemic group (28.6%) than it was in the control group (6.5%), and the median homeostasis model assessment (HOMA) score for hypertriglyceridaemic Miniature Schnauzers (4.9) was significantly higher than that for control dogs (2.8).

The association between hyperlipidaemia, insulin resistance and type 2 diabetes mellitus is not clear in cats. In a study of 142 cats in Japan (including 25 cats with naturally occurring hypertriglyceridaemia and 117 healthy control cats), cats with naturally occurring hypertriglyceridaemia were found to have significantly increased serum insulin and decreased serum adiponectin concentrations compared with controls, indicating insulin resistance (Hatano et al., 2010). In another study, experimentally induced severe hyperlipidaemia (mean serum triglyceride concentration 33.7 ± 17.2 mmol/l) was found to induce insulin resistance, as assessed by glucose clamps (Nichii et al., 2012). In contrast, in a previous study, lipid infusion for 10 days did not affect insulin sensitivity in cats (Zini et al., 2010). One possible explanation for the conflicting results between these two experimental studies might be that in the earlier study the hyperlipidaemia was milder (2.8–6.5 mmol/l) than in the later study. Therefore, although results from different studies might be conflicting, there is some evidence that both naturally occurring and experimentally induced hyperlipidaemia in cats might be associated with insulin resistance, as is the case in humans and dogs. The role of hyperlipidaemia in the pathogenesis of diabetes mellitus in dogs and cats remains to be determined.

Hyperthyroidism

In humans with hyperthyroidism, total cholesterol and LDL cholesterol are often decreased. This is the result of excess concentrations of thyroid hormones leading to increased expression of hepatic LDL receptors, resulting in accelerated clearance of circulating LDL. In addition, evidence from experimental animal models suggests that thyroid hormones increase the conversion of cholesterol into bile acids and increase biliary secretion of bile acids and cholesterol. Finally, thyroid hormones reduce intestinal absorption of dietary cholesterol. Thyroid hormones also increase CETP, LCAT, hepatic lipase and hormone-sensitive lipase activities.

Despite the important role of thyroid hormones in lipoprotein metabolism, serum cholesterol and triglyceride concentrations are usually within reference limits in most cats with hyperthyroidism. Lipoprotein profiles in cats with hyperthyroidism have not been investigated.

Hypersomatotropism

In humans, hypertriglyceridaemia is commonly associated with hypersomatotropism (approximately 30% of patients), while hypercholesterolaemia is less common.

Growth hormone increases the activity of hormone-sensitive lipase in adipose tissue, leading to increased hydrolysis of triglycerides. This leads to an increased release of free fatty acids in the blood, which reach the liver and are used for VLDL synthesis. Subsequently, increased release of VLDL in the blood leads to hypertriglyceridaemia. In addition, growth hormone excess leads to decreased activity of lipoprotein lipase, resulting in decreased clearance of triglycerides from the blood. Growth hormone also affects the activity of several enzymes such as LCAT, choline/ethanolamine phosphotransferase and hepatic lipase, which in turn affect lipoprotein metabolism in various ways. Finally, insulin resistance and abnormal glucose metabolism are commonly seen in affected human patients and likely contribute to lipid abnormalities.

Hypercholesterolaemia and/or hypertriglyceridaemia are seen in cats and dogs with hypersomatotropism but are attributed mainly to concurrent uncontrolled, or poorly controlled, diabetes mellitus.

Growth hormone deficiency

Lipid abnormalities are relatively common in humans with growth hormone deficiency. These include increases in both serum cholesterol and triglyceride concentrations. It should be noted that growth hormone deficiency leads to increased adiposity, which might also account, at least partially, for lipid abnormalities in these patients.

Growth hormone increases the expression of hepatic LDL receptors. Therefore, in growth hormone deficiency, there is decreased expression of LDL receptors in the liver, leading to decreased clearance of LDL from the blood and hypercholesterolaemia. In addition, in affected human patients, there is increased hepatic synthesis of VLDL and decreased VLDL clearance, both of which contribute to hypertriglyceridaemia. Treatment with growth hormone typically resolves lipid abnormalities in human patients.

Lipid abnormalities (hypercholesterolaemia and/or hypertriglyceridaemia) may be seen in dogs and cats with growth hormone deficiency. However, some of these animals have concurrent secondary hypothyroidism, which may account, at least partially, for these abnormalities.

Diagnostic approach to dogs and cats with hyperlipidaemia

Hyperlipidaemia is typically diagnosed by measurement of fasting serum triglyceride and/or cholesterol concentrations (Figure 7.3). As hyperlipidaemia is most commonly secondary, it can serve as an important diagnostic clue to aid identification of the primary disease; it is often the only abnormality in dogs and cats with primary hyperlipidaemia. Thus, measurement of serum cholesterol and, especially, triglyceride concentration should be part of every routine chemistry profile. Unfortunately, measurement of serum triglyceride concentration is often not included in a routine chemistry profile and has to be specifically requested by the clinician. Moderate and severe hypertriglyceridaemia (but not mild hypertriglyceridaemia or hypercholesterolaemia) can be suspected based on inspection of serum or plasma that has a turbid or lactescent appearance. However, even in these cases, measurement of serum triglyceride and cholesterol concentrations is mandatory in order to reach an accurate assessment of the severity and spectrum of hyperlipidaemia. In some cases, use of a meal challenge to diagnose postprandial hyperlipidaemia might be necessary, although experience with such a test is limited.

After hyperlipidaemia has been diagnosed, the next step is to determine whether the animal has a primary or a secondary lipid disorder. If hyperlipidaemia is secondary, the underlying condition should be diagnosed and treated. Thus, specific diagnostic investigations should be performed in order to diagnose or rule out specific diseases that can cause secondary hyperlipidaemia. If secondary hyperlipidaemia is excluded, a tentative diagnosis of a primary lipid disorder is made.

Firstly, a detailed history should be obtained and a physical examination performed. This is crucial because dogs and cats with secondary hyperlipidaemia typically show clinical signs of the primary disease (e.g. polyuria and polydipsia in animals with diabetes mellitus or hypercortisolism, or reduced activity and hair loss in animals with hypothyroidism), which can help prioritize the selection of diagnostic tests. Animals with primary hyperlipidaemia may or may not have clinical signs. Dogs and cats with hyperlipidaemia should have at least a complete blood count, chemistry panel and urinalysis performed. Additional diagnostic tests include measurement of serum total and free T4, thyrotropin (thyroid-stimulating hormone), glucose and bile acid concentrations, measurement of urine glucose concentration (if not previously performed), determination of pancreas-specific lipase and urine protein:creatinine, and a low-dose dexamethasone suppression test or another test to confirm or exclude hypercortisolism. A more general and wide selection of tests might be necessary for animals that have vague or no clinical signs.

If a primary lipid disorder is suspected following an appropriate diagnostic investigation, there is little more that can be done to identify the precise cause. Tests that have occasionally been used to further characterize or investigate the cause of primary hyperlipidaemia in dogs include the chylomicron test, lipoprotein electrophoresis or ultracentrifugation, or a heparin response test as described above (see 'Definitions and measurement of serum lipid concentrations'). Many of these tests are not used routinely in clinical cases and their availability is limited. Genetic testing for specific inherited lipid disorders is currently not available in dogs or cats.

Treatment guidelines for hyperlipidaemia

Treatment of secondary hyperlipidaemia relies on successful treatment of the underlying disorder, after which hyperlipidaemia usually resolves. Treatment of primary or persistent secondary hypertriglyceridaemia is clinically important. In most cases, treatment should initially be pursued with dietary management, while drug therapy can be initiated later if deemed necessary. Although the management of hypercholesterolaemia appears to be of lesser clinical importance in dogs and cats than in humans, and there are no studies evaluating the need for treatment of hypercholesterolaemia in these species, severe hypercholesterolaemia may require treatment.

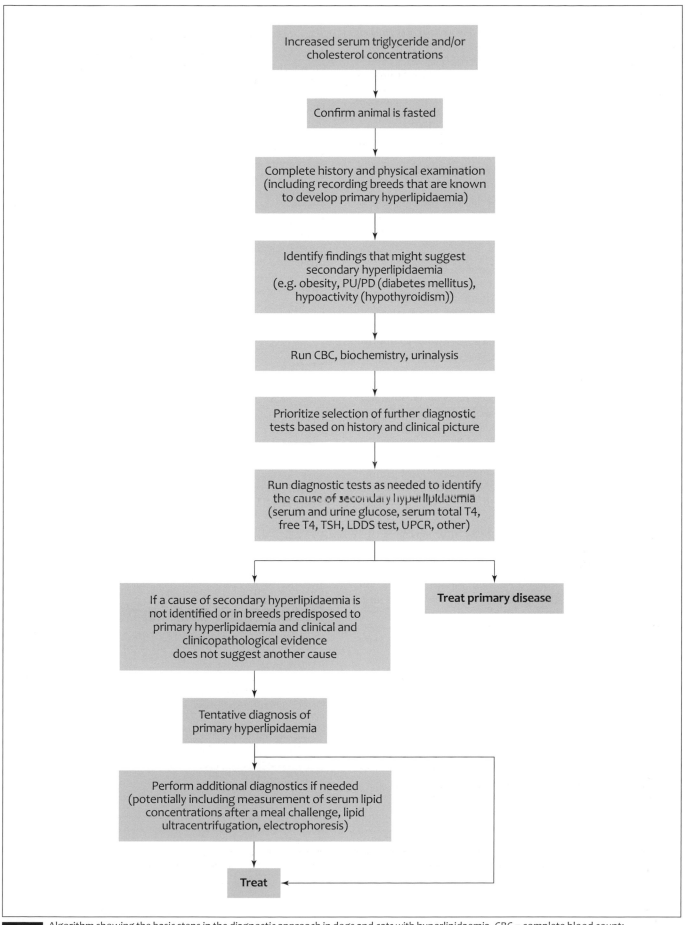

7.3 Algorithm showing the basic steps in the diagnostic approach in dogs and cats with hyperlipidaemia. CBC = complete blood count; LDDS = low-dose dexamethasone suppression; PU/PD = polyuria and polydipsia; T4 = thyroxine; TSH = thyroid-stimulating hormone; UPCR = urine protein:creatinine.

Low-fat diets

Typically, the first step in the management of primary or persistent secondary hyperlipidaemia is dietary modification. The most commonly used and likely most effective dietary option for hyperlipidaemia in dogs and cats is feeding a low-fat diet. It is generally recommended that diets containing less than 25 g of total fat per 1000 kcal (metabolizable energy) be used. Home-made low-fat diets have not been systematically evaluated for the management of hyperlipidaemia in dogs and cats. If such diets are used, care should be taken to make sure that they are balanced, especially when intended for long-term feeding, and that the minimum requirements are met for all nutrients, including essential fatty acids.

Dietary supplements

Omega-3 fatty acids

Polyunsaturated fatty acids of the n-3 series (omega-3 fatty acids: eicosapentaenoic acid (EPA) and docosahexaenoic acid (DHA)) are abundant in marine fish. Omega-3 fatty acid supplementation has been shown to lower serum triglyceride concentrations in experimental animals and humans, including cases of primary hypertriglyceridaemia. However, studies evaluating the efficacy and safety of omega-3 fatty acid supplementation in dogs or cats with hyperlipidaemia are lacking. Omega-3 fatty acids may be used in dogs and cats at doses ranging from 200 to 300 mg/kg orally q24h, and their effect on serum triglyceride concentrations is dose dependent.

Niacin

Niacin (nicotinic acid) is a form of vitamin B3 that has been used successfully for the treatment of hyperlipidaemia in humans for many years. Clinical trials regarding the efficacy and safety of niacin in dogs and cats with primary hypertriglyceridaemia are lacking and clinical experience is limited. As is often the case in humans, niacin administration in dogs and cats may be associated with side effects such as erythema and pruritus, which may require discontinuation of therapy. Long-term risk for myotoxicity and hepatotoxicity may also exist. Niacin may be administered to dogs and cats at a dose of 50–100 mg/day. Both the therapeutic effects and side effects of niacin are dose dependent, and it is therefore recommended that niacin is started at a low dose and slowly titrated upward (every 4 weeks) based on the results of follow-up serum cholesterol and triglyceride concentrations. It should be used with caution in diabetic animals because it can increase blood glucose concentration, especially when used at higher doses. Serum liver enzyme activities should be monitored with long-term use.

Lipid-lowering drugs

Some animals with primary hyperlipidaemia may not respond sufficiently to dietary modification, or faster and more predictable lowering of serum lipid concentrations may be required. In these cases, medical treatment is required. No studies have evaluated the efficacy and safety of most lipid-lowering drugs in dogs and cats and, therefore, evidence-based recommendations cannot be made for their use.

Fibrates

Fibrates (fibric acid derivatives) are weak agonists of peroxisome proliferator-activated receptor-alpha (PPARα), a nuclear transcription factor that regulates lipid and lipoprotein synthesis and catabolism. Gemfibrozil is one of the most commonly used fibrates in humans and has also been used anecdotally in dogs and cats with hypertriglyceridaemia. In dogs, it can be administered at 10 mg/kg orally q12h. In the author's experience, similar to what has been reported in humans, many dogs with primary hyperlipidaemia do not respond well to treatment with gemfibrozil. Bezafibrate, another fibric acid derivative, may be both more effective and associated with fewer adverse effects in the treatment of humans and dogs with hyperlipidaemia. Bezafibrate (4–10 mg/kg q24h) has been evaluated for the treatment of hyperlipidaemia of various causes (both primary and secondary) in dogs and was found to be highly effective in reducing serum triglyceride and cholesterol concentrations. Fenofibrate (10 mg/kg q24h) has also been evaluated in the treatment of severe hypertriglyceridaemia (both primary and secondary) in dogs and was found to be highly effective, leading to normalization of serum triglyceride concentrations. No studies have evaluated the safety and efficacy of fibrates in cats and clinical experience has been extremely limited. Periodic testing of serum triglyceride concentration and liver enzyme activities is recommended.

Statins

Statins (beta-hydroxy beta-methylglutaryl-CoA reductase inhibitors) are among the most potent and commonly used lipid-lowering drugs, and constitute first-line therapy for the treatment of hypercholesterolaemia in humans. Statins are mainly cholesterol-lowering drugs (in humans they specifically lower LDL cholesterol) with less potent effects on triglyceride metabolism. This makes them less than ideal for cases with hypertriglyceridaemia as the main lipid abnormality. Statins have been associated with myopathy, rhabdomyolysis and hepatotoxicity in humans. In animals in which statins are used, serum hepatic enzyme activities should be periodically monitored for potential hepatotoxicity.

References and further reading

Crenshaw KL and Peterson ME (1996) Pretreatment clinical and laboratory evaluation of cats with diabetes mellitus: 104 cases (1992–1994). *Journal of the American Veterinary Medical Association* **209**, 943–949

Dixon RM, Reid SW and Mooney CT (1999) Epidemiological, clinical, haematological and biochemical characteristics of canine hypothyroidism. *Veterinary Record* **145**, 481–487

Hatano Y, Mori N, Asada M *et al.* (2010) Hypertriglyceridemia with increased plasma insulin concentrations in cats. *Research in Veterinary Science* **88**, 458–460

Hess RS, Kass PH and Van Winkle TJ (2003) Association between diabetes mellitus, hypothyroidism or hyperadrenocorticism, and atherosclerosis in dogs. *Journal of Veterinary Internal Medicine* **17**, 489–494

Huang HP, Yang HL, Liang SL, Lien YH and Chen KY (1999) Iatrogenic hyperadrenocorticism in 28 dogs. *Journal of the American Animal Hospital Association* **35**, 200–207

Kluger EK, Caslake M, Baral RM, Malik R and Govendir M (2010) Preliminary postprandial studies of Burmese cats with elevated triglyceride concentrations and/or presumed lipid aqueous. *Journal of Feline Medicine and Surgery* **12**, 621–630

Kluger EK, Hardman C, Govendir M *et al.* (2009) Triglyceride response following an oral fat tolerance test in Burmese cats, other pedigree cats and domestic crossbred cats. *Journal of Feline Medicine and Surgery* **11**, 82–90

Ling GV, Stabenfeldt GH, Comer KM, Gribble DH and Schechter RD (1979) Canine hyperadrenocorticism: pretreatment clinical and laboratory evaluation of 117 cases. *Journal of the American Veterinary Medical Association* **174**, 1211–1215

Nishii N, Maeda H, Murahata Y, Matsuu A and Hikasa Y (2012) Experimental hyperlipemia induces insulin resistance in cats. *Journal of Veterinary Medical Science* **74**, 267–269

Xenoulis PG, Cammarata PJ, Walzem RL *et al.* (2013) Novel lipoprotein density profiling in healthy dogs of various breeds, healthy miniature schnauzers, and miniature schnauzers with hyperlipidemia. *BMC Veterinary Research* **9**, 47

Xenoulis PG, Cammarata PJ, Walzem RL, Suchodolski JS and Steiner JM (2020) Serum triglyceride and cholesterol concentrations and lipoprotein profiles in dogs with naturally occurring pancreatitis and healthy control dogs. *Journal of Veterinary Internal Medicine* **34**, 644–652

Xenoulis PG, Levinski MD, Suchodolski JS and Steiner JM (2011a) Serum triglyceride concentrations in Miniature Schnauzers with and without a history of probable pancreatitis. *Journal of Veterinary Internal Medicine* **25**, 20–25

Xenoulis PG, Levinski MD, Suchodolski JS and Steiner JM (2011b) Association of hypertriglyceridemia with insulin resistance in healthy Miniature Schnauzers. *Journal of the American Veterinary Medical Association* **238**, 1011–1016

Xenoulis PG and Steiner JM (2010) Lipid metabolism and hyperlipidemia in dogs. *Veterinary Journal* **183**, 12–21

Xenoulis PG and Steiner JM (2015) Canine hyperlipidaemia. *Journal of Small Animal Practice* **56**, 595–605

Xenoulis PG, Suchodolski JS, Levinski MD and Steiner JM (2008) Serum liver enzyme activities in healthy Miniature Schnauzers with and without hypertriglyceridemia. *Journal of the American Veterinary Medical Association* **232**, 63–67

Valentin SY, Cortright CC, Nelson RW *et al.* (2014) Clinical findings, diagnostic test results, and treatment outcome in cats with spontaneous hyperadrenocorticism: 30 cases. *Journal of Veterinary Internal Medicine* **28**, 481–487

Zini E, Osto M, Konrad D *et al.* (2010) 10-day hyperlipidemic clamp in cats: effects on insulin sensitivity, inflammation, and glucose metabolism-related genes. *Hormone and Metabolic Research* **42**, 340–347

Chapter 8

The effect of endocrine disease on the skin

Rosario Cerundolo

Introduction

In some animals with endocrinopathies, the dermatological (skin/coat) changes are the first signs noticed by the owners. A subtle, sparse hair loss not related to seasonal moulting should prompt investigation to find the underlying cause. In an adult dog, these clinical signs are likely caused by either a hormonal or a hereditary disorder with late onset. Unfortunately, their clinical presentation may be similar and to differentiate them a number of factors need to be considered during history taking, physical examination and diagnostic investigations.

None of these cases presents with the label of being an endocrine disease. Dogs and cats suffering from endocrine diseases are often presented because the owners have noticed unusual metabolic or dermatological clinical signs. It is up to the experienced veterinary surgeon (veterinarian) to recognize those clinical signs and decide on the appropriate diagnostic tests that will help rule endocrine disease in or out.

The purpose of this chapter is to provide tips and clues on how to recognize skin and coat changes that may be caused by an endocrinopathy. Detailed information on the pathogenesis of, and metabolic disorders caused by, endocrinopathies is provided in other relevant chapters. Greater details on dermatological conditions and tests are available in the *BSAVA Manual of Canine and Feline Dermatology*.

Hypercortisolism

Spontaneous hypercortisolism is a common and well recognized disorder in middle-aged and older dogs. Clinical signs are insidious in onset and slowly progressive, and typically include a combination of both metabolic and dermatological features. Excess cortisol concentrations cause inhibition of hair growth and subsequent hair follicle and skin atrophy. Therefore, the most common dermatological signs include hair loss affecting the trunk (Figure 8.1) skin thinning, comedones and calcinosis cutis. Lack of hair regrowth after clipping for a routine diagnostic procedure is also common. Similar clinical signs are caused by the administration of exogenous glucocorticoids (Figures 8.2 and 8.3). Medical treatment of hypercortisolism normally leads to hair regrowth within a month with normalization of skin thickness. Usually, calcinosis cutis takes several months to resolve once the excessive steroid production is controlled or external administration is withdrawn.

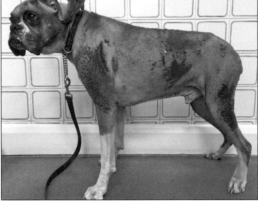

8.1 Generalized alopecia in a 10-year-old male neutered Boxer with hypercortisolism.

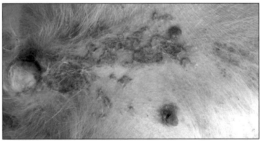

8.2 Calcinosis cutis presenting in the inguinal area of a 5-year-old neutered Maltese bitch treated long term with oral steroids for meningoencephalitis of unknown origin.

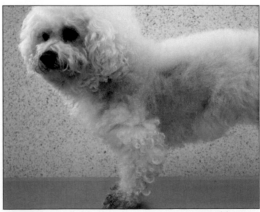

8.3 Localized area of hair loss in a 14-year-old neutered Bichon Frise bitch treated long term with hydrocortisone aceponate spray to control pruritus.

Hypothyroidism

Hypothyroidism is one of the most common canine endocrinopathies but it is also the one most frequently misdiagnosed. Hypothyroidism occurs most commonly in mid- to large-sized purebred dogs of middle/adult age. It is characterized by a plethora of clinical signs affecting the skin and other organ systems. Thyroid hormones are required for initiation and acceleration of anagen hair follicles and, therefore, deficiency induces perpetuation of the resting stage (telogen) of the hair follicle. The most common cutaneous signs include partial to generalized hair loss (Figure 8.4), often with pigmentation of the nose, trunk and tail (Figure 8.5). Comedones can occur in alopecic areas (Figure 8.6). However, none of the clinical signs is pathognomonic for hypothyroidism, and their progression is generally gradual and insidious. Dermatological changes improve within 1–3 months once the dog is successfully supplemented with levothyroxine, but full resolution may take a further 2–3 months (see Chapter 18).

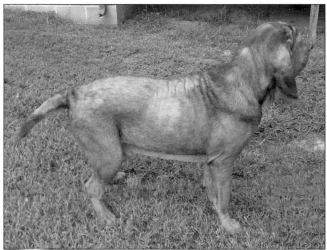

8.4 Generalized hair loss in a 6-year-old male neutered Bloodhound with hypothyroidism.

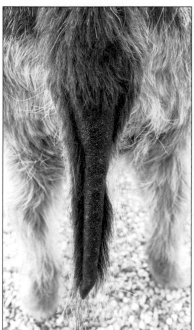

8.5 Alopecia and cutaneous hyperpigmentation of the tail of an 8-year-old male neutered Border Terrier with hypothyroidism.

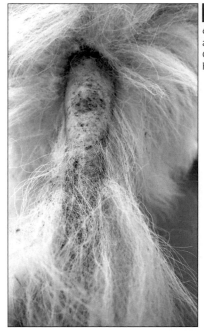

8.6 Alopecia with numerous comedones along the tail of a 5-year-old male neutered German Shepherd Dog with hypothyroidism.

Sex hormone imbalance

Sex hormone imbalance is uncommon in those countries where dogs are routinely neutered and common where neutering is not routinely carried out. These conditions are frequently associated with cutaneous lesions, which may be the predominant changes observed. The cause-and-effect relationship between sex hormone imbalances and cutaneous changes has been known for some time but the mechanism underlying the distribution of the cutaneous lesions is still not fully understood. Differences in the peripheral distribution of hormone receptors or abnormal peripheral conversion of the sex hormones may play a role in the clinical presentation.

Involvement of the sex hormones has been proven in only two clinical conditions: hyperoestrogenism and hyperandrogenism. Both conditions are usually caused by an autonomously secreting tumour originating from the testes or ovaries. The sex hormones can influence not just the skin but also sebaceous glands and hair follicles.

Increased oestrogen concentrations inhibit hair growth, while hyperandrogenism causes increased epidermal thickness, cutaneous pigmentation, sebaceous gland size and sebum production. The circumanal glands and the tail gland are anatomical areas composed of hepatoid cells that are androgen responsive.

Hyperoestrogenism in bitches

Hyperoestrogenism may occur spontaneously in bitches as a result of cystic or neoplastic ovaries. It can also be iatrogenic in animals treated with oestrogens for management of mismating or urinary incontinence. There is a progressive alopecia beginning in the perineal and genital areas that progresses to the caudal aspects of the thighs, the ventral aspect of the abdomen, the flanks and the neck (Figure 8.7). Affected areas demonstrate hyperpigmentation, lichenification and seborrhoea; a ceruminous otitis externa may also be present. Pruritus is usually secondary to bacterial and/or yeast infections and might require topical antiseptic therapy or systemic antibiotics. There are

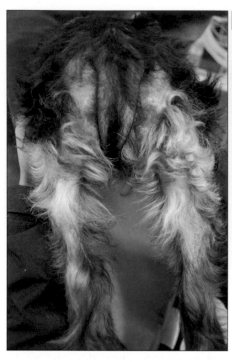

8.7 Alopecia of the thighs and the tail in a 5-year-old neutered Cocker Spaniel bitch treated with oestriol tablets for the past 3 months for urinary incontinence.

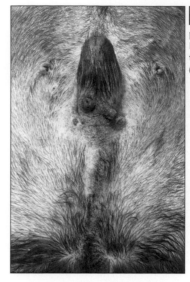

8.9 Linear cutaneous erythema on the prepuce of a 10-year-old male Field Spaniel with a Sertoli cell tumour.
(Courtesy of Dr Julie Pradel)

enlarged nipples and vulva, with a serosanguineous vulvar discharge that simulates that of oestrus. Normally, the dermatological changes resolve within 1–2 months of successful treatment of the underlying disorder.

Hyperoestrogenism in dogs with testicular tumours

Hyperoestrogenism occurs more commonly in dogs with Sertoli cell tumours than in those with either an interstitial cell tumour or a seminoma. The affected testicle may be in the scrotum or retained in the abdomen, and cryptorchidism is considered a predisposing factor. Affected dogs exhibit alopecia of the perineal and genital regions progressing to the thighs, flanks, ventral abdomen and ventral neck (Figure 8.8). A linear cutaneous erythema or melanosis may be present on the ventral aspect of the prepuce up to and over the scrotal area (Figure 8.9). The skin is often thin, mildly seborrhoeic and hyperpigmented. There is a pendulous prepuce and gynaecomastia (Figure 8.10). Normally, the dermatological changes resolve within 1–2 months of treatment of the hyperoestrogenism.

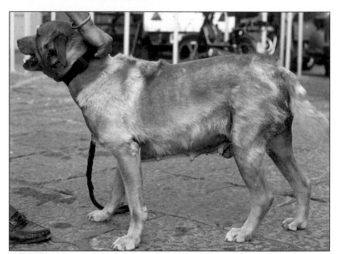

8.10 A 9-year-old male crossbreed dog with a Sertoli cell tumour, with hair loss, gynaecomastia and a pendulous prepuce.

Hypertestosteronism in dogs with testicular tumours

Hypertestosteronism may occur in dogs with an interstitial cell tumour of the testicle. It has also been reported in a neutered bitch associated with adrenocorticotropic hormone-dependent hypercortisolism (Dow *et al.*, 1988). Affected animals exhibit perianal gland and tail gland hyperplasia, which presents as a thick, alopecic, crusted and greasy area with possible secondary infection. Macular hyperpigmentation of the perineal area, tail gland and scrotum may occur. Normally, the dermatological changes resolve within 1–2 months following treatment.

Transdermal oestradiol gel-induced alopecia

Contact with the skin of people who use a transdermal oestradiol gel, most commonly as treatment for postmenopausal symptoms, represents a possible cause of non-inflammatory alopecia in dogs. Such cases may have increased baseline oestradiol concentrations and most exhibit signs of feminization with alopecia (Figure 8.11). Hair regrowth restarts within 1 month once the contact with the transdermal oestradiol gel is avoided.

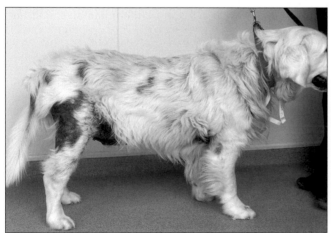

8.8 Alopecia and cutaneous hyperpigmentation in a 12-year-old male Golden Retriever with a Sertoli cell tumour.

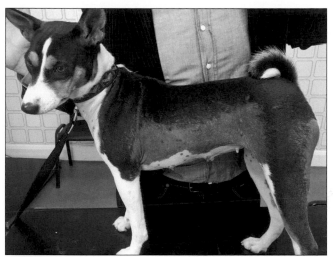

8.11 A 1-year-old Basenji bitch with hair loss caused by continuous contact with the owner's legs. The owner was using a transdermal oestrogen gel.

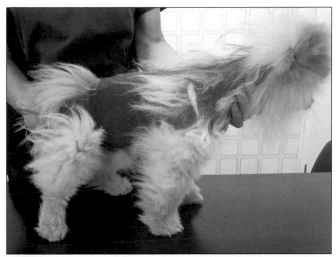

8.13 A 1-year-old male neutered Pomeranian with alopecia X with dramatic alopecia and cutaneous hyperpigmentation.

Alopecia X

Alopecia X is a form of canine adult-onset alopecia that is also known as growth hormone-responsive alopecia, castration-responsive dermatosis and congenital adrenal hyperplasia-like syndrome. The diversity of names is merely descriptive and based upon the differences in endocrine findings and/or clinical responses to various therapeutic modalities. It is known to primarily affect Nordic breeds but also some other breeds such as the Miniature Poodle. It has been postulated to be an endocrine disorder characterized by an abnormally functioning pituitary–adrenal axis. Specifically, the abnormality is thought to involve the pathway for cortisol production, with increased production of 17-alpha-hydroxyprogesterone and a slight increase of cortisol, although this remains to be proven. It manifests clinically as progressive, symmetrical, truncal, non-pruritic hair loss with variable hyperpigmentation occurring in both males and females between 1 and 5 years of age. Initially, alopecia may involve only the primary or guard hairs, giving the dog a 'puppy coat' appearance (Figure 8.12) before becoming completely bald (Figure 8.13). Affected dogs

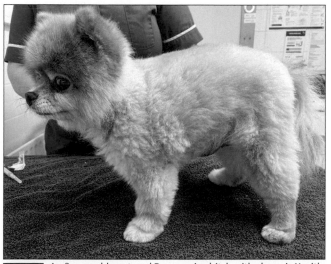

8.12 An 8-year-old neutered Pomeranian bitch with alopecia X with patchy hair loss around the neck, lack of primary hairs and presence of a woolly coat.

are clinically healthy and routine haematology and biochemistry values all remain with their respective reference intervals. Various therapeutic modalities have been suggested, with different outcomes. Castration appears to temporarily normalize the coat but alopecia may recur after a couple of years. Oral supplementation with melatonin is safe and might be helpful in approximately half of affected dogs but is not always freely available. Trilostane, given as if treating hypercortisolism, appears to promote hair regrowth. Deslorelin implants have also been effective in promoting hair regrowth in some breeds such as Keeshonds and Chow Chows. Some breeds appear to respond better to one therapeutic approach than to another. Interestingly, the trauma associated with skin biopsy may initiate hair regrowth at that site.

Seasonal flank alopecia

This flank alopecia, also known as canine recurrent flank alopecia, is often a seasonal, cyclical type of alopecia that occurs over the flanks and mid-lateral thorax of dogs, sometimes affecting the rump, and that results in marked hyperpigmentation (Figure 8.14). The most commonly affected breeds are the Boxer, Bulldog, Airedale Terrier, Labrador Retriever and Schnauzer. It may recur predictably each year or may skip a year. It may progress to permanent alopecia or disappear forever after one or more seasons. Most dogs living in northern latitudes lose hair in the autumn/winter and regrow it in the spring/summer. This pattern has suggested that daylight changes may play a role in this condition by modifying the melatonin/prolactin concentrations. The diagnosis is supported by breed predisposition, characteristic clinical signs and history of cyclic recurrence in long-standing cases. Other endocrinopathies must be ruled out (especially if the dog is presented during the first episode). Histopathology will help to confirm this condition. Specific treatment is unnecessary in most cases as this is a purely aesthetic problem and the hairs will usually spontaneously regrow. However, in cases with protracted alopecia, permanent alopecia or predictable seasonality, melatonin has been useful in preventing recurrence and might hasten hair regrowth. Melatonin downregulates oestrogen receptor expression in the skin and hair follicles, is an anagen inducer and suppresses prolactin production.

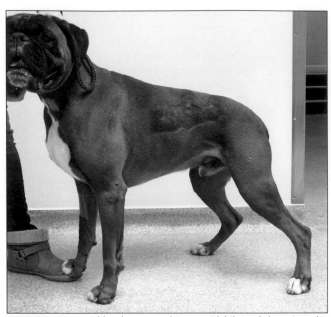

8.14 A 4-year-old male neutered Boxer with bilateral alopecia and cutaneous hyperpigmentation over the flank. The coat grew back spontaneously after a couple of months.

Clinical approach

Hair loss is undoubtedly one of the most common dermatological features of endocrine disease. A methodical approach and an accurate diagnosis are therefore essential for the successful management of these cases. The diagnostic approach to follow when presented with an affected animal is summarized in Figure 8.15. This includes identifying breed predisposition, sex and reproductive status, taking a detailed history, completing a physical and dermatological examination and, finally, exploring the most appropriate diagnostic tests.

Signalment

Some dog breeds are predisposed to hereditary dermatological conditions that appear similar to endocrine disease and that can also appear late in life. Irish Water Spaniels, Portuguese Water Dogs, Spanish Water Dogs, Chesapeake Bay Retrievers, Curly Coated Retrievers and

- Breed predisposition
- Sex and reproductive status
- History
  - Age of onset
  - Presence of pruritus
  - Signs of internal/systemic disease
  - Initial location of alopecia and progression
  - Response to previous therapy
- Physical and dermatological examination
- Routine dermatological tests (skin scrapings, trichogram, cytology)
- Routine haematology, biochemistry and urinalysis
- Endocrine tests
  - Thyroid function evaluation: T4, TSH, free T4, thyroglobulin autoantibodies
  - Hypothalamic–pituitary–adrenal axis function evaluation: adrenocorticotropic hormone response test, low-dose dexamethasone suppression test, urine cortisol:creatinine
  - Sex hormone measurements in intact dogs
- Skin biopsy

8.15 Diagnostic approach to dogs with dermatological problems caused by a suspected endocrinopathy. T4 = thyroxine; TSH = thyroid-stimulating hormone.

Weimaraners are predisposed to an adult-onset type of symmetrical/generalized alopecia called follicular dysplasia; Dachshunds and many terrier breeds have a hereditary predisposition to hair loss in typical patterns. Certain breeds are also more predisposed to specific endocrine disorders.

Cats behave differently to dogs and while symmetrical alopecia of the trunk is well recognized, it is not associated with sex or thyroid hormone imbalances. Most cases are in fact self-induced alopecia likely caused by an underlying allergy.

Sex status

Sex status should be considered because intact male or female dogs may develop tumours of the gonads. Excess hormone production can lead to hair loss and secondary skin changes and infections (see 'Sex hormone imbalance', above).

Coat colour

Consideration of coat colour is useful as some forms of alopecia are linked to specific coat colour (e.g. Rottweilers (follicular lipidosis affecting tan/mahogany areas); dogs with black coats (black hair follicular dysplasia); dogs with a dilute coat colour, such as blue coat Dobermanns, Dachshunds and Yorkshire Terriers (colour dilution alopecia)).

History

Taking a detailed history of the case before carrying out the physical examination is a vital step in the diagnostic work-up. It is important to consider asking the questions listed in Figure 8.16.

The age of onset may point toward one endocrinopathy or another, as hypothyroidism is more common in middle-aged dogs while hypercortisolism affects middle-to-old aged dogs.

A history of excessive weight gain and lethargy might suggest hypothyroidism; the presence of polyphagia, polyuria and polydipsia might suggest hypercortisolism.

- Is the owner aware of the littermates or parents showing similar clinical signs?
- What type of environment does the animal live in?
- Are other animals or humans that live in the same environment showing any skin/coat lesions?
- Has the owner seen any ectoparasites?
- Is the animal showing any systemic clinical signs or has it been affected by other illnesses? It is important to ask if there has been any change in urine output or water/food intake, any sign of respiratory or gastrointestinal disorder, or any change in physical activity level.
- Has the animal recently undergone any surgical intervention, blood loss, pregnancy or a stressful event?
- How long has the disease been present and how has it progressed?
- Is the animal pruritic: any scratching, licking, chewing or rubbing?
- At what age did the hair loss or the skin lesions start?
- Has the alopecia been waxing and waning?
- On which part of the body did the problem start?
- Has the alopecia or skin lesion slowly progressed and spread to other parts of the body?
- Is the alopecia related to the season of the year or oestrous cycle?
- Has there been any response to the previous/current therapy?
- Is the animal currently undergoing treatment for a different illness or has it received any such treatment in recent months?

8.16 Questions to consider asking in order to obtain a detailed history of the case.

Unfortunately, there are cases where the above classical clinical signs are not present or are subtle, and animals may present solely with dermatological problems.

The presence of pruritus should be carefully evaluated, as it normally suggests an ectoparasitic or allergic aetiology. However, endocrinopathies that are normally non-inflammatory may become pruritic if complicated by a secondary bacterial/yeast infection; hair regrowth may not be complete unless these infections are properly controlled. Re-evaluation of these cases after an appropriate course of topical antiseptics and/or systemic antibiotic therapy may be helpful.

Most endocrinopathies and inflammatory disorders tend to be progressive and generalized without intermittent remission.

A dog's response to previous therapy for a skin disorder, or a lack of response, is helpful in the diagnostic process: for example, failure of hair regrowth after 3–5 months of appropriate thyroid hormone supplementation suggests that hypothyroidism is an unlikely cause of alopecia.

Long-term glucocorticoid therapy may cause iatrogenic hypercortisolism and hair cycle arrest in dogs. Oestrogens may also interfere with the hair cycle. Dogs receiving chemotherapy (doxorubicin and cyclophosphamide) may develop hair follicle dystrophy resulting in hair loss and simulating an endocrine alopecia; this is more commonly seen in Miniature Poodles, Labrador Retrievers and Golden Retrievers.

Physical examination

A general physical examination should be undertaken before dermatological examination; this should help rule out concurrent diseases or systemic conditions that may affect the skin and coat. For example, the presence of a pendulous abdomen and/or panting should raise suspicion of hypercortisolism, whilst the presence of lethargy, hypothermia and bradycardia may suggest hypothyroidism. Gynaecomastia, a pendulous prepuce and an enlarged testicle may indicate a Sertoli cell tumour.

Dermatological examination

The skin and the coat condition should be carefully examined. Primary or secondary lesions should be identified. The possibility of secondary/concurrent bacterial/yeast infections or ectoparasitic infestations should be borne in mind. Their presence may be a coincidence or an indication that the immune system is compromised.

The dermatological examination should first concentrate on signs of follicular inflammation and infection, helping to differentiate non-inflammatory diseases. However, there may be cases of endocrinopathies with secondary bacterial infections that need to be properly diagnosed and treated during the endocrine diagnostic work-up.

There are specific clinical presentations for some endocrinopathies that need to be carefully evaluated:

- Alopecia with thinning of the skin, presence of comedones and prominent subcutaneous vessels is consistent with hypercortisolism. Calcium deposits along dermal collagen fibres (calcinosis cutis) are pathognomonic for hypercortisolism
- Discoloration of the coat (leucotrichia) is not uncommon in dogs with hypercortisolism

- Alopecia, thickened (myxoedema) and hyperpigmented skin, and comedones without inflammation are often present in dogs with hypothyroidism
- Hyperpigmentation is common in dogs with alopecia X
- Well demarcated, hyperpigmented skin of the alopecic areas is commonly seen in dogs with canine recurrent flank alopecia and the affected area of the skin often feels cold.

The severity of hair loss should be recorded to allow documentation of progression or resolution of the disease.

Endocrine disease is usually associated with hairs that are mainly in telogen because there is a hair follicle cycle arrest. Consequently, the areas of the body that are subject to continuous friction (e.g. the bridge of the nose, lateral neck, thighs and tail) may undergo fracture of the hairs, with subsequent hair loss. Interestingly, the head and distal extremities of dogs are largely unaffected, or less severely affected, than other parts of the body. This most likely reflects the differences in hair genetics or variation in hormone receptor numbers at different body locations. Specific factors to consider when examining the coat are listed in Figure 8.17.

- Is the hair missing or just broken?
- Is the coat around the alopecic area normal?
- Is the hair easily epilated?
- Is the hair easily broken by just touching the coat?
- Is the coat normal or does it look dry, greasy, matted or dirty?
- Are the primary and/or secondary hairs missing?
- Is the hair thinner than normal in some areas of the body?
- Has the hair density changed?
- Has the coat colour changed?

8.17 Specific factors to consider when examining coat condition.

Diagnostic tests

Routine dermatological investigations (Figure 8.18) carried out at the time of the initial visit should rule out the presence of ectoparasites and fungal or bacterial infections.

Trichogram

Under physiological conditions, a trichogram will reveal hair shafts in anagen (growing) and in telogen (resting) phases. Telogen hairs are easily epilated and anagen hairs can be pulled out only by applying traction. Dogs with endocrinopathies tend to have high numbers of hair follicles in the telogen stage, where the root of the hair has a spear shape, and an altered ratio of anagen to telogen hairs.

Examining the hair tips of plucked hairs with a microscope may help to differentiate broken hair shafts or split ends from the fine-peaked ends of normal hairs. This is often the best way to differentiate alopecia caused by self-trauma compared with hormonal alopecia. Furthermore, the hair shaft can reveal clumped melanin and thus will draw attention towards colour dilution alopecia or black hair follicular dysplasia. Microscopic examination of plucked hairs mounted on a glass slide with mineral oil can be used to search for ectoparasites and fungal arthrospores or hyphae within or along the hair shaft. Hair shafts may be covered by keratinosebaceous material (follicular casts), suggesting abnormalities within the hair follicle and with sebum production.

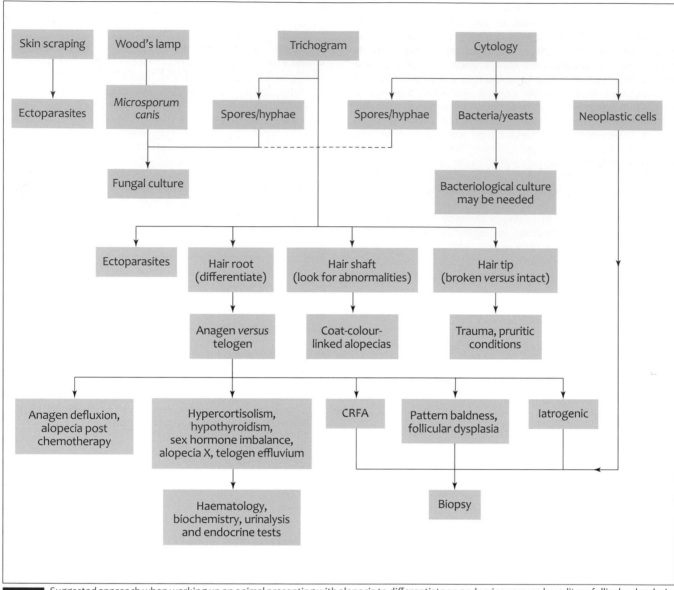

8.18 Suggested approach when working up an animal presenting with alopecia to differentiate an endocrine *versus* a hereditary follicular dysplasia condition. CRFA = canine recurrent flank alopecia.

Clinicopathological investigations

Specific laboratory tests, such as routine haematology, biochemistry, urinalysis and endocrine tests, are often required for a definitive diagnosis in cases of suspected endocrinopathy. These will not be discussed in detail, as they are covered in other relevant chapters on specific endocrine disorders.

Skin biopsy

Skin biopsy is indicated in cases where the diagnosis cannot be readily confirmed by any other means. As a general rule, multiple biopsy specimens should be collected from alopecic areas. Skin biopsy is useful to confirm or rule out alopecia linked to coat colour, recurrent flank alopecia and follicular dysplasias: the so-called 'endocrine impersonators'. Skin biopsy is impractical for the diagnosis of

endocrine diseases, since these conditions result in similar changes in the skin and hair follicles, which are difficult to differentiate. Occasionally, the histopathological changes observed in skin biopsy specimens are subtle and only experienced dermatopathologists are capable of evaluating them clearly.

Summary

The work-up in dogs suspected of having an endocrine disease may be complex. The previously common assumption that symmetrical or generalized alopecia were the most common signs of an endocrine disease should be reconsidered. Furthermore, there are a number of congenital/genetic diseases affecting specific canine breeds, and some neoplastic diseases, that may simulate an endocrine disease. Changes in coat density represent no risk to the animal when caused by a hereditary alopecic condition, as these are simply aesthetic problems.

It has been common In the past to supplement dogs and cats presenting with alopecia with thyroid hormones without confirming the hypothyroidism; therapeutic trials should be avoided unless hypothyroidism is confirmed. A methodical approach and an accurate diagnosis are therefore essential not only to restore a normal skin and coat but also for the successful management of an endocrine disorder.

References and further reading

Brunner MAT, Jagannathan V, Waluk DP *et al.* (2017) Novel insights into the pathways regulating the canine hair cycle and their deregulation in alopecia X. *PLoS ONE* **12**, e0186469

Cerundolo R, Lloyd DH, Vaessen MMAR *et al.* (2007) Alopecia in pomeranians and miniature poodles in association with high urinary corticoid: creatinine ratios and resistance to glucocorticoid feedback. *Veterinary Record* **160**, 393–397

Credille KM, Slater MR, Moriello KA *et al.* (2001) The effects of thyroid hormones on the skin of beagle dogs. *Journal of Veterinary Internal Medicine* **15**, 539–546

Daminet S and Paradis M (2000) Evaluation of thyroid function in dogs suffering from recurrent flank alopecia. *Canadian Veterinary Journal* **41**, 699–703

Dow SW, Olson PN, Rosychuk RA and Withrow SJ (1988) Perianal adenomas and hypertestosteronemia in a spayed bitch with pituitary-dependent hyperadrenocorticism. *Journal of the American Veterinary Medical Association* **192**, 1439–1441

Jackson HA and Marsella R (2021) *BSAVA Manual of Canine and Feline Dermatology, 4th edn.* BSAVA Publications, Gloucester

Wiener DJ, Rüfenacht S, Koch HJ *et al.* (2015) Estradiol-induced alopecia in five dogs after contact with a transdermal gel used for the treatment of postmenopausal symptoms in women. *Veterinary Dermatology* **26**, 393–e91

Zur G and White SD (2011) Hyperadrenocorticism in 10 dogs with skin lesions as the only presenting clinical signs. *Journal of the American Animal Hospital Association* **47**, 419–427

Chapter 9

Control of water balance and investigation of polyuria and polydipsia

Robert E. Shiel

Introduction

Polydipsia is defined as a water intake of more than 100 ml/kg/day in dogs and 50 ml/kg/day in cats. Polyuria is defined in both species as a urine output of more than 50 ml/kg/day. However, the identification of polyuria and polydipsia (PU/PD) can be challenging because values in individual healthy animals are variable and owners can struggle to quantify water intake and urine output.

Polyuria and polydipsia are components of many diseases, including several common endocrinopathies. Often, the cause is readily apparent after physical examination and routine clinicopathological investigations. However, for more complex cases, an awareness of the underlying pathophysiology and a logical approach are necessary to determine the underlying cause. This chapter will provide an overview of the diagnostic investigation of PU/PD in dogs and cats. Many of the endocrinopathies included here are covered in greater detail in their relevant chapters.

Physiology

The ability to regulate water balance is essential for life, particularly in the face of restricted water intake. There are two main components of water balance: water intake and water excretion.

Water intake

Water intake is regulated by thirst, which is thought to originate within the lamina terminalis of the forebrain but is dependent upon a complex neural network. Plasma osmolality is the principal stimulus of the thirst response. This response is seen after a 2–3% increase in osmolality. Decreased blood volume and pressure and a variety of anticipatory signals also stimulate or modulate this response.

Water intake is affected by multiple additional factors (Figure 9.1). High environmental temperatures and exercise increase evaporative heat loss from panting; the resulting dehydration stimulates thirst. In addition, high environmental temperatures may directly stimulate, and cold temperatures inhibit, thirst responses. Lactating animals have increased water intake to compensate for fluid loss in milk. The effect of food and diet must also be considered. Anorexic animals drink less water, likely due to the decreased requirement to excrete solutes derived

- Environmental temperature
- Exercise
- Food intake
- Feeding practices
- Diet
  - Water content
  - Protein content
  - Salt content
  - Digestibility
- Water source

9.1 Factors affecting water intake in healthy dogs and cats.

from metabolism of food. Animals fed diets high in carbohydrate or fat drink less water because these nutrients generate less solute for urinary excretion and more metabolic water compared with protein. Conversely, diets high in protein or salt lead to increased renal solute and obligate water loss, and feeding highly digestible foods can result in increased urine volume and relatively higher water excretion in urine than faeces. Several diets are manipulated to increase urinary water loss as part of the prevention of urolithiasis.

Dogs will drink more water when fed a dry diet and less when fed a wet diet to maintain a similar overall total water intake. By contrast, cats are more efficient at conserving water, likely reflecting their desert origins. A cat's natural diet consists of small prey containing 70–75% water, and they can maintain hydration when fed a meat-only diet for extended periods. This is made possible by their capacity to produce very concentrated urine and to tolerate low levels of dehydration without stimulation of a thirst response. The water content of canned pet food is similar to or higher than that of a cat's natural diet. Therefore, cats fed a wet diet may not drink additional water, and water intake whilst receiving dry food may remain less than observed in a comparably sized dog. *Ad libitum* feeding also increases water intake. The type of water source may also influence water intake, particularly in cats, with individual animals preferring still or flowing sources. Dogs tend to drink less during the night compared with cats, likely reflecting typical nocturnal activity levels. As a result of all of these factors, normal water intake in healthy animals is highly variable.

Water excretion

Water excretion is predominantly controlled by the hormone arginine vasopressin (AVP), which is released from the posterior pituitary gland. The ability to resorb water and concentrate urine is dependent on the following:

- The ability to synthesize and secrete adequate AVP in response to appropriate stimuli
- The ability of renal tubular cells to bind AVP and induce expression of luminal aquaporin-2 channels
- The presence of an osmotic gradient between the tubular lumen and renal medulla. This is dependent upon hypotonicity within the distal tubular lumen, established by the absorption of most filtered solute within the more proximal segments, as well as hypertonicity within the medullary interstitium due to high concentrations of sodium and urea as a result of differential permeability of individual nephron segments
- An adequate number of functional nephrons. Renal concentrating ability is decreased following loss of approximately two thirds of functional nephrons, and therefore can precede the development of azotaemia.

Synthesis of arginine vasopressin

Arginine vasopressin is a nine-amino-acid peptide similar in structure to oxytocin. It is synthesized as preproarginine vasopressin within hormone-specific neurons in the hypothalamic supraoptic and paraventricular nuclei. This precursor protein consists of a signal peptide, AVP, a hormone-specific neurophysin and a glycoprotein known as copeptin. The signal peptide is cleaved, and the prohormone undergoes folding and assembly. The prohormone is transported to the axon terminals in the posterior pituitary. Neurophysin and copeptin residues are cleaved from AVP during transport, but all three are stored together in secretory granules within the posterior pituitary until released by an appropriate stimulus. All three molecules are released in unison but circulate independently. Circulating AVP has a half-life of approximately 15 minutes.

Stimuli for arginine vasopressin release

The principal stimulus for release of AVP is an increase in plasma osmolality, which is detected by osmoreceptor cells within the hypothalamus. These cells are believed to lie within the organum vasculosum of the lamina terminalis and in the anterior hypothalamus. They are surrounded by a highly fenestrated capillary network and are considered to lie outside the blood–brain barrier. Increases of as little as 1% in plasma osmolality result in AVP release and water resorption in the renal collecting tubule. Although AVP concentrations may increase dramatically in response to hyperosmolality, minor increases in AVP concentration are sufficient to produce near-maximal urine concentration (Figure 9.2). Therefore, clinical signs of AVP deficiency are often not apparent until late in the disease process. The maximal urine concentration achieved is dependent upon the magnitude of the renal interstitial concentration gradient.

The production of AVP also occurs in response to decreased blood volume or pressure. Decreased blood pressure is detected by high-pressure baroreceptors in the carotid sinus and aortic arch. Decreased blood volume is detected by low-pressure receptors in the atria and pulmonary veins. Afferent fibres from these areas are carried by cranial nerves IX and X to the brainstem. It has been suggested that input from these receptors exerts a tonic inhibitory effect on AVP secretion. Reduced stimulation of these receptors in response to decreased blood volume or pressure leads to increased AVP secretion, whereas increased receptor stimulation (increased blood volume/pressure) leads to decreased AVP secretion. The combined vasoconstrictive and water-retentive effects of AVP contribute to restoration of blood volume and pressure. However, a 10–15% decrease in blood volume or pressure is necessary before AVP secretion is stimulated (Figure 9.3). Therefore, the renin–angiotensin–aldosterone and sympathetic systems are considered to be the principal means by which blood volume and pressure are maintained.

Several additional physiological factors affect AVP secretion. The act of drinking stimulates a volume-dependent oropharyngeal response that inhibits AVP secretion. Non-specific factors such as nausea, pain, emotion and exercise can also stimulate AVP release.

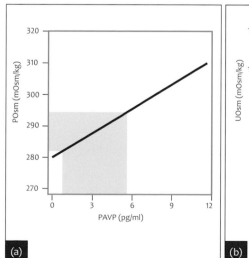
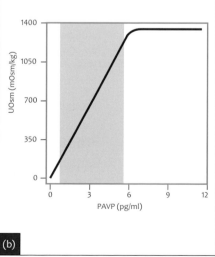
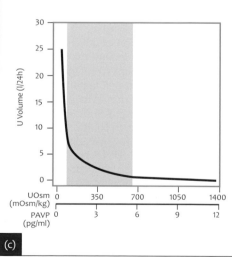

9.2 Relationships between plasma osmolality (POsm), plasma arginine vasopressin (PAVP) concentration, urine osmolality (UOsm) and urine volume (U Volume). (a) Small changes in plasma osmolality are associated with relatively large increases in PAVP concentration. (b) Urine osmolality is increased proportional to the PAVP concentration, until maximal urine-concentrating ability is reached (plateau). The height of this plateau is dependent upon the renal medullary concentration gradient. (c) Urine volume rapidly decreases in response to increases in PAVP concentration. The shaded areas represent the reference interval for PAVP in healthy dogs.
(Reproduced from Robinson and Verbalis (2008) with permission from the publisher. © Elsevier)

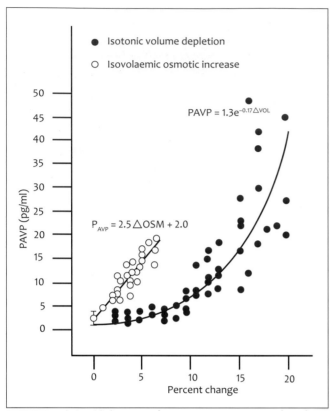

$$P_{AVP} = 1.3e^{-0.17\triangle VOL}$$

$$P_{AVP} = 2.5\triangle OSM + 2.0$$

- ● Isotonic volume depletion
- ○ Isovolaemic osmotic increase

9.3 Relationship between plasma arginine vasopressin (PAVP) and blood volume (VOL) or plasma osmolality (OSM) in rats. Plasma hypertonicity serves as the primary stimulus for AVP release; very small changes are associated with significant linear increases in AVP secretion. A greater degree of volume depletion is required to promote AVP release, which is exponential, and the magnitude of release may exceed that due to osmolality changes.
(Reproduced from Dunn *et al.* (1973) with permission from the publisher)

Biological effects of arginine vasopressin

Once released, AVP has several functions, which are exerted through a range of different receptors. Control of water homeostasis is mediated via V2 receptors located in the basolateral membrane of principal cells in the renal collecting tubules. Binding of AVP to V2 receptors causes increased expression of aquaporin-2 water channels within the apical cell membrane, thereby increasing water permeability and resorption from the tubular lumen. Water then passes through the cell, exiting the basolateral membrane via constitutively expressed aquaporin-3 and -4 channels, to the hypertonic renal medullary interstitium, from where it is returned to the circulation. Aquaporin-2 molecules are re-internalized when AVP dissociates from the receptor, thereby returning tubular permeability to its resting state. This process allows rapid regulation of water homeostasis in response to minor alterations in plasma osmolality. More prolonged stimulation of receptors also increases the synthesis and total number of aquaporin-2 molecules. The overall effect is increased resorption of water, decreased urine volume and eventual return of plasma osmolality to normal values. Conversely, decreased AVP secretion leads to decreased aquaporin-2 expression and increased diuresis. Arginine vasopressin and V2 receptors also regulate urea absorption in the inner medullary collecting duct, thereby directly contributing to the maintenance of the renal interstitial concentration gradient (Figure 9.4).

Binding of AVP to vascular endothelial V2 receptors stimulates the release of von Willebrand factor and coagulation factor VIII. Several other receptors are responsible for the additional metabolic effects of AVP, including:

- The V1a receptor, which is involved in vascular wall contraction, glycogenolysis and platelet aggregation
- The V3 receptor (also termed the V1b receptor), which is expressed within the anterior pituitary and mediates the stimulatory effect of AVP on adrenocorticotropic hormone (ACTH) secretion.

Arginine vasopressin has also been identified as a neurotransmitter in other areas of the brain and has an important role in behavioural responses. Many other tissues express AVP receptors, and their full biological role is not yet understood.

Pathophysiology

Polyuria and polydipsia can occur when any of the above physiological mechanisms are disturbed. The approach can be simplified by dividing the causes into two categories: primary polydipsia and primary polyuria. The latter can be subdivided into central diabetes insipidus (CDI), nephrogenic diabetes insipidus and osmotic diuresis. In reality, multiple mechanisms are involved in many individual diseases, and not all causes fall neatly within these categories. Nevertheless, disease classification in this way facilitates the diagnostic approach to clinical cases.

Primary polydipsia

Primary (or dipsogenic) polydipsia is the term used to describe an increase in thirst that drives excess water consumption. Secondary polyuria occurs to excrete the increased water load. Psychogenic polydipsia is a common differential for primary polydipsia in humans, named due to its frequent identification in patients with schizophrenia and other psychiatric disorders in the absence of structural brain disease. In dogs, an association has been made with a variety of behavioural abnormalities, but this is not well defined. Altered osmoreceptor or neurohormonal regulation of thirst centres is suspected in some cases of primary polydipsia. In most dogs, an underlying cause is not identified, although structural brain disease is not consistently excluded. Primary polydipsia has also been reported to contribute to the PU/PD observed in hyperthyroidism and liver disease in both dogs and cats, and as a rare feature of gastrointestinal disease in dogs through uncertain mechanisms.

Primary polyuria
Central diabetes insipidus

Central diabetes insipidus is a rare disorder characterized by reduced ability to secrete AVP in response to appropriate stimuli. This is most commonly due to neoplastic, traumatic or inflammatory diseases affecting synthesis or release of AVP, or may be induced by certain drugs (Figure 9.5). Profound PU/PD are the usual responses to complete CDI because distal tubular cells remain impermeable to water, resulting in excretion of hypotonic urine. Partial CDI is also reported but less well characterized. In this disorder, some AVP secretory ability remains, but less than necessary for maximal urine concentration.

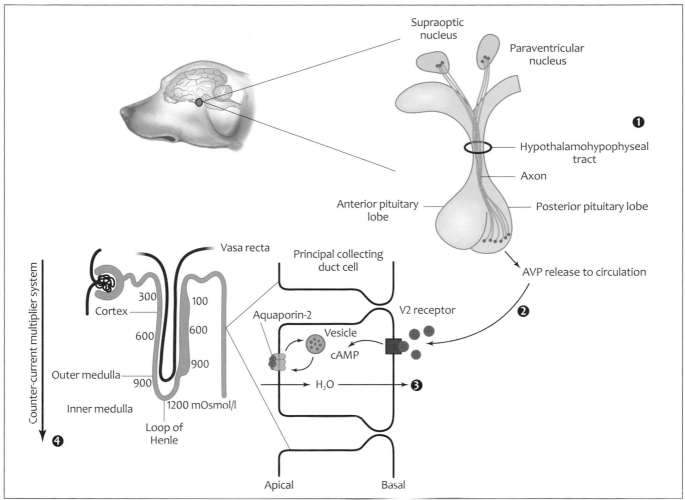

9.4 Arginine vasopressin (AVP) production and action in the kidney. 1 = AVP is synthesized in the hypothalamus as a preprohormone and stored in vesicles within the posterior pituitary. Secretion of AVP from the posterior pituitary is stimulated by increasing plasma osmolality sensed by the osmoreceptors in the hypothalamus or by decreased total circulating plasma volume sensed as a change in pressure within the atria, veins and the carotid sinus. 2 = Circulating AVP acts primarily in the distal tubule and the collecting ducts of the kidney. Arginine vasopressin interacts with its receptor (V2) and, via a cascade of events, facilitates the transient insertion of water channels (aquaporin-2), which increases the permeability of these epithelial cells to water. By an independent pathway, AVP also regulates urea transport within the inner medullary collecting duct. AVP causes an increase in transepithelial transport of urea, which is important for maintenance of the urea gradient. 3 = The fluid in the distal tubule is dilute, allowing passive movement of water from the tubule to the hypertonic medullary interstitium along an osmotic gradient. 4 = Maintenance of the osmotic gradient is dependent on the counter-current multiplier system between the loop of Henle and the vasa recta blood supply, which concentrates solutes (urea and sodium) within the medullary interstitium. cAMP = cyclic adenosine monophosphate.
(Reproduced from the BSAVA Manual of Canine and Feline Nephrology and Urology)

Decreased AVP release
• Glucocorticoids
• Alpha-adrenergic agonists
• Phenytoin
• Tetracycline

Decreased AVP responsiveness
• Glucocorticoids
• Barbiturates
• Alpha-adrenergic agonists
• Methoxyflurane

9.5 Drugs associated with decreased release of, or responsiveness to, arginine vasopressin (AVP).

Nephrogenic diabetes insipidus

Nephrogenic diabetes insipidus includes the most common causes of PU/PD. Both primary and secondary nephrogenic diabetes insipidus are characterized by reduced renal responsiveness to AVP. The degree of impact on urinary concentrating ability is variable; for example, some dogs with hypercortisolism or hypercalcaemia have marked hyposthenuria and profound PU/PD, while others are much less affected. Similarly, the typical magnitude of PU/PD varies between the individual causative diseases. This likely reflects differences in disease severity and the underlying mechanisms whereby the response to AVP is disrupted.

Primary nephrogenic diabetes insipidus is an inherited resistance to the effects of AVP. This disorder is well characterized in human medicine and is usually associated with mutations of the V2 receptor or, less commonly, aquaporin-2 genes. Primary nephrogenic diabetes insipidus has been suspected in several cases of PU/PD in young dogs, but never characterized at the molecular level in this species.

By contrast, secondary nephrogenic diabetes insipidus is relatively common and believed to be a cause of PU/PD in several diseases, including hypercalcaemia, hypercortisolism, hypoadrenocorticism, hyperthyroidism, pyelonephritis, pyometra and liver disease. Secondary nephrogenic diabetes insipidus is also responsible for the polyuric effects of several drugs, including glucocorticoids and barbiturates (Figure 9.5).

Osmotic diuresis

Osmotic diuresis is caused by disruption of the osmotic gradient between the hypotonic tubular lumen and the hypertonic renal interstitium. This leads to an inability to resorb water despite adequate AVP-induced permeability of tubular cells. Osmotic diuresis is most commonly caused by the presence of increased solute concentrations within the tubular lumen, such as occurs with glucosuria in diabetes mellitus, primary renal glucosuria and Fanconi syndrome. Post-obstructive diuresis may also cause PU/PD by this mechanism. Although less well defined, diets high in salt or protein and the syndrome of inappropriate antidiuresis (SIAD) may also lead to increased excretion of solute and associated obligate water loss.

Conditions that decrease renal medullary tonicity also disrupt the osmotic gradient. Hypoadrenocorticism and liver disease may decrease sodium and urea concentrations, respectively. Severely restricted protein diets may have a similar effect. Renal medullary washout, associated with intravenous fluid therapy or secondary to PU/PD of any cause, has also been demonstrated to decrease medullary tonicity, although this mechanism has been questioned in human medicine (Sadowski and Dobrowolski, 2003). Chronic kidney disease (CKD) can also be classified as a form of osmotic diuresis because affected kidneys lack the capacity to produce hypotonic tubular fluid or achieve renal medullary hypertonicity.

Other mechanisms

Finally, there are several mechanisms and causes that are poorly defined. Pressure diuresis may contribute to PU/PD in dogs during the polyuric phase of acute kidney injury, or with phaeochromocytoma or erythrocytosis. The presence of PU/PD has also been described in dogs with splenic haemangiosarcoma and intestinal leiomyosarcoma, but mechanisms have not been described and other causes of PU/PD were not always excluded. Leptospirosis can cause PU/PD through hepatic or renal injury, but it has been suggested that polyuria can occur in the absence of such effects due to decreased tubular responsiveness to AVP, based upon experimental studies. A single case has been described in a dog with such atypical leptospirosis in which persistent hyposthenuria preceded clinical or clinicopathological evidence of organ dysfunction, but other potential causes were not completely excluded (Etish et al., 2014). Hypersomatotropism typically causes PU/PD because of the development of diabetes mellitus, but the occurrence of mild to moderate PU/PD in some affected dogs without concurrent glucosuria led to the suggestion that nephrogenic diabetes insipidus was responsible.

As mentioned above, the classification of PU/PD using categories is somewhat artificial. For example, liver failure can cause primary polydipsia, decrease AVP release, induce secondary nephrogenic diabetes insipidus through direct mechanisms as well as decreased cortisol degradation, and decrease medullary hypertonicity through decreased urea synthesis. Similarly, although kidney disease is often classified as a cause of osmotic diuresis, the reduced number of functional nephrons as well as downregulation of V2 receptors also contribute, and the contributory role of hypokalaemia or hypercalcaemia in cases in which these occur is not known.

Pyometra and pyelonephritis are recognized causes of PU/PD, thought to be mediated through bacterial endotoxin-induced downregulation of V2 receptors, although pyelonephritis may also have direct effects on kidney function secondary to inflammation and infection. In humans, there is a reported association between interstitial cystitis and polyuria, possibly due to primary polydipsia. Polyuria is not thought to occur in dogs and cats with bacterial cystitis alone, which may reflect lower circulating plasma endotoxin concentrations in individuals with acute uncomplicated cystitis compared with other endotoxin-mediated mechanisms.

Differential diagnosis

The differentials for PU/PD are listed in Figure 9.6. Most are described predominantly in dogs. Some are also commonly recognized causes in cats, particularly kidney disease, hyperthyroidism and diabetes mellitus. The occurrence of PU/PD in several of the other diseases is poorly characterized or not reported in the cat. Polyuria and polydipsia are not described in the small number of non-diabetic cats with hypersomatotropism, suggesting that nephrogenic diabetes insipidus is not a major contributor. Likewise, most cats with hypercortisolism have concurrent diabetes mellitus. Although PU/PD have been described in a small number of non-diabetic affected cats, this species appears more resistant to the effects of glucocorticoids compared with dogs; a relatively higher dose or duration of administration of exogenous glucocorticoids is necessary to induce PU/PD. Both hypokalaemia and hypercalcaemia are common in cats with CKD, and therefore it is difficult to determine their relative contribution to PU/PD. However, PU/PD are rarely reported

---

Primary polydipsia
Primary polyuria
- Central diabetes insipidus [a, b]
- Primary nephrogenic diabetes insipidus
- Secondary nephrogenic diabetes insipidus
  - Hypercortisolism [a]
  - Hypercalcaemia [a]
  - Hypoadrenocorticism [a]
  - Liver disease [a]
  - Hyperthyroidism [b]
  - Pyometra/Escherichia coli endotoxaemia [a]
  - Pyelonephritis [a, b]
  - Hypokalaemia
  - Erythrocytosis
  - Hyperaldosteronism
  - Hypersomatotropism
  - Leptospirosis
  - Drug administration (e.g. glucocorticoids, phenobarbital) [a]
- Osmotic diuresis
  - Diabetes mellitus [a, b]
  - Fanconi syndrome
  - Primary renal glucosuria
  - Post-obstructive diuresis [a, b]
  - Chronic kidney disease [a, b]
  - Syndrome of inappropriate diuresis
  - High-salt or high-protein diet [a]
  - Drug administration (e.g. mannitol)
- Decreased medullary tonicity
  - Renal medullary washout
  - Low-protein diet
- Other/unknown mechanisms
  - Polyuric phase of acute kidney injury
  - Phaeochromocytoma
  - Splenic haemangiosarcoma
  - Intestinal leiomyosarcoma

9.6 Differential diagnoses for polyuria and polydipsia. Multiple mechanisms are responsible for the polyuria and polydipsia in several diseases. [a] = most important differentials in dogs; [b] = most important differentials in cats.

in cats with idiopathic hypercalcaemia or hypokalaemic myopathy. It is not known whether these observed differences between dogs and cats are due to true pathophysiological differences or to difficulties of owner recognition of all but the most severe PU/PD in cats.

Diagnosis

In many cases, differentiating between the causes of PU/PD is straightforward if other classical signs of the underlying disease are present. However, often the underlying cause is not clear, and it is important to prioritize the differentials with the particular case in mind according to the following information.

Confirm polyuria and polydipsia are truly present

Clearly, before embarking on a lengthy and costly investigation of PU/PD, it is necessary to ensure that excessive drinking and urination are truly present. Owners may confuse polyuria with pollakiuria, nocturia, incontinence or other forms of inappropriate urination. An appropriate increase in thirst associated with a dietary change, such as switching to dry food, can be considered abnormal by owners. Conversely, owners can fail to identify PU/PD when they are truly present, especially when various sources of water are available, multiple animals are present within the household or animals have unsupervised outdoor access. This is particularly common in cats, where PU/PD are often unrecognized even in those with consistently low urine specific gravity (SG) values. Therefore, confirming PU/PD requires objective measurement of water intake or urinary output, or assessment of markers of urine-concentrating ability.

In some cases, the presence of PU/PD is without question. However, in equivocal cases, the first step is usually measurement of water intake at home by the owners over a 24-hour period. A measured quantity of water should be provided, and intake calculated by subtraction of the residual volume. Water should be available *ad libitum* and replaced as often as necessary, while making certain that spillage does not occur. It is necessary to ensure no access to alternative water sources, limit unsupervised outdoor access and separate animals from multi-pet households. Such changes can influence drinking behaviours and mask polydipsia, particularly in cats. This is compounded in cats by their ability to suppress thirst despite mild dehydration. Similarly, measurement of water intake in hospital is often unreliable because drinking patterns usually differ from those in the home environment.

Measurement of urine output is rarely feasible. However, it may be possible to weigh the litter of indoor cats from single-cat households. Excess drinking with normal urine volume may be seen in animals with gastrointestinal fluid losses.

Urine-concentrating ability can also be assessed by measuring urine osmolality or SG. Osmolality is the number of osmotically active particles per kilogram of fluid. Specific gravity refers to the weight of the fluid of interest expressed as a ratio to that of an equal volume of water. As a result, SG is affected by both the number of particles and their mass. Nevertheless, a good correlation has been reported between both measurements in healthy dogs and cats (Ayoub *et al.*, 2013; Di Bella *et al.*, 2014). In dogs, urine

osmolality can be estimated by multiplying the last two digits of the SG by 36. For example, a urine SG of 1.020 corresponds to an approximate osmolality of 720 mOsm/kg. However, a poorer correlation has been described in human urine samples with pathological changes such as ketonuria, bilirubinuria, haemoglobinuria or glucosuria, as well as in samples containing mannitol or iodinated contrast media (Imran *et al.*, 2010). In healthy cats, urine osmolality can be estimated using the equation:

**Urine osmolality (mOsm/kg) =
1.25(Urea) + 1.1(Sodium) + 67(Glucose)**

No adjustments are required when the biochemical parameters are measured using standard international units (i.e. mmol/l). If conventional units are used (i.e. mg/dl), the glucose value should be divided by 18 and the urea value by 2.8. The performance of this formula has not been assessed in the presence of illness (Bouzouraa *et al.*, 2021). Facilities to measure urine osmolality are not widely available in practice. Therefore, the following section will focus on the use of SG.

The SG of urine samples from healthy animals can vary, influenced by many of the factors affecting water intake described above. In dogs, higher urine SG values are common in the morning, reflecting decreased water intake overnight. In cats, this diurnal pattern is not apparent. Concentrating ability significantly decreases with age but the magnitude of decline is small in healthy animals. Cats fed wet food have lower values compared with those fed dry food, while dogs fed dry food tend to drink larger volumes to compensate, resulting in less effect on urine SG. Water intake and urine SG can also be affected by altered drinking patterns in hospital. Therefore, the presence of PU/PD is best assessed using urine samples collected at home. In cats, the use of non-absorbent cat litter can facilitate collection. In dogs, collection of early morning samples can be useful to assess urine-concentrating ability. The analysis of multiple samples is beneficial to identify animals that intermittently have the ability to concentrate urine.

In healthy dogs, urine SG values vary widely, ranging from 1.001 to 1.065, and averaging 1.033. Although also variable in cats, values are typically higher, with an average of 1.050 and 90% of values greater than 1.035 (Rishniw and Bicalho, 2014). In this study, approximately 20% of apparently healthy adult cats with lower values were more than 9 years old and had underlying kidney disease or hyperthyroidism. For this reason, identification of low urine SG values in cats may prompt additional investigations even in the absence of owner-reported PU/PD, particularly in older cats. In most cases, urine SG values greater than 1.030 in dogs and 1.035 in cats do not support the presence of PU/PD. However, in some diseases, urine SG values can increase if water is not provided. This is expected with primary polydipsia but can also occur with other diseases. For example, specific gravity values as high as 1.035 are reported in dogs with hypercortisolism when water is withheld.

Signalment

The list of potential causes of PU/PD can be rapidly refined by consideration of the signalment. Congenital conditions are more likely in younger animals, while neoplastic conditions, including many hyperfunctional endocrine disorders, are more likely in older animals. Breed-associated conditions should be considered, such as hypercalcaemia due to primary hyperparathyroidism in Keeshonds or renal dysplasia in Boxers. Although sex predispositions are reported for many disorders, in most cases this cannot be used to refine the differential list, with a few notable exceptions such as pyometra.

History

The history should be thorough enough to identify features that could allow prioritization of the differential list. For example, appetite may be increased in animals with hypercortisolism, hyperthyroidism or diabetes mellitus. The history should also explore the diet, particularly for content and any change, and recently administered drugs. This should include details of any treats because these can be high in salt, and some dried chicken jerky treats have been associated with acquired Fanconi-like syndrome. Likewise, non-prescribed drugs should also be considered. Glucocorticoid activity has been demonstrated in some herbal medicines, and owners may administer systemic or topical agents that were not recently dispensed, or not prescribed for that animal. Administered medications may also impact the interpretation or choice of subsequent tests. In some cases, the history will provide an almost certain cause of PU/PD, negating the need for further investigations, for example in cases of post-obstructive diuresis or following the administration of some medications.

Physical examination

A thorough physical examination must be performed in all cases. For many conditions, PU/PD are among a constellation of presenting clinical signs, some of which will make certain diagnoses more likely. Dogs with hypercortisolism commonly display abdominal distension, hepatomegaly, fat redistribution, alopecia, and loss of elasticity and thinning of the skin. Clearly, naturally occurring hypercortisolism would be a major differential in an older dog exhibiting these signs, provided glucocorticoids had not been recently administered. Hyperthyroidism is usually associated with palpable goitre, severe hypokalaemia with muscle weakness, pyelonephritis with abdominal pain, and advanced CKD is often accompanied by poor body and muscle condition scores. Even if an underlying cause is immediately suspected, it is important to avoid pattern recognition. For example, while hyperthyroidism can cause PU/PD, they are not present in all cases and are usually not severe. However, concurrent hyperthyroidism and CKD are common in older cats.

It should also be recognized that PU/PD can be the predominant or only clinical features in many diseases, including primary polydipsia, CDI, hypercalcaemia, diabetes mellitus, early CKD and pyometra. Likewise, PU/PD can be the only notable features of hypercortisolism in some dogs. This may be particularly true in large breeds because the volumes of water intake and urine are more noticeable or inconvenient to their owners.

The refinement of the differential list based upon the signalment, history and physical examination is essential to ensure appropriate tests are prioritized. Care should be taken not to group all clinical features and focus the investigation too early because such a pattern-recognition-based approach can result in differentials being overlooked, particularly in complex cases with more than one disease.

Routine clinicopathological tests

Regardless of the cause of PU/PD, comprehensive haematology, biochemistry and urinalysis are recommended as part of the initial clinicopathological assessment.

Serum or plasma biochemistry should include all of the parameters necessary to refine the differential list, including sodium, potassium, chloride, calcium, cholesterol, glucose, and a comprehensive range of liver and kidney parameters. If the sample is not rapidly processed, the serum or plasma should ideally be separated as rapidly as possible, or a fluoride oxalate tube used, to ensure an accurate glucose concentration is determined. Glucose can also be measured using a hand-held glucometer. Total calcium is routinely included on most biochemistry panels; however, ionized calcium should also be measured when possible. Ionized calcium is the only biologically active fraction, and therefore only animals with ionized hypercalcaemia have associated PU/PD. Approximately one third of dogs with ionized hypercalcaemia have total calcium concentrations within the reference interval (Robin et al., 2020; Tørnqvist-Johnsen et al., 2020). Simple corrections of total calcium for hypoproteinaemia are not reliable, and although more complex predictive models are available based upon routine biochemical values, ionized hypercalcaemia may still be missed in approximately 20% of cases (Robin et al., 2020).

Routine biochemistry parameters can also be used to calculate osmolality. Direct measures of osmolality, such as freezing point depression or vapour pressure osmometry, are more accurate but not widely available. In both dogs and cats, the following formula is sufficient:

Serum or plasma osmolality (mOsm/kg) = 2(Sodium) + Glucose + Urea

No adjustments are required when the biochemical parameters are measured using standard international units (i.e. mmol/l). If conventional units are used (i.e. mg/dl), the glucose value should be divided by 18 and the urea value by 2.8. Older formulae included potassium, but this can lead to overestimation of osmolality (Dugger et al., 2013, 2014). Reference intervals of 290–310 mOsm/kg in dogs and 290–330 mOsm/kg in cats are commonly used.

The main value of calculating osmolality is to support a diagnosis of primary polydipsia. In such cases, osmolality is close to or below the lower reference limit because of increased water intake and subsequent dilutional effects. However, the effects on osmolality can be rapidly reversed if water is not available or drinking patterns are altered as a result of attending a veterinary surgery, for example. Also, decreased osmolality can be seen in several other disorders, primarily those associated with hyponatraemia, including hypoadrenocorticism, SIAD, and some liver and kidney diseases.

Although urinalysis may have already been performed to help confirm the presence of PU/PD, it is important that this is repeated at the same time as blood testing. Assessment of SG at this time may aid differentiation between renal and prerenal azotaemia, and pathological findings may contribute to the assessment of organ dysfunction. Marked hyposthenuria (urine SG <1.008) is most commonly encountered in dogs with hypercortisolism, hypercalcaemia, primary polydipsia or CDI. In cats, CDI and hyperthyroidism are the most common causes. In animals with most forms of osmotic diuresis (see Figure 9.6), excess tubular solute drives water loss, therefore hyposthenuria should not occur unless a comorbidity is responsible. The presence of hyposthenuria allows exclusion of CKD.

The presence of glucose in the urine may cause an increase in SG. However, the effect is minimal, with the addition of 10 g of glucose per litre (equivalent to a strong positive on most dipsticks) expected to change the SG of water by only 0.003–0.005. The effect in urine is a little more variable. Although the effects of marked glucosuria are minimal around the values used to support the presence of PU/PD in both dogs and cats, these effects could interfere with differentiation between isosthenuria and hyposthenuria due to greater effects in more dilute urine (Behrend et al., 2019).

With some exceptions, the presence of glucosuria suggests that blood glucose concentrations exceed the renal resorptive threshold (10–12 mmol/l in dogs and 14–16 mmol/l in cats) or that renal tubular dysfunction is present. Increased blood glucose concentrations may be due to stress hyperglycaemia or diabetes mellitus.

The basic clinical and routine clinicopathological features may allow a rapid diagnosis without the need for further extensive investigations. For example, hypercalcaemia may be identified and whilst the underlying cause may have to be investigated, no further evaluation of PU/PD is necessary. Supportive clinicopathological abnormalities may also be seen in animals with many conditions including hypercortisolism, hypoadrenocorticism, diabetes mellitus and kidney and liver disease. Many other diseases may be excluded. Thus, the results provide the platform for subsequent investigations.

In interpreting results, care should be taken to consider the effects and consequences of PU/PD. Water consumption may be decreased in animals presenting to a veterinary surgery because of water restriction during travel or altered drinking patterns in hospital. This may lead to dehydration, as well as clinicopathological changes such as relative erythrocytosis, prerenal azotaemia, hypernatraemia or hyperproteinaemia. Differentiation between prerenal and renal azotaemia can be challenging in cases with primary polyuria because urine concentration is impaired. This is a particular problem in animals with hypoadrenocorticism and hypercalcaemia in which azotaemia is common and can be severe. Urine-concentrating ability may also be impaired in cases of primary polydipsia because of medullary washout. As a result, attempts should be made to ensure that water is not restricted prior to testing. Decreased urea or potassium concentrations may be observed in animals as a consequence of PU/PD.

Urine culture

Urine culture is often recommended in animals with PU/PD. The sample should be collected by cystocentesis unless there is a contraindication present, such as coagulopathy. The presence of a positive culture could be supportive of pyelonephritis, one of the causes of PU/PD. Although definitive diagnosis of this disease requires pyelocentesis, a presumptive diagnosis is commonly made based upon the presence of a positive urine culture collected by cystocentesis, as well as supportive clinical, clinicopathological and diagnostic imaging findings.

Positive urine bacterial cultures are associated with several other causes of PU/PD and are described in up to approximately half of dogs with hypercortisolism and one third with diabetes mellitus. Positive bacterial cultures are also reported in approximately one in four cats with CKD and one in eight cats with diabetes mellitus. The significance of positive urine cultures is not always clear. The most recent International Society for

Companion Animal Infectious Diseases (ISCAID) guidelines recommend that urine culture should not be performed in dogs or cats that do not display lower urinary tract signs, including those with hypercortisolism or diabetes mellitus, because treatment may not be necessary and could promote antimicrobial resistance (Weese et al., 2019). Conversely, proponents of treatment argue that clinical signs of urinary tract infection may not be readily apparent in animals, especially those with immuno-suppressive diseases such as hypercortisolism. It is recommended that the decision to test and treat bacteriuria in small animals is supported by careful review of the history and physical examination for signs indicative of urinary tract infection rather than subclinical bacteriuria.

Additional diagnostic tests

The choice of additional diagnostic tests depends upon the differential diagnoses that are considered likely based upon the animal's age and signalment, history and physical examination, and following analysis of routine clinicopathological results.

Tests of endocrine function

As detailed in Figure 9.6, there are a number of endocrine causes of PU/PD. Diabetes mellitus may be suspected based upon concurrent hyperglycaemia and glucosuria. However, measurement of fructosamine or glycated haemoglobin may be necessary for confirmation, particularly in cats. Adrenal function tests include the ACTH response test, low-dose dexamethasone suppression test, determination of urine cortisol:creatinine, or measurement of aldosterone, renin or catecholamines, depending upon the suspected underlying disease. In particular, hypercortisolism is important to exclude in dogs because PU/PD are the most frequently reported clinical signs and may occur in the absence of other compatible features. Total thyroxine (T4) measurement is initially performed for the diagnosis of hyperthyroidism. Given the high prevalence of feline hyperthyroidism in many countries, this test is performed early in the diagnostic process in older cats. Serum insulin-like growth factor-1 concentrations can be measured to confirm hypersomatotropism, although severe PU/PD are usually seen only in animals that develop secondary diabetes mellitus. Measurement of parathyroid hormone (PTH) or PTH-related protein may be necessary as part of the investigation of hypercalcaemia.

Tests of liver and kidney function

Liver dysfunction may be supported by decreased concentrations of liver products (albumin, urea, cholesterol and glucose) with or without evidence of hepatocellular injury. In some cases, PU/PD are the predominant signs with limited or no routine serum biochemical abnormalities. Bile acid stimulation testing or blood ammonia measurement may be used to confirm liver dysfunction; the former should not be performed in animals with hyperbilirubinaemia. In animals with CKD, urine-concentrating ability is reduced after loss of approximately two thirds of functional nephrons, whereas azotaemia occurs after loss of 75%. Therefore, loss of urine-concentrating ability often precedes the development of azotaemia. Identification of kidney disease in these cases is challenging. Measurement of symmetric dimethylarginine is useful because concentrations increase earlier, often preceding the development of azotaemia by several months. In very early cases, calculation of glomerular filtration rate may be necessary as the gold-standard method of documenting decreased renal function, for example, using plasma iohexol clearance. In animals with suspected tubulopathy, investigation of aminoaciduria, fractional excretion of electrolytes and assessment of acid–base status are indicated.

Diagnostic imaging

Abdominal ultrasonography is commonly performed early in the investigation of PU/PD. Abnormalities may be identified in animals with diseases affecting the liver, kidney, adrenal glands, spleen, uterus, lymph nodes or gastrointestinal tract. Dilation of the renal pelvis (pyelectasia) with anechoic fluid can be seen in polyuric animals regardless of the cause. Therefore, this change should not be automatically attributed to pyelonephritis, in which pyelectasia is described as the most common finding (Bouillon et al., 2018). If the appearance of the fluid within the renal pelvis is corpuscular, pyelonephritis is more likely. Anechoic fluid can be seen with both causes. Additional changes consistent with pyelonephritis include ureteral dilation, decreased corticomedullary definition, altered renal size, renal hyperechogenicity or pyelonephrosis. However, some animals have no ultrasonographic abnormalities.

Other abdominal imaging modalities, particularly computed tomography, may be useful to further characterize abnormalities or assist surgical planning. In animals with CDI or primary polydipsia, advanced brain imaging modalities such as magnetic resonance imaging may help to identify the underlying cause.

Additional tests

As described above, atypical leptospirosis may be a cause of PU/PD in the absence of clinicopathological evidence of hepatic or renal injury due to secondary nephrogenic diabetes insipidus affecting medullary collecting ducts. The prevalence of this form of infection is not known, but it is likely to be rare because many cases would be expected to progress to organ dysfunction. Antigen-based detection methods such as polymerase chain reaction (PCR) are more useful in early or acute infections and, given the likely renal localization of organisms, urine testing may be most appropriate. Dark-field microscopy, blood-based PCR, in-house antibody tests or microscopic agglutination tests may also aid the diagnosis. However, the diagnosis is complicated by the recognition of leptospiral antigen in up to over 10% of asymptomatic dogs and the uncertain pathogenicity of some serovars (Rojas et al., 2010; Spangler et al., 2020).

Water intake is affected by the protein and salt content of food and its digestibility. In some cases, dogs with PU/PD appear to respond to a dietary change despite receiving an apparently balanced commercial diet. A dietary change can be attempted as a therapeutic trial in these cases, provided there is no contraindication.

Tests used to differentiate central diabetes insipidus and primary polyuria

The modified water deprivation test can be used to differentiate CDI, primary polydipsia and primary nephrogenic diabetes insipidus in dogs. This test should only be performed when all other relevant differential diagnoses have been excluded. Failure to exclude all other causes, particularly hypercortisolism, will likely lead to results that are challenging to interpret. The test comprises three main stages: gradual water restriction; complete water deprivation; and administration of desmopressin. This test is described in depth in Chapter 10. The modified water deprivation test is usually not performed in cats due to the rarity of primary polydipsia and primary nephrogenic diabetes insipidus in this species. A desmopressin response test can be performed as an alternative but may be associated with adverse effects in dogs with primary polydipsia.

References and further reading

Ayoub JA, Beaufrere H and Acierno MJ (2013) Association between urine osmolality and specific gravity in dogs and the effect of commonly measured urine solutes on that association. American Journal of Veterinary Research 74, 1542–1545

Behrend EN, Botsford AN, Mueller SA et al. (2019) Effect on urine specific gravity of the addition of glucose to urine samples of dogs and cats. American Journal of Veterinary Research 80, 907–911

Bouillon J, Snead E, Caswell J et al. (2018) Pyelonephritis in dogs: retrospective study of 47 histologically diagnosed cases (2005–2015). Journal of Veterinary Internal Medicine 32, 249–259

Bouzouraa T, Rannou B, Cappelle J et al. (2021) Formula for the estimation of urine osmolality in healthy cats. Research in Veterinary Science 135, 121–126

Di Bella A, Maurella C, Witt A et al. (2014) Relationship and intra-individual variation between urine-specific gravity and urine osmolarity in healthy cats. Comparative Clinical Pathology 23, 535–538

Dugger DT, Epstein SE, Hopper K et al. (2014) A comparison of the clinical utility of several published formulae for estimated osmolality of canine serum. Journal of Veterinary Emergency and Critical Care 24, 188–193

Dugger DT, Mellema MS, Hopper K et al. (2013) Comparative accuracy of several published formulae for the estimation of serum osmolality in cats. Journal of Small Animal Practice 54, 184–189

Dunn FL, Brennan TJ, Nelson AE and Robertson GL (1973) The role of blood osmolality and volume in regulating vasopressin secretion in the rat. Journal of Clinical Investigation 52, 3212–3219

Elliott J, Grauer GF and Westropp JL (2017) BSAVA Manual of Canine and Feline Nephrology and Urology, 3rd edn. BSAVA Publications, Gloucester

Etish JL, Chapman PS and Klag AR (2014) Acquired nephrogenic diabetes insipidus in a dog with leptospirosis. Irish Veterinary Journal 67, 7

Imran S, Eva G, Christopher S et al. (2010) Is specific gravity a good estimate of urine osmolality? Journal of Clinical Laboratory Analysis 24, 426–430

Rishniw M and Bicalho R (2015) Factors affecting urine specific gravity in apparently healthy cats presenting to first opinion practice for routine evaluation. Journal of Feline Medicine and Surgery 17, 329–337

Robin E, Cuq B, Sharman MJ et al. (2020). The multivariate predictive model to estimate ionized calcium concentration from serum biochemical results in dogs: external validation. Veterinary Clinical Pathology 49, 48–58

Robinson A and Verbalis J (2008) Posterior pituitary. In: Williams' Textbook of Endocrinology, 11th edn, ed. HM Kronenberg, S Melmed, KS Polonsky and PR Larsen, pp. 263–296. Saunders Elsevier, Philadelphia

Rojas P, Monahan AM, Schuller S et al. (2010) Detection and quantification of leptospires in urine of dogs: a maintenance host for the zoonotic disease leptospirosis. European Journal of Clinical Microbiology & Infectious Diseases 29, 1305–1309

Sadowski J and Dobrowolski L (2003) The renal medullary interstitium: focus on osmotic hypertonicity. Clinical and Experimental Pharmacology and Physiology 30, 119–124

Spangler D, Kish D, Beigel B et al. (2020) Leptospiral shedding and seropositivity in shelter dogs in the Cumberland Gap Region of Southeastern Appalachia. PLoS ONE 15, e0228038

Tørnqvist-Johnsen C, Schnabel T, Gow AG et al. (2020) Investigation of the relationship between ionised and total calcium in dogs with ionised hypercalcaemia. Journal of Small Animal Practice 61, 247–252

Weese JS, Blondeau J, Boothe D et al. (2019) International Society for Companion Animal Infectious Diseases (ISCAID) guidelines for the diagnosis and management of bacterial urinary tract infections in dogs and cats. The Veterinary Journal 247, 8–25

Chapter 10

Central diabetes insipidus

Robert E. Shiel

Introduction

Arginine vasopressin (AVP) is the principal hormone responsible for water homeostasis. Loss of normal AVP control can be caused either by reduced circulating concentrations of AVP or by an inadequate renal response, termed central and nephrogenic diabetes insipidus, respectively. Both conditions are characterized by the presence of marked polyuria and polydipsia (PU/PD). Central diabetes insipidus (CDI) and primary nephrogenic diabetes insipidus are rare in dogs and cats. The following discussion focuses on these two disorders, but as primary polydipsia is closely related and is the main differential for CDI, a brief description is also included where relevant. Causes of secondary nephrogenic diabetes insipidus are detailed in Chapter 9.

Central diabetes insipidus is the clinical syndrome that results from deficiency of AVP. Complete deficiency of this hormone is most common. However, partial diabetes insipidus, characterized by a subnormal AVP response, has been reported in a small number of animals. Central diabetes insipidus has been reported in both dogs and cats but is an uncommon diagnosis in both species. True estimates of prevalence are not available, largely because the condition is frequently misdiagnosed, resulting from failure to identify other more common causes of PU/PD.

Aetiology

As outlined in Chapter 9, AVP is produced within hormone-specific neurons in the hypothalamus, transported via axons to the posterior pituitary, and stored until there is an appropriate signal for its release. Abnormalities in any of these areas can result in the development of CDI. Pituitary tumours often extend dorsally, and prolonged compression of the overlying hypothalamus can cause irreversible damage to the supraoptic and paraventricular nuclei. If more than 90% of the cells within these nuclei are destroyed, CDI can develop. Likewise, severe hypothalamic lesions can result in permanent CDI by directly destroying AVP-producing cells or by altering osmoreceptor regulation of secretion. Lesions affecting the distal pituitary stalk or posterior pituitary alone commonly result in only transient CDI. This may be because of the low concentrations of AVP required to maintain plasma osmolality, and sufficient AVP release from fibres ending in the median eminence and proximal pituitary stalk.

Proximal transection of the pituitary stalk can result in the death of AVP-producing neurons by retrograde degeneration, and permanent CDI.

The recognized causes of CDI in dogs and cats are listed in Figure 10.1. Neoplasia is the most common cause in dogs, of which chromophobe adenoma, chromophobe adenocarcinoma and craniopharyngioma appear to be most common. Rare reports of primary focal B-cell lymphoma, meningioma or pro-opiomelanocortin-secreting tumours and metastatic tumours have also been documented. Trauma-induced CDI is the most common cause in cats and has also been reported in dogs. This cause may be under-recognized because animals with significant neurological impairment may not be capable of drinking, with any observed signs related solely to hypernatraemia. Severe hypernatraemia (>154 mmol/l) has been reported in almost 7% of dogs following head trauma, and CDI may be the cause in at least some cases (Riese et al., 2018). Trauma-induced CDI may be transient or permanent. In humans, the response to traumatic stalk transection follows a triphasic pattern: acute CDI develops within 24 hours due to axon shock, followed by an antidiuretic period associated with unregulated AVP release from storage granules in the posterior pituitary gland, and eventual development of transient or permanent CDI. This triphasic response has not been specifically described in dogs or cats.

In dogs, the development of transient or permanent CDI has been reported as a complication of hypophysectomy, primarily performed for the treatment of adrenocorticotropic hormone (ACTH)-dependent hypercortisolism (Hanson et al., 2005). Transient CDI is common in these dogs and often resolves within 2 weeks of surgery. Clinical signs of CDI may persist for a longer period. Lifelong desmopressin therapy is not necessary in most of these cases, but may be required for months to years, with a median duration of approximately 4 months (Meij et al., 1998; Hanson et al., 2005). The likelihood of developing CDI is higher in dogs with enlarged pituitary glands

- Idiopathic
- Head trauma
- Hypophysectomy
- Pituitary or hypothalamic neoplasia
- Inflammation
- Developmental neurological structural defects
- Infection
- Cysts

10.1 Causes of central diabetes insipidus in dogs and cats.

(pituitary to brain area ratio >0.31). In cats, CDI was originally reported as an uncommon complication of hypophysectomy for the treatment of ACTH-dependent hypercortisolism, although only a small number of cases were included (Meij *et al.*, 2001). In a more recent report of hypophysectomy for the management of feline hypersomatotropism, long-term administration of desmospressin was required in over 70% of cases (Fenn *et al.*, 2021). Recognition of transient CDI may be challenging because both dogs and cats are routinely administered desmopressin in the post-surgery period.

Several cases of CDI have been described in association with neuroinflammatory diseases, including hypophysitis and hypothalamitis, which may be focal or part of a more diffuse inflammatory response. Visceral larva migrans and structural developmental disorders causing CDI are rarely reported. In some cases of CDI, an underlying cause cannot be identified. These are generally termed idiopathic in dogs and cats, although several 'idiopathic' cases have been characterized at a molecular level in humans. Mutations in the signal peptide and hormone-specific neurophysin can result in impaired secretion of AVP. No such mutations have been investigated in dogs or cats. However, juvenile-onset CDI has been described in two Afghan Hound littermates without any apparent underlying structural defect (Post *et al.*, 1989).

Clinical features

Clinical features of CDI can occur at any age, and there is no apparent breed or sex predisposition. Polyuria and polydipsia are commonly the only presenting signs in affected animals. The onset of clinical signs is variable, ranging from acute to chronic over several weeks or months. The presence of additional systemic clinical features should prompt thorough investigation for other potential causes of PU/PD (see Chapter 9). In many cases, water intake and urine volume are markedly increased, up to 5–20 times normal values. Polydipsia can be so severe that water intake is preferred over food, resulting in weight loss. Some animals may drink any liquid available, including their own urine. Excessive water consumption can lead to vomiting, especially when large volumes of water are made available following a period of water restriction. Polyuria can result in nocturia and loss of house training. Urinary incontinence has been reported in several cases. This may be associated with overflow incontinence, due to large volumes of urine, or may represent owner misinterpretation of nocturia. Clinical signs are less marked in animals with partial CDI.

Neurological signs

In dogs with underlying pituitary or hypothalamic disease, additional neurological clinical signs may develop because of involvement or compression of adjacent tissue. In the largest case series of CDI in dogs, 7 of 10 animals developed neurological signs prior to death or euthanasia, including ataxia, seizures, obtundation, altered behaviour, impaired vision and tremors (Harb *et al.*, 1996). Neurological signs can also be present in dogs and cats following head trauma or can develop as a result of multifocal or extensive inflammatory, infectious and developmental structural central nervous system disease.

Concurrent endocrinopathies

Multiple endocrine abnormalities in addition to CDI can occur in association with congenital or acquired lesions affecting the pituitary gland. Concurrent CDI, pituitary dwarfism and likely secondary hypothyroidism were reported in a young German Shepherd Dog with suspected congenital structural abnormalities (Ramsey *et al.*, 1999). Central hypothyroidism, secondary hypoadrenocorticism and/or decreased growth hormone production have also been described in association with traumatic and neoplastic causes. Cortisol and thyroid hormone deficits also develop following hypophysectomy, due to the removal of thyrotropin (thyroid-stimulating hormone (TSH))- and ACTH-secreting cells within the anterior pituitary. These changes are predictable and replacement therapy should be commenced before the development of clinical signs of such endocrinopathies (Hanson *et al.*, 2005). As chromophobe adenomas and adenocarcinomas are known to result in CDI, signs of hypercortisolism may be present concurrently with CDI. In such cases, dogs will present with dermatological and metabolic changes associated with hypercortisolism. However, CDI should be specifically investigated only if PU/PD persist despite adequate control of hypercortisolism.

Signs associated with hypertonicity

Severe and sudden water restriction in animals with CDI can lead to the syndrome of hypertonic dehydration. This can also be seen in animals with trauma-induced CDI that are incapable of drinking due to other injuries, or in those with decreased water intake due to involvement of thirst-regulatory pathways. Hypertonicity occurs because water is lost from the circulation but electrolytes are conserved. This causes markedly increased plasma osmolality and a fluid shift from the intracellular to extracellular compartments, preserving normal extracellular and vascular volume. Thus, substantial cellular dehydration can develop without the typical clinical signs of volume depletion. Affected animals can exhibit anorexia, weakness, disorientation, ataxia and seizures. In head trauma cases, vigilance and monitoring of serum sodium concentrations and urine output are necessary to distinguish signs of developing CDI and hypernatraemia from those associated with other neurological injuries.

Conversely, neurological signs can develop in animals given free access to water following a period of chronic dehydration and hypernatraemia. In this case, neurological signs are due to cerebral oedema caused by a fluid shift from the extracellular to intracellular compartments. Clinically, these disorders can be difficult to distinguish in a dog or cat with suspected CDI and neurological signs. However, an accurate history and measurement of sodium concentrations and/or serum osmolality can help to differentiate these two syndromes.

Differential diagnosis
Primary nephrogenic diabetes insipidus

Primary nephrogenic diabetes insipidus is a rare disorder, characterized by the inability of renal tubular cells to respond to adequate plasma concentrations of AVP in the absence of an acquired cause of AVP resistance. In humans, primary nephrogenic diabetes insipidus is usually caused by mutations of the genes encoding either the V2 receptor (*AVPR2*) or aquaporin-2 (*AQP2*). A congenital form of nephrogenic diabetes insipidus has been described in Siberian Huskies, associated with a 10-fold reduction in the responsiveness of renal tubular cells to AVP (Luzius *et al.*, 1992). A mutation of the V2 receptor gene was suspected. Clinical signs were reported only in male dogs, presumably because of the presence of this gene on the X chromosome. This condition has not been described in cats.

Primary polydipsia

Primary polydipsia is characterized by excessive water intake that in turn drives secondary polyuria (see Chapter 9). This can result from altered function of the thirst centres within the brain, or altered stimulation of these centres by osmoregulatory, neural or hormonal stimuli. In humans, primary polydipsia is most commonly described associated with various types of psychosis, especially schizophrenia. In dogs, it is often a manifestation of a behavioural problem, particularly in young dogs, and has also been described in association with gastrointestinal disease in this species. Primary polydipsia can also contribute to the PU/PD observed in hyperthyroidism and hepatic insufficiency. Isolated primary polydipsia appears to be rare in cats, with only a single suspected case described (Long *et al.*, 2015).

Diagnosis

There is no single confirmatory test for CDI in dogs. The diagnosis cannot be made until most other causes of PU/PD have been thoroughly excluded (see Chapter 9). Prior to consideration of CDI in adult animals, the only remaining differential diagnoses should be CDI and primary polydipsia. If PU/PD are present from an early age, primary nephrogenic diabetes insipidus should also be considered. Only at this point can a modified water deprivation test, hypertonic saline infusion test or desmopressin trial be considered to distinguish between these conditions. Incorrect conclusions may be drawn from these tests if the preceding diagnostic work-up has been inadequate because withholding water or administering desmopressin may cause urine concentration in animals with a variety of other diseases.

Routine clinicopathological features

No significant haematological or biochemical abnormalities are consistently observed in dogs or cats with CDI, provided water is not restricted. If any significant abnormalities are evident, they are more likely to be associated with another disease causing PU/PD, which should be further investigated. In animals with CDI, serum urea concentrations are frequently reduced as a result of renal medullary solute washout and the loss of AVP-dependent urea resorption in the renal tubule. Decreases can be more marked than in other polyuric conditions because of the severity of polyuria. If water has been restricted, primary water loss can result in increased haematocrit, hyperproteinaemia, hypernatraemia and pre-renal azotaemia. Severe hypernatraemia and serum hyperosmolality are present in cases of hypertonic dehydration. Serum osmolality can be measured directly or calculated using the formula described in Chapter 9. Serum osmolality

reference intervals in dogs and cats are approximately 290–310 and 290–330 mOsm/kg, respectively. Calculation of osmolality can also be useful to support primary polydipsia: reduced values can be seen, provided the polydipsia is severe and water has not been withheld prior to collection of blood.

Urinalysis

Urine specific gravity (SG) values <1.030 in dogs and <1.035 in cats are consistent with PU/PD, but much lower values are detected in animals with CDI. Indeed, the only consistent clinicopathological feature in dogs with CDI is the presence of hyposthenuria or, less commonly, isosthenuria. Severe hyposthenuria (SG 1.000–1.006) is typically detected in dogs with complete CDI. In cats, hyposthenuria is usually slightly less extreme (1.005–1.008). Common differentials for such marked hyposthenuria include hypercortisolism, hypoadrenocorticism and primary polydipsia in dogs, hyperthyroidism in cats, and liver disease, hypercalcaemia and CDI in both species. In some cases, isosthenuria has been noted at presentation, presumably as a result of partial CDI (Harb *et al.*, 1996).

Urine culture is a routine part of the diagnostic investigation of PU/PD. Approximately 25% of dogs with CDI have positive urine bacteriological cultures at presentation (Harb *et al.*, 1996). However, when a positive urine culture is identified in an animal with PU/PD, pyelonephritis should be excluded as a potential cause before investigating CDI. Owners should also be questioned to attempt to distinguish between subclinical bacteriuria and urinary tract infection.

Diagnostic imaging

Abdominal ultrasonography is commonly performed as part of the diagnostic investigation of PU/PD. In dogs and cats with CDI, renal pyelectasia may be observed. This is a response to severe polyuria; increased urine flow within the renal pelvis leads to increased pressure and subsequent dilation. The fluid within the renal pelvis should be anechoic. The presence of hyperechoic material should increase suspicion of pyelonephritis.

Computed tomography or magnetic resonance imaging (MRI) can be performed to identify developmental or acquired structural lesions within the hypothalamus and/or pituitary gland (Figure 10.2). This is most commonly performed following the confirmation and initial treatment of CDI. By contrast, in humans, MRI findings can be used

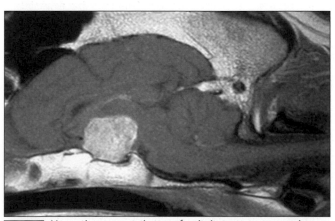

10.2 Magnetic resonance image of a pituitary macrotumour in a 10-year-old dog with central diabetes insipidus, central hypothyroidism and secondary hypoadrenocorticism.

to aid diagnosis. In healthy patients, a hyperintense signal on MRI can be identified within the sella turcica, thought to represent secretory granules containing AVP or oxytocin within the neurohypophysis. The presence of this bright spot is identified in approximately 80% of healthy humans but is absent in the majority of people with CDI. This feature has been used to evaluate human neurohypophyseal function. Although the intensity of the posterior pituitary on T1-weighted MRI images is directly proportional to AVP content in dogs (Teshima *et al.*, 2008), this has not been evaluated in dogs or cats as a diagnostic test.

Water deprivation test

The traditional water deprivation test involves the sudden and complete withdrawal of water and subsequent assessment of urine and plasma osmolality and urine SG. In theory, urine will become concentrated in animals with primary polydipsia, but will remain dilute (despite increasing plasma osmolality and hypernatraemia) in dogs with both CDI and nephrogenic diabetes insipidus. This test is not recommended because it can result in rapid alterations of

water and electrolyte status that can be life-threatening. This is a particular risk in practices lacking an in-house laboratory capable of measuring osmolality and electrolyte concentrations. Renal medullary washout may limit urine-concentrating capacity, regardless of the cause of polyuria and the animal's capability of producing AVP. In addition, animals with partial CDI may have results that are difficult to distinguish from both nephrogenic diabetes insipidus and primary polydipsia.

Modified water deprivation test

The modified water deprivation test is used to differentiate between CDI, nephrogenic diabetes insipidus and primary polydipsia (Mulnix *et al.*, 1976). However, it is time-consuming, unpleasant for the animal, and results can be difficult to interpret. A summary of the protocol is provided in Figure 10.3. The test is rarely performed in cats because of practical difficulties performing the test, such as urinary catheterization, accurate weighing and repeated blood sampling. Furthermore, primary nephrogenic diabetes insipidus has never been reported in cats, and only a

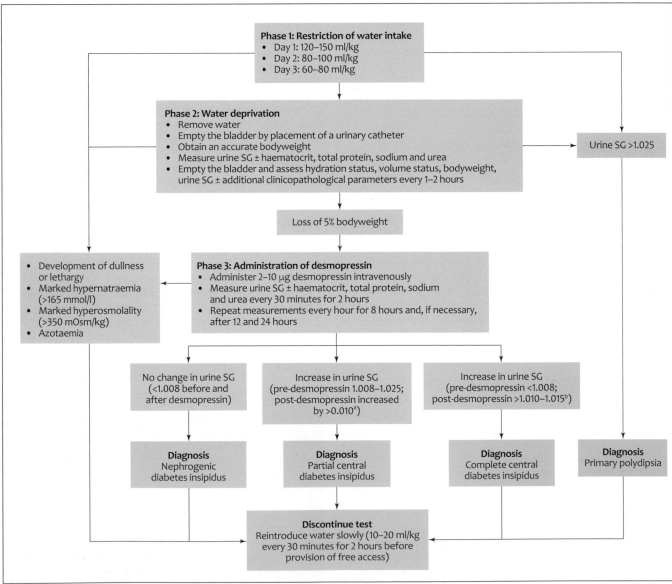

10.3 Performance and interpretation of the modified water deprivation test. SG = specific gravity. [a] = this response may also be seen in animals with secondary nephrogenic diabetes insipidus – consider completion of prior investigations; [b] = interpret in conjunction with magnitude of change, typically >0.010.
(Modified from Ettinger *et al.*, 2016)

single possible case of primary polydipsia has been described. Therefore, the test only confirms the already almost certain diagnosis of CDI in most cases.

Stage 1: Gradual restriction of water intake

Renal medullary washout can occur in animals with PU/PD regardless of the cause. As described in Chapter 9, the magnitude of the renal medullary concentration gradient determines maximal urine-concentrating ability. Therefore, in the presence of renal medullary washout, water resorption cannot occur even if adequate concentrations of AVP and functional V2 receptors are present. The first step of the modified water deprivation test is gradual water restriction over 3–5 days. In theory, this allows for re-establishment of the renal medullary concentration gradient. This part of the test can be performed in the home environment. However, owners must be aware of the need for rapid veterinary intervention if their animal becomes depressed or dehydrated. This is more likely in those cases initially presenting with very severe PU/PD. The veterinary surgeon (veterinarian) must also be confident of owner compliance and restricted access of the animal to other sources of water. As a consequence, hospitalization during this period may be preferred. Typically, in a 3-day water restriction protocol, water is restricted to 120–150 ml/kg on the first day, 80–100 ml/kg on the second day and 60–80 ml/kg on the third day, offered in small but frequent amounts. Owners should monitor their pet's bodyweight and demeanour, and the animal should be examined by the veterinary surgeon immediately if dullness or other adverse effects develop.

Stage 2: Complete water deprivation

Water is completely withheld during the second part of the test for a variable period of time. Due to the need for intensive monitoring and repeated testing, this stage of the test is performed under direct veterinary supervision. The animal is catheterized, the bladder emptied and urine SG or osmolality measured. An indwelling urinary catheter may be placed to avoid repeated catheterization. An accurate bodyweight is obtained immediately after emptying the bladder. Baseline total protein, sodium and haematocrit can also be determined at this time. Clinical signs, bodyweight, urine SG or osmolality and occasionally clinicopathological parameters (haematocrit, total protein, sodium and urea concentrations) are monitored every 1–2 hours until a predefined endpoint is reached. This can be:

- Urine SG >1.025
- Roughly 5% of bodyweight is lost
- Presence of dullness and/or azotaemia
- Sodium concentration >165 mmol/l
- Serum osmolality >350 mOsm/kg.

At each time point, the bladder is completely emptied by catheterization.

The time taken to achieve 5% weight loss is variable. In dogs with complete CDI, it is usually rapid, occurring within 3–10 hours of water restriction. In dogs with primary polydipsia or partial CDI, it can take considerably longer. The test is usually commenced early in the morning to increase the probability that it will be completed by the end of the working day. Nevertheless, overnight continuation of the test is necessary in some cases. If direct overnight supervision is not possible, maintenance water requirements (2.5–3.0 ml/kg/hour) can be provided and the test resumed the following morning.

Animals should be closely monitored during the modified water deprivation test to prevent excessive fluid loss. Pure water loss is most common in animals with diabetes insipidus, and hypertonic dehydration can rapidly develop during the water restriction phase. As described above, significant cellular dehydration and associated signs can develop before typical signs of extracellular dehydration develop. For this reason, monitoring bodyweight is a more sensitive marker for pure water loss than assessing clinical hydration status. Given that the endpoint is a decrease of only 5% bodyweight, scales must be sufficiently accurate to detect small changes. Monitoring serum sodium concentrations is particularly useful in dogs with severe PU/PD, in which rapid water loss and hypernatraemia can develop. Total protein and haematocrit can also be monitored over time. Total protein has been shown to be more reliable than haematocrit, presumably due to the effects of splenic contraction on the latter parameter. Adequate urine concentration during this stage (SG >1.025) is consistent with primary polydipsia, and the test is discontinued. No significant urine concentration occurs with complete CDI or nephrogenic diabetes insipidus. A moderate response (SG 1.008–1.015) is consistent with partial CDI.

Stage 3: Administration of synthetic analogues of arginine vasopressin

If urine SG remains below 1.025 despite loss of 5% bodyweight, the synthetic AVP analogue desmopressin (1-deamino-8-D-arginine vasopressin) is administered. Maintenance volumes of fluid (2.5–3.0 ml/kg/hour) can be given orally in small amounts during this stage of the test. Large single volumes should be avoided because rapid alterations of plasma sodium concentration and osmolality may precipitate neurological signs. This is a particular risk in animals in which severe hypernatraemia (>165 mmol/l) has developed. In addition, animals may drink excessively and vomit. It is preferable to administer desmopressin by the intravenous route to ensure a maximal response. Urine SG or osmolality is monitored every 2 hours for 8–10 hours after administration of desmopressin, and if necessary after 12 and 24 hours. The maximal response to desmopressin typically occurs within 4–8 hours but can take up to 24 hours in some animals. Water should be gradually reintroduced following completion of the modified water deprivation test. This prevents excessive overconsumption of water and associated vomiting or rapid alterations in plasma osmolality.

The typical response in complete CDI is an increase in urine SG from the severe hyposthenuric range to above 1.015. In nephrogenic CDI, the urine should remain dilute. Unfortunately, interpretation of results between these two extremes is more complicated. Partial concentration, with a further increase following desmopressin administration, is seen with partial CDI. However, intermediate results can also occur in some animals with complete CDI or primary polydipsia, likely due to incomplete restoration of the renal medullary concentration gradient during the first stage of the test, or altered expression of renal AVP receptors or the sensitivity or osmotic threshold for AVP release, as a consequence of chronic overhydration or dehydration. Furthermore, abnormal AVP responses to hypertonic saline infusion have been demonstrated in young dogs with suspected primary polydipsia, suggesting that the classical distinction between these disorders is not always appropriate (van Vonderen et al., 2004a). Other causes of PU/PD can be associated with almost any response during the modified water deprivation test, emphasizing the need for extensive prior investigations.

Measurement of plasma arginine vasopressin

Assays for the measurement of plasma AVP concentration have been validated for use in the dog. Measurement of this hormone is problematic because it is very sensitive to proteolysis and requires immediate chilling, separation and freezing of samples. In addition, its measurement is offered by few veterinary laboratories and, even then, inconsistently. In theory, measurement of AVP can allow differentiation of CDI and nephrogenic diabetes insipidus; low concentrations are expected in the former condition and high concentrations in the latter. However, the interpretation of basal AVP concentrations can be difficult. Arginine vasopressin is secreted in a pulsatile fashion, with wide inter-individual variation in the number of pulses, pulse duration and pulse amplitude, even in healthy dogs (van Vonderen et al., 2004b). This is further compounded by the effects of chronic over- and under hydration on the sensitivity and osmotic threshold for AVP release (van Vonderen et al., 2004a).

Hypertonic saline infusion test

The hypertonic saline infusion test was once considered the gold-standard method for differentiating CDI, nephrogenic diabetes insipidus and primary polydipsia. The test is performed by administering 20% sodium chloride intravenously via the jugular vein for 2 hours at a rate of 0.03 ml/kg/minute. Plasma osmolality is measured every 20 minutes and samples are stored for measurement of AVP. In theory, a decreased or absent AVP response is consistent with CDI. A normal or exaggerated AVP response with failure to concentrate urine is indicative of nephrogenic diabetes insipidus, whereas a normal AVP response with appropriate urine concentration indicates primary polydipsia. However, the ability of the hypertonic saline infusion test to differentiate these disorders has been questioned (van Vonderen et al., 2004a). Dogs with urine osmolality changes consistent with primary polydipsia can display exaggerated, subnormal or non-linear responses to hypertonic saline infusion, which suggests that the conditions are not always discrete clinical entities.

The test is not commonly performed in practice because an osmometer must be available on site to monitor urine and plasma osmolality. In addition, the administration of a hypertonic solution can precipitate hypertonic dehydration, particularly in animals that cannot mount an appropriate protective antidiuretic or thirst response.

Response to therapy

A simple alternative to the provocative testing protocols described above is the assessment of the clinical response to trial desmopressin therapy. This can also be used in situations where other tests have failed to yield a definitive diagnosis. It is the most common method used to confirm CDI in cats, due to the rarity of primary polydipsia and primary nephrogenic diabetes insipidus in this species.

The average 24-hour water intake is determined by the owner at home over a period of 2–3 days before the test is commenced. Therapeutic doses of desmopressin (see below) are administered, typically via the conjunctival sac. Treatment is continued over a period of 5–7 days, during which time the owner continues to monitor water intake. Water consumption dramatically decreases in dogs with both complete and partial CDI. As expected, dogs with primary polydipsia and nephrogenic diabetes insipidus usually fail to respond.

Desmopressin therapy is associated with minimal adverse effects when administered to healthy dogs. However, administration of desmopressin to a dog with persistent primary polydipsia can prevent appropriate secondary polyuria, leading to water intoxication and severe hypervolaemic hyponatraemia, a complication that has been reported in one dog (Plickert et al., 2018). Clinical signs of hyponatraemia are described in Chapter 11. In such cases, water should be withheld and desmopressin treatment immediately discontinued. The resultant diuresis should rapidly improve electrolyte and osmolality values.

Additional tests

Urinary aquaporin-2 excretion has been demonstrated to reflect exposure of renal tubular cells to AVP in healthy dogs, following hypotonic and hypertonic saline infusions (van Vonderen et al., 2004c). Further studies are required to determine whether this test can be applied in a clinical setting. In humans, copeptin can be assessed as a stable surrogate marker of AVP concentration. No copeptin assays have been validated for use in either dogs or cats, and interpretation of results would likely be complicated by the same factors that affect AVP.

Treatment

Central diabetes insipidus

Treatment of CDI may not be necessary, provided the animal has continuous access to water and the owner is willing to accept uncontrolled PU/PD. Water restriction should not be attempted because this can result in rapid cellular dehydration and hyperosmolality. The underlying cause should be treated if possible, for example, in the case of neuroinflammatory diseases. However, such treatment may not restore the ability to secrete AVP.

Synthetic arginine vasopressin analogues

The synthetic AVP analogue desmopressin is successful in controlling the clinical signs of CDI in most cases. This drug has little effect on V1a receptors and therefore does not induce significant vasoconstriction. It is available in several forms: a sterile solution for intravenous administration (4 μg/ml), a solution for intranasal use (100 μg/ml) and as tablets or oral lyophilisates (0.05–0.24 mg). Most commonly in dogs, the intranasal solution is administered at an empirical dose of 1–4 drops (approximately 1.5–4.0 μg/drop) into the conjunctival sac or nose 1–3 times daily. Injectable desmopressin can be administered subcutaneously at a dose of 2–5 μg once or twice daily. Subcutaneous administration of the nasal preparation has been described anecdotally, but the preparation is not sterile or specifically authorized for this route, and adverse skin reactions can occur. Oral formulations can be used at an initial dose of 0.1 mg once or twice daily. However, absorption of desmopressin and response to oral therapy are very variable between cases, making this route less effective in some animals. In cats, conjunctival treatment is successful but is not tolerated by many in the long term. Adequate control of clinical signs in cats has also been reported with 4 μg desmopressin administered subcutaneously q24h, or 25–50 μg orally q8–12h (Aroch et al., 2005). Although the pharmacokinetics of desmopressin vary depending upon the method of administration, both intranasal and oral routes have been reported to control clinical signs of CDI in humans. It is therefore recommended that the mode of administration should be based upon the ability of the owner to administer the drug by a particular route and the observed response. Additional factors, such as high cost of the oral medication, should also be considered.

The response to desmopressin is usually rapid. Some owners elect to treat animals only at night to prevent nocturia. The absorption and duration of action of desmopressin are very variable between animals. The dose and dosing frequency should be tailored to whatever achieves best control in an individual animal. The dosing frequency is often spaced to allow a slight return of polyuria between administrations – this helps to avoid adverse reactions.

Adverse effects are rare with desmopressin therapy. Hyponatraemia is very uncommon, presumably because maximal antidiuresis is not persistent with recommended treatment protocols. Desmopressin has little activity at V1a receptors and increased blood pressure has not been documented following desmopressin administration.

Other treatments

In humans, drugs such as thiazide diuretics and chlorpropamide are occasionally prescribed for the control of CDI. Use of these drugs has been described in experimental and naturally occurring canine cases; however, their use is rarely necessary given the high success of desmopressin therapy. They are more commonly used for the management of primary nephrogenic diabetes insipidus in this species (see below). Dietary therapy of CDI is ineffective as the sole method of treatment, but restricted-sodium and -protein diets decrease obligate water loss and may be beneficial in cases that are difficult to stabilize by desmopressin therapy alone.

Treatment of hypertonic dehydration

Hypertonic dehydration should be managed immediately. In affected animals, the underlying disorder is pure water loss; therefore, therapy is aimed at replacing this deficit. If the animal is capable of drinking, oral fluid should be offered. If this is not possible (e.g. the dog is obtunded or vomiting), intravenous fluid administration should be commenced. Hypotonic fluids, either 5% dextrose or 0.45% saline, can be administered.

Hypernatraemia of acute onset can be treated rapidly. However, hypernatraemia should be corrected slowly if it has been present for longer than 24 hours or if the duration is unknown. In these cases, organic osmolytes may have formed and rapid reduction of serum osmolality could result in cerebral oedema. The decline in serum sodium concentration should not exceed 0.5 mmol/l/hour.

Primary polyuria and primary nephrogenic diabetes insipidus

Treatment of primary polyuria involves restriction of water intake or treatment of the underlying behavioural or medical cause. Clinical signs can resolve spontaneously in some cases.

The treatment of primary nephrogenic diabetes insipidus can be challenging. In human medicine, a limited response to desmopressin therapy has been reported when defects are partial, but most patients do not respond. Chlorpropamide (5–40 mg/kg orally q24h) increases the responsiveness of renal tubular principal cells to AVP and may have additional direct antidiuretic effects in the loop of Henle. In humans, it is more commonly used for the treatment of partial CDI. There is limited information on its use in dogs and cats, but results appear variable and commonly disappointing. Adverse effects include hypoglycaemia. Natriuretic agents, such as thiazide diuretics, are occasionally used in the management of CDI in humans. The principle of their use is that extracellular volume contraction will lead to decreased glomerular filtration rate and increased sodium and water resorption in the proximal tubule. This results in decreased water delivery to the distal tubule, and consequently decreased water loss. Thiazides may also directly increase aquaporin-2 expression in renal tubule principal cells. Thiazide diuretics have been shown to have a variable antidiuretic effect in dogs with CDI, reducing urine output by 50% in some cases but being ineffective in others. The recommended dose of hydrochlorothiazide in dogs is 2.5–5.0 mg/kg orally q12h. A diet restricted in sodium and protein is often recommended to decrease obligate water loss.

Prognosis

The majority of dogs and cats with CDI respond adequately to desmopressin therapy. The long-term prognosis is dependent upon the underlying cause. Idiopathic and trauma-associated cases can be managed successfully for several years. Animals with pituitary or hypothalamic neoplasia may deteriorate due to progressive neurological signs.

References and further reading

Aroch I, Mazaki-Tovi M, Shemesh O, Sarfaty H and Segev G (2005) Central diabetes insipidus in five cats: clinical presentation, diagnosis and oral desmopressin therapy. *Journal of Feline Medicine and Surgery* **7**, 333–339

Ettinger SJ, Feldman EC and Côté E (2016) *Textbook of Veterinary Internal Medicine: Diseases of the Dog and the Cat, 8th edn.* Saunders, Philadelphia

Fenn J, Kenny PJ, Scudder CJ *et al.* (2021) Efficacy of hypophysectomy for the treatment of hypersomatotropism-induced diabetes mellitus in 68 cats. *Journal of Veterinary Internal Medicine* **35**, 823–833

Hanson JM, Hoofd MM, Voorhout G *et al.* (2005) Efficacy of transsphenoidal hypophysectomy in treatment of dogs with pituitary-dependent hyperadrenocorticism. *Journal of Veterinary Internal Medicine* **19**, 687–694

Harb MF, Nelson RW, Feldman EC, Scott-Moncrieff JC and Griffey SM (1996) Central diabetes insipidus in dogs: 20 cases (1986–1995). *Journal of the American Veterinary Medical Association* **209**, 1884–1888

Long CT, Williams M, Savage M *et al.* (2015) Probable primary polydipsia in a domestic shorthair cat. *Journal of Feline Medicine and Surgery Open Reports* **1**, doi: 10.1177/2055116915615370

Luzius H, Jans DA, Grunbaum EG *et al.* (1992) A low affinity vasopressin V2-receptor in inherited nephrogenic diabetes insipidus. *Journal of Receptors and Signal Transduction Research* **12**, 351–368

Meij BP, Voorhout G, van den Ingh TSGAM *et al.* (1998) Results of transsphenoidal hypophysectomy in 52 dogs with pituitary-dependent hyperadrenocorticism. *Veterinary Surgery* **27**, 246–261

Meij BP, Voorhout G, van den Ingh TSGAM and Rijnberk A (2001) Transsphenoidal hypophysectomy for treatment of pituitary-dependent hyperadrenocorticism in 7 cats. *Veterinary Surgery* **30**, 72–86

Mulnix JA, Rijnberk A and Hendriks HJ (1976) Evaluation of a modified water-deprivation test for diagnosis of polyuric disorders in dogs. *Journal of the American Veterinary Medical Association* **169**, 1327–1330

Plickert HD, Pagitz M and Luckschander-Zeller N (2018) Desmopressin acetate-induced water intoxication in a dog with psychogenic polydipsia. *Veterinary Record Case Reports* **6**, e000606

Post K, McNeill JR, Clark EG, Dignean MA and Olynyk GP (1989) Congenital central diabetes insipidus in two sibling Afghan hound pups. *Journal of the American Veterinary Medical Association* **194**, 1086–1088

Ramsey IK, Dennis R and Herrtage ME (1999) Concurrent central diabetes insipidus and panhypopituitarism in a German shepherd dog. *Journal of Small Animal Practice* **40**, 271–274

Riese F, Rohn K, Hoppe S and Tipold A (2018) Hypernatremia and coagulopathy may or may not be useful clinical biomarkers in dogs with head trauma: a retrospective study. *Journal of Neurotrauma* **35**, 2820–2826

Teshima T, Hara Y, Masuda H *et al.* (2008) Relationship between arginine vasopressin and high signal intensity in the pituitary posterior lobe on T1-weighted MR images in dogs. *Journal of Veterinary Medical Science* **70**, 693–699

van Vonderen IK, Kooistra HS, Timmermans-Sprang EP, Meij BP and Rijnberk A (2004a) Vasopressin response to osmotic stimulation in 18 young dogs with polyuria and polydipsia. *Journal of Veterinary Internal Medicine* **18**, 800–806

van Vonderen IK, Wolfswinkel J, Oosterlaken-Dijksterhuis MA, Rijnberk A and Kooistra HS (2004b) Pulsatile secretion pattern of vasopressin under basal conditions, after water deprivation, and during osmotic stimulation in dogs. *Domestic Animal Endocrinology* **27**, 1–12

van Vonderen IK, Wolfswinkel J, van den Ingh TSGAM *et al.* (2004c) Urinary aquaporin-2 excretion in dogs: a marker for collecting duct responsiveness to vasopressin. *Domestic Animal Endocrinology* **27**, 141–153

Chapter 11

The syndrome of inappropriate antidiuresis

Robert E. Shiel

Introduction

Arginine vasopressin (AVP) is the principal hormone regulating water balance within the body. In the syndrome of inappropriate antidiuresis (SIAD), the secretion and/or effects of AVP are increased in the absence of appropriate triggers, leading to hyponatraemia, decreased plasma osmolality and associated neurological dysfunction. The condition is also known as the syndrome of inappropriate antidiuretic hormone secretion (SIADH), but the term SIAD has been proposed to be more accurate because AVP concentrations are not consistently increased in all cases.

Prevalence

In human medicine, hyponatraemia is common in hospitalized patients and is associated with increased morbidity and mortality. In approximately one third of these patients, SIAD is identified as the underlying cause. Although hyponatraemia is also common in hospitalized dogs and cats, SIAD is very rare. In total, fewer than 20 cases of SIAD have been reported in dogs and only three in cats, with most confined to single case reports. However, it is possible that the condition is underrecognized.

Pathophysiology

Inappropriate activation of V2 receptors causes increased tubular absorption of water, plasma volume expansion and dilutional hyponatraemia. However, this is likely to be the driving mechanism of hyponatraemia in only the initial stages of the disease, with restoration of euvolaemia in most affected individuals resulting from reduced V2 receptor binding capacity and aquaporin-2 expression and enhanced natriuresis. This increase in urinary sodium excretion is one of the essential diagnostic requirements of SIAD, is thought to be the major factor responsible for hyponatraemia in chronic disease and may contribute to polyuria and polydipsia (PU/PD) in the later stages of disease through osmotic diuresis. Signs relating to activation of V1a and V1b receptors, such as hypertension or hypercortisolism, respectively, are not described.

Sodium is the main contributor to plasma osmolality. The development of clinical signs in SIAD is dependent upon the magnitude of hypo-osmolality and the speed with which it develops. As plasma osmolality decreases, intracellular fluid becomes relatively hypertonic and an osmotic gradient is established that causes entry of water into cells. Brain tissue is most affected because of its limited capacity to expand due to enclosure within the cranial vault. If severe brain swelling occurs, this can lead to herniation of cerebral tissue beneath the tentorium cerebelli (caudal transtentorial herniation) and compression of the brainstem. Resultant signs of brainstem dysfunction include ataxia, cranial nerve deficits, reduced level of consciousness and death. To protect against this event, brain cells contain low molecular weight organic compounds termed organic osmolytes. The intracellular concentrations of organic osmolytes can increase or decrease in response to hypernatraemia and hyponatraemia, respectively, thereby reducing the osmotic gradient between the intracellular and extracellular fluid. However, these responses take 24–48 hours to develop. As a result, relatively large alterations in plasma osmolality can be associated with minimal clinical signs, provided they develop slowly, whereas acute severe hyponatraemia is often associated with more severe clinical signs. If plasma osmolality decreases to a sufficiently low level, this protective mechanism is no longer sufficient and cellular overhydration and associated signs occur.

Aetiology

In humans, the causes of SIAD are well characterized and most can be divided into four main aetiological groups: neoplasia, pulmonary disease, central nervous system disorders and drug-related. Congenital causes are also recognized but are very rare. Many drugs are capable of inducing SIAD, including selective serotonin reuptake inhibitors, phenothiazines and vinca alkaloids. Mechanisms include stimulation of excessive AVP release from the posterior pituitary, ectopic hormone production or potentiation of the renal effects of AVP.

In dogs, SIAD has been reported in association with presumptive dirofilariasis, aspiration pneumonia, babesiosis, liver disease, granulomatous amoebic meningoencephalitis, hydrocephalus, and sarcomas affecting the thalamic and hypothalamic regions (Breitschwerdt and Root, 1979; Houston et al., 1989; Brofman et al., 2003; Shiel et al., 2009; Kang and Park 2011; Bowles et al., 2015; Barrot et al., 2017; Martínez and Torrente 2017; Gójska-Zygner et al., 2019). The syndrome has been produced experimentally in dogs by caval constriction and obstruction, and has been reported as a potential complication of transsphenoidal hypophysectomy in this species (Meij et al., 1998). Several cases have been described as idiopathic; however, diagnostic investigations were not always comprehensive. In cats, the condition has been associated with vinblastine toxicity, liver disease and cystic Rathke's pouch (Cameron and Gallagher, 2010; Grant et al., 2010; DeMonaco et al., 2014). Although several of the causes of SIAD are similar to those described in humans, the number of affected animals is small, and the diagnosis is questionable in some cases because not all diagnostic criteria were fulfilled. Congenital forms have not been described in small animals.

Clinical features

Given the wide range of suspected underlying causes, no overall age, breed or sex predispositions are expected. Dogs and cats with naturally occurring SIAD have ranged in age from 12 weeks to 8 years, and 3 to 11 years, respectively. Four dogs with presumed idiopathic SIAD have ranged in age from 1 to 8 years.

Most clinical features of SIAD are related to severe hyponatraemia (usually <125 mmol/l). It is possible that less severely affected dogs display clinical signs, but it is known that the symptoms of mild hyponatraemia in humans are vague and non-specific. Clinical signs reported in dogs include weakness, lethargy, nausea, tremor, seizures and coma. Polyuria and polydipsia have been reported in several dogs but are not consistent features. Clinical signs may wax and wane in severity because of varying concentrations of AVP over time and may spontaneously resolve because of reduced water intake secondary to lethargy or nausea. Clinical signs may also relate to the underlying disease.

Diagnosis

In dogs and cats, SIAD is initially suspected due to the presence of hyponatraemia, particularly when other causes are not apparent and there is a poor response to intravenous fluid therapy. Causes of hyponatraemia are listed in Figure 11.1. Marked hyperlipidaemia and hyperproteinaemia can result in pseudohyponatraemia, an artefactual decrease in sodium that is due to the decrease in the aqueous content of plasma. This is more common when sodium concentrations are assessed by flame photometry than with ion-specific electrode techniques. Indeed, hyponatraemia related to such measurements may be responsible for the controversial inclusion of hypothyroidism as a relatively common cause of hyponatraemia, as it is frequently associated with hyperlipaemia. In accord with this, hypothyroidism as a cause of hyponatraemia in humans is considered to be rare (Liamis et al., 2017). Hyponatraemia may also be an appropriate response to hyperosmolality caused by increased concentrations of other effective osmoles such as glucose or mannitol. The remaining causes of hyponatraemia can be largely classified based on their association with hypervolaemia, hypovolaemia or euvolaemia.

The diagnosis of SIAD in humans is based upon confirming the essential Bartter–Schwartz criteria (Cuesta and Thompson, 2016):

- Decreased effective serum osmolality (<275 mOsm/kg)
- Inappropriately concentrated urine for the degree of plasma osmolality (>100 mOsm/kg)

Hypovolaemic hyponatraemia
• Hypoadrenocorticism
• Administration of certain drugs (e.g. loop diuretics)
• Gastrointestinal disease
• Body cavity effusions
Hypervolaemic hyponatraemia
• Congestive heart failure
• Nephrotic syndrome
• Kidney failure
• Liver failure
• Cerebral salt wasting syndrome
Euvolaemic hyponatraemia
• Syndrome of inappropriate antidiuresis
• Primary polydipsia
• Hypotonic fluid administration
Other
• Pseudohyponatraemia
○ Hypertriglyceridaemia
○ Hyperproteinaemia
• Hyperosmolality
○ Hyperglycaemia
○ Mannitol administration
• Exercise-associated hyponatraemia

11.1 Causes of hyponatraemia in the dog and cat.

- Clinical euvolaemia
- Increased sodium excretion (urinary sodium concentration >30 mmol/l)
- Normal kidney, adrenal and thyroid function.

Measurement of AVP concentrations is not useful because values are not consistently increased in SIAD patients, and increased values can occur with most causes of hypovolaemic and hypervolaemic hyponatraemia.

In dogs and cats, all of the essential criteria should be fulfilled. However, optimal cut-off values have not been described for osmolality or urinary sodium concentrations, and fractional excretion of sodium is commonly measured in place of urinary sodium concentration. Hypoadrenocorticism (see Chapters 28 and 31) should be excluded. Urine and plasma osmolality should be measured concurrently to allow correct interpretation of results. Direct osmometry is advised. Although plasma osmolality can be estimated from sodium, glucose and urea concentrations, as described in Chapter 9, this will not identify the presence of unmeasured osmoles. Likewise, urine osmolality can be estimated from urine specific gravity (SG), but this is less accurate.

The importance of assessing volume status cannot be overemphasized because many of the other essential criteria for diagnosis of SIAD are present in hypovolaemic and hypervolaemic hyponatraemic cases. However, it can be difficult to classify volume status accurately. In human medicine, physical examination alone has less than 50% accuracy to distinguish between euvolaemic and hypovolaemic states (Cuestro and Thompson, 2016). Therefore, exclusion of other common causes of hyponatraemia is recommended even if there is no evidence of altered blood volume on physical examination. In addition, in human medicine, it is common to assess the response to intravenous sodium chloride therapy to aid differentiation between hypovolaemic and euvolaemic hyponatraemia. Such treatment would be expected to improve hypovolaemic hyponatraemia without causing harm in SIAD patients. However, rapid increases in sodium concentration must be avoided to prevent osmotic demyelination syndrome, as discussed below.

Routine haematology and remaining serum biochemistry results are often unremarkable but may reflect the underlying disease process. Urinalysis results are variable. Decreased urine SG can be detected in animals with PU/PD. However, urine SG and osmolality are inappropriately high compared with plasma values. Diagnostic imaging is advised to investigate pulmonary, central nervous system and neoplastic causes of SIAD.

Treatment

Management of hyponatraemia

In the absence of severe neurological signs, euvolaemic hyponatraemia is managed differently to both hypervolaemic and hypovolaemic causes. Hypervolaemic hyponatraemia is typically managed with judicious diuretic therapy, and hypovolaemic hyponatraemia with isotonic saline at a rate deemed appropriate to correct the fluid and electrolyte deficits. By contrast, isotonic saline will have little effect if SIAD is present; natriuresis and water excretion will occur, and plasma osmolality will be largely unaltered.

The first-line therapy for asymptomatic SIAD is moderate water restriction. This includes water obtained from food and other sources. In humans, water requirements are calculated from total urine output plus insensible losses, and fluid intake is restricted to below this volume. In dogs, this is more complex due to difficulties in measuring total urine output in non-catheterized animals and the variable presence of PU/PD. Water restriction is aimed at improving clinical signs rather than restoring sodium concentrations to the reference interval. Salt should not be restricted because ongoing natriuresis increases the risk of negative total body sodium balance. The response to fluid restriction can take several days.

In a chronically hyponatraemic animal, a rapid increase in the plasma sodium concentration results in dehydration of cerebral tissue due to the inability of cells to produce organic osmolytes at a sufficient rate to counteract the newly formed osmotic gradient. This can result in a syndrome known as central pontine myelinosis or osmotic demyelination syndrome – a condition with high neurological morbidity and mortality. Clinical signs typically develop several days after osmolality changes occur. The severity of signs may improve over time, but they are often permanent. In most cases of SIAD, the hyponatraemia is chronic or the duration is not known. As a result, hyponatraemia should be corrected with care.

Symptomatic hyponatraemia can develop in animals with severe or rapidly developing hyponatraemia and may require more aggressive management. This can be accomplished by the judicious administration of hypertonic saline. The aim of this treatment is to increase the sodium concentration sufficiently to resolve the clinical signs, not to return the sodium concentration to the reference interval (for further information see the *BSAVA Manual of Canine and Feline Emergency and Critical Care*). The increase in serum sodium concentration should be carefully monitored, and the rate limited to a maximum of 0.5 mmol/l/h. Slightly higher rates may be used in seizuring or comatose animals at immediate risk of transtentorial herniation, but alterations in osmolality should still not exceed 12 mmol/l in the first 24 hours.

Additional therapies

The underlying cause should be removed if possible and potential causative medications discontinued. In human medicine, there are a number of selective V2 receptor antagonists available for the treatment of SIAD. These drugs are known as vaptans and include conivaptan and tolvaptan. There has been a single case report on the use of one such drug (OPC-31260) in a dog with idiopathic SIAD (Fleeman *et al.*, 2000). Administration at a dose of 3 mg/kg orally q12h resulted in aquaresis and increased plasma osmolality, with good control of clinical signs over a follow-up period of 3 years. No deleterious effects were observed. Other drugs include demeclocycline, a tetracycline derivative that induces resistance to the renal effects of AVP, and urea, which increases free water clearance and decreases natriuresis. Both drugs have considerable adverse effects, and neither has been used in affected dogs or cats.

References and further reading

Barrot AC, Bédard A and Dunn M (2017) Syndrome of inappropriate antidiuretic hormone secretion in a dog with a histiocytic sarcoma. *Canadian Veterinary Journal* **58**, 713–715

Bowles KD, Brainard BM and Coleman KD (2015) Syndrome of inappropriate antidiuretic hormone in a bulldog with aspiration pneumonia. *Journal of Veterinary Internal Medicine* **29**, 972–976

Breitschwerdt EB and Root CR (1979) Inappropriate secretion of antidiuretic hormone in a dog. *Journal of the American Veterinary Medical Association* **175**, 181–186

Brofman PJ, Knostman KA and DiBartola SP (2003) Granulomatous amebic meningoencephalitis causing the syndrome of inappropriate secretion of antidiuretic hormone in a dog. *Journal of Veterinary Internal Medicine* **17**, 230–234

Cameron K and Gallagher A (2010) Syndrome of inappropriate antidiuretic hormone secretion in a cat. *Journal of the American Animal Hospital Association* **46**, 425–432

Cuesta M and Thompson CJ (2016) The syndrome of inappropriate antidiuresis (SIAD). *Best Practice & Research: Clinical Endocrinology & Metabolism* **30**, 175–187

DeMonaco SM, Koch MW and Southard TL (2014) Syndrome of inappropriate antidiuretic hormone secretion in a cat with a putative Rathke's cleft cyst. *Journal of Feline Medicine and Surgery* **16**, 1010–1015

Fleeman LM, Irwin PJ, Phillips PA and West J (2000) Effects of an oral vasopressin receptor antagonist (OPC-31260) in a dog with syndrome of inappropriate secretion of antidiuretic hormone. *Australian Veterinary Journal* **78**, 825–830

Gójska-Zygner O, Bartosik J, Górski P and Zygner W (2019) Hyponatraemia and syndrome of inappropriate antidiuretic hormone secretion in non-azotaemic dogs with babesiosis associated with decreased arterial blood pressure. *Journal of Veterinary Research* **63**, 339–344

Grant IA, Karnik K and Jandrey KE (2010) Toxicities and salvage therapy following overdose of vinblastine in a cat. *Journal of Small Animal Practice* **51**, 127–131

Houston DM, Allen DG, Kruth SA *et al.* (1989) Syndrome of inappropriate antidiuretic hormone secretion in a dog. *Canadian Veterinary Journal* **30**, 423–425

Kang MH and Park HM (2011) Syndrome of inappropriate antidiuretic hormone secretion concurrent with liver disease in a dog. *Journal of Veterinary Medical Science* **74**, 645–649

King LG and Boag A (2018) *BSAVA Manual of Canine and Feline Emergency and Critical Care, 3rd edn.* BSAVA Publications, Gloucester

Liamis G, Filippatos TD, Liontos A and Elisaf MS (2017) Hypothyroidism-associated hyponatremia: mechanisms, implications and treatment. *European Journal of Endocrinology* **176**, R15–R20

Martínez R and Torrente C (2017) Syndrome of inappropriate antidiuretic hormone secretion in a mini-breed puppy associated with aspiration pneumonia. *Topics in Companion Animal Medicine* **32**, 146–150

Meij BP, Voorhout G, van den Ingh TSGAM *et al.* (1998) Results of transsphenoidal hypophysectomy in 52 dogs with pituitary-dependent hyperadrenocorticism. *Veterinary Surgery* **27**, 246–261

Shiel RE, Pinilla M and Mooney CT (2009) Syndrome of inappropriate antidiuretic hormone secretion associated with congenital hydrocephalus in a dog. *Journal of the American Animal Hospital Association* **45**, 249–252

Chapter 12

Pituitary dwarfism

Annemarie M.W.Y. Voorbij and Hans S. Kooistra

Introduction

Growth retardation, or failure to grow, is defined as not growing at the anticipated rate or to a normal extent, resulting in dwarfism. Several endocrine and non-endocrine disorders may lead to dwarfism or growth retardation. This chapter will concentrate on congenital growth hormone (also known as somatotropin) deficiency.

Normal pituitary development

The hypophysis cerebri, or pituitary gland, is a small appendage attached to the diencephalon at the ventral midline. The term 'hypophysis cerebri' is derived from the Greek 'hypo', meaning under, and 'physis', meaning growth, together describing its presence on the undersurface of the brain. The term 'pituitary' is derived from the word 'pituita', which is Latin for mucus or phlegm, as originally the pituitary gland was thought to be the source of nasal exudates. The pituitary gland is also called the 'master gland' because, despite its small size, it plays a major regulatory role in the endocrine system. The pituitary gland is composed of two major parts:

- The adenohypophysis, also called the anterior lobe, consisting of the pars distalis and the pars intermedia
- The neurohypophysis, also called the posterior lobe or pars nervosa.

During embryogenesis, the adenohypophysis develops from Rathke's pouch, which arises from the roof of the primitive mouth adjacent to the primordium of the ventral diencephalon (Figure 12.1). At the roof of the primitive oral cavity, the ectoderm thickens and invaginates upwards to form a pouch. Eventually, the pouch will completely detach from the oral cavity. The cells of the anterior wall of Rathke's pouch proliferate and form the anterior lobe. The posterior wall of Rathke's pouch is closely apposed to the neural tissue of the neurohypophysis and forms the pars intermedia. The neurohypophysis, or posterior lobe, is derived from neural ectoderm from the base of the developing diencephalon.

The development of the adenohypophysis is a highly differentiated process that is tightly regulated by the coordinated actions of numerous transcription factors (for a review, see Zhu et al., 2007). These factors are not only involved in the formation of the adenohypophysis, but also regulate endocrine cell specification.

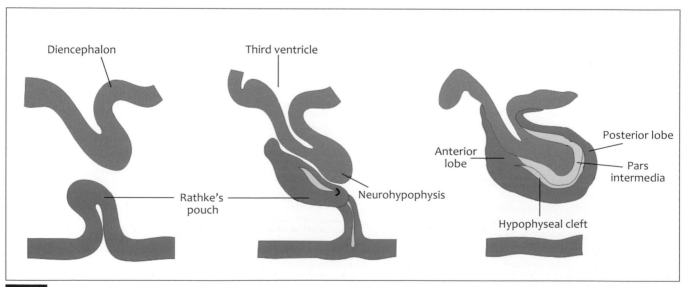

12.1 Schematic representation of canine and feline pituitary gland development.

Following proliferation of the progenitor cells that form the adenohypophysis, different endocrine cell phenotypes arise in a distinct temporal fashion and undergo highly selective differentiation. Corticotropic cells are the first to differentiate from the pituitary progenitor cells (Figure 12.2). In later stages, the pituitary progenitor cells differentiate into thyrotropes, somatolactotropes and gonadotropes. The mature anterior lobe is populated by at least five highly differentiated types of endocrine cells that are classified according to the tropic hormones they produce:

- **Somatotropic cells** – secrete growth hormone (GH)
- **Lactotropic cells** – secrete prolactin (PRL)
- **Thyrotropic cells** – secrete thyrotropin (thyroid-stimulating hormone (TSH))
- **Gonadotropic cells** – secrete luteinizing hormone (LH) and follicle-stimulating hormone (FSH)
- **Corticotropic cells** – synthesize the precursor molecule pro-opiomelanocortin (POMC), which gives rise to adrenocorticotropic hormone (ACTH) and related peptides such as alpha-melanocyte stimulating hormone (α-MSH).

In dogs and cats, the somatotropic cells account for 50% or more of the anterior lobe cells. The other cell types each represent approximately 5–15% of the endocrine cells (Rijnberk and Kooistra, 2010).

Regulation and effects of growth hormone secretion

Growth hormone is a single-chain polypeptide containing 190 amino acids. The amino acid sequence of GH varies considerably between species, but the amino acid sequence of canine GH is identical to that of porcine GH (Ascacio-Martínez and Barrera-Saldaña, 1994). Like other pituitary hormones, GH is secreted in rhythmic pulses with intervening troughs. Pituitary GH secretion is regulated mainly by the opposing actions of the stimulatory hypothalamic peptide growth hormone-releasing hormone (GHRH) and the inhibitory hypothalamic peptide somatostatin (Figure 12.3). The GH pulses predominantly reflect the pulsatile delivery of GHRH, whereas GH concentrations between pulses are primarily under somatostatin control.

Growth hormone release can also be elicited by synthetic GH secretagogues. These GH secretagogues exert their effect on GH release by acting through receptors different from those for GHRH. The endogenous ligand for these receptors is ghrelin (Kojima et al., 1999). The main source of circulating ghrelin is the stomach. Ghrelin is a potent stimulator of pituitary GH release, and in young dogs it is a more potent GH secretagogue than GHRH (Bhatti et al., 2002). The main function of ghrelin, however, is stimulation of food intake. Fasting and food intake are associated with higher and lower circulating ghrelin concentrations, respectively (Bhatti et al., 2006a). In addition, ghrelin also accelerates gastric and intestinal emptying.

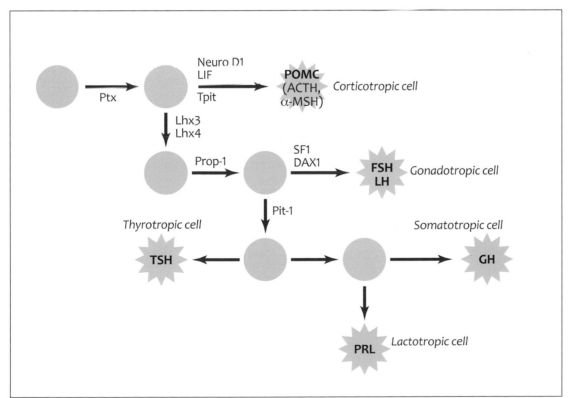

12.2 Simplified model of the differentiation of anterior lobe cell lineages. Each type of endocrine cell is labelled with the hormone(s) it synthesizes. Steps in precursor cell differentiation and some of the involved transcription factors are indicated. ACTH = adrenocorticotropic hormone; DAX1 = dosage-sensitive sex reversal-adrenal hypoplasia congenita critical region on the X chromosome 1; FSH = follicle-stimulating hormone; GH = growth hormone; LH = luteinizing hormone; Lhx3/4 = LIM-domain transcription factors 3 and 4; LIF = leukaemia inhibiting factor; α-MSH = alpha-melanocyte-stimulating hormone; Neuro D1 = neurogenic differentiation factor D1; Pit-1 = pituitary transcription factor 1; POMC = pro-opiomelanocortin; PRL = prolactin; Prop-1 = prophet of Pit-1; Ptx = pituitary homeobox; SF1 = steroidogenic factor 1; Tpit = T-box pituitary transcription factor; TSH = thyroid-stimulating hormone.

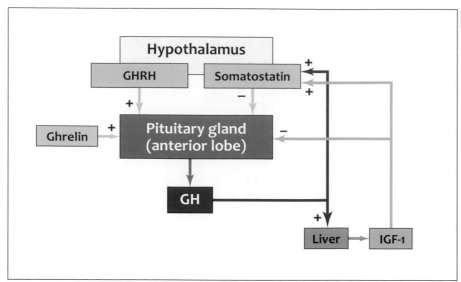

12.3 The pituitary secretion of growth hormone (GH) is under inhibitory (somatostatin) and stimulatory (GH-releasing hormone, GHRH) hypothalamic control and is also modulated by negative feedback control by insulin-like growth factor-1 (IGF-1) and GH itself. + = stimulation; – = inhibition.
(Redrawn after Rijnberk and Kooistra, 2010)

The effects of GH can be divided into two main categories, rapid catabolic actions and slow (long-lasting) anabolic actions:

- The acute catabolic actions are mainly due to insulin antagonism and result in enhanced lipolysis, gluconeogenesis and restricted glucose transport across the cell membrane. The net effect of these catabolic actions is promotion of hyperglycaemia
- The slow anabolic effects are mainly mediated via insulin-like growth factor-1 (IGF-1).

Insulin-like growth factor-1

Insulin-like growth factor-1 is produced in many different tissues, and in most it has a local (paracrine or autocrine) growth-promoting effect. The main source of circulating IGF-1 is the liver. The sequence of IGF-1 is approximately 50% identical to that of insulin. In contrast to insulin, circulating IGF-1 is bound to specific binding proteins (IGFBPs). As a result of this binding, the half-life is prolonged, which contributes to its long-term growth-promoting actions. Insulin-like growth factor-1 is an important regulator of body size through stimulation of protein synthesis, chondrogenesis and growth.

There is some evidence to suggest that the biological effects of GH and IGF-1 are not entirely distinct. There is increasing evidence that GH exerts its growth-promoting effect not only via IGF-1 but also by a direct effect on target cells. There is also evidence that GH may be the major determinant of body size. It appears that young dogs of large breeds go through a longer period of high GH release (i.e. juvenile hypersomatotropism) compared with young dogs of small breeds (Favier et al., 2001). On the other hand, there is a strong linear correlation between plasma IGF-1 concentrations and body size. Furthermore, an IGF-1 single-nucleotide polymorphism haplotype has been reported as an important factor in determining final body size in dogs (Sutter et al., 2007).

Insulin-like growth factor-1 exerts an inhibitory effect on GH release by stimulating the release of somatostatin and by a direct inhibitory influence at the level of the pituitary gland. In addition, GH itself has a negative feedback effect at the hypothalamic level (see Figure 12.3).

Pathophysiology

Any defect in the development of the pituitary gland may result in a form of isolated or combined pituitary hormone deficiency. Congenital GH deficiency, or pituitary dwarfism, is the most striking example of pituitary hormone deficiency. Congenital GH deficiency has been described in several dog breeds, including the German Shepherd Dog (GSD), Czechoslovakian Wolfdog and Saarloos Wolfdog, but only rarely in cats. The condition is encountered most often as a simple autosomal recessive inherited abnormality in GSDs. Genealogical investigations in this breed indicate that the original mutation occurred sometime around 1940, with several champion dogs suggested as likely carriers (Andresen and Willeberg, 1976). German Shepherd Dogs with dwarfism have a combined deficiency of GH, TSH and PRL, as well as impaired release of gonadotropins. By contrast, ACTH secretion is preserved in these animals (Figure 12.4) (Kooistra et al., 2000).

Originally, congenital GH deficiency in GSDs was ascribed to pressure atrophy of the anterior lobe of the pituitary gland by cyst formation in Rathke's pouch (Müller-Peddinghaus et al., 1980). Indeed, most dwarfs in this breed have pituitary cysts (Kooistra et al., 2000). However, at a young age, these dwarfs sometimes have no detectable or only a small pituitary cyst, which is unlikely to be responsible for pressure atrophy (Kooistra et al., 2000). Also, the preservation of ACTH secretion in GSD dwarfs argues against cyst formation in Rathke's pouch as the primary cause of pituitary dwarfism. The cyst formation in Rathke's pouch is currently considered a consequence of the underlying genetic defect rather than the cause of pituitary dwarfism in affected dogs.

Genetic studies have revealed that the disorder in GSDs is due to a mutation in *LHX3* (Voorbij et al., 2011). This gene encodes a member of the LIM homeodomain protein family of DNA-binding transcription factors. Molecular defects in the *LHX3* gene in humans and mice result in a deficit of all adenohypophysis hormones except for ACTH, identical to the endocrine phenotype of affected GSDs. Analysis of intron 5 of *LHX3* revealed that affected dogs have a deletion of one of six 7-basepair repeats. This small intron size is associated with defective splicing of *LHX3* (Voorbij et al., 2011).

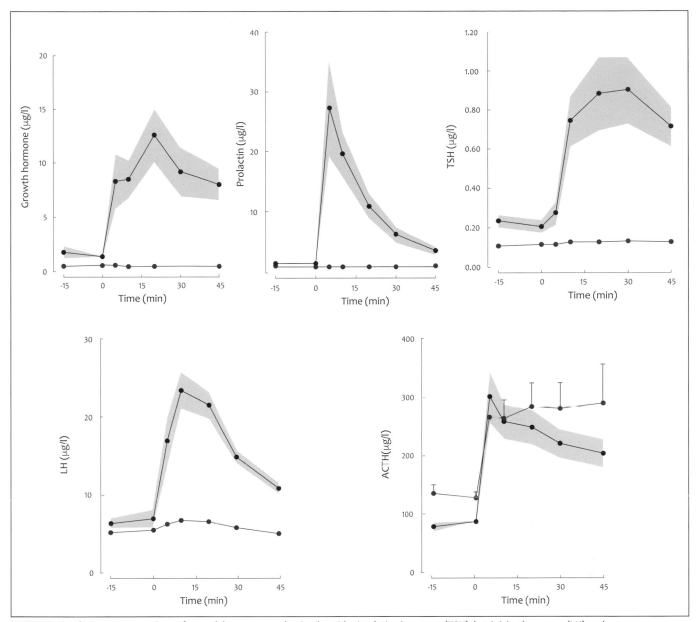

12.4 Circulating concentrations of growth hormone, prolactin, thyroid-stimulating hormone (TSH), luteinizing hormone (LH) and adrenocorticotropic hormone (ACTH) before and after the combined injection of four hypothalamic releasing hormones (corticotropin-, growth hormone-, TSH- and gonadotropin-releasing hormones) in eight German Shepherd Dogs (●) with pituitary dwarfism (mean + standard error). The mean values for eight healthy Beagles are given for comparison (●); the shaded areas represent the standard error.

The genetic defect causing congenital GH deficiency in GSDs is also the cause of pituitary dwarfism in Saarloos and Czechoslovakian Wolfdogs (Voorbij *et al.*, 2014). Both are GSD–wolf crossbreeds, and GSDs have been used in their breeding in an attempt to harden the breed. Screening of a large group of clinically healthy Saarloos and Czechoslovakian Wolfdogs revealed a high percentage of carriers of the mutated allele, of 31% and 21%, respectively (Voorbij *et al.*, 2014). These results clearly demonstrate that pituitary dwarfism is a relevant disorder in these breeds and emphasize the need for genetic screening. Pituitary dwarfism and the associated DNA defects most likely render the individuals so adversely affected that they die either *in utero* or shortly after birth, which would explain why dwarfs are only seen occasionally. The same genetic defect has recently been described in Tibetan Terriers with pituitary dwarfism (Thaiwong *et al.*, 2021). The relationship of this ancient breed to GSDs is not clear.

Congenital GH deficiency may also be due to genetic defects other than *LHX3* mutation. For example, recently, a 6-month-old Chihuahua bitch was reported with pituitary dwarfism. The deficiency in this Chihuahua was ascribed to a 6-basepair deletion in exon 5 of the GH gene, *GH1* (Iio *et al.*, 2020). An intronic mutation in the gene *POU1F1* has been described as a cause of pituitary dwarfism in the Karelian Bear Dog (Kyöstilä *et al.*, 2021).

Clinical features

Pituitary dwarfism can lead to a wide range of clinical manifestations, which are not shared by all dwarfs (Voorbij and Kooistra, 2009). During the first weeks of their lives, pituitary dwarfs may be of normal size, but after this period they grow more slowly than their littermates. Pituitary dwarfs are usually presented to the veterinary surgeon (veterinarian) at 2–5 months of age because of proportionate growth retardation, retention of lanugo or secondary hairs, and lack of primary or guard hairs (Figure 12.5). The

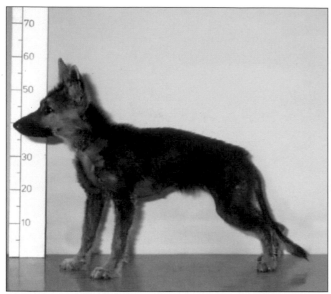

12.5 A 6-month-old German Shepherd Dog bitch with growth retardation, retention of secondary hairs (puppy coat) and lack of primary hairs due to pituitary dwarfism.

lanugo hairs are easily epilated and there is gradual development of truncal alopecia, beginning at the points of wear and sparing the head and the extremities. The skin becomes progressively hyperpigmented and scaly, and secondary bacterial infections are common. Dwarfs usually have a pointed muzzle, resembling that of a fox (Figure 12.6).

As pituitary dwarfism is an autosomal inherited disorder, there is an equal distribution between males and females. In male dwarfs, unilateral or bilateral cryptorchidism is a common feature. In female dwarfs, persistent oestrus is often observed. Persistent oestrus in affected dwarfs is characterized by swelling of the vulva, attractiveness to male dogs and bloody vaginal discharge, frequently of more than 4 weeks' duration. Circulating progesterone concentration remains low, often below 3 nmol/l, indicating that ovulation does not occur due to the absence of an LH surge.

The *LHX3* mutation is also associated with malformations of the atlantoaxial joint, leading to instability and dynamic compression of the cervical spinal cord (Voorbij *et al.*, 2015). Physical examination may reveal a continuous heart murmur due to a patent ductus arteriosus (Kooistra *et al.*, 2000).

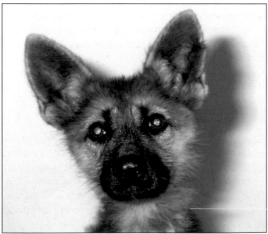

12.6 German Shepherd Dog dwarf with the characteristic pointed muzzle typical of affected animals.

Initially, pituitary dwarfs are usually bright and alert. With time, the animals develop inappetence and become less active. This situation usually becomes evident at 2–3 years of age and has been ascribed to secondary hypothyroidism and impaired kidney function (Rijnberk and Kooistra, 2010).

Differential diagnosis

Although the clinical signs of pituitary dwarfism may be very obvious, other endocrine and non-endocrine causes of growth retardation have to be excluded. Juvenile-onset (congenital) hypothyroidism may be the most important differential diagnosis, but other endocrine causes such as juvenile diabetes mellitus, iatrogenic hypercortisolism resulting from exogenous glucocorticoid administration, and even hypoadrenocorticism should be considered.

With regard to non-endocrine causes, malnutrition, gastrointestinal disorders, exocrine pancreatic insufficiency, liver disease (e.g. portosystemic shunting), kidney disease, heart failure and skeletal disorders may be the cause of growth retardation. In addition, the apparently dwarf animal may simply be a small individual within the normal biological variation, or the result of an unexpected or unwanted mating.

Diagnosis

Routine clinicopathological features

Although the clinical signs of pituitary dwarfism may be obvious, the diagnosis has to be substantiated. Usually, no significant abnormalities are noted on routine laboratory examination, except perhaps for an increased plasma creatinine concentration. Growth hormone deficiency is associated with maldevelopment of the glomeruli, and kidney function may be impaired because of a functionally decreased glomerular filtration rate as a result of the deficiencies of GH and thyroid hormones. However, it may not be apparent initially.

Thyroid hormones

Frequently, there is evidence of secondary hypothyroidism because pituitary dwarfism is often the result of combined pituitary hormone deficiency. Consequently, a circulating total thyroxine concentration below the reference interval is a common feature in pituitary dwarfs. However, instead of the increased plasma TSH concentration expected with primary hypothyroidism, TSH concentrations are often at or close to the lower limit of the TSH assay because of decreased pituitary TSH secretion.

Growth hormone

Direct information regarding the function of the somatotropic cells can be obtained by measuring circulating GH concentrations. However, as GH is secreted in a pulsatile fashion, and the basal circulating GH concentrations may also be low in healthy animals, a definitive diagnosis of GH deficiency cannot be based upon a low circulating GH concentration alone. As the amino acid sequence of GH varies between species, concentrations should be determined by a species-specific assay. Unfortunately, such assays for measuring canine and feline GH are not widely available.

Insulin-like growth factor-1

Growth hormone deficiency results in a low circulating IGF-1 concentration (see Figure 12.3). The amino acid sequence of IGF-1 is less species specific than that of GH and therefore IGF-1 can be determined using a hetero-logous (human) assay (Rijnberk and Kooistra, 2010). Moreover, circulating IGF-1 has a long half-life and the secretion of IGF-1 is not episodic. As a result, measure-ment of the plasma IGF-1 concentration can be used to assess the GH status of an animal indirectly.

Circulating IGF-1 concentrations are low in pituitary dwarfs, even when age and body size are taken into account. The mean (± standard error) plasma IGF-1 con-centration in GSD dwarfs has been reported to be 62 ± 10 ng/ml, which is considerably lower than the mean plasma IGF-1 concentrations in healthy adult (280 ± 23 ng/ml) and immature (345 ± 50 ng/ml) GSDs (Kooistra et al., 2000). Nevertheless, IGF-1 measurements do not pro-vide such a definitive diagnosis as do the measurements of GH after stimulation.

Pituitary function tests

Given the problems of basal GH analysis, a definitive diagnosis of pituitary dwarfism using GH measurement should only be based on the results of a stimulation test. For this purpose, intravenous GH stimulants such as GHRH (1 µg/kg) or alpha-adrenergic drugs, such as cloni-dine (10 µg/kg) or xylazine (100 µg/kg), can be used. Growth hormone concentrations are determined immedi-ately before and 20–30 minutes after administration of the stimulant.

In healthy dogs, circulating GH concentrations should increase at least two- to four-fold after stimulation. In dogs with pituitary dwarfism there is no significant increase in circulating GH concentrations (see Figure 12.4). Administration of xylazine or clonidine may result in seda-tion, bradycardia, hypotension or vomiting. The ghrelin stimulation test is a possible alternative. A circulating GH concentration greater than 5 µg/l 20 minutes after intra-venous administration of 2 µg/kg human ghrelin excludes pituitary dwarfism (Bhatti et al., 2006b).

To test the secretory capacity of the other hormone-secreting pituitary cells, the adenohypophysis can be concurrently stimulated with intravenous corticotropin-releasing hormone (CRH, 1 µg/kg), thyrotropin-releasing hormone (TRH, 10 µg/kg) and gonadotropin-releasing hormone (GnRH, 10 µg/kg) (Meij et al., 1996). The results of this combined adenohypophyseal function test in healthy dogs and GSDs with pituitary dwarfism are depicted in Figure 12.4.

Diagnostic imaging

Diagnostic imaging of the pituitary area (using computed tomography or magnetic resonance imaging) often reveals the presence of pituitary cysts in dogs with congenital GH deficiency (Figure 12.7). In the majority of young dogs with pituitary dwarfism, the pituitary gland is quite small despite the presence of cysts (Kooistra et al., 2000). This is compatible with pituitary hypoplasia. The size of the cysts gradually enlarges during life (Kooistra et al., 1998). When large cysts are present, the pituitary size may also increase. It is important to note that pituitary cysts are not unusual in healthy dogs, especially in brachycephalic breeds. Consequently, the presence of pituitary cysts is not synonymous with pituitary dwarfism.

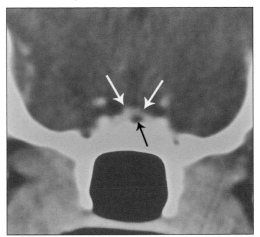

12.7 Contrast-enhanced computed tomography image of the pituitary area of a German Shepherd Dog dwarf at 6 months of age with a pituitary gland of normal size (height 3.6 mm; width 4.3 mm). A radiolucent area with a diameter of 1.5 mm is visible in the pituitary gland, suggestive of a cyst (arrowed).

Genetic testing

Identification of the *LHX3* mutation causing pituitary dwarf-ism in GSDs, Saarloos and Czechoslovakian Wolfdogs resulted in the development of a DNA test (Voorbij et al., 2011, 2014). The availability of this diagnostic test not only allows confirmation of the clinical diagnosis in affected dogs, but also enables breeders to select against the trait by identifying carriers of the *LHX3* mutation. If all breeding animals were genetically tested for the presence of the *LHX3* mutation, and an appropriate breeding policy imple-mented, this disease could be eradicated completely.

Treatment

Unfortunately, canine GH is not available for therapeutic use. Attempts have been made to treat canine dwarfs with human GH. However, because of the differences between canine and human GH, antibody formation may preclude its use (Van Herpen et al., 1994). Administration of porcine GH does not result in antibody formation, because of the simi-larity of porcine and canine GH (Ascacio-Martínez and Barrera-Saldaña, 1994), but legislation forbids its use in most European countries.

The recommended subcutaneous dose for porcine GH is 0.1–0.3 IU/kg three times per week. This treatment may result in GH excess and consequently side effects such as diabetes mellitus may develop. Therefore, three-weekly monitoring of the circulating concentrations of GH and glucose is recommended. Long-term dose rates should be based on measurements of circulating IGF-1 concentra-tions. Whether or not administration of porcine GH will lead to linear growth is dependent on the status of the growth plates when treatment is initiated. A beneficial response in the skin and hair coat usually occurs within 6–8 weeks after the start of therapy. The hairs that grow back are mainly lanugo hairs; growth of guard hairs is variable.

Progestins are capable of inducing expression of the GH gene in the canine mammary gland and subsequent secretion of GH into the systemic circulation (Selman et al., 1994). This has raised the possibility of progestin treatment for GH deficiency. Treatment of young dwarfs with medro-xyprogesterone acetate at 2.5–5.0 mg/kg s.c., initially at 3-week intervals and subsequently at 6-week intervals, has resulted in some increase in body size and the development of a complete adult hair coat. Parallel with the physical improvements, circulating IGF-1 concentrations increase sharply, whereas GH concentrations increase but do not exceed the upper limit of the reference interval (Kooistra *et al.*, 1998). Similarly, proligestone treatment of pituitary dwarfs has been reported to result in the development of an adult hair coat, bodyweight gain and increased plasma IGF-1 concentration (Knottenbelt and Herrtage, 2002). Progestin treatment may be associated with several side effects, including:

- Recurrent periods of pruritic pyoderma
- Skeletal maldevelopment
- Development of mammary tumours
- Hypersomatotropism
- Diabetes mellitus
- Cystic endometrial hyperplasia.

As with treatment using porcine GH, monitoring of circulating concentrations of GH, IGF-1 and glucose is important. In bitches, an ovariohysterectomy should be performed before progestin treatment is initiated. Thyroid hormone supplementation should be started as soon as there is any evidence of secondary hypothyroidism.

Prognosis

The long-term prognosis for dwarfs is usually poor without appropriate treatment. By 3–5 years of age, affected animals are usually bald, thin and dull. These changes are usually due to:

- Progressive loss of pituitary function
- Continuing expansion of pituitary cysts
- Progressive kidney disease.

At this stage, owners usually request euthanasia for their dog, if they have not done so long before (Rijnberk and Kooistra, 2010). Although the prognosis improves significantly when dwarfs are adequately treated with either porcine GH or progestins (and thyroid hormone supplementation), it remains guarded.

References and further reading

Andresen E and Willeberg P (1976) Pituitary dwarfism in German shepherd dogs: additional evidence of simple, autosomal recessive inheritance. *Nordisk Veterinaermedicin* **28**, 481–486

Ascacio-Martínez JA and Barrera-Saldaña HA (1994) A dog growth hormone cDNA codes for a mature protein identical to pig growth hormone. *Gene* **143**, 277–280

Bhatti SF, Hofland LJ, Van Koetsveld P *et al.* (2006b) Effects of food intake and food withholding on plasma ghrelin concentrations in healthy dogs. *American Journal of Veterinary Research* **67**, 1557–1563

Bhatti SFM, De Vliegher SP, Mol JA, Van Ham LML and Kooistra HS (2006a) Ghrelin-stimulation test in the diagnosis of canine pituitary dwarfism. *Research in Veterinary Science* **81**, 24–30

Bhatti SFM, De Vliegher SP, Van Ham L and Kooistra HS (2002) Effects of growth hormone-releasing peptides in healthy dogs and in dogs with pituitary-dependent hyperadrenocorticism. *Molecular and Cellular Endocrinology* **197**, 97–103

Favier RP, Mol JA, Kooistra HS and Rijnberk A (2001) Large body size in the dog is associated with transient GH excess at a young age. *Journal of Endocrinology* **170**, 479–484

Iio A, Maeda S, Yonezawa T, Momoi Y and Motegi T (2020) Isolated growth hormone deficiency in a Chihuahua with a *GH1* mutation. *Journal of Veterinary Diagnostic Investigation* **32**, 733–736

Knottenbelt CM and Herrtage ME (2002) Use of proligestone in the management of three German shepherd dogs with pituitary dwarfism. *Journal of Small Animal Practice* **43**, 164–170

Kojima M, Hosoda H, Date Y *et al.* (1999) Ghrelin is a growth-hormone-releasing acylated peptide from stomach. *Nature* **402**, 656–660

Kooistra HS, Voorhout G, Selman PJ and Rijnberk A (1998) Progestin-induced growth hormone (GH) production in the treatment of dogs with congenital GH deficiency. *Domestic Animal Endocrinology* **15**, 93–102

Kooistra HS, Voorhout G, Mol JA and Rijnberk A (2000) Combined pituitary hormone deficiency in German shepherd dogs with dwarfism. *Domestic Animal Endocrinology* **19**, 177–190

Kyöstilä K, Niskanen JE, Arumilli M *et al.* (2021) Intronic variant in *POU1F1* associated with canine pituitary dwarfism. *Human Genetics* **140**, 1553–1562

Meij BP, Mol JA, Hazewinkel HAW, Bevers MM and Rijnberk A (1996) Assessment of a combined anterior pituitary function test in beagle dogs: rapid sequential intravenous administration of four hypothalamic releasing hormones. *Domestic Animal Endocrinology* **13**, 161–170

Müller-Peddinghaus R, El Eltebry MF, Siefert J and Ranke M (1980) Hypophysärer Zwergwuchs beim Deutschen Schäferhund. *Veterinary Pathology* **17**, 406–421

Rijnberk A and Kooistra HS (2010) Hypothalamus-pituitary system. In: *Clinical Endocrinology of Dogs and Cats, 2nd edition*, ed. A Rijnberk and HS Kooistra, pp. 13–54. Schlütersche Verlagsgesellschaft mbH & Co, Hannover

Selman PJ, Mol JA, Rutteman GR, van Garderen E and Rijnberk A (1994) Progestin-induced growth hormone excess in the dog originates in the mammary gland. *Endocrinology* **134**, 287–292

Sutter NB, Bustamante CD, Chase K *et al.* (2007) A single *IGF1* allele is a major determinant of small size in dogs. *Science* **316**, 112–115

Thaiwong T, Corner S, La Forge S and Kiupel M (2021) Dwarfism in Tibetan Terrier dogs with an *LHX3* mutation. *Journal of Veterinary Diagnostic Investigation* **33**, 740–732

Van Herpen H, Rijnberk A and Mol JA (1994) Production of antibodies to biosynthetic human growth hormone in the dog. *Veterinary Record* **134**, 171

Voorbij AMWY and Kooistra HS (2009) Pituitary dwarfism in German Shepherd dogs. *Journal of Veterinary Clinical Sciences* **2**, 4–11

Voorbij AMWY, Leegwater PA and Kooistra HS (2014) Pituitary dwarfism in Saarloos and Czechoslovakian wolfdogs is associated with a mutation in *LHX3*. *Journal of Veterinary Internal Medicine* **28**, 1770–1774

Voorbij AMWY, Meij BP, van Bruggen LWL *et al.* (2015) Atlanto-axial malformation and instability in dogs with pituitary dwarfism due to an *LHX3* mutation. *Journal of Veterinary Internal Medicine* **29**, 207–213

Voorbij AMWY, Van Steenbeek FG, Vos-Loohuis M *et al.* (2011) A contracted DNA repeat in *LHX3* intron 5 is associated with aberrant splicing and pituitary dwarfism in German shepherd dogs. *PLoS ONE* **6**, e27940

Zhu X, Gleiberman AS and Rosenfeld MG (2007) Molecular physiology of pituitary development: signaling and transcriptional networks. *Physiological Reviews* **87**, 933–963

Chapter 13

Hypersomatotropism

Stijn Niessen

Introduction

Growth hormone (GH), or somatotropin, is a single-chain polypeptide hormone that is synthesized, stored, and secreted by the somatotropic cells within the pars distalis of the anterior pituitary gland. In health, GH is secreted in a well regulated pulsatile fashion, stimulated by GH-releasing hormone (GHRH) and inhibited by somatostatin. Growth hormone itself, as well as GH-induced insulin-like growth factor-1 (IGF-1), also provides its own negative feedback. This is described in greater detail in Chapter 12.

Specific pathological conditions in the dog and cat can result in excess production of GH. This is called hypersomatotropism and, if present chronically, can cause a broad range of clinical signs reflecting the many different biological functions of this hormone. Ultimately, chronic excess exposure to GH can lead to the clinical syndrome of acromegaly. In the last two decades, hypersomatotropism has become increasingly recognized, particularly in diabetic but also occasionally in non-diabetic cats. Both predisposing genetic factors (*AIP* gene mutations) and environmental factors (organohalogenated contaminants) have been implicated in the possible increase in prevalence of hypersomatotropism in the cat (Dirtu *et al.*, 2013; Scudder *et al.*, 2017).

Growth hormone exerts its effects both directly and indirectly. The indirect actions of GH are mediated by IGF-1, which is predominantly produced by the liver, provided there is sufficient portal insulin. Insulin-like growth factor-1 has anabolic effects, increasing protein synthesis and soft tissue and skeletal growth. By contrast, the direct effects of GH are predominantly catabolic and include lipolysis and restricted cellular glucose transport. Extensive research has shown that GH is an important modulator of insulin sensitivity through a wide variety of mechanisms. Excessive GH concentrations can therefore induce insulin resistance as well as overt diabetes mellitus.

Aetiology

In the vast majority of cases, the pathogenesis of GH excess is different in cats than it is in dogs.

Dogs

In bitches, hypersomatotropism is almost exclusively caused by excess progesterone or progestins that induce overproduction of GH by mammary tissue (Concannon *et al.*, 1980; Eigenmann and Venker-van Haagen, 1981; Eigenmann *et al.*, 1983). Mature intact bitches may develop hypersomatotropism spontaneously because of the high endogenous progesterone concentrations of dioestrus (Eigenmann and Venker-van Haagen, 1981; Eigenmann *et al.*, 1983). Alternatively, hypersomatotropism may result from attempts to suppress oestrus through the administration of long-acting progestins (e.g. medroxyprogesterone acetate). Pregnancy has also been reported to result in hypersomatotropism in at least two bitches that developed diabetes mellitus during pregnancy (Norman *et al.*, 2006; Fall *et al.*, 2010).

With either endogenous progesterone or exogenous progestin excess, GH excess occurs because of induction of expression of the gene encoding GH in the mammary gland (Selman *et al.*, 1994a; Mol *et al.*, 1996). As the mammary- and pituitary-expressed genes are identical, GH secreted by the mammary gland is biochemically identical to pituitary GH. Additionally, cases of mammary-tumour-induced GH oversecretion have also been described in the dog (Murai *et al.*, 2012).

Three suspected cases and one confirmed case of hypersomatotropism due to a GH-secreting pituitary tumour have been described in dogs and represent a rare exception to the above-described predominant aetiology (Lucksch, 1923; King *et al.*, 1962; Fracassi *et al.*, 2007; Zublena *et al.*, 2018). Additionally, hypothyroidism-induced excess GH secretion and the clinical syndrome of acromegaly, including diabetes mellitus, has been reported in one dog (Johnstone *et al.*, 2014).

Cats

In cats, as in humans, hypersomatotropism is most often caused by an adenoma of the GH-secreting somatotropes in the pars distalis of the pituitary gland (Niessen, 2010; Scudder *et al.*, 2018). Hyperplasia, rather than adenoma, is also recognized as a cause in a minority of cats with hypersomatotropism (Niessen *et al.*, 2007b; Niessen, 2010; Scudder *et al.*, 2018). This hyperplasia might represent a pre-adenomatous change or a separate disease process. Hypersecretion of multiple hormones (including hyperprolactinaemia) represents a minority of acromegalic disease in humans. One cat with a double pituitary adenoma causing both hypercortisolism and hypersomatotropism has been described (Meij *et al.*, 2004). As in dogs, administration of progestins to cats can induce expression of the mammary GH gene and thereby stimulate the local production of GH in the mammary gland (Mol *et al.*, 1996). As in dogs, this mammary-expressed gene was found to be identical to the pituitary-expressed gene, as well as being driven by the same promoter (Mol *et al.*, 2000). However, this local production of GH has never been shown to lead to high circulating GH concentrations or the clinical state of acromegaly in cats (Peterson, 1987; Niessen, 2010).

Clinical features

Many of the clinical and laboratory features in dogs and cats with hypersomatotropism are similar but there are some notable differences.

Signalment

In dogs and cats, naturally occurring hypersomatotropism is a disease of middle to old age with no apparent breed predisposition. A large group of cats with hypersomatotropism had a median age of approximately 12 years (range 6–17 years) (Niessen *et al.*, 2015).

In contrast to humans, where hypersomatotropism has no sex predilection, affected cats are more likely to be male, with a reported ratio of 7:1 (Niessen *et al.*, 2007a, 2015). Virtually all dogs with naturally occurring hypersomatotropism are entire bitches (Eigenmann and Venker-van Haagen, 1981; Eigenmann *et al.*, 1983). Interestingly, all four reported dogs with hypersomatotropism and a functional pituitary adenoma were male.

History and physical examination

Not all of the expected changes or signs associated with hypersomatotropism are consistently present in all affected animals, especially when the clinician's index of suspicion is high and the disease is encountered early. Cats with hypersomatotropism can be (at least initially) morphologically indistinguishable from cats without the disease, and this may at least partly explain the apparent 'underdiagnosis' of this endocrinopathy (Niessen *et al.*, 2007a, 2010, 2015).

Additionally, it is increasingly recognized that, as in humans, hypersomatotropism is not always associated with diabetes mellitus. Alternative presentations in cats have included seizures, polyphagia and weight gain, upper respiratory stridor and stertor, and hypertrophic changes to the myocardium (Fletcher *et al.*, 2016; Steele *et al.*, 2021).

The historical and physical examination findings from the largest series of cats with hypersomatotropism are presented in Figure 13.1 (Niessen *et al.*, 2007a, 2015).

Most common owner-reported historical findings
• Polyuria
• Polydipsia
• Polyphagia (often extreme)
• Weight gain
• Lameness
• Central nervous system signs
• Increase in paw size
• Broad facial features
• Abdominal enlargement
• Plantigrade stance – hindlimbs (diabetic neuropathy)

13.1 Historical and physical examination findings of feline hypersomatotropism. (continues) ▶

(Data from Niessen *et al.*, 2007a, 2015)

Most common clinician-reported physical examination findings
• Abdominal organomegaly (liver and kidneys)
• Broad facial features
• Respiratory stridor
• Prognathia inferior with increased distance between upper and lower canine teeth
• Multiple limb lameness
• Systolic cardiac murmur
• Clubbed (enlarged) paws
• Central nervous system signs
• Gallop rhythm
• Plantigrade stance – hindlimbs
• Periods of open-mouth breathing and tachypnoea when stressed (due to congestive heart failure)

13.1 (continued) Historical and physical examination findings of feline hypersomatotropism.

(Data from Niessen *et al.*, 2007a, 2015)

In humans, the earliest recognizable signs of acromegaly are soft tissue swelling and hypertrophy of the face and extremities. Both dogs and cats with hypersomatotropism have been reported to show mandibular enlargement resulting in prognathism, widened interdental spaces, thickening of the bony ridges of the skull, large paws, and soft tissue swelling of the head and neck (Niessen *et al.*, 2007b) (Figures 13.2 and 13.3).

Growth hormone-induced proliferation of connective tissue may cause the body to increase in size, most frequently manifested as marked weight gain and enlargement of the abdomen and face. The increase in bodyweight can occur despite the presence of the catabolic state of unregulated diabetes mellitus. Weight gain should therefore prompt consideration of hypersomatotropism as a concurrent disorder, especially in poorly regulated diabetic cats. In dogs, the skin may become thickened and develop excessive folds, particularly around the head and neck.

Hypertrophy of all organs in the body (e.g. heart, liver, kidneys and tongue) has also been described with hypersomatotropism, especially in cats (Figure 13.4).

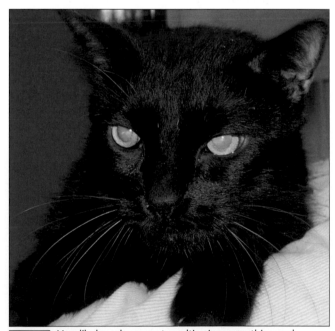

13.2 Mandibular enlargement resulting in prognathism and thickening of the bony ridges of the skull in a cat with hypersomatotropism. While a typical finding, this is not seen in all cats with hypersomatotropism.

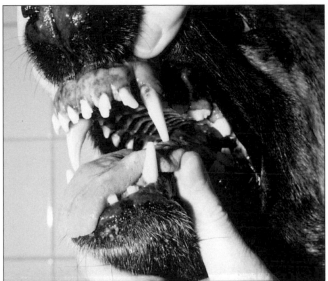

13.3 Widening of interdental spaces due to chronic exposure to excess growth hormone in a dog with hypersomatotropism.

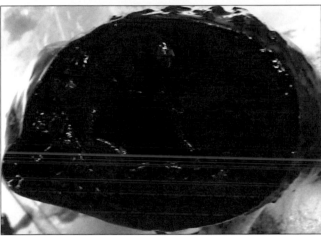

13.4 Cross-section of the heart from a cat with hypersomatotropism, showing generalized myocardial hypertrophy.

Diabetes mellitus

Diabetes mellitus remains a commonly recognized clinical manifestation of hypersomatotropism in cats (Niessen *et al.*, 2007a, 2010, 2015). The largest screening study to date, which included 1221 diabetic cats in the UK, found that approximately 25% were suffering from hypersomatotropism-induced diabetes mellitus (Niessen *et al.*, 2015). Diabetes mellitus is also common in affected dogs and, even in the absence of overt disease, carbohydrate intolerance may be apparent (Eigenmann and Venker-van Haagen, 1981; Fracassi *et al.*, 2007).

Extensive research has shown that GH is an important inhibitor of insulin sensitivity and thus evokes a compensatory increase in insulin production. In a proportion of cats, this chronic overproduction of insulin results in accelerated islet apoptosis and so-called 'islet exhaustion'. The combination of decreased insulin-secreting capacity and insulin resistance leads to hyperglycaemia and glucosuria and accompanying clinical signs of diabetes mellitus, including polyuria and polydipsia (PU/PD) and polyphagia, in some cats. Although polyphagia is a recognized sign of uncontrolled diabetes mellitus, the excess GH is also likely to play an important role in this phenomenon. This is substantiated by the frequent observation of persistent, and often extreme, polyphagia, despite apparent reasonable control of the diabetes mellitus, in cats with hypersomatotropism treated with insulin only.

Respiratory signs

In dogs with hypersomatotropism, soft tissue proliferation in the oropharyngeal region may be so profound that they exhibit panting, exercise intolerance and inspiratory stridor due to compression of the upper airway (Eigenmann *et al.*, 1983; Fracassi *et al.*, 2007; Zublena *et al.*, 2018). In cats, inspiratory stridor due to upper airway narrowing occurs relatively frequently (>50%) (Niessen *et al.*, 2007a, 2015; Niessen, 2010; Fletcher *et al.*, 2016). Dyspnoea may also develop in cats with long-standing untreated hypersomatotropism as a result of pulmonary oedema or pleural effusion from assumed GH-induced cardiac failure (Fletcher *et al.*, 2016; Steele *et al.*, 2021).

Orthopaedic signs

In some cats with hypersomatotropism, articular changes (associated with degenerative arthritis) are severe and crippling. Radiographic evidence includes:

- An increase in joint space secondary to thickening of the articular cartilage
- Cortical thickening
- Osteophyte proliferation
- Periarticular periosteal reaction
- Joint collapse.

A similar arthropathy has not been observed in dogs.

Both cats and dogs with hypersomatotropism may develop mandibular prognathism with an underbite of the lower incisors. The spacing between the teeth may increase, a common change in dogs (see Figure 13.3). In cats, an increase in the distance between the upper and lower canine teeth might be observed. Computed tomography (CT) studies have shown an overall thickening of the skull bones and widening of the facial structure (Lamb *et al.*, 2014).

Cardiovascular signs

Recent studies have confirmed the impact of excess GH on the feline myocardium, causing changes virtually indistinguishable from idiopathic hypertrophic cardiomyopathy (HCM) without the use of histopathology (Borgeat *et al.*, 2018). Effective treatment of hypersomatotropism may result in normalization of the myocardium. Therefore, consideration should be given to screening cats presenting with HCM for underlying hypersomatotropism. One study estimated the prevalence of hypersomatotropism among such cats as just under 7% (Steele *et al.*, 2021). Radiographic findings may be normal or may include mild to severe cardiomegaly, pleural effusion and pulmonary oedema. Echocardiography frequently reveals left ventricular and septal hypertrophy but can also be normal; electrocardiogram findings are generally unremarkable. Similar cardiac changes have not been observed in dogs with hypersomatotropism.

Hypertension, which is common in humans with hypersomatotropism, has thus far not proven to be more prevalent than would be expected in a group of age-matched control cats (Niessen *et al.*, 2007a; Borgeat *et al.*, 2018).

Neurological signs

In cats, central nervous system (CNS) signs can develop as a result of expansion of the pituitary tumour beyond the sella turcica. These can include epileptic seizures (Fletcher *et al.*, 2016). However, this presentation is uncommon as the tumours tend to be both benign and slow growing, and overt neurological signs are rare even when a large pituitary tumour is compressing and invading the hypothalamus (Niessen *et al.*, 2007a, 2015). The vast majority of dogs with hypersomatotropism do not have pituitary tumours and CNS signs do not occur. They are, however, possible in those rare dogs with pituitary tumours.

Kidney disease

Polyuria and polydipsia are common signs of hypersomatotropism in cats and dogs and appear to develop primarily because of the associated diabetic state. An increased prevalence of kidney disease has not been proven in cats or dogs with hypersomatotropism. A case of non-diabetic canine hypersomatotropism with extreme PU/PD during dioestrus has been described (Schwedes, 1999). Transient central diabetes insipidus was demonstrated by documenting an inadequate rise of arginine vasopressin concentration after water deprivation and stimulation with hypertonic saline. Clinical signs, except for bony changes, completely disappeared in this dog following ovariohysterectomy. The relationship between CDI and excess GH is unclear.

Reproductive signs

In dogs with progesterone-induced hypersomatotropism, concomitant mammary gland nodules, cystic endometrial hyperplasia or pyometra may develop (Concannon *et al.*, 1980). The pathogenesis of the mammary gland nodules involves progesterone-induced GH production by the mammary gland tissue; GH then acts locally in an autocrine or paracrine manner to promote mammary tumorigenesis by stimulating proliferation of susceptible mammary epithelial cells. By contrast, the pathogenesis of the uterine changes of cystic endometrial hyperplasia probably involves a direct effect of the progesterone excess rather than GH, since uterine production of GH does not occur in dogs (Kooistra *et al.*, 1997).

Iatrogenic hypoadrenocorticism

Dogs with hypersomatotropism caused by the chronic administration of progestins may develop iatrogenic hypoadrenocorticism, characterized by low serum cortisol concentrations (both basal and adrenocorticotropic hormone (ACTH)-stimulated cortisol) and atrophy of the adrenal cortex. The intrinsic glucocorticoid-like activity of these progestins suppresses ACTH secretion, causing the secondary hypoadrenocorticism (Selman *et al.*, 1994b). Cats may also develop iatrogenic hypoadrenocorticism secondary to progestins, but they do not develop hypersomatotropism.

Pancreatic disease

Pancreatic disease has previously been reported in feline hypersomatotropism. Specific macroscopic and microscopic lesions described have included pancreatic enlargement, cysts, diffuse hyperplasia with fibrous tissue and lymphoid follicles (Figure 13.5). It remains to be determined

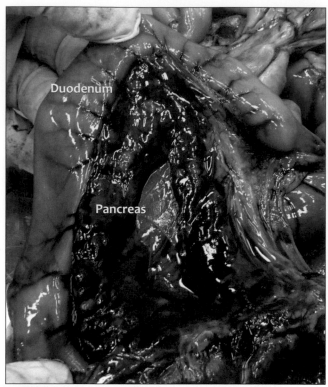

13.5 Macroscopic abnormalities, specifically pancreatic enlargement and cysts, in a pancreas from a cat with hypersomatotropism.

if pancreatic disease is indeed more common in cats with hypersomatotropism. This is especially true in view of the relatively small number of cases reported thus far, together with the potentially high prevalence of pancreatic disease, based on increased feline pancreas-specific lipase concentrations found in the general diabetic cat population (Forcada *et al.*, 2008). Pathology of the pancreas could represent a secondary effect of long-term insulin-resistant diabetes mellitus or direct effects of excess GH and IGF-1.

Other neoplastic disorders

An association between hypersomatotropism and colorectal cancer is reported in humans. Since relatively few cases of feline hypersomatotropism have been described thus far, it is difficult to estimate the prevalence of neoplasia in cats with hypersomatotropism. Nevertheless, cats with hypersomatotropism have had pharyngeal or oesophageal neoplasia on post-mortem examination. Further investigation of a definitive link is required.

Diagnosis

Diagnosis is dependent on demonstrating excess production of GH and/or IGF-1 concentrations in animals with appropriate clinical signs.

- Hypersomatotropism should be suspected in bitches receiving progestins and intact bitches that develop diabetes mellitus or laryngeal stridor during dioestrus or pregnancy (Eigenmann and Venker-van Haagen, 1981; Eigenmann *et al.*, 1983; Norman *et al.*, 2006; Fall *et al.*, 2008, 2010).
- Screening for hypersomatotropism should be discussed with owners whose cats have been diagnosed with

diabetes mellitus, given the high prevalence of hypersomatotropism among diabetic cats.

- Hypersomatotropism should be suspected in any cat that has insulin-resistant diabetes mellitus (i.e. persistent hyperglycaemia despite total daily insulin doses of >1.5 IU/kg/injection on a twice-daily regimen) or poorly controlled diabetes mellitus (Niessen *et al.*, 2007a).
- Hypersomatotropism should also be at least considered in older cats presenting with HCM, upper respiratory stridor, unexplained polyphagia, weight gain or a pituitary tumour.
- Hypersomatotropism should also be considered in male dogs presenting with supportive signs.

Routine clinicopathological features

Routine biochemistry and haematology are not useful in providing support for hypersomatotropism, apart from the possible changes associated with diabetes mellitus.

Growth hormone and IGF-1 concentrations

Confirmation of the diagnosis ideally requires demonstration of a high circulating GH concentration. An in-house radioimmunoassay using ovine GH standards and antibodies was partially validated for cats and results proved useful in distinguishing healthy cats from cats with hypersomatotropism, with no overlap between the two groups (Niessen *et al.*, 2007a). A confirmed case of hypersomatotropism with a GH concentration less than 10 ng/ml has yet to be described. Additionally, stability studies demonstrated that feline GH concentrations remained stable in circumstances similar to overnight transport at room temperature, making estimation of serum feline GH concentrations a potentially practical method of confirming a diagnosis. Unfortunately, this assay is not currently widely available. A species specific canine assay is also not widely available.

Measurement of serum IGF-1 concentrations contributes to the diagnosis of hypersomatotropism by indirectly evaluating the GH concentration. The IGF-1 concentration reflects the magnitude of GH secretion over the previous 24 hours and has been reported to be high in both dogs and cats with hypersomatotropism (Middleton *et al.*, 1985; Abrams-Ogg *et al.*, 1993; Berg *et al.*, 2007; Niessen *et al.*, 2007b, 2015). An abnormally high serum IGF-1 concentration strongly suggests hypersomatotropism, but the disease should not be excluded if values are within the upper half of the reference interval. Portal insulin is necessary for hepatic IGF-1 production, which means that IGF-1 concentrations can be falsely low in a diabetic cat with hypersomatotropism before or at the start of insulin therapy. However, with 2–4 weeks of insulin treatment, IGF-1 concentrations may increase into the diagnostic range. In addition, increased serum IGF-1 concentrations have been reported in insulin-treated diabetic cats without hypersomatotropism, and thus false-positive test results can also occur (Lewitt *et al.*, 2000; Niessen *et al.*, 2007b).

If circulating GH or IGF-1 concentrations cannot be measured, most dogs with hypersomatotropism are tentatively diagnosed on the basis of a characteristic set of clinical features in an animal with a history of recent dioestrus or pregnancy, or exposure to progestins, together with an improvement in clinical signs after withdrawal of progestins, cessation of gestation or ovariohysterectomy.

If circulating IGF-1 concentration cannot be measured, diagnosing feline hypersomatotropism probably represents a bigger challenge. Documentation of a pituitary mass by CT or magnetic resonance imaging adds further support for the diagnosis, with the latter being a more sensitive method for this particular condition (Abrams-Ogg *et al.*, 1993; Elliott *et al.*, 2000; Niessen *et al.*, 2007b) (Figure 13.6). However, normal intracranial imaging does not preclude a diagnosis of feline hypersomatotropism and the demonstration of a pituitary tumour does not provide evidence of function (Niessen *et al.*, 2007b, 2015).

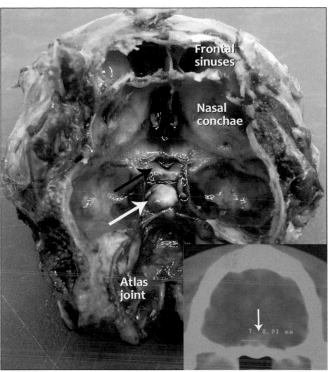

13.6 Post-mortem examination and computed tomographic findings in a cat with hypersomatotropism. The white arrows indicate the enlarged pituitary gland. The black arrow indicates the optic chiasm, illustrating the potential, albeit rare, for visual abnormalities to occur when a large pituitary tumour is present.

Differential diagnoses

In dogs, the signalment, history and physical examination findings are usually suggestive of hypersomatotropism. In cats, other common causes of diabetes mellitus or poor glycaemic control must be considered. These include:

- Concurrent endocrinopathies (hyperthyroidism, hypercortisolism)
- Iatrogenic hormone administration (corticosteroids)
- Other diseases (obesity, neoplasia, kidney disease, cardiovascular disease)
- Stress hyperglycaemia mimicking true insulin resistance
- Management-associated causes (incorrect insulin administration or storage, use of inactive insulin preparations, hypoglycaemia-induced hyperglycaemia, short duration of insulin action)
- Infectious disease (urinary tract infection, dental disease)
- Inflammatory disease (pancreatitis, inflammatory bowel disease, gingivostomatitis).

In cats, differentiation of hypersomatotropism from pituitary-dependent hypercortisolism is particularly important because both diseases can cause insulin resistance despite poorly controlled diabetes mellitus. Furthermore, a pituitary tumour and positive tests for hypercortisolism can be detected in both conditions. Successful differentiation can be achieved through careful assessment for specific clinical differences. For example, broad facial features, clubbed paws, arthropathy, prognathia inferior and particularly severe insulin resistance are features of hypersomatotropism, while frail skin, fur changes, bruising and less severe insulin resistance are more suggestive of hypercortisolism. Endocrine testing, including measurement of feline GH and/or IGF-1 concentrations, may also aid differentiation.

However, similar myocardial hypertrophy is present in cats with hypersomatotropism and idiopathic HCM, as well as secondary to hyperthyroidism or hypertension. Nasal and nasopharyngeal polyps, neoplasia and nasopharyngeal stenosis can mimic the upper respiratory stridor and stertor seen in some feline cases of hypersomatotropism.

Treatment

Dogs

In dogs, progesterone/progestin-induced hypersomatotropism is treated by ovariohysterectomy or discontinuation of progestin-based medication (Eigenmann and Venker-van Haagen, 1981; Eigenmann et al., 1983). Circulating GH concentrations will normalize rapidly after ovariohysterectomy, or more slowly after withdrawal of progestin-based medication. This will be accompanied by resolution of the soft tissue proliferation and signs of respiratory stridor; however, the skeletal changes may persist.

The insulin requirement for GH-induced diabetes mellitus will also decline, but the reversibility of the diabetes depends on the insulin reserve of the pancreatic islet beta cells. Consequently, it is advisable to start insulin therapy as soon as possible in an effort to preserve beta cell function and maximize the chances of diabetic remission.

Should ovariohysterectomy not be immediately possible or permitted, or if a long-acting exogenous progestin has been administered, treatment with aglepristone, a progesterone receptor antagonist, has been suggested (Bhatti et al., 2006).

Treatment with the somatostatin analogue pasireotide, in addition to radiotherapy, has proven successful in one dog with pituitary-adenoma-induced hypersomatotropism (Zublena et al., 2018). Hypophysectomy is also possible in these cases.

Cats

In cats, three potential treatment modalities are available: hypophysectomy, medical therapy and radiotherapy. Of these, hypophysectomy is currently considered to be the most effective.

Hypophysectomy

Experience with and access to transsphenoidal hypophysectomy in cats has expanded significantly in recent years. The largest study to date included 68 cats with hypersomatotropism (Fenn et al., 2021). Fifty-eight cats (85%) were alive 4 weeks postoperatively, with 10 (15%) postoperative deaths. Complications included hypoglycaemia (n = 9), electrolyte imbalances (n = 9) and transient congestive heart failure (n = 5). Improved glycaemic control was achieved in 95% of cases. Diabetic remission occurred in 71%, with insulin administration discontinued

after a median of 9 (range 2–120) days. Four weeks after surgery, serum IGF-1 concentrations were significantly lower in cats that achieved diabetic remission (median 20 (15–708) ng/ml) compared with those that did not (324 (15–1955) ng/ml). Post hypophysectomy, cats require long-term oral levothyroxine and glucocorticoid supplementation. Desmopressin treatment is required in over 70% of cases. Overall median survival time was 853 days (range 1–1740). Similar results were confirmed by another study of a smaller number of cats (van Bokhorst et al., 2021). Cryohypophysectomy has been described in two cases to date; however, this technique requires further evaluation and longer-term follow-up before it can be confidently recommended (Abrams-Ogg et al., 2002; Blois et al., 2008).

Medical therapy

Medical treatment options have also become available in recent years. The somatostatin analogue pasireotide has thus far proven most effective. A fast and significant decrease in serum IGF-1, as well as diabetic remission, has been documented with the use of this drug in some cats (Scudder et al., 2015; Gostelow et al., 2017). The long-acting preparation is administered once monthly by subcutaneous injection. Of eight treated cats in one study, three entered diabetic remission, with significant decreases in both IGF-1 concentration and insulin dose. Adverse events include loose stools, hypoglycaemia and worsening polyphagia. Other somatostatin analogues, including octreotide and lanreotide, have not proven useful in the clinical setting, which might relate to the somatostatin receptor subtype expressed in cats with hypersomatotropism (Scudder et al., 2018).

Given the expense of pasireotide, the cheaper dopamine receptor agonist cabergoline has also been evaluated. An initial study showed no effect in cats with hypersomatotropism in the UK, whereas three affected cats in Argentina demonstrated significant improvement (Miceli et al., 2021; Scudder et al., 2021).

Radiation therapy

The reported response to radiation therapy ranges from poor to excellent (Goossens et al., 1998; Kaser-Hotz et al., 2002; Dunning et al., 2009). A good response is mainly characterized by shrinkage of the pituitary tumour. However, disadvantages of this treatment are not inconsiderable and include limited availability, extended time in hospital, frequent anaesthesia, high expense, unpredictable outcome and frequent persistence of a high IGF-1 concentration (and its biological consequences) despite decreased GH concentrations (so-called GH–IGF-1 discordance, a phenomenon also recognized in humans) (Niessen, 2010). Radiotherapy should therefore be mainly considered when there are contraindications for surgery, such as the presence of a large macroadenoma, or when surgery is not available.

Prognosis

Dogs

In dogs with progestin-induced GH excess, the prognosis is excellent if the source can be eliminated. Diabetes mellitus resulting from GH excess is sometimes reversible.

Even in dogs where the diabetic state persists after discontinuation of the progestin excess, the insulin resistance that commonly accompanies hypersomatotropism will resolve, and the diabetes mellitus will be much easier to control. In two cases with suspected hypersomatotropism in pregnancy, maternal hyperglycaemia was proposed to have contributed to fetal death (Norman *et al.*, 2006). Too few cases of pituitary-adenoma-induced canine hypersomatotropism have been described to determine prognosis. Hypothyroidism-induced hypersomatotropism is reversible with adequate thyroid hormone supplementation, and remission of associated diabetes mellitus is possible if it had developed.

Cats

In cats, even without definitive treatment for hypersomatotropism and with unstable diabetes mellitus, the short-term prognosis is relatively good. The insulin-resistant diabetes mellitus can generally be managed satisfactorily with large doses of insulin, divided daily. Reported survival times of both aggressively and conservatively managed cats with hypersomatotropism vary enormously. Some cats survive for only a few months and others live for many years and die from causes unlikely to be related to hypersomatotropism. Use of a standardized and validated tool for measuring quality of life for diabetic cats may be useful in objective assessment that could guide a productive discussion on the benefits of additional therapies (Niessen *et al.*, 2010).

References and further reading

Abrams-Ogg A, Holmberg DL, Stewart WA and Claffey FP (1993) Acromegaly in a cat: diagnosis by magnetic resonance imaging and treatment by cryohypophysectomy. *Canadian Veterinary Journal* **34**, 682–685

Abrams-Ogg A, Holmberg DL, Quinn RF *et al.* (2002) Blindness now attributed to enrofloxacin therapy in a previously reported case of a cat with acromegaly treated by cryohypophysectomy. *Canadian Veterinary Journal* **43**, 53–54

Berg RI, Nelson RW, Feldman EC *et al.* (2007) Serum insulin-like growth factor-I concentration in cats with diabetes mellitus and acromegaly. *Journal of Veterinary Internal Medicine* **21**, 892–898

Bhatti SF, Duchateau L, Okkens AC *et al.* (2006) Treatment of growth hormone excess in dogs with the progesterone receptor antagonist aglépristone. *Theriogenology* **66**, 797–803

Blois SL and Holmberg DL (2008) Cryohypophysectomy used in the treatment of a case of feline acromegaly. *Journal of Small Animal Practice* **49**, 596–600

Borgeat K, Niessen SJM, Wilkie L *et al.* (2018) Time spent with cats is never wasted: lessons learned from feline acromegalic cardiomyopathy, a naturally occurring animal model of the human disease. *PLoS ONE* **13**, 0194342

Concannon P, Altszuler N, Hampshire J, Butler WR and Hansel W (1980) Growth hormone, prolactin, and cortisol in dogs developing mammary nodules and an acromegaly-like appearance during treatment with medroxyprogesterone acetate. *Endocrinology* **106**, 1173–1177

Dirtu AC, Niessen SJ, Jorens PG and Covaci A (2013) Organohalogenated contaminants in domestic cats' plasma in relation to spontaneous acromegaly and type 2 diabetes mellitus: a clue for endocrine disruption in humans? *Environment International* **57–58**, 60–67

Dunning MD, Lowrie CS, Bexfield NH, Dobson JM and Herrtage ME (2009) Exogenous insulin treatment after hypofractionated radiotherapy in cats with diabetes mellitus and acromegaly. *Journal of Veterinary Internal Medicine* **23**, 243–249

Eigenmann JE and Venker-van Haagen AJ (1981) Progestagen-induced and spontaneous canine acromegaly due to reversible growth hormone overproduction: clinical picture and pathogenesis. *Journal of the American Animal Hospital Association* **17**, 813

Eigenmann JE, Eigenmann RY, Rijnberk A *et al.* (1983) Progesterone-controlled growth hormone overproduction and naturally occurring canine diabetes and acromegaly. *Acta Endocrinologica* **104**, 167–176

Elliott DA, Feldman EC, Koblik PD, Samii VF and Nelson RW (2000) Prevalence of pituitary tumors among diabetic cats with insulin resistance. *Journal of the American Veterinary Medical Association* **216**, 1765–1768

Fall T, Hedhammar Å, Wallberg A *et al.* (2010) Diabetes mellitus in elkhounds is associated with diestrus and pregnancy. *Journal of Veterinary Internal Medicine* **24**, 1322–1328

Fall T, Johanssen Kreuger S, Juberget Å *et al.* (2008) Gestational diabetes mellitus in 13 dogs. *Journal of Veterinary Internal Medicine* **22**, 1296–1300

Fenn J, Kenny PJ, Scudder CJ *et al.* (2021) Efficacy of hypophysectomy for the treatment of hypersomatotropism-induced diabetes mellitus in 68 cats. *Journal of Veterinary Internal Medicine* **35**, 823–833

Fletcher JM, Scudder CJ, Kiupel M *et al.* (2016) Hypersomatotropism in 3 cats without concurrent diabetes mellitus. *Journal of Veterinary Internal Medicine* **30**, 1216–1221

Forcada Y, German AJ, Noble PJM *et al.* (2008) Determination of fPLI concentrations in cats with diabetes mellitus. *Journal of Feline Medicine and Surgery* **10**, 480–487

Fracassi F, Gandini G, Diana A *et al.* (2007) Acromegaly due to a somatroph adenoma in a dog. *Domestic Animal Endocrinology* **32**, 43–54

Goossens MM, Feldman EC, Nelson RW *et al.* (1998) Cobalt 60 irradiation of pituitary gland tumors in three cats with acromegaly. *Journal of the American Veterinary Medical Association* **213**, 374–376

Gostelow R, Scudder C, Keyte S *et al.* (2017) Pasireotide long-acting release treatment for diabetic cats with underlying hypersomatotropism. *Journal of Veterinary Internal Medicine* **31**, 355–364

Gunn-Moore D (2005) Feline endocrinopathies. *Veterinary Clinics of North America: Small Animal Practice* **35**, 171–210

Johnstone T, Terzo E and Mooney CT (2014) Hypothyroidism associated with acromegaly and insulin-resistant diabetes mellitus in a Samoyed. *Australian Veterinary Journal* **92**, 437–442

Kaser-Hotz B, Rohrer CR, Stankeova S *et al.* (2002) Radiotherapy of pituitary tumours in five cats. *Journal of Small Animal Practice* **43**, 303–307

King JM, Kavanaugh JF and Bentinck-Smith J (1962) Diabetes mellitus with pituitary neoplasms in a horse and in a dog. *Cornell Veterinarian* **52**, 133–145

Kooistra HS, Okkens AC, Mol JA *et al.* (1997) Lack of association of progestin-induced cystic endometrial hyperplasia with GH gene expression in the canine uterus. *Journal of Reproduction and Fertility (Supplement)* **51**, 355–361

Lamb CR, Ciasca TC, Mantis P *et al.* (2014) Computed tomographic signs of acromegaly in 68 diabetic cats with hypersomatotropism. *Journal of Feline Medicine and Surgery* **16**, 99–108

Lewitt MS, Hazel SJ, Church DB *et al.* (2000) Regulation of insulin-like growth factor-binding protein-3 ternary complex in feline diabetes mellitus. *Journal of Endocrinology* **166**, 21–27

Lichtensteiger CA, Wortman JA and Eigenmann JE (1986) Functional pituitary acidophilic adenoma in a cat with diabetes mellitus and acromegalic features. *Veterinary Pathology* **23**, 518–521

Lucksch F (1923) Über Hypophysentumoren beim Hunde. *Tierärztliche Archiv* **3**, 1–16

Meij BP, Van der Vlugt-Meijer RH, van den Ingh IS and Rijnberk A (2004) Somatotroph and corticotroph pituitary adenoma (double adenoma) in a cat with diabetes mellitus and hyperadrenocorticism. *Journal of Comparative Pathology* **130**, 209–215

Miceli DD, Vidal PN, Pompili GA *et al.* (2021) Diabetes mellitus remission in three cats with hypersomatotropism after cabergoline treatment. *Journal of Feline Medicine and Surgery Open Reports* **7**, 20551169211018991

Middleton DJ, Culvenor JA, Vasak E and Mintohadi K (1985) Growth hormone-producing pituitary adenoma, elevated serum somatomedin C concentration and diabetes mellitus in a cat. *Canadian Veterinary Journal* **26**, 169–171

Mol JA, Lantinga-van Leeuwen I, van Garderen E and Rijnberk A (2000) Progestin-induced mammary growth hormone (GH) production. *Advances in Experimental Medicine and Biology* **480**, 71–76

Mol JA, van Garderen E, Rutteman GR and Rijnberk A (1996) New insights in the molecular mechanism of progestin-induced proliferation of mammary epithelium: induction of the local biosynthesis of growth hormone (GH) in the mammary glands of dogs, cats and humans. *Journal of Steroid Biochemistry and Molecular Biology* **57**, 67–71

Murai A, Nishii N, Morita T and Yuki M (2012) GH-producing mammary tumors in two dogs with acromegaly. *Journal of Veterinary Medical Science* **74**, 771–774

Niessen SJ (2010) Feline acromegaly: an essential differential diagnosis for the difficult diabetic. *Journal of Feline Medicine and Surgery* **12**, 15–23

Niessen SJ, Forcada Y, Mantis P *et al.* (2015) Studying cat (*Felis catus*) diabetes: beware of the acromegalic imposter. *PLoS ONE* **10**, e0127794

Niessen SJ, Khalid M, Petrie G and Church DB (2007a) Validation and application of a radioimmunoassay for ovine growth hormone in the diagnosis of acromegaly in cats. *Veterinary Record* **160**, 902–907

Niessen SJ, Petrie G, Gaudiano F *et al.* (2007b) Feline acromegaly: an underdiagnosed endocrinopathy? *Journal of Veterinary Internal Medicine* **21**, 899–905

Niessen SJ, Powney S, Guitian J *et al.* (2010) Evaluation of a quality-of-life tool for cats with diabetes mellitus. *Journal of Veterinary Internal Medicine* **24**, 1098–1105

Norman EJ, Wolsky KJ and MacKay GA (2006) Pregnancy-related diabetes mellitus in two dogs. *New Zealand Veterinary Journal* **54**, 360–364

Peterson ME (1987) Effects of megestrol acetate on glucose tolerance and growth hormone secretion in the cat. *Research in Veterinary Science* **42**, 354–357

Schwedes CS (1999) Transient diabetes insipidus in a dog with acromegaly. *Journal of Small Animal Practice* **40**, 392–396

Scudder CJ, Gostelow R, Forcada Y *et al.* (2015) Pasireotide for the medical management of feline hypersomatotropism. *Journal of Veterinary Internal Medicine* **29**, 1074–1080

Scudder CJ, Hazuchova K, Gostelow R *et al.* (2021) Pilot study assessing the use of cabergoline for the treatment of cats with hypersomatotropism and diabetes mellitus. *Journal of Feline Medicine and Surgery* **23**, 131–137

Scudder CJ, Mirczuk SM, Richardson KM *et al.* (2018) Pituitary pathology and gene expression in acromegalic cats. *Journal of the Endocrine Society* **16**, 181–200

Scudder CJ, Niessen SJ, Catchpole B *et al.* (2017) Feline hypersomatotropism and acromegaly tumorigenesis: a potential role for the AIP gene. *Domestic Animal Endocrinology* **59**, 134–139

Selman PJ, Mol JA, Rutteman GR and Rijnberk A (1994b) Progestin treatment in the dog. II. Effects on the hypothalamic–pituitary–adrenocortical axis. *European Journal of Endocrinology* **131**, 422–430

Selman PJ, Mol JA, Rutteman GR, van Garderen E and Rijnberk A (1994a) Progestin-induced growth hormone excess in the dog originates in the mammary gland. *Endocrinology* **134**, 287–292

Steele MM, Borgeat K, Payne JR *et al.* (2021) Increased insulin-like growth factor 1 concentrations in a retrospective population of non-diabetic cats diagnosed with hypertrophic cardiomyopathy. *Journal of Feline Medicine and Surgery* **23**, 952–958

van Bokhorst KL, Galac S, Kooistra HS *et al.* (2021) Evaluation of hypophysectomy for treatment of hypersomatotropism in 25 cats. *Journal of Veterinary Internal Medicine* **35**, 834–842

Zublena F, Tamborini A, Mooney CT *et al.* (2018) Radiotherapy and pasireotide treatment of a growth hormone producing pituitary tumor in a diabetic dog. *Canadian Veterinary Journal* **59**, 1089–1093

Chapter 14

Control of calcium metabolism and investigation of hypo- and hypercalcaemia

Barbara J. Skelly

Introduction

A number of vital homeostatic mechanisms are necessary to maintain circulating ionized calcium concentrations within a narrow range. The ubiquitous role of calcium explains why it is subject to such close regulation. It has functions within both intracellular and extracellular compartments that include: maintaining the skeleton; preserving the integrity of plasma membranes; acting as a cofactor to proteins enabling coagulation, adhesion and enzyme function; activating exocytosis; contraction of muscles; and propagation of action potentials in some nerve cells. Calcium is an intracellular second messenger, often acting through binding to receptors such as calmodulin, with roles in mitosis, apoptosis, metabolism and gene expression.

A large proportion of total body calcium exists in bone. This can be released when dietary calcium is scarce or in response to greater physiological need. Calcium also exists within the circulation in the following fractions in healthy dogs and cats:

- Protein-bound, predominantly to albumin (~30–40%)
- Complexed to other ions, including citrate and bicarbonate (~10%)
- Ionized (~55%).

As the biologically active fraction, only the ionized calcium concentration is specifically controlled. The relative distribution of calcium between the three fractions is changeable and reflects other variables: chiefly, the acid–base balance of the extracellular fluid and the concentration of albumin and other proteins. The protein-bound and complexed fractions act as a buffer, aiding regulation of ionized calcium concentrations. Fluctuations in protein concentrations, commonly found in many medical conditions, do not have an impact on the accurate measurement of ionized calcium, and ionized calcium is therefore diagnostically more useful.

Key components of calcium homeostasis

Several factors can affect circulating calcium concentrations, including:

- Parathyroid hormone (PTH)
- Parathyroid hormone-related protein (PTHrP)
- Calcitonin
- Vitamin D
- The calcium-sensing receptor (CaSR)
- The major effector organs – kidney, small intestine and skeletal bone
- The supply of dietary calcium.

These components interact and exert effects on each other in classic positive and negative feedback loops (Figure 14.1).

Parathyroid hormone

Parathyroid hormone, a small polypeptide of 84 amino acids, is synthesized in the parathyroid glands, which are situated within and adjacent to thyroid tissue in the neck (Figure 14.2). There are four separate glands; an internal (caudal) and an external (cranial) gland is associated with each thyroid lobe. Each gland is roughly the same size, and all respond to stimuli to produce PTH. As endocrine glands, they are ductless and histologically consist of cords or nests of cells arranged around capillaries. The chief cells (also called principal cells) of the parathyroid gland synthesize PTH, while the oxyphil cells (which are not numerous in the cat or dog) have no known function.

> ### The main functions of PTH
> - To stimulate calcium resorption through the kidneys and to reduce calciuria.
> - To stimulate mobilization of skeletal calcium through the action of osteoclasts.
> - To activate vitamin D, which in turn increases calcium absorption through the gastrointestinal tract.
> - To enhance phosphate excretion.

Parathyroid hormone has a half-life of minutes before the majority is broken down by the liver and excreted via the kidneys. The PTH molecules are inactivated when the critical N-terminal portions are excised, creating relatively large C-terminal fragments that have longer half-lives than complete PTH. These fragments are the cause of inaccuracies in the measurement of PTH, particularly when using older assays.

Tiny fluctuations in calcium concentrations are continuously assessed by the CaSR of the chief cells. There is an inverse sigmoidal relationship between calcium and PTH

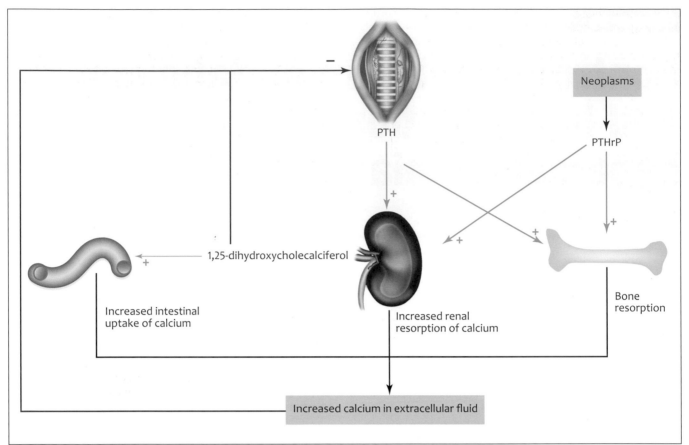

14.1 The interactive hormones that lead to an increase in extracellular calcium. Increased calcium concentrations and 1,25-dihydroxycholecalciferol (calcitriol, active vitamin D) exert negative feedback to reduce parathyroid hormone (PTH) secretion. Parathyroid hormone-related potein (PTHrP) can function in the same way as PTH but is thought to have minimal effects on vitamin D synthesis. + = stimulation; − = inhibition.

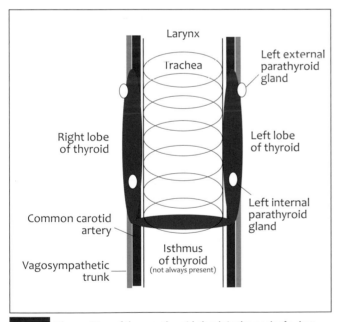

14.2 The position of the parathyroid glands in the neck of a dog.

that is mediated by the CaSR. High calcium concentrations suppress, and low concentrations stimulate, PTH secretion. The set-point of calcium homeostasis is the calcium concentration that corresponds to the midpoint on the curve between minimal and maximal PTH secretory rates. PTH cannot be suppressed completely and there is always some low level of production. Many diseases characterized by hypercalcaemia arise because the calcium set-point is raised, meaning that there is a drive to generate a higher calcium concentration through the synthesis and release of PTH.

Calcium exerts an active effect on the rates of synthesis and degradation of PTH. Thus, a system exists for the minute-by-minute regulation of PTH concentration that is able to fine-tune the calcium concentration in the extracellular fluid.

Parathyroid hormone-related protein

Like PTH, PTHrP is a small peptide hormone that has a role in fetal development and early infancy, but production ceases in adulthood. Parathyroid hormone-related protein binds to the same receptors as PTH and has the same basic biological activity. Although PTHrP is homologous to PTH in the N-terminal part of the molecule, the remainder of the peptide is different and, as a consequence, it does not cross-react with PTH in assays. Parathyroid hormone-related protein has become a useful biomarker in screening hypercalcaemic animals for suspected malignancies. Although low concentrations of PTHrP do not rule out malignancy, a concentration above the reference interval significantly increases the index of suspicion for neoplasia. Thus, PTHrP is used routinely as part of a diagnostic work-up for dogs and cats with hypercalcaemia.

Calcitonin

Calcitonin is produced and released from the parafollicular cells, or C-cells, of the thyroid gland when hypercalcaemia is induced, either exogenously or endogenously. It functions as an antagonistic hormone to PTH, primarily through inhibiting the function of osteoclasts, whilst also mildly enhancing renal calcium excretion and, over the longer term, reducing intestinal uptake of calcium. Like PTH, the secretion of calcitonin is mediated by CaSR activation (Felsenfeld and Levine, 2015). In humans, malignancy of the parafollicular cells is known as medullary thyroid carcinoma, or C-cell carcinoma. These tumours can be associated with hypercalcitoninaemia. Hypocalcaemia is rare in dogs with medullary thyroid carcinoma (Feldman et al., 2015).

Vitamin D

Unlike humans, dogs and cats have no ability to synthesize vitamin D in their skin and they rely on sufficient dietary intake. This is commonly in the form of cholecalciferol (vitamin D3) of animal origin but may also include ergocalciferol (vitamin D2) of plant origin or synthetic forms of vitamin D. These forms of vitamin D need to go through two stages of activation before they are biologically active. The first stage, which is an uncontrolled and non-rate-limiting step, occurs in the liver to form 25-hydroxycholecalciferol (calcifediol). The final, rate-limiting step occurs in the kidneys, where 1,25-dihydroxycholecalciferol (calcitriol, active vitamin D) is produced through the action of the enzyme CYP27B1 (1-alpha-hydroxylase) (Figure 14.3). Parathyroid hormone has a permissive effect on this conversion, whereas calcium and phosphate inhibit the enzyme.

Biologically active vitamin D increases calcium and phosphate uptake through the gastrointestinal tract. Vitamin D also has a positive effect on PTH-mediated renal calcium resorption and, at high circulating concentrations,

can induce bone calcium release (de Brito Galvao et al., 2013). As the serum calcium concentration increases, PTH secretion is inhibited and activation of vitamin D is reduced.

Either endogenously produced or exogenously supplied vitamin D can cause significant hypercalcaemia. Generally, an investigation of vitamin D is initiated if PTH and PTHrP have been found to be within or below their respective reference intervals. Further information on vitamin D is provided in Chapter 17.

The calcium-sensing receptor

The CaSR is located on the surface of parathyroid cells and kidney cells, where it responds to variations in the concentration of extracellular calcium. This receptor allows regulation of PTH secretion and renal tubular calcium resorption in response to alterations in extracellular calcium concentrations. Loss-of-function and gain-of-function *CASR* mutations have been reported in over 200 human diseases, causing hypercalcaemia or hypocalcaemia, respectively, although neither has been reported in dogs or cats.

Phosphate

Phosphate is provided by dietary sources, particularly meat protein, and its uptake from the gastrointestinal tract is increased by 1,25-dihydroxycholecalciferol. Parathyroid hormone stimulates phosphate release from bone by increasing osteoclastic activity, but also promotes renal excretion of phosphate. The net effect is that a high concentration of PTH increases the calcium concentration and lowers the phosphate concentration in the circulation.

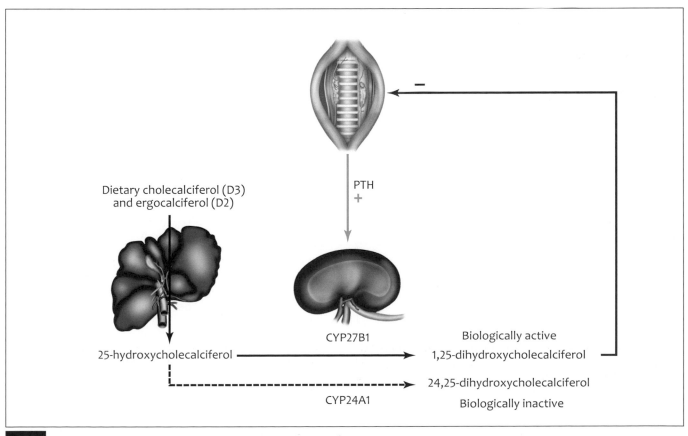

14.3 Synthesis and control of vitamin D. PTH = parathyroid hormone; + = stimulation; − = inhibition.

Diagnostic tests for investigating calcium disorders

Clinicopathological tests

Calcium

Accurate measurement of circulating calcium concentrations is necessary. Total calcium concentration is routinely measured as part of a full biochemistry profile but ionized calcium usually needs to be specifically requested and is often performed only if total calcium is abnormal. When total calcium was used to predict ionized calcium concentrations, diagnostic discordance was calculated to be 27% in dogs and 40% in cats (Schenck and Chew, 2005, 2010). Sensitivity was lower than specificity for diagnosis of ionized hypercalcaemia, with only two thirds of affected dogs and one third of cats displaying total hypercalcaemia. Approximately two thirds of dogs and almost 90% of cats with ionized hypocalcaemia had total hypocalcaemia. However, the sensitivity for detection of clinically significant hypocalcaemia may be higher, at least in hypoalbuminaemic dogs (De Witte *et al.*, 2021). Correction calculations are not recommended, although a multivariate predictive model has been proposed to allow factors other than total calcium and albumin alone to contribute to the prediction of ionized calcium in situations where direct measurement is not possible (Hodgson *et al.*, 2019).

Phosphate

The concentration of phosphate ions in the extracellular fluid is linked to the concentration of calcium, and the correct interpretation of phosphate concentrations can help to determine the pathophysiological mechanism behind measured hyper- or hypocalcaemia. The mechanisms leading to hypophosphataemia are shown in Figure 14.4.

By contrast, hyperphosphataemia usually reflects decreased renal excretion and is associated with acute and chronic kidney disease (CKD). Less frequently, hyperphosphataemia occurs because of significant cell lysis (e.g. tumour lysis syndrome or reperfusion injury) or vitamin D toxicosis. In the latter, typically both calcium and phosphate concentrations are increased.

Mechanism	Cause
Shift to intracellular space	• Insulin therapy • Parenteral nutrition • Intravenous glucose/dextrose • Respiratory alkalosis • Metabolic alkalosis • Salicylate toxicity
Increased urinary excretion	• Diabetes mellitus/ketoacidosis • **Hypercortisolism** • Eclampsia • **Hyperparathyroidism** • Renal tubular defects • Diuresis
Decreased gastrointestinal absorption	• Decreased intake • **Malabsorption** • Vomiting or diarrhoea • **Phosphate binders** • **Hypovitaminosis D**
Other	• Laboratory error • Hypothermia • Idiopathic

14.4 Mechanisms leading to the development of hypophosphataemia. Causes in bold have a significant effect on extracellular calcium concentrations.

Parathyroid hormone

Parathyroid hormone concentrations should be interpreted alongside ionized calcium concentrations (Figure 14.5):

- Physiologically, concentrations of PTH should be high during hypocalcaemia and low during hypercalcaemia
- Failure of PTH to increase during ionized hypocalcaemia suggests hypoparathyroidism
- Increased concentrations of PTH in the context of ionized hypercalcaemia suggest hyperparathyroidism.

Ionized calcium concentration	PTH concentration	Diagnosis
Low	High	Normal physiological response
Low	Low	Parathyroid suppression or insufficiency
High	High	Hyperparathyroidism
Within reference interval	High	Physiological compensation/ secondary hyperparathyroidism

14.5 Interpretation of PTH with ionized calcium concentrations.

Parathyroid hormone is found in the blood as the biologically active hormone together with a large number of inactive carboxyl-terminal fragments of variable length that result from hormone degradation. Two-site assays, with antibodies directed against the carboxyl- and amino-terminal ends of the molecule, are used to reduce interference from smaller fragments. Most modern PTH assays detect either 'intact' (7–84) or 'whole' (1–84) PTH. The intact PTH assay measures biologically active 1–84 PTH as well as shorter C-terminal fragments, most of which are thought to be the large 7–84 inactive fragment. By contrast, the whole PTH assay measures only biologically active hormone by inclusion of an antibody targeting the first four amino acids of the molecule. Whole and intact PTH assays are used commercially in dogs and cats but performance is variable, not all have been fully validated and the availability of individual assays is inconsistent. A point-of-care chemiluminescent intact human PTH assay (Immulite Turbo Intact PTH, Siemens) was validated for use in dogs, but anecdotal reports suggest that it is no longer suitable (Mooney *et al.*, 2019). A solid-phase, two-site chemiluminescent enzyme-labelled immunometric assay for human use (Immulite intact PTH, Siemens) is not recommended for use in dogs due to its ability to detect only markedly increased PTH values (Mooney *et al.*, 2019). A canine intact PTH enzyme-linked immunosorbent assay (ELISA) (Canine intact PTH, Immunotopics) is widely used despite incomplete validation. A dual intact and whole PTH immunoradiometric assay (IRMA) (Duo PTH Kit, Scantibodies Laboratory) has been used and validated in dogs (Estepa *et al.*, 2003). A variety of other assays are available for research use, with variable validation. Therefore, results must be interpreted with knowledge of the assay used.

In theory, measurement of whole PTH concentrations should provide a more accurate result, as it excludes all degraded hormone. However, in humans with primary hyperparathyroidism, there is limited diagnostic value from using whole over intact PTH assays, and excellent correlation between results from whole and intact PTH assays has also been described in dogs (Mooney *et al.*, 2019). The impact of other diseases, particularly kidney disease, on the relative concentrations of whole and intact PTH warrants further study. Parathyroid hormone is unstable, necessitating special sample-handling requirements.

Increased PTH concentrations can occur when ionized calcium concentrations are within the reference interval; secondary renal, nutritional and adrenal hyperparathyroidism have been described.

Parathyroid hormone-related protein

Concentrations of PTHrP can be increased in animals with certain neoplastic diseases, and measurement is common during the investigation of hypercalcaemia due to the high frequency of underlying neoplasia in affected animals.

Parathyroid hormone-related protein is measured by two-site IRMA and by N-terminal radioimmunoassay. There are several circulating forms of PTHrP that have biological activity, including intact PTHrP (amino acids 1–141), an N-terminal fragment (1–36) and an N-terminal plus mid-region fragment (1–86). The roles of the different forms are not completely understood. Like PTH, PTHrP is not stable, and it is measured preferentially in plasma using EDTA as an anticoagulant. The reference interval for PTHrP is <0.5 pmol/l in both the dog and cat.

Diagnostic imaging

Dogs and cats that are presented for investigation of hypercalcaemia or hypocalcaemia may have some form of diagnostic imaging performed. This usually involves radiographic assessment of the thorax and ultrasound examination of the abdomen. Abdominal radiographs may also be informative. Advanced imaging techniques (computed tomography and magnetic resonance imaging) can also be valuable. Imaging studies may identify enlargement of organs, including lymph nodes and lymphoreticular organs in the thoracic or abdominal cavity, calcium-containing uroliths in the urinary tract, evidence for pancreatitis, and features such as demineralization and fractures in the skeletal system or soft tissue mineralization in other organs. Focused imaging of the neck is also indicated in animals with suspected primary hyperparathyroidism but is less valuable in assessing for hypoparathyroidism.

Hypercalcaemia

The differential diagnoses for hypercalcaemia, categorized by pathophysiological classification, are shown in Figure 14.6. When hypercalcaemia is discovered, a logical approach to the investigation should be based upon the signalment, history and physical examination as well as relevant clinicopathological and diagnostic imaging data.

Signalment

The age, breed and sex of the animal can influence decision-making when investigating hypercalcaemia. Hyperparathyroidism has an insidious onset and a diagnosis is often reached when the animal is over 10 years old. Chronic kidney disease can result from congenital kidney pathology, for which there are specific breed predispositions, or can be a consequence of ageing. Whilst the frequency of neoplastic diseases generally increases with age, and anal sac adenocarcinoma occurs in later life, lymphoma can affect an animal of any age, even the very young. Immune-mediated diseases such as hypoadrenocorticism most commonly occur in young to middle-aged animals and females are somewhat predisposed. Keeshonds have an inherited form of primary hyperparathyroidism and certain other breeds are known to be predisposed to other causes of hypercalcaemia, for example hypoadrenocorticism (Poodles, Nova Scotia Duck Tolling Retrievers), lymphoma (Boxers, Bernese Mountain Dogs) and anal sac adenocarcinoma (Cocker Spaniels).

Although the signalment may help to prioritize differential diagnoses, it should be noted that most animals develop hypercalcaemia as a spontaneous manifestation of disease (see Figure 14.6), and not as an inherited, familial or breed-related disorder.

Clinical features

The clinical signs of hypercalcaemia are shown in Figure 14.7. Mild hypercalcaemia rarely produces any clinical signs. Even moderate to severe hypercalcaemia, if it develops insidiously, can be tolerated by individual animals remarkably well. Clinical signs are often subtle. This likely

Cause	Characteristics
Parathyroid disease	
Primary hyperparathyroidism	Increased PTH, tCa and iCa, decreased or low-normal PO$_4$
Neoplasia	
Malignancy (lymphoma, anal sac adenocarcinoma, thymoma, multiple myeloma)	Decreased PTH, increased tCa and iCa, decreased or low-normal PO$_4$, PTHrP may be increased
Kidney disease	
Chronic kidney disease	Increased PTH, increased or reference interval tCa, usually reference interval iCa, increased PO$_4$
Acute kidney injury	Hypercalcaemia documented in majority of reported cases
Osteolytic	
Non-malignant skeletal lesions (osteomyelitis, hypertrophic osteodystrophy, disuse osteoporosis) (uncommon)	Decreased PTH, increased tCa and iCa, reference interval or increased PO$_4$
Calcium overdose	
Excess calcium administration (supplementation (calcium carbonate) or calcium-containing phosphate binders)	Decreased PTH, increased tCa and iCa, reference interval or increased PO$_4$

14.6 Differential diagnoses for hypercalcaemia. Note that where increased or decreased parathyroid hormone (PTH) is noted, concentrations may not be outside the reference limits but rather inappropriately high or low for the concurrent ionized calcium concentration. iCa = ionized calcium; PO$_4$ = phosphate; PTHrP = parathyroid hormone-related protein; tCa = total calcium. (continues) ▶

Cause	Characteristics
Vitamin D dependent	
Iatrogenic (e.g. cod liver oil supplementation)	Decreased PTH, increased tCa, iCa and PO_4
Plants (calcitriol glycosides found in nightshade, jessamine and other plants)	Vitamin D may be increased depending on which form has been ingested and what is measured
Rodenticide toxicity (cholecalciferol)	
Anti-psoriasis creams (calcipotriol, calcipotriene and maxacalcitol)	
Granulomatous disease	
Granulomatous lymphadenitis	Can be difficult to characterize because of the often unknown aetiology of hypercalcaemia
Fungal disease (rare in UK)	Documented to be due to increased vitamin D but could also be PTHrP mediated
Angiostrongylus vasorum infection	
Mycobacterial disease	
Implant-induced granulomatous disease	
Mechanism unknown	
Hypoadrenocorticism	Reference interval or decreased PTH and 1,25-dihydroxycholecalciferol PTHrP within reference interval
Feline idiopathic hypercalcaemia	Decreased PTH PTHrP within reference interval
Non-pathological	
Immature, growing animal	Both calcium and phosphate higher than in adults
Lipaemia	Causes increased tCa
Laboratory error	

14.6 (continued) Differential diagnoses for hypercalcaemia. Note that where increased or decreased parathyroid hormone (PTH) is noted, concentrations may not be outside the reference limits but rather inappropriately high or low for the concurrent ionized calcium concentration. ASA = anal sac adenocarcinoma; iCa = ionized calcium; PO_4 = phosphate; PTHrP = parathyroid hormone-related protein; tCa = total calcium.

Mild hypercalcaemia (<3.3 mmol/l)
• Mild polyuria and polydipsia
• May be no signs

Moderate hypercalcaemia (3.4–3.8 mmol/l)
• Polyuria and polydipsia
• Lethargy
• Gastrointestinal signs – vomiting, diarrhoea or constipation

Severe hypercalcaemia (>3.9 mmol/l)
• Polyuria and polydipsia
• More severe lethargy
• Reluctance to move
• Bone pain or pain when eating (dependent on cause)
• Gastrointestinal signs

14.7 Clinical signs of mild, moderate and severe hypercalcaemia.

accounts for the large number of hypercalcaemic animals that are identified serendipitously.

It can be useful to distinguish between animals that are hypercalcaemic and well, and those that are hypercalcaemic and clinically ill. Well animals are usually diagnosed with diseases that are slow to develop and better tolerated, such as primary hyperparathyroidism, whilst ill animals are more likely to have some form of neoplasia where calcium concentrations increase more rapidly and are less well tolerated. An exception to this may be in hypercalcaemic animals that develop urolithiasis with resultant signs of urinary tract disease or obstruction. This is commonly reported in primary hyperparathyroidism and is discussed further in Chapter 16. Owners of pets with neoplastic diseases may mention other related clinical signs, such as straining to defecate or ribbon-like faeces in dogs with anal sac neoplasia. Animals, most commonly

dogs, with vitamin D toxicosis may have mild general malaise and polyuria and polydipsia, or may be seriously unwell because of associated kidney damage.

Physical examination may yield more specific information that allows differential diagnoses to be narrowed further. Lymphoma is a major differential for hypercalcaemia, particularly in an unwell animal, so careful palpation of all superficial lymph nodes is mandatory. In addition, abdominal palpation may reveal hepatosplenomegaly or enlarged abdominal lymph nodes. Multiple myeloma can cause lameness, reluctance to move and generalized bone pain. Anal sac adenocarcinoma can be identified by palpation of the emptied anal sacs. Rectal examination of dogs with this suspected diagnosis may also identify palpably enlarged retroperitoneal lymph nodes. Dogs, and rarely cats, with hypoadrenocorticism may have non-specific physical examination findings but noticeable bradycardia if they are significantly hyperkalaemic.

Specific diseases causing hypercalcaemia
Primary hyperparathyroidism

Primary hyperparathyroidism is discussed in detail in Chapter 16. One of the important first steps when investigating PTH-dependent disease is to differentiate between primary and, particularly renal, secondary hyperparathyroidism. Figure 14.8 details their clinicopathological differences. Both syndromes are characterized by increased or high reference interval PTH concentrations; however, in primary hyperparathyroidism, increased renal phosphate excretion causes hypophosphataemia or low reference interval phosphate concentrations, while in renal secondary hyperparathyroidism, reduced renal excretion often results in hyperphosphataemia. Furthermore, both total and ionized calcium concentrations are above the

Parameter	Primary hyperparathyroidism	Renal secondary hyperparathyroidism
Total calcium	↑	↓ or within reference interval or ↑
Ionized calcium	↑	↓ or within reference interval or ↑
Phosphate	↓	↑
PTH	↑ or high reference interval	↑ or high reference interval
PTHrP	Within reference interval	Within reference interval or ↑

14.8 Clinicopathological features of primary and secondary hyperparathyroidism. ↑ = increased; ↓ = decreased; PTH = parathyroid hormone; PTHrP = parathyroid hormone-related protein.

reference interval in primary hyperparathyroidism, whereas they may be low, within reference interval or, rarely, increased in renal secondary hyperparathyroidism. This method of differentiation is complicated when hypercalcaemia due to hyperparathyroidism has caused kidney damage, or when there is kidney disease of another cause concurrent with primary hyperparathyroidism. Under these circumstances, phosphate excretion is impaired and is no longer helpful for differentiation.

Kidney disease

Dogs and cats with CKD suffer disruption to their calcium and phosphate homeostatic mechanisms. In most cases, this manifests as a progressive rise in phosphate concentrations throughout the course of the disease. Changes in calcium concentrations can occur but are less predictable.

Total calcium concentrations can be increased, decreased or within the reference interval. Ionized calcium concentrations can be increased in either acute or, more commonly, CKD. Ionized hypercalcaemia is more common in cats and is reported to occur in approximately 30% of cases with CKD, compared with approximately 10% in dogs (Schenck and Chew, 2005, 2010).

Phosphate is an important regulator of calcium homeostasis as a specific inhibitor of CYP27B1, the renal enzyme that converts 25-hydroxycholecalciferol into the active 1,25-dihydroxycholecalciferol. High concentrations of phos-phate, 1,25-dihydroxycholecalciferol and PTH stimulate osteocytic release of fibroblast growth factor 23 and this is also responsible for inhibiting CYP27B1 as well as increasing CYP24A1 (24-hydroxylase) activity. These mechanisms effectively remove vitamin D-mediated increases in calcium and phosphate absorption through the gastrointestinal tract and increase reliance on PTH-mediated mechanisms to maintain calcium concentrations (Figure 14.9). This phenomenon is called renal secondary hyperparathyroidism. Ultimately, loss of functional kidney tissue contributes to the decline in CYP27B1 activity as the ability to synthesize this enzyme is lost as kidney function declines.

Some dogs and cats with acute kidney injury are hypercalcaemic. The development of hypercalcaemia is unexpected, as a rapid build-up of phosphate due to a sudden lack of excretion would naturally lead to a reduction in calcium concentration. In one retrospective study of hypercalcaemia in dogs, kidney disease was identified as the underlying cause in 17% of cases, of which 89% had CKD and only 11% had acute kidney injury (Messinger et al., 2009). Dogs with grape and raisin

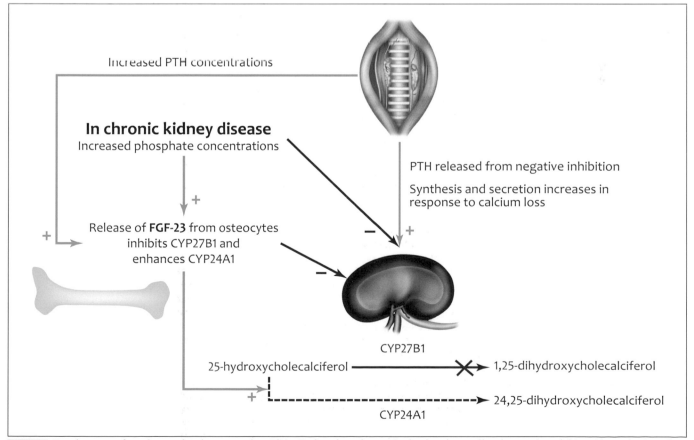

14.9 Development of renal secondary hyperparathyroidism. Reduced renal excretion leads to hyperphosphataemia and this, with synthesis and release of fibroblast growth factor 23 (FGF-23), inhibits the activity of CYP27B1 so that 1,25-dihydroxycholecalciferol (calcitriol, active vitamin D) is not synthesized. PTH = parathyroid hormone; + = stimulation; − = inhibition.

toxicity appear to be at particular risk of hypercalcaemia. In a retrospective study of 43 dogs with such toxicity, over 60% were hypercalcaemic (Eubig et al., 2005). There are fewer reports of cats ingesting raisins or grapes. Although it seems as if this species is also at risk of kidney damage, it is unknown if cats are as likely to develop hypercalcaemia. Leptospirosis may cause hypercalcaemia in dogs, although hypocalcaemia is also reported and outcomes may be dependent upon the serovar responsible for disease.

Malignant neoplasia

Malignant neoplasia is the most common cause of hypercalcaemia in both dogs and cats. The most common cancers known to cause hypercalcaemia in dogs are lymphoma and anal sac adenocarcinoma, although many other forms of cancer are sporadically reported. In a recent study of 1,641 dogs and 119 cats with ionized hypercalcaemia, an underlying malignancy was identified in >40% and >30% of cases, respectively, representing the single most common cause of persistent or pathological hypercalcaemia in each species (Coady et al., 2019). In dogs, lymphoma was identified as the most common underlying cause, in 37.7% of these malignancy-associated cases, with anal sac adenocarcinoma in 11.8% and an unidentified tumour in 22.2%. In cats, lymphoma was also the most frequently identified malignant cause (40% of cases).

Of lymphoma cases, T-cell phenotypes are most likely to lead to hypercalcaemia. Parathyroid hormone-related protein has been implicated in the aetiology of malignancy-associated hypercalcaemia, but it is not the only cause. Therefore, a reference interval PTHrP concentration does not exclude malignancy. The finding of increased PTHrP does, however, necessitate further investigation to attempt to identify the site of the presumed malignancy. When PTHrP was first reported in cats it was commonly found to be associated with carcinomas; six of seven cats with various carcinomas had malignancy-associated hypercalcaemia and increased PTHrP concentration (Bolliger et al., 2002).

Vitamin D ingestion

Although relatively uncommon, vitamin D ingestion can be a cause of severe hypercalcaemia and frequently leads to kidney damage and soft tissue calcification. Simply supplementing dogs with cod liver or salmon oil has been associated with severe hypercalcaemia. This appears to be a rather idiosyncratic reaction, as some dogs seem more sensitive than others to supplements. As with all nutraceuticals, marine oil supplements that are designed for human consumption are often used and, because they are not prescription-controlled products and are viewed as 'natural', some owners do not suspect the possibility of doing harm. Giving prescription vitamin D products (calcitriol or alfacalcidol) or non-prescription vitamin D2 or D3 supplements can also potentially result in hypercalcaemia.

Vitamin D-containing psoriasis creams (calcipotriene, calcipotriol and maxacalcitol) are the most common medications ingested by animals that are subsequently presented for hypercalcaemia. These creams are applied to the skin and are often found to be palatable by dogs. Owners do not perceive that chronic low-grade ingestion through licking will cause problems, and careful history-taking is required in dogs and cats that display the resulting hypercalcaemia (total and ionized) as well as hyperphosphataemia in the absence of kidney disease. Vitamin D intoxication rapidly causes kidney damage, so azotaemia is a common finding and may distract from the real cause of the changes.

Granulomatous disease

A range of granulomatous diseases have been associated with hypercalcaemia in small animals, chiefly in dogs. Occasionally, increased vitamin D concentrations are implicated, as has been described in cases of angiostrongylosis (Boag et al., 2005), granulomatous lymphadenitis (Mellanby et al., 2006) and gastric pythiosis (LeBlanc et al., 2008). However, an increased PTHrP concentration was also reported to mediate hypercalcaemia in two dogs with schistosomiasis (Fradkin et al., 2001). The mechanism through which 1,25-dihydroxycholecalciferol production escapes regulation in activated macrophages within granulomatous tissue is described in human medicine, although it is speculated that increased vitamin D concentrations are not always identified in the circulation. In cats, hypercalcaemia has been reported in cases of histoplasmosis and other granulomatous diseases, but reports are more sparse than for dogs.

Hypoadrenocorticism

Hypercalcaemia has been described in dogs with hypoadrenocorticism. Initial reports estimated a frequency of hypercalcaemia of approximately 30%, when assessing only total calcium concentration (Peterson et al., 1996). In one study, over half of affected dogs had ionized hypercalcaemia, total hypercalcaemia or both (Adamantos and Boag, 2008). Although most studies suggest that mild to moderate hypercalcaemia is most commonly encountered, severe hypercalcaemia can occasionally occur, with total calcium concentrations >3.80 mmol/l and ionized calcium concentrations >1.7 mmol/l reported. Hypercalcaemia of this magnitude should prompt a thorough search for a secondary cause but can be found to resolve with treatment for hypoadrenocorticism alone. Hypercalcaemia can occur in dogs with both mineralocorticoid and glucocorticoid deficiency or glucocorticoid deficiency alone.

Despite attempts to identify the underlying aetiology and mechanism of hypercalcaemia (Gow et al., 2009), no convincing explanation has been reached. The pathophysiology is presumed to be multifactorial, involving blood volume contraction, metabolic acidosis and enhanced intestinal absorption of calcium. Decreased urinary excretion of calcium may also be a factor, as glucocorticoids are calciuric. The degree of hypercalcaemia is not associated with the severity of the other electrolyte changes (sodium and potassium) and, therefore, is difficult to predict.

Feline idiopathic hypercalcaemia

Feline idiopathic hypercalcaemia was first noticed in 1990 and quickly became more widely recognized. Affected cats show either no clinical signs or most commonly a combination of gastrointestinal (vomiting, anorexia and weight loss) and urinary (urolithiasis) signs. Despite thorough investigation, the aetiology is unknown. The PTH concentration is usually below the reference interval whilst PTHrP, phosphate, 24,25-dihydroxycholecalciferol and precursor vitamin D concentrations are within their respective reference intervals (Midkiff et al., 2000).

Chronic kidney disease is not present initially, although cats with idiopathic hypercalcaemia can incur kidney damage through prolonged hypercalcaemia. Diagnosis is thus by exclusion of any of the other defined causes of hypercalcaemia. The use of alendronate to treat cats with idiopathic hypercalcaemia is widespread and doses of 5–20 mg/cat once weekly are seemingly well tolerated (Hardy *et al.*, 2015).

Hypocalcaemia

The differential diagnoses for hypocalcaemia are shown in Figure 14.10.

Signalment

There are few strong breed associations for any of the diseases that commonly lead to hypocalcaemia. Small numbers of dogs with primary hypoparathyroidism have been reported, but possible breed predispositions in Toy Poodles, Miniature Schnauzers, Labrador Retrievers and Scottish Terriers have been suggested in an early case series of 28 dogs from the USA (Bruyette and Feldman, 1988). This may not reflect breed distribution in the UK. Eclampsia is described most frequently in small-breed dogs and can also occur in cats. Pancreatitis is common in terrier breeds, Cocker Spaniels, Cavalier King Charles Spaniels and Miniature Schnauzers, but can occur in a range of other breeds.

Cause	Mechanism and characteristics
Laboratory, sampling and interpretive errors	
Laboratory error	Technical errors
Improper sample handling	EDTA and fluoride oxalate tubes chelate calcium Sample exposure to air may increase pH and decrease ionized calcium concentration
Hypoproteinaemia	Approximately 45% of calcium is bound to protein Indicated by low total calcium concentration whilst ionized calcium is within reference interval
Reproductive	
Eclampsia	Lactation-mediated calcium loss in milk leads to decreased ECF concentrations
Renal and urinary	
Acute kidney injury and chronic kidney disease	Multifactorial Difficult to predict outcome case by case
Ethylene glycol toxicity	Oxalate metabolites from breakdown of ethylene glycol precipitate with calcium Renal tubular damage inhibits calcium uptake
Bicarbonate therapy	Bicarbonate binds calcium and is lost through urinary excretion
Feline obstructive lower urinary tract disease	Rapid increase in circulating phosphate caused by post-renal obstruction leads to hypocalcaemia
Critical illness	
Acute pancreatitis	Originally thought to be due to fatty acids precipitating calcium but may be caused by glucagon-stimulated calcitonin release
Sepsis	Inappropriate response to low calcium concentrations thought to be due to endotoxins
Parathyroid dependent	
Hypoparathyroidism (irreversible)	Primary idiopathic (immune mediated) Iatrogenic (removal of parathyroid glands) Spontaneous infarction of parathyroid adenoma
Hypoparathyroidism (reversible)	Following treatment for primary hyperparathyroidism
Magnesium deficiency	Magnesium is required for release of, and end-organ response to, PTH Termed functional hypoparathyroidism
Driven by hyperphosphataemia	
Nutritional secondary hyperparathyroidism	Diet high in phosphate (meat based) causes secondary hypocalcaemia and activates PTH release
Tumour lysis syndrome	Cell lysis releases phosphate, which causes hypocalcaemia
Phosphate enemas or excess supplementation	Increased circulating phosphate causes hypocalcaemia
Vitamin D dependent	
Hypovitaminosis D	Reduced dietary intake Intestinal malabsorption leading to low calcium, low vitamin D and low magnesium concentrations
Rickets	Vitamin D-dependent rickets Hereditary vitamin D-resistant rickets
Calcitonin dependent	
C-cell tumour of the thyroid	Leads to calcitonin overproduction and hypocalcaemia (rare)
Other	
Soft tissue trauma or rhabdomyolysis	May be related to calcium deposition in damaged tissue but can be complicated by development of acute kidney injury
Blood transfusion	Citrated anticoagulants chelate calcium

14.10 Differential diagnoses for hypocalcaemia. ECF = extracellular fluid; EDTA = ethylenediaminetetraacetic acid; PTH = parathyroid hormone.

Clinical features

The clinical signs of hypocalcaemia are listed in Figure 14.11. Mild hypocalcaemia is not associated with any specific sign. As the severity of hypocalcaemia worsens, or if a sudden drop in calcium concentration occurs, clinical signs develop, starting with apparent unease and panting before progressing to muscle tremors and hypocalcaemic tetany.

Signs associated with neuromuscular excitability
• Muscle fasciculations or tremors
• Face rubbing
• Hypersensitivity to external stimuli
• Stiff, stilted gait
• Tetanic seizures
• Respiratory arrest
Behavioural changes
• Agitation
• Anxiety
• Aggression
• Vocalization
Other
• Panting
• Pyrexia
• Bradycardia or tachycardia
• Cataracts
• Prolapse of third eyelid (cats)
• Prolonged QT interval on electrocardiogram

14.11 Clinical signs of hypocalcaemia.

Specific diseases associated with hypocalcaemia

Of all of the differential diagnoses listed in Figure 14.10, relatively few are associated with significant clinical signs of hypocalcaemia. Symptomatic hypocalcaemia is most commonly associated with primary hypoparathyroidism, protein-losing enteropathy and eclampsia. Nutritional secondary hyperparathyroidism and rickets most commonly present with bone pain, distorted growth and pathological fractures. Kidney disease and critical illness rarely cause neuromuscular or other specific signs attributable to hypocalcaemia.

Reproductive causes

Eclampsia (puerperal tetany) is described most commonly during the first 4 weeks postpartum in small-breed dogs with large litters, but it can also occur in larger breeds, before whelping and in queens. Its development is associated with either inadequate peripartum nutrition or excessive dietary calcium supplementation during gestation. The latter is thought to suppress PTH secretion so that, when required, skeletal calcium mobilization and intestinal uptake are delayed.

Kidney and lower urinary tract disease

Hypocalcaemia in CKD may be caused by increased serum phosphate concentrations and decreased renal production of 1,25-dihydroxycholecalciferol. Phosphate forms complexes with serum calcium and deposits it into bone and other tissues, while the lack of active vitamin D causes hypocalcaemia by decreasing gastrointestinal absorption of calcium.

Hypocalcaemia can also occur in acute kidney injury. One mechanism leading to both acute kidney injury and hypocalcaemia is seen in cases of ethylene glycol toxicity, where oxalate metabolites of the toxin complex with calcium, leading to renal tubular deposition of insoluble calcium oxalate and proximal tubular necrosis. Calcium oxalate crystals can also be found in the urine, which is useful diagnostically. The hypocalcaemia is rarely sufficient to require specific therapy. In acute kidney injury of other aetiologies, hypocalcaemia is a consequence of a rapid rise in phosphate concentration, as in CKD.

Postrenal azotaemia, such as obstructive feline lower urinary tract disease (FLUTD), can cause hypocalcaemia that is related to the speed and magnitude of the increase in phosphate concentration. Hypocalcaemia in this situation can lead to a greater risk of clinical signs related to the cardiac and nervous systems in response to other electrolyte disturbances, particularly hyperkalaemia.

Critical illness

Hypocalcaemia in critical illness and sepsis has been recognized in dogs and cats more frequently since the measurement of ionized calcium became commonplace. Mechanisms are probably multifactorial and include altered parathyroid gland function, vitamin D variations, enhanced calciuresis, hypomagnesaemia and the effect of inflammatory cytokines (Kelly and Levine, 2013). An experimental study using lipopolysaccharide-induced endotoxaemia demonstrated that hypovitaminosis D was responsible for hypocalcaemia and that PTH concentrations increased in response (Holowaychuk et al., 2012). A subsequent study demonstrated increased procalcitonin concentrations, raising the possibility that calcitonin is involved in mediating hypocalcaemia, or at least may be a biomarker of sepsis in dogs, as in humans (Easley et al., 2020).

The impact of hypocalcaemia varies from case to case. Hypocalcaemia at presentation at a critical care facility has been linked to a longer stay in intensive care but not a worse prognosis (Holowaychuk et al., 2009), whilst a similar study reported both longer hospitalization and higher mortality (Luschini et al., 2010). Management of hypocalcaemia in this situation and its impact on prognosis is still debated, although symptomatic hypocalcaemia clearly needs to be treated.

Parathyroid hormone-dependent causes

Irreversible, reversible and functional hypoparathyroidism are covered in detail in Chapter 15. Primary hypoparathyroidism is presumed to be caused by immune-mediated destruction of parathyroid tissue in a way that is analogous to the destruction of adrenal tissue in hypoadrenocorticism. This process is almost always irreversible. The disease is rare in dogs and extremely rare in cats, where very few cases have been reported. Dogs usually have an array of neuromuscular signs that progress to tetanic seizure with stress, exercise or excitement. Parathyroid hormone concentrations are low to undetectable, and total and ionized calcium concentrations are low. Functional hypoparathyroidism can occur secondary to magnesium depletion because magnesium is a necessary cofactor for PTH synthesis and release. This appears to occur rarely but should be considered when there is a coexisting disease that would be expected to lead to magnesium depletion.

Nutritional secondary hyperparathyroidism

Nutritional secondary hyperparathyroidism is a state of metabolic dysregulation induced by a diet in which calcium and phosphate are not in the appropriate ratio (recommended 1–1.2:1). This condition usually occurs when a meat-only diet is fed. It has been described in cats, particularly exotic breeds that, anecdotally, are attributed characteristics that require them to be fed a specific and limited diet (Taylor-Brown *et al.*, 2016). Dogs can also be affected, particularly large and giant breeds due to increased demand for calcium associated with delayed closure of growth plates and prolonged duration of their growth phase. Animals may have an ionized hypocalcaemia and associated clinical signs that include muscle twitching and seizures, bone pain, stiffness and neurological signs secondary to spinal fractures.

Vitamin D deficiency

Hypovitaminosis D may be caused by dietary deficiency but more commonly occurs in severe malabsorptive disorders such as inflammatory bowel disease or protein-losing enteropathy caused by intestinal lymphangiectasia. The mechanism of hypocalcaemia involves impaired fat absorption in the small intestine leading to reduced uptake of vitamin D, a fat-soluble vitamin. Hypomagnesaemia may also have a role as it has been documented in severely diarrhoeic animals and magnesium depletion is known to cause functional hypoparathyroidism. Hypocalcaemia has been associated with a negative outcome in gastrointestinal disease but the effect of supplementation to alter outcome has not been evaluated (Allenspach *et al.*, 2017).

Rickets: Rickets can occur when there is dietary calcium deficiency, vitamin D deficiency or mutations leading to an inability to activate or respond to vitamin D during growth. Rickets is a differential diagnosis for young animals presenting with lameness, bony malformation, pain when moving and hypocalcaemia. The bone pathology is most pronounced in the most rapidly growing bones, such as the radius, tibia, metacarpals and metatarsals.

Rickets is rarely reported in the cat and dog but there are case reports of animals with various acquired and congenital forms of the disease, as described in Chapter 17.

Summary

Both hyper- and hypocalcaemia are caused by a diverse range of conditions, and a logical and methodical approach is required. Using problem-based differential diagnoses to direct case work-up should yield results, although there are still a number of syndromes where our knowledge remains imperfect.

References and further reading

Adamantos S and Boag A (2008) Total and ionised calcium concentrations in dogs with hypoadrenocorticism. *Veterinary Record* **163**, 25–26

Allenspach K, Rizzo J, Jergens AE and Chang YM (2017) Hypovitaminosis D is associated with negative outcome in dogs with protein losing enteropathy: a retrospective study of 43 cases. *BMC Veterinary Research* **13**, 96

Boag AK, Murphy KF and Connolly DJ (2005) Hypercalcaemia associated with *Angiostrongylus vasorum* in three dogs. *Journal of Small Animal Practice* **46**, 79–84

Bolliger AP, Graham PA, Richard V *et al.* (2002) Detection of parathyroid hormone-related protein in cats with humoral hypercalcemia of malignancy. *Veterinary Clinical Pathology* **31**, 3–8

Bruyette DS and Feldman EC (1988) Primary hypoparathyroidism in the dog: report of 15 cases and review of 13 previously reported cases. *Journal of Veterinary Internal Medicine* **2**, 7–14

Coady M, Fletcher DJ and Goggs R (2019) Severity of ionized hypercalcemia and hypocalcemia is associated with etiology in dogs and cats. *Frontiers in Veterinary Science* **6**, 276

de Brito Galvao JF, Nagode LA, Schenck PA and Chew DJ (2013) Calcitriol, calcidiol, parathyroid hormone, and fibroblast growth factor-23 interactions in chronic kidney disease. *Journal of Veterinary Emergency and Critical Care* **23**, 134–162

De Witte F, Klag A and Chapman P (2021) Adjusted calcium concentration as a predictor of ionized hypocalcaemia in hypoalbuminemic dogs. *Journal of Veterinary Internal Medicine* **35**, 2249–2255

Easley F, Holowaychuk MK, Lashnits EW *et al.* (2020) Serum procalcitonin concentrations in dogs with induced endotoxemia. *Journal of Veterinary Internal Medicine* **34**, 653–658

Estepa JC, Lopez I, Felsenfeld AJ *et al.* (2003) Dynamics of secretion and metabolism of PTH during hypo- and hypercalcaemia in the dog as determined by the 'intact' and 'whole' PTH assays. *Nephrology Dialysis Transplantation* **18**, 1101–1107

Eubig PA, Brady MS, Gwaltney-Brant SM *et al.* (2005) Acute renal failure in dogs after the ingestion of grapes or raisins: a retrospective evaluation of 43 dogs (1992–2002). *Journal of Veterinary Internal Medicine* **19**, 663–674

Feldman EC, Nelson RW, Reusch CE, Scott-Moncrieff JCR and Behrend EN (2015) *Canine and Feline Endocrinology, 4th edn.* Elsevier Saunders, St. Louis

Felsenfeld AJ and Levine BS (2015) Calcitonin, the forgotten hormone: does it deserve to be forgotten? *Clinical Kidney Journal* **8**, 180–187

Fradkin JM, Braniecki AM, Craig TM *et al.* (2001) Elevated parathyroid hormone-related protein and hypercalcemia in two dogs with schistosomiasis. *Journal of the American Animal Hospital Association* **37**, 349–355

Gow AG, Gow DJ, Bell R *et al.* (2009) Calcium metabolism in eight dogs with hypoadrenocorticism. *Journal of Small Animal Practice* **50**, 426–430

Hardy BT, de Brito Galvao JF, Green TA *et al.* (2015) Treatment of ionized hypercalcemia in 12 cats (2006–2008) using PO-administered alendronate. *Journal of Veterinary Internal Medicine* **29**, 200–206

Hodgson N, McMichael MA, Jepson RE and Le Boedec K (2019) Development and validation of a multivariate predictive model to estimate serum ionized calcium concentration from serum biochemical profile results in cats. *Journal of Veterinary Internal Medicine* **33**, 1943–1953

Holowaychuk MK, Birkenheuer AJ, Li J *et al.* (2012) Hypocalcemia and hypovitaminosis D in dogs with induced endotoxemia. *Journal of Veterinary Internal Medicine* **26**, 244–251

Holowaychuk MK, Hansen BD, DeFrancesco TC and Marks SL (2009) Ionized hypocalcemia in critically ill dogs. *Journal of Veterinary Internal Medicine* **23**, 509–513

Kelly A and Levine MA (2013) Hypocalcemia in the critically ill patient. *Journal of Intensive Care Medicine* **28**, 166–177

LeBlanc CJ, Echandi RL, Moore RR, Souza C and Grooters AM (2008) Hypercalcemia associated with gastric pythiosis in a dog. *Veterinary Clinical Pathology* **37**, 115–120

Luschini MA, Fletcher DJ and Schoeffler GL (2010) Incidence of ionized hypocalcemia in septic dogs and its association with morbidity and mortality: 58 cases (2006–2007). *Journal of Veterinary Emergency and Critical Care* **20**, 406–412

Mellanby RJ, Mellor P, Villiers EJ *et al.* (2006) Hypercalcaemia associated with granulomatous lymphadenitis and elevated 1,25 dihydroxyvitamin D concentration in a dog. *Journal of Small Animal Practice* **47**, 207–212

Messinger JS, Windham WR and Ward CR (2009) Ionized hypercalcemia in dogs: a retrospective study of 109 cases (1998–2003). *Journal of Veterinary Internal Medicine* **23**, 514–519

Midkiff AM, Chew DJ, Randolph JF, Center SA and DiBartola SP (2000) Idiopathic hypercalcemia in cats. *Journal of Veterinary Internal Medicine* **14**, 619–626

Mooney CT, Shiel RE, Fawcett K, Matthews E and Gunn E (2019) A comparison of canine whole and intact parathyroid hormone concentrations as measured by different assays. *Journal of Small Animal Practice* **60**, 507–513

Peterson ME, Kintzer PP and Kass PH (1996) Pretreatment clinical and laboratory findings in dogs with hypoadrenocorticism: 225 cases (1979–1993). *Journal of the American Veterinary Medical Association* **208**, 85–91

Schenck PA and Chew DJ (2005) Prediction of serum ionized calcium concentration by use of serum total calcium concentration in dogs. *American Journal of Veterinary Research* **66**, 1330–1336

Schenck PA and Chew DJ (2010) Prediction of serum ionized calcium concentration by serum total calcium measurement in cats. *Canadian Journal of Veterinary Research* **74**, 209–213

Taylor-Brown F, Beltran E and Chan DL (2016) Secondary nutritional hyperparathyroidism in Bengal cats. *Veterinary Record* **179**, 287–288

Chapter 15

Hypoparathyroidism

Barbara J. Skelly

Introduction

Hypoparathyroidism is rare in dogs and extremely rare in cats. In dogs, the disease most frequently results from immune-mediated destruction of the parathyroid glands. Although this aetiology is also described in cats, it is rare, and few cases are reported (Peterson *et al.*, 1991). Hypoparathyroidism is characterized by low circulating ionized and total calcium concentrations in combination with a low parathyroid hormone (PTH) concentration and an increased phosphate concentration.

Anatomy and physiology

The anatomy of the parathyroid glands is described and illustrated in Chapter 14. In summary, there are two parathyroid glands (external and internal) associated with each thyroid lobe. They are responsible for the synthesis and release of PTH, which is pivotal in calcium homeostasis. Calcium regulation in the body is governed by the activities of PTH, 1,25-dihydroxycholecalciferol (calcitriol, active vitamin D) and calcitonin. The activities and effects of PTH and 1,25-dihydroxycholecalciferol are explained in Chapter 14.

In hypoparathyroidism, the absence of adequate PTH means that there is:

- Reduced skeletal mobilization of calcium
- Urinary calcium net excretion (calciuresis)
- Reduced phosphate excretion
- Reduced vitamin D activation within the kidney.

Signalment

Hypoparathyroidism most commonly affects middle-aged bitches and entire male cats. In a series of 735 dogs with hypoparathyroidism, 62% were female and 38% were male (Refsal *et al.*, 2001). In cats, the age range may be somewhat younger at between 5 months and 7 years of age (Gunn-Moore, 2005). No breed predisposition has been observed (Feldman, 2015). In dogs, terrier breeds (particularly West Highland White and Scottish Terriers), Miniature and Standard Schnauzers, Border Collies and Dachshunds may be more commonly affected, and in Australia and New Zealand, the St Bernard appears to be predisposed (Kornegay *et al.*, 1980; Jones and Alley, 1985; Refsal *et al.*, 2001; Russell *et al.*, 2006).

Aetiology and pathophysiology

The mechanisms through which parathyroid-dependent hypocalcaemia develops are shown in Figure 15.1.

Hypoparathyroidism (naturally occurring)
• Primary (idiopathic)
• Spontaneous infarction of parathyroid adenoma
Hypoparathyroidism (iatrogenic)
• Following treatment for hyperparathyroidism
• Secondary to trauma or surgery (especially bilateral thyroidectomy)
Functional hypoparathyroidism (reversible)
• Magnesium dysregulation/deficiency

15.1 Mechanisms through which parathyroid-dependent hypocalcaemia develops.

Naturally occurring primary hypoparathyroidism

Permanent hypoparathyroidism is typically caused by inflammatory destruction of the parathyroid glands, presumably due to an immune-mediated mechanism. Thus, hypoparathyroidism is similar to other endocrinopathies caused by underproduction of a hormone due to immune-mediated damage (including some forms of diabetes mellitus, hypoadrenocorticism and hypothyroidism). When affected parathyroid glands are examined, an inflammatory cell infiltrate is identified, consisting mainly of lymphocytes with some plasma cells and neutrophils. Affected glands are fibrotic, have an increase in the number of small capillaries and a loss of normal secretory cells (Bruyette and Feldman, 1988; Peterson *et al.*, 1991). In one review of 17 cases, gross and histopathological examinations of the parathyroid glands were only performed in two dogs (Russell *et al.*, 2006). In both cases, the gross and histopathological appearance of the parathyroid glands were normal, suggesting either that another mechanism was responsible for hypoparathyroidism or that gross and microscopic changes correlate weakly with functional activity.

A further, rare cause of naturally occurring hypoparathyroidism has been reported in two dogs. In these cases, parathyroid gland tumours caused hypercalcaemia, but spontaneous infarction occurred and resulted in acute hypocalcaemia (Rosol *et al.*, 1988).

Iatrogenic hypoparathyroidism

When an animal with primary hyperparathyroidism is treated, the source of PTH is suddenly removed. As a result, the remaining glands, which tend to be small and hypofunctional, must increase hormone secretion to maintain calcium homeostasis. This is discussed in Chapter 16 and has been the subject of a number of recent publications (Dear *et al.*, 2017, Armstrong *et al.*, 2018). Previously, animals with severe or prolonged hypercalcaemia have been considered more at risk of post-treatment hypocalcaemia. Recent studies have questioned this assumption and the supplementation of calcium and vitamin D to all dogs with severe pre-treatment hypercalcaemia is no longer recommended. It is necessary to monitor these dogs closely to avoid a hypocalcaemic crisis, usually between 3 and 5 days following surgery or ablation, but only those that are symptomatically hypocalcaemic require calcium and vitamin D supplementation.

The recalcification of the skeleton that occurs after parathyroidectomy in human patients with hyperparathyroidism is referred to as 'hungry bone syndrome'. This is caused by a rapid increase in bone remodelling. Hypocalcaemia can occur if the rate of skeletal mineralization exceeds the rate of osteoclast-mediated bone resorption. This syndrome can be associated with severe and diffuse bone pain. A similar phenomenon may be seen in dogs but is not well characterized.

In cats, postoperative hypocalcaemia typically occurs 1–3 days after bilateral thyroidectomy. This can be common, depending on the surgical technique chosen, but is rarer than it used to be as techniques have been modified to minimize the risk of parathyroid damage. Chapter 19 discusses postoperative hypocalcaemia in cats in greater detail. Eucalcaemia can be maintained as long as one functional parathyroid gland remains.

A recent case report details the occurrence of hypoparathyroidism in a Chihuahua that had suffered severe ventral circumferential cervical lacerations when attacked by another dog. After management including debridement and flushing it was found that the right thyroid lobe was missing and the left lobe was damaged. No parathyroid glands were visualized and the dog displayed clinical signs suggestive of hypocalcaemia 72 hours after the initial trauma. The dog received calcium, magnesium and vitamin D supplementation but this was successfully discontinued after 4 months and the dog was able to maintain calcium concentrations thereafter (Wolf *et al.*, 2020).

Functional hypoparathyroidism

Severe hypomagnesaemia can cause decreased secretion of PTH, a state known as functional hypoparathyroidism (Schenck, 2005). Magnesium and calcium depletion is reported in dogs, particularly Yorkshire Terriers, with small intestinal malabsorption. The primary cause of hypocalcaemia appears to be mediated through intestinal vitamin D malabsorption (Kimmel *et al.*, 2000; Bush *et al.*, 2001). However, functional hypoparathyroidism induced by hypomagnesaemia may contribute in some cases. It is recommended, therefore, that the concentration of ionized magnesium is checked in dogs and cats with reduced parathyroid function.

Clinical features

The clinical signs of hypoparathyroidism are listed in Figure 15.2 and are caused by the presence of hypocalcaemia. The differential diagnoses for hypocalcaemia are described in greater detail in Chapter 14.

The severity of clinical signs depends on the magnitude of the hypocalcaemia and the rapidity with which it develops. Most animals do not show clinical signs until the total calcium concentration falls below 1.5 mmol/l and the ionized calcium concentration falls below approximately 0.8 mmol/l. These numbers vary according to the acid–base balance of the animal, as the presence of alkalosis reduces the ionized component and makes clinical signs more likely at a higher total calcium concentration. Clinical signs are more likely if the calcium concentration has decreased rapidly (e.g. over hours to days in the case of surgical removal of a parathyroid adenoma) compared with the slow development of hypocalcaemia seen with idiopathic primary hypoparathyroidism.

Primary hypoparathyroidism is likely to result in severe hypocalcaemia and is the most likely cause of symptomatic hypocalcaemia in the dog and cat without evidence of eclampsia, urinary tract obstruction or chronic enteropathy.

The signs of hypocalcaemia are intermittent and may be induced by exercise, excitement or stress. The reasons for this are twofold: the requirement for calcium increases during muscular activity and therefore a deficit is most apparent at this time, and panting leads to rapid alkalinization of the blood (respiratory alkalosis) and induces a fall in the proportion of ionized calcium available. The most obvious signs to be precipitated in this way are those associated with the neuromuscular system, such as muscle tremors or fasciculation.

Neuromuscular signs

Since calcium plays such an important role in nervous and neuromuscular transmission, it would be intuitive to assume that hypocalcaemia would cause reduced muscle

Signs associated with neuromuscular excitability
• Muscle fasciculations or tremors
• Face rubbing
• Biting and licking at paws or body
• Hypersensitivity to external stimuli
• Stiff, stilted gait
• Ataxia
• Tetanic seizures
• Respiratory arrest
• Weakness
Behavioural changes
• Agitation
• Anxiety
• Vocalization
• Aggression
Cardiac changes
• Lengthening of ST segment and QT interval on electrocardiogram
• Tachycardia or bradycardia
• Myocardial failure
• Hypotension
Other
• Panting
• Hyperthermia
• Cataracts
• Third eyelid prolapse in cats

15.2 Clinical features of hypoparathyroidism.

and nerve excitability. This is not the case, however, and the classic signs of hypocalcaemia revolve around hyperexcitability in the form of muscle tremors, muscle cramping and rigidity, and tetanic seizures (Gagliardo *et al.*, 2021). The mechanism involves the ability of calcium to alter the threshold potential; hypercalcaemia raises the threshold while hypocalcaemia lowers it and allows an impulse to be propagated more readily.

Signs are often initially observed around the facial muscles but may then progress to whole body involvement and seizures. Champing was frequently reported in one case series as a manifestation of the increased excitability of the muscles of mastication (Russell *et al.*, 2006). In the same case series, facial pruritus was recorded in 4 of 17 dogs (24%). Seizures caused by hypocalcaemia are, unlike epileptic seizures, most frequent during periods of activity, not rest. Animals retain consciousness and do not tend to urinate. The seizures often resolve spontaneously and do not respond to anticonvulsant therapy. Interestingly, the stress and excitement of a visit to a veterinary surgeon (veterinarian) and the physical examination may precipitate overt neuromuscular signs of hypocalcaemia such as muscle tremors, cramping or seizures. In addition, affected animals may resent handling and become aggressive because they are in pain.

Gastrointestinal signs

Some reports of hypoparathyroid dogs list gastrointestinal signs as frequent. Russell *et al.* (2006) reported vomiting and inappetence as common features in a case series, but the aetiopathogenesis of these signs is not clear.

Ocular signs

Cataracts (Figure 15.3) may be found in animals with chronic and relatively severe hypocalcaemia, and are described as bilaterally symmetrical punctate to linear opacities in the anterior and posterior subcapsular region of the lens (Feldman, 2015). The mechanism of cataract formation is unclear. Typically, in human hypoparathyroidism, progression is halted if the serum calcium concentration is stabilized. In one review of canine cases, however, three were described as developing cataracts after the initiation of therapy (Bruyette and Feldman, 1988). Other ocular manifestations reported in hypoparathyroid dogs include blepharospasm, blepharitis and keratoconjunctivitis sicca (Jones and Alley, 1985). These findings

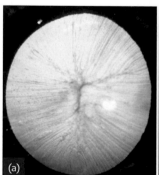 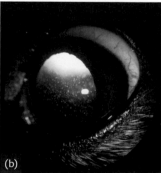

15.3 (a) Lens of a Border Collie with hypoparathyroidism. There are marked linear opacities in the anterior and posterior subcapsular cortex as well as anterior and posterior suture lines. Visual acuity would be expected to be affected, although this dog was still able to negotiate obstacles. (b) Punctate opacities in the lens of a dog with hypoparathyroidism.
(a, Courtesy of David Williams; b, Courtesy of David Gould)

were reported in one hypoparathyroid St Bernard and it was unclear whether they were necessarily manifestations of the primary disease or concurrent, independent ocular changes. Cataracts are frequently reported in feline cases and are of similar appearance to those of other species (Peterson *et al.*, 1991, Bassett, 1998).

Cardiovascular signs

In humans, severe hypocalcaemia can cause a prolongation of the QT interval on an electrocardiogram and either sudden death, because of the development of arrhythmia, or congestive heart failure. Severe chronic hypocalcaemia is described as a cause of dilated cardiomyopathy and consequent heart failure in humans. This is most frequently reported in infants with rickets, but may also affect older patients with hypoparathyroidism (Brown *et al.*, 2009; Mavroudis *et al.*, 2010). Cardiac manifestations of hypocalcaemia secondary to hypoparathyroidism are uncommon in dogs and are not emphasized in the two largest case series (Bruyette and Feldman, 1988; Russell *et al.*, 2006). There is, however, a report of a hypoparathyroid cat that presented with concurrent myocardial failure that was attributed to prolonged hypocalcaemia (Lie and MacDonald, 2013).

Diagnosis
Routine clinicopathological features

Total hypocalcaemia is expected in dogs with hypoparathyroidism. However, hypocalcaemia can occur in other diseases and can also be a manifestation of hypoalbuminaemia. This is discussed in greater detail in Chapter 14.

Ionized calcium

Ionized hypocalcaemia is also expected in dogs with hypoparathyroidism. The measurement of ionized calcium allows a more accurate assessment of calcium homeostasis to be made, particularly in animals with concurrent disease or hypoalbuminaemia. Without the measurement of ionized calcium, it is difficult to base diagnoses on the interpretation of total calcium alone and even calculations to correct for alterations in circulating protein or albumin concentrations do not improve diagnostic accuracy. This is discussed in greater detail in Chapter 14. Samples for the measurement of ionized calcium should be protected from air exposure and analysed rapidly to ensure accurate results.

Confirmation of hypoparathyroidism

A definitive diagnosis of primary hypoparathyroidism is based on the following:

- Low total calcium concentration (<1.5 mmol/l)
- Low ionized calcium concentration (<0.8 mmol/l)
- Low concurrent PTH concentration, using an appropriate assay (see Chapter 14). In primary hypoparathyroidism, PTH is expected to be below or within the lower half of the reference interval despite the presence of hypocalcaemia
- High reference interval to increased phosphate concentration
- Adequate kidney function.

Parathyroid hormone increases calcium resorption in the kidney whilst also enhancing phosphate loss; hyperphosphataemia is thus a feature of hypoparathyroidism.

As kidney disease is a differential diagnosis for both hypocalcaemia and hyperphosphataemia, renal parameters should be assessed. However, renal secondary hyperparathyroidism is frequently present in cases of kidney disease so, although calcium concentrations may be reduced, PTH can be within the high end of or above the reference interval.

In animals with hypoparathyroidism, the fractional excretion of calcium is increased in the face of hypocalcaemia, whilst the fractional excretion of phosphate is decreased. Urinary fractional excretion values can be measured relatively easily but can be difficult to interpret due to the wide variability in values both between and within individuals. In one case series, fractional excretion did not correlate well with final diagnosis (Russell *et al.*, 2006).

Diagnostic imaging

Radiography or ultrasonography of hypoparathyroid dogs is unhelpful. The parathyroid glands may be atrophied, but they can be difficult to find even in healthy individuals.

Treatment

The treatment of acute, subacute and chronic hypocalcaemia is summarized in Figure 15.4.

Treatment of acute hypocalcaemia

Intravenous calcium salts are the initial treatment of choice. Calcium gluconate or calcium borogluconate is most frequently recommended, as calcium chloride solutions are caustic when extravasated or given intravenously. The following are guidelines.

- 0.5–1.5 ml/kg of 10% calcium gluconate administered slowly intravenously over 20–30 minutes until clinical signs have subsided and the animal is considered to be stable (equivalent to 4.65–13.95 mg elemental calcium/kg, as 10% calcium gluconate solution contains 9.3 mg elemental calcium per ml). Electrocardigraphy may be used to monitor cardiac effects and the infusion should be stopped if there is ST segment elevation or QT shortening, or if arrhythmias develop. In an emergency

situation, however, calcium can be administered slowly and the heart rate auscultated or the pulse monitored by digital palpation, stopping the infusion if bradycardia develops. A one-off dose of intravenous calcium will relieve clinical signs only in the short term (minutes to hours) and they are likely to recur in a hypoparathyroid dog or cat. A continuous rate infusion is therefore recommended for adequate control of calcium concentrations until oral medication has begun to take effect. A continuous rate infusion of 6.5–10 ml/kg/day 10% calcium gluconate can be used (equivalent to an approximate elemental calcium dose of 60–90 mg/kg/day or 2.50–3.75 mg/kg/h) until oral therapy has reached maximum effect. As a guide, the elemental dose of calcium required is approximated using 25–40 ml of 10% calcium gluconate, diluted in 250 ml of 0.9% saline and infused at a rate of 2.5 ml/kg/h.

- The commonly available solution of 200 mg/ml calcium borogluconate contains the equivalent of approximately 15 mg/ml elemental calcium. It therefore contains approximately 1.6 times more elemental calcium than 10% calcium gluconate and can be administered as described above, using an appropriate dose adjustment to account for the higher calcium content.
- 10% calcium chloride solution contains three times the elemental calcium per ml (27.2 mg/ml elemental calcium) as 10% calcium gluconate solution. Thus, the initial dose is reduced by one third to 0.16–0.5 ml/kg of 10% calcium chloride. This solution is extremely irritating if injected perivascularly and should be administered using a catheter only.
- It is useful to calculate the dose required and then dilute the solution (in 0.9% saline) to increase the volume; this will make it easier to achieve a slow administration rate.
- Precipitation may occur if calcium solutions are mixed with bicarbonate-containing solutions.

The use of subcutaneous calcium supplementation is controversial. Sterile abscess formation and skin sloughing (Figure 15.5) have been reported (Feldman, 2015); however, some authors still recommend that calcium gluconate is given by this route, as it is least likely to cause a problem. 10% calcium gluconate diluted 1:1 with 0.9% saline may be given subcutaneously with no adverse effects, but even diluted calcium gluconate can cause dramatic skin sloughing in some cases. For this reason, only the intravenous and oral routes of administration are recommended.

	Drug	Dose	Precautions
Acute	10% calcium gluconate 10% calcium borogluconate 10% calcium chloride*	0.5–1.5 ml/kg over 20–30 minutes 0.3–0.6 ml/kg over 20–30 minutes 0.16–0.5 ml/kg over 20–30 minutes	Monitor heart by auscultation, pulse palpation or electrocardiography for bradycardia, shortened QT interval and ST segment elevation
Subacute	10% calcium gluconate 10% calcium borogluconate 10% calcium chloride*	6.5–10 ml/kg over 24 hours in 0.9% NaCl 6–9 ml/kg over 24 hours in 0.9% NaCl 3–5 ml/kg over 24 hours in 0.9% NaCl	Do not give subcutaneously
Chronic	Calcium carbonate Calcium gluconate Calcium lactate Calcitriol Alfacalcidol Dihydrotachysterol	25–50 mg/kg of elemental calcium 20–30 ng/kg/day orally, divided into two doses 10–30 ng/kg q24h 0.02–0.03 mg/kg q24h reducing to 0.01–0.02 mg/kg q24–48h as required	Can be stopped once vitamin D dose is appropriate Time to maximum effect <4 days Time to maximum effect <4 days Time to maximum effect <7 days

15.4 Treatment of acute, subacute and chronic hypocalcaemia. 1 mg of elemental calcium = 10.75 mg calcium gluconate = 7.7 mg calcium lactate = 2.5 mg calcium carbonate. * Calcium chloride is extremely irritant compared with calcium gluconate and calcium borogluconate. It is recommended that calcium chloride is not used except when there is no alternative in a life-threatening situation and that a minimum dilution of 1:2 in 0.9% saline is used.

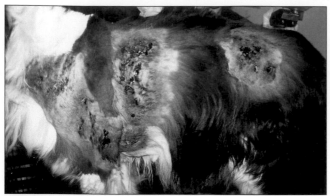

15.5 Dramatic skin sloughing in a Border Collie that had received calcium gluconate subcutaneously in several sites.
(Courtesy of Andria Cauvin)

Treatment of chronic hypocalcaemia

- Calcitriol is the active form of vitamin D and does not require further metabolism for efficacy. It has a rapid onset of action (1–4 days) and a short half-life. Toxic effects would be expected to resolve in 2–7 days. Calcitriol comes in capsules of 0.25 or 0.5 μg. The dose rate used is 20–30 ng/kg/day orally, divided into two doses, but may be decreased to 5–15 ng/kg/day in the long term. This product is not authorized for veterinary use and availability is not guaranteed.
- Alfacalcidol (1-hydroxycholecalciferol) requires 25-hydroxylation by the liver before it is active. This process occurs rapidly in a relatively unregulated fashion so this does not significantly alter the time to maximal effect compared with calcitriol. The drug is available as 0.25, 0.5 and 1 μg capsules and also as drops (2 μg/ml), which are useful in small dogs and cats. A dose of 10–30 ng/kg q24h is used. However, these doses have some flexibility and may be titrated upwards or downwards to suit the individual animal. This product is not authorized for veterinary use.
- Dihydrotachysterol is a useful vitamin D supplement because it is available in a liquid formulation as a 0.25 mg/ml solution. This synthetic analogue is hydroxylated in the liver but does not require hydroxylation within the kidney to become active. The onset of action occurs within 24 hours and peak activity is reached within 7 days. The dose rate used is 0.02–0.03 mg/kg q24h for initial treatment. The dose can be reduced for longer-term management to 0.01–0.02 mg/kg q24–48h or as required. This product is not authorized for veterinary use. Compared with the vitamin D preparations above, it takes longer for maximal effect and has a more prolonged half-life that requires consideration when overdosed.
- It must be remembered that vitamin D2 and D3 will take a lot longer to reach a steady state (weeks) compared with calcitriol and alfacalcidol (days). The same is true of dose alterations, which can take unpredictable lengths of time to again reach a steady calcium concentration. Rapid changes in medication, either increases or decreases in dose, need to be avoided unless hypercalcaemia occurs. Vitamin D-associated hypercalcaemia should be avoided because it can frequently lead to kidney damage and soft tissue calcification (see Chapter 14).

The dose of elemental calcium required per day as an oral supplement is 25–50 mg/kg/day (divided into two or three doses), although higher doses may be used initially. However, calcium preparations vary in the amount of elemental calcium they contain and doses must be adjusted to take this into consideration: 1 mg elemental calcium = 10.75 mg calcium gluconate = 7.7 mg calcium lactate = 2.5 mg calcium carbonate.

The following are guidelines for different preparations:

- Calcium gluconate at 250–500 mg/kg/day divided into two or three doses
- Calcium lactate at 200–380 mg/kg/day divided into two or three doses
- Calcium carbonate 62.5–125 mg/kg/day divided into two doses.

Early calcium supplementation is helpful to ensure high intestinal luminal calcium concentrations that will encourage passive calcium absorption over the period of time it takes for vitamin D to begin to have an effect.

Long-term management and prognosis

Once an animal has been stabilized on a dose of vitamin D, calcium supplementation can usually be stopped and the diet relied upon as a source of calcium. The long-term prognosis is good, but regular monitoring is advisable, particularly if other medical conditions occur that may have an impact on the intestinal absorption of calcium, for example, chronic diarrhoea. Hypercalcaemia should also be avoided, as this will have a negative impact on kidney function if allowed to persist long term. In humans with hypoparathyroidism managed using vitamin D and calcium, 50% were found to suffer from chronic kidney disease or nephrocalcinosis when followed up (Mitchell et al., 2012). The aim should be to keep calcium concentrations within the low end of the reference interval to avoid excessive calciuria, as renal calcium resorption will be impaired due to the ongoing lack of PTH. To do this effectively is difficult and the approach varies from case to case. Sometimes, increasing calcium supplementation and lowering the vitamin D dose works better in humans, but in dogs, where panting on exercise or excitement is frequent, very low resting calcium concentrations can lead to clinical signs during such times.

References and further reading

Armstrong AJ, Hauptman JG, Stanley BJ et al. (2018) Effect of prophylactic calcitriol administration on serum ionized calcium concentrations after parathyroidectomy: 78 cases (2005–2015). *Journal of Veterinary Internal Medicine* **32**, 99–106

Bassett JR (1998) Hypocalcemia and hyperphosphatemia due to primary hypoparathyroidism in a six-month-old kitten. *Journal of the American Animal Hospital Association* **34**, 503–507

Brown J, Nunez S, Russel M and Spurney C (2009) Hypocalcemic rickets and dilated cardiomyopathy: case reports and review of literature. *Pediatric Cardiology* **30**, 818–823

Bruyette DS and Feldman EC (1988) Primary hypoparathyroidism in the dog: report of 15 cases and review of 13 previously reported cases. *Journal of Veterinary Internal Medicine* **2**, 7–14

Bush WW, Kimmel SE, Wosar MA and Jackson MW (2001) Secondary hypoparathyroidism attributed to hypomagnesemia in a dog with protein-losing enteropathy. *Journal of the American Veterinary Medical Association* **219**, 1732–1734

Dear JD, Kass PH, Della Maggiore AM and Feldman EC (2017) Association of hypercalcemia before treatment with hypocalcemia after treatment in dogs with primary hyperparathyroidism. *Journal of Veterinary Internal Medicine* **31**, 349–354

Feldman EC (2015) Hypocalcaemia and primary hypoparathyroidism. In: *Canine and Feline Endocrinology, 4th edn*, ed. EC Feldman, RW Nelson, CE Reusch, JCR Scott-Moncrieff and EN Behrend, pp. 625–648. Elsevier Saunders, St. Louis

Gagliardo T, Ruggeri R, Di Paola A *et al.* (2021) Clinical features of muscle cramp in 14 dogs. *Journal of Veterinary Internal Medicine* **35**, 372–377

Gunn-Moore D (2005) Feline endocrinopathies. *Veterinary Clinics of North America: Small Animal Practice* **35**, 171–210

Jones BR and Alley MR (1985) Primary idiopathic hypoparathyroidism in St. Bernard dogs. *New Zealand Veterinary Journal* **33**, 94–97

Kimmel SE, Waddell LS and Michel KE (2000) Hypomagnesemia and hypocalcemia associated with protein-losing enteropathy in Yorkshire terriers: five cases (1992–1998). *Journal of the American Veterinary Medical Association* **217**, 703–706

Kornegay JH, Greene CE, Martin C, Gorgacz EJ and Melcon DK (1980) Idiopathic hypocalcemia in four dogs. *Journal of the American Animal Hospital Association* **16**, 723–734

Lie AR and MacDonald KA (2013) Reversible myocardial failure in a cat with primary hypoparathyroidism. *Journal of Feline Medicine and Surgery* **15**, 932–940

Mavroudis K, Aloumanis K, Stamatis P *et al.* (2010) Irreversible end-stage heart failure in a young patient due to severe chronic hypocalcemia associated with primary hypoparathyroidism and celiac disease. *Clinical Cardiology* **33**, E72–E75

Mitchell DM, Regan S, Cooley MR *et al.* (2012) Long-term follow-up of patients with hypoparathyroidism. *Journal of Clinical Endocrinology and Metabolism* **97**, 4507–4514

Peterson ME, James KM, Wallace M, Timothy SD and Joseph RJ (1991) Idiopathic hypoparathyroidism in five cats. *Journal of Veterinary Internal Medicine* **5**, 47–51

Refsal KR, Provencher-Bolliger AL, Graham PA and Nachreiner RF (2001) Update on the diagnosis and treatment of disorders of calcium regulation. *Veterinary Clinics of North America: Small Animal Practice* **31**, 1043–1062

Rosol TJ, Chew DJ, Capen CC and Sherding RG (1988) Acute hypocalcemia associated with infarction of parathyroid gland adenomas in two dogs. *Journal of the American Veterinary Medical Association* **192**, 212–214

Russell NJ, Bond KA, Robertson ID, Parry BW and Irwin PJ (2006) Primary hypoparathyroidism in dogs: a retrospective study of 17 cases. *Australian Veterinary Journal* **84**, 285–290

Schenck PA (2005) Serum ionized magnesium concentrations in dogs and cats with hypoparathyroidism (abstract). *Journal of Veterinary Internal Medicine* **19**, 462

Schenck PA and Chew DJ (2003) What's new in assessing calcium disorders – Part 1. *Proceedings of the 21st ACVIM Forum, Charlotte, NC, USA, 4–7 June, 2003*, 517–518

Schenck PA and Chew DJ (2005) Prediction of serum ionized calcium concentration by use of serum total calcium concentration in dogs. *American Journal of Veterinary Research* **66**, 1330–1336

Schenck PA, Chew DJ and Brooks CL (1995) Effects of storage on serum ionized calcium and pH values in clinically normal dogs. *American Journal of Veterinary Research* **56**, 304–307

Wolf J, Vigani A and Schaer M (2020) Trauma-induced primary hypoparathyroidism following severe bite wound injury to the neck in a dog. *Journal of Veterinary Emergency and Critical Care* **30**, 331–335

Chapter 16

Hyperparathyroidism

Barbara J. Skelly

Introduction

Primary hyperparathyroidism is uncommon in dogs and rare in cats but must still be considered as a possible cause for hypercalcaemia, particularly in older, relatively asymptomatic dogs. It develops when one or more of the parathyroid glands begin to function autonomously. Hyperparathyroidism may also develop through non-endocrine disruptions to calcium homeostasis, such as those caused by kidney disease, hypercortisolism or nutritional imbalances.

Anatomy

The anatomy of the parathyroid gland is described in Chapter 14. In summary, there are two parathyroid glands associated with each thyroid lobe. The external (cranial) glands may be visualized as a small pale spherical object at the cranial pole of each thyroid lobe (Figure 16.1). The internal (caudal) parathyroid glands are not easily visualized unless they are significantly enlarged. Parathyroid tissue can be ectopic and such tissue is usually situated alongside the trachea. Histologically, parathyroid tissue consists of nests of cells around capillaries (Figure 16.2).

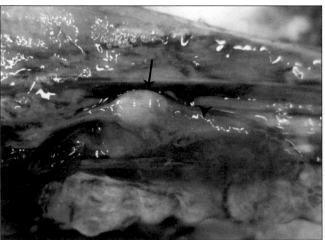

16.1 Gross pathological specimen showing the anatomical position of a parathyroid gland (arrowed) at the cranial pole of the thyroid gland (arrowhead). Normal glands are small and difficult to see but this specimen is from a dog that had parathyroid disease and a single enlarged, pale gland.
(Courtesy of Fernando Constantino-Casas)

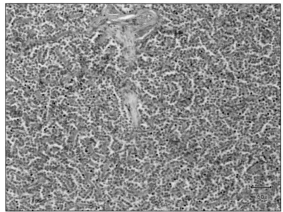

16.2 Histological appearance of the parathyroid gland from a healthy dog, showing cords or nests of cells around capillaries. Haematoxylin and eosin stain; bar = 50 μm.
(Courtesy of Fernando Constantino-Casas)

Physiology

The release of parathyroid hormone (PTH) is mediated by activation or inactivation of the calcium-sensing receptor (CaSR) by hypercalcaemia or hypocalcaemia, respectively.

Parathyroid hormone acts directly on bone and the kidneys, and indirectly on the gastrointestinal tract to increase calcium mobilization or reuptake. Negative feedback occurs from increased serum calcium concentrations such that PTH secretion is switched off once the required calcium concentration is reached. See Chapter 14 for a more detailed discussion of PTH.

Primary hyperparathyroidism

Hyperparathyroidism is defined by increased secretion of PTH and is one of the differential diagnoses for hypercalcaemia (see Chapter 14). Primary hyperparathyroidism is characterized by hypercalcaemia and an increased or high reference interval PTH concentration with no other identifiable underlying cause.

Prevalence

Primary hyperparathyroidism is an uncommon disease in dogs. It is very rare in cats, with only a few case reports (Kallet et al., 1991; Savary et al., 2000; Parker et al., 2015).

Aetiology

Primary hyperparathyroidism is caused by adenoma or, less commonly, carcinoma or adenomatous hyperplasia of one or more of the parathyroid glands. As a consequence, affected glands function autonomously, independent of the effects of serum calcium concentration. Hyperplasia may not affect each gland uniformly and, although most frequently associated with secondary disease, it has been described as a cause of primary hyperparathyroidism in cats and dogs.

In humans, primary hyperparathyroidism is a feature of several inherited disorders, including familial parathyroid syndromes and multiple endocrine neoplasia. In dogs, the Keeshond is the only breed known to have an inherited form of hyperparathyroidism. The mode of inheritance has been evaluated and two studies have described the investigation of the disease using a candidate gene strategy (Goldstein *et al.*, 2007; Skelly and Franklin, 2007). Affected dogs develop an autosomal dominant form of primary hyperparathyroidism that has partial, age-dependent penetrance. This means that a Keeshond need have only one copy of the mutated allele to develop the disease, and all dogs carrying the mutation will go on to develop the disease if they live long enough. No dogs have been identified that have two copies of the mutated allele and it is speculated that this would be incompatible with survival to birth. A genetic test is available for primary hyperparathyroidism in Keeshonds (Cornell University, see 'Useful websites', below) but, as yet, the mutation or the identity of the gene involved has not been published. This test enables breeders to limit their use of mutation-carrying animals and choose replacement breeding stock that are negative for the disease-causing mutation.

Signalment

Primary hyperparathyroidism is a disease of older dogs (mean age 11.2 years, range 6–17 years). There is no sex predisposition but there is a breed predilection in that Keeshonds are over-represented. In one review of cases, Keeshonds were found to have the highest breed-associated odds ratio, of 50.7 (Refsal *et al.*, 2001). Neonatal hyperparathyroidism has been reported in a litter of German Shepherd Dogs (Thompson *et al.*, 1984) but there have been no other reports since.

Clinical features

The clinical signs of hyperparathyroidism are summarized in Figure 16.3.

Primary hyperparathyroidism is not a dramatic disease; rather, it is slow in development and insidious in nature. As such, changes are subtle and can occur over a long time period. As affected dogs tend to be older, many of the clinical signs are attributed to ageing changes and owners do not seek veterinary advice until late in the course of the disease. It is frequently a disease that is identified serendipitously. In one study of 210 cases, 42% of dogs were identified as having primary hyperparathyroidism when they were presented for other reasons, such as routine geriatric checks or after pre-anaesthetic blood work was performed for procedures such as dental treatment (Feldman *et al.*, 2005). The most common reason for seeking veterinary advice was for the investigation of clinical signs related to urolithiasis or urinary tract infection (50% of the 210 cases). Urolithiasis can also present as acute urinary outflow obstruction in a dog with primary hyperparathyroidism.

Kidney and lower urinary tract signs
• Polyuria
• Polydipsia
• Urinary incontinence
• Stranguria
• Pollakiuria
• Urolithiasis

Neuromuscular signs
• Lethargy
• Exercise intolerance
• Shivering
• Muscle twitching

Gastrointestinal signs
• Vomiting
• Inappetence
• Constipation

Other
• Dental pain
• Difficulty eating
• Stiff gait
• Lameness

16.3 Clinical signs of hyperparathyroidism.

Polyuria and polydipsia were noticed by less than 10% of owners of dogs with primary hyperparathyroidism, a surprisingly small number given that calcium acts as an antagonist to arginine vasopressin in the collecting ducts of the kidney and thereby inhibits the urinary concentrating mechanism. The result is that affected dogs are polyuric with secondary compensatory polydipsia.

The presence of hypercalcaemia can also affect the kidneys in other ways. Dogs that are hypercalcaemic are at an increased risk of developing kidney failure. It is difficult to understand the underlying mechanism and why some dogs are affected and others are spared. Calculating the calcium–phosphate product has been suggested to predict the likelihood of kidney failure developing; dogs with primary hyperparathyroidism and a low phosphate concentration have a relatively low calcium–phosphate product and are thought to be less likely to develop kidney failure. In a case series of 210 dogs, the risk of kidney failure was deemed to be low (Feldman *et al.*, 2005), while in a smaller case series from the UK, approximately 25% of dogs developed kidney insufficiency (Gear *et al.*, 2005). In the latter study, the calcium–phosphate product was a poor predictor of kidney damage.

The phosphate concentration should be decreased or at the low end of the reference interval in a dog with primary hyperparathyroidism. If it is not, the presence of kidney disease should be considered, even in the absence of overt azotaemia. In these cases, closer monitoring should be implemented and a more guarded prognosis can be given.

It is interesting to examine the genetically homogeneous Keeshond population and the prevalence of kidney disease in dogs that have primary hyperparathyroidism. Some dogs left untreated die of other causes with normal kidney function despite having prolonged, and in some cases severe (>4.0 mmol/l), hypercalcaemia. Others succumb to kidney failure with much more modest hypercalcaemia, while some develop large nephroliths (Figure 16.4). It is clear that predicting long-term outcomes with and without treatment is fraught with problems. When managing affected dogs, it is recommended to treat promptly and err on the side of caution.

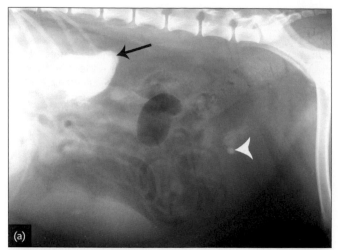

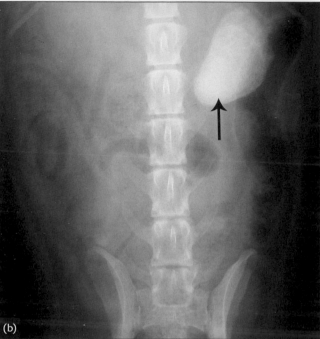

16.4 (a) Lateral and (b) ventrodorsal abdominal radiographs of a dog showing a large nephrolith in the left kidney (arrowed) and multiple smaller uroliths within the lower urinary tract (arrowhead).

Physical examination findings are few and non-specific, and may include stiffness and gait abnormalities, dull mentation, weakness and muscle wastage. In dogs, little information is gathered from palpation of the ventral neck area because any parathyroid abnormalities are usually beyond the most sensitive palpation skills. In cats, a ventral cervical mass is sometimes reported (Parker *et al.*, 2015), although most palpable masses are subsequently identified as enlarged cystic lesions associated with adenomatous glands. Any masses in this area must also be differentiated from thyroid enlargement, which is much more common.

Urolithiasis

Urolith formation is common in dogs with hyperparathyroidism due to the increased quantity of calcium filtered by the kidney and lost in urine. Calcium-containing uroliths are also reported in cats. Although PTH causes increased calcium uptake from the renal tubules, in cases of primary hyperparathyroidism there is overt hypercalciuria,

presumably because the amount of filtered calcium exceeds tubular uptake capacity. Conditions in urine are such that there is an increased tendency for calcium salts to precipitate within the urinary tract. Dogs with primary hyperparathyroidism have hypercalciuria but also have increased phosphate excretion. Urine is therefore supersaturated with both calcium and phosphate, and it is unsurprising that this leads to calcium phosphate precipitation and stone formation. The prevalence of calcium oxalate urolithiasis is also increased in dogs with primary hyperparathyroidism. Dietary oxalate uptake from the gastrointestinal tract is reduced when there is abundant intraluminal calcium because calcium oxalate is not absorbable from the intestine. If intestinal calcium absorption increases, oxalate absorption will also increase and the kidney will filter higher amounts of both calcium and oxalate, again leading to supersaturation in the urine.

Clinicopathological features

The critical parameters to measure in animals with primary hyperparathyroidism include total and ionized calcium, phosphate, PTH and parathyroid hormone-related protein (PTHrP).

Calcium and phosphate

Hypercalcaemia, both total and ionized, is a defining feature of primary hyperparathyroidism. The degree of hypercalcaemia is largely dependent on the duration of disease before its identification. Keeshonds from families with primary hyperparathyroidism generally start to show mild hypercalcaemia (<3.3 mmol/l) when they are 6–8 years of age and this gradually worsens over subsequent years. Some untreated dogs continue to have increased calcium concentrations until severe hypercalcaemia is reached (>4.0 mmol/l). It is not clear how reproducible this pattern is between breeds, but the disease appears to be slow and insidious in development in all dogs.

If the hypercalcaemia is PTH-mediated, hypophosphataemia should also be evident, provided kidney function is normal. Other biochemical parameters may be unremarkable. Urea, creatinine and symmetric dimethylarginine concentrations may be increased, along with phosphate concentrations, due to pre-existing kidney damage or prerenal factors. This complicates diagnosis, in that the changes associated with primary hyperparathyroidism with secondary kidney failure can mimic those of primary kidney disease with secondary hyperparathyroidism and hypercalcaemia (see Chapter 14).

Haematological parameters show no consistent changes, although anaemia of chronic disease may be identified, particularly if hypercalcaemia has been present for some time.

Parathyroid hormone

In dogs with primary hyperparathyroidism, a PTH concentration above the reference interval or inappropriately high for the concurrent serum calcium concentration (i.e. usually in the upper half of the reference interval) is expected. There is less information on the appropriate PTH reference interval in cats, and unexpectedly higher values for whole compared with intact PTH have been reported, possibly reflecting differences in antibody affinities at the amino terminal of the PTH molecule (Pineda *et al.*, 2012). As a result, a definitive diagnosis of primary hyperparathyroidism can be more challenging in the cat.

Parathyroid hormone-related protein

Parathyroid hormone-related protein should be low or undetectable in animals meeting the criteria for diagnosis of primary hyperparathyroidism. If this is not the case, the animal should be carefully reassessed for the presence of neoplasia.

Diagnostic imaging

Ultrasonography of the ventral neck is the most useful imaging modality for investigating parathyroid adenomas, with 90–95% positively identified by experienced imagers (Feldman, 2005). A high-frequency transducer (7.5–10 MHz) is required for adequate resolution. In healthy dogs and cats, the parathyroid glands are so small that they are rarely recognized. When enlarged due to adenomatous, hyperplastic or carcinomatous disease, they are identified as small (2–20 mm), round to oval, hypoechoic nodules within thyroid tissue (Figure 16.5).

Scintigraphy using technetium (^{99m}Tc) sestamibi has been used in dogs as an aid to parathyroid identification but, unlike in humans, it lacks sensitivity and specificity, and is therefore unreliable.

Abdominal radiographs may be useful as they may reveal calcium-containing renal or cystic calculi. These may be present without associated clinical signs.

Pathology

Three different types of pathological change are reported from autonomously secreting parathyroid glands: carcinoma, adenoma and hyperplasia. To some extent the subdivision is subjective and may vary between pathologists

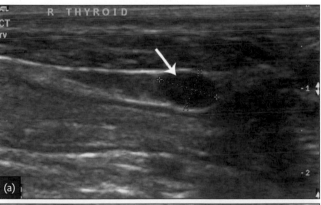

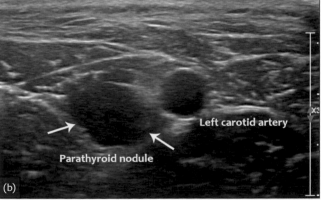

16.5 (a) Ultrasonographic image showing the typical appearance of a parathyroid adenoma (arrowed). (b) Transverse image through the cervical region showing a large, irregular parathyroid nodule (arrowed) that was later identified as a parathyroid carcinoma.
(Courtesy of Lorraine Peschard)

since, in common with many functional endocrine tumours, differentiation is difficult, especially when only one gland is excised and examined. In parathyroid carcinomas where malignant criteria are identified, metastatic disease is rare. Disease recurrence, where there is involvement of another gland, is possible with all three pathological classifications.

Treatment
Pre-treatment management of hypercalcaemia

Once hypercalcaemia has been recognized, it is important to institute treatment to lower calcium concentrations whilst other diagnostic tests are underway. Kidney damage caused by persistent hypercalcaemia due to primary hyperparathyroidism is uncommon but difficult to predict. All affected animals must therefore be considered at risk if they are significantly hypercalcaemic.

Fluid therapy is the cornerstone of the management of hypercalcaemia. Induction of diuresis using 0.9% sodium chloride at rates of 5 ml/kg/h, or higher, increases renal calcium loss and lowers circulating calcium concentrations. Fluid therapy should aim to correct any dehydration and then additionally expand the extracellular fluid volume so that the glomerular filtration rate is increased. Sodium chloride is the fluid of choice because extra sodium ions induce diuresis and are able to compete with calcium and reduce tubular calcium resorption. When an animal is considered to be optimally hydrated, furosemide (2 mg/kg q8–12h) can potentiate renal calcium loss by reducing tubular calcium resorption still further. When using sodium chloride at high rates, particularly coupled with furosemide use, serum potassium must be monitored to avoid inducing hypokalaemia.

If this treatment is not sufficient to lower serum calcium concentrations, other medications can be used. These include:

- Glucocorticoids
- Bisphosphonates
- Calcitonin
- Plicamycin
- Cinacalcet.

Glucocorticoids: The use of glucocorticoids (approximately 1 mg/kg once daily) to lower serum calcium concentrations should be restricted to those cases where there is a clear diagnosis and a delay to rational treatment. They are most effective when used in cases of hypercalcaemia of malignancy due to lymphoma as they cause rapid tumour lysis and reduced production of the mediators of hypercalcaemia (e.g. PTHrP). When glucocorticoids are used before a diagnosis is confirmed, there is a real risk of masking and complicating the diagnosis of lymphoma and potentially reducing the response to future chemotherapy. Glucocorticoids work by increasing renal calcium loss, decreasing intestinal calcium uptake, decreasing bone resorption and antagonising the effects of vitamin D. They do not have a great effect in cases of primary hyperparathyroidism or neoplasms other than lymphomas, and do not significantly lower calcium concentrations.

Bisphosphonates: Bisphosphonates are potent inhibitors of bone resorption and act through inhibition of osteoclastic activity and induction of osteoclast apoptosis. Several different bisphosphonates have been used in both dogs and cats, but clodronate, alendronate, etidronate, pamidronate and zoledronate are most commonly reported. Although clodronate, alendronate and etidronate can be used orally, this route of administration is not very effective; however, absorption can be improved by administration on an empty stomach. The oral bisphosphonates can be irritant and have been reported to cause oesophagitis. An intravenous infusion of pamidronate is more reliable and can be used in both dogs and cats (1.3–2.0 mg/kg in 150 ml of 0.9% saline, given over 2 hours (Hostutler *et al.*, 2005)). Pamidronate is approximately 100 times more potent than etidronate. The average response lasts approximately 3 weeks, although this is often shorter and can be longer in individual dogs. The dose can be repeated as required. This drug is generally well tolerated (Hostutler *et al.*, 2005) but can cause gastrointestinal side effects and hypocalcaemia, particularly if an overdose is given. Medication-related osteonecrosis of the jaw is a reported side effect of bisphosphonates in humans and has been reported in a cat and a dog. The cat developed osteonecrosis as a consequence of long-term management of idiopathic hypercalcaemia using both pamidronate and alendronate at increasing doses over a 4-year period (Larson *et al.*, 2019), and the dog was receiving zoledronate for osteosarcoma-related bone pain (Lundberg *et al.*, 2016). Pamidronate has been used frequently to treat humans with hypercalcaemia of malignancy but availability can be problematic. A newer, more potent bisphosphonate, zoledronic acid, is now superseding pamidronate as the drug of choice. Zoledronic acid is 100–850 times more active than pamidronate and can be infused more rapidly but has not yet been used extensively. It is recommended at a dose of 0.1–0.25 mg/kg diluted in 45–100 ml of 0.9% saline administered intravenously over 15–30 minutes. The onset of action of bisphosphonates is 24–48 hours, so they are not useful in a situation where there is life-threatening hypercalcaemia that must be reduced rapidly.

Calcitonin: Salmon calcitonin is available commercially to treat hypercalcaemia. Like bisphosphonates, it inhibits osteoclastic activity and also the renal resorption of calcium. It is useful as an emergency treatment to decrease calcium concentrations. A disadvantage of this treatment is that after an initial intravenous infusion (4 IU/kg), treatment must continue at least daily (4–8 IU/kg s.c. q12–24h) (Nelson and Elliott, 2003). Calcitonin therapy can cause anorexia and vomiting. It is an expensive treatment and is rarely used. Animals may become resistant to the effects of calcitonin after a few days of treatment.

Plicamycin (mithramycin): There are few reports of plicamycin being used in dogs. A dose rate of 25 μg/kg in 5% dextrose administered intravenously over 2–4 hours every 2–4 weeks has been suggested (Schenck *et al.*, 2006). This drug is no longer recommended in humans or animals due to the potential for development of adverse effects. In dogs, these effects include pain during infusion, shivering, hyperthermia and mild gastrointestinal upset. Fatal hepatocellular necrosis has also been reported related to the use of high doses in dogs with malignancies.

Cinacalcet: Cinacalcet is a CaSR analogue that is especially useful in conditions where the calcium set-point has been altered. If the CaSR has become less sensitive to extracellular calcium, a higher than normal calcium concentration is maintained. This process can be interrupted by the use of cinacalcet, a calcimimetic. In human medicine, this drug is used in familial hypercalciuric hypercalcaemia

and renal secondary hyperparathyroidism. In the future, it may have a role in dogs and cats, for example, in feline idiopathic hypercalcaemia or some forms of hyperparathyroidism, but its use has not been adequately investigated in these species.

Definitive treatment options

Surgical parathyroidectomy: Surgery is the treatment of choice at many referral institutions and is also preferred if the parathyroid nodule is greater than 12 mm in size (Rasor *et al.*, 2007). Good visualization of the thyroid glands is essential during surgical exploration of the neck and this is achieved using a ventral midline cervical approach. Parathyroid adenomas are usually easily identified compared with normal parathyroid glands because they are larger than normal and are paler than the surrounding dark red thyroid tissue. When the internal parathyroid glands are affected, they can be identified by palpation and may be visible through the ventral or dorsal aspect of the thyroid gland. Preoperative localization of the abnormal glands by ultrasonography or computed tomography aids surgical identification.

Parathyroid adenomas can be removed either by dissection of the enlarged gland from the adjacent thyroid tissue or by partial or unilateral thyroidectomy, where the parathyroid and part of the thyroid gland are removed *en bloc*. The intraoperative appearance of a parathyroid adenoma is illustrated in Figure 16.6. In cases of primary hyperparathyroidism, usually only one gland is affected. If more than one gland is found to be enlarged, then up to three glands may be removed at one time. At least one parathyroid gland should be left *in situ* so that calcium homeostasis can be maintained. If multiple glands are enlarged, it is more likely that the glands are hyperplastic rather than adenomatous and, therefore, secondary rather than primary hyperparathyroidism is suspected. This method of diagnostic differentiation is not infallible, however, and multiple gland involvement has also been reported in primary hyperparathyroidism.

Percutaneous, ultrasound-guided ethanol ablation: In order for parathyroid nodules to be effectively treated using ethanol injection, they must be successfully identified by ultrasound examination and must also be larger than 3 mm in diameter so that a 27 G needle can be inserted accurately. Animals must be under general anaesthesia.

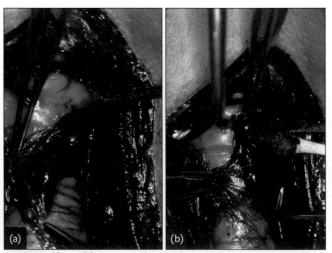

16.6 (a) and (b) Removal of a parathyroid adenoma. The thyroid (dark red) is visible overlying the trachea with a smaller, paler, parathyroid nodule (at the tip of the cotton bud in (b)).
(Courtesy of Ed Friend)

The technique works because ethanol induces coagulative necrosis and thrombosis in the parathyroid nodule. The success of this technique is operator dependent, in that skill is needed for accurate needle placement and injection so that the carotid artery and vagosympathetic trunk, which pass close by, are not compromised.

Percutaneous, ultrasound-guided heat ablation: This technique is the least frequently used, mainly because few institutions offer this therapy (Pollard *et al.*, 2001, Rasor *et al.*, 2007). The technique depends on inserting a needle into a parathyroid nodule and causing thermal necrosis at the needle tip. To do this, the animal is anaesthetized and positioned on an electrocautery ground pad, a 20 G catheter is inserted into the affected parathyroid gland and radiofrequency is applied at 10–20 W until the entire gland becomes hyperechoic.

Pre- and post-treatment considerations

When the three techniques for treating primary hyperparathyroidism were compared, ethanol ablation was the least successful, with a positive outcome achieved in 13/18 (72%) procedures compared with 45/48 (94%) for surgery and 44/49 (90%) for heat ablation (Rasor *et al.*, 2007). However, a success rate of greater than 90% using ethanol ablation in 30 dogs has also been reported (Schaefer and Goldstein, 2009). This technique has also recently been described as effective in a cat (Riehl *et al.*, 2019).

When primary hyperparathyroidism is treated successfully using one of the three techniques described above, PTH and therefore calcium concentrations should drop rapidly (usually over 6–12 hours) and, in some circumstances, a hypocalcaemic crisis may be encountered. In these cases, intravenous supplementation of calcium is required (see Chapter 15).

In theory, when a parathyroid adenoma is functioning autonomously, the remaining parathyroid glands may atrophy and become unable to support normal calcium homeostasis once the adenoma is removed. It has been suggested that long-standing hypercalcaemia of high magnitude was more likely to lead to parathyroid atrophy and postoperative hypocalcaemia. The evidence to support this is controversial. Although a recent study has shown that preoperative ionized calcium concentration is predictive for the development of postoperative hypocalcaemia, most other studies suggest that calcium and vitamin D supplementation are rarely needed, no matter the magnitude of pre-treatment hypercalcaemia (Milovancev and Schmiedt, 2013; Dear *et al.*, 2017; Armstrong *et al.*, 2018; Burkhardt *et al.*, 2021). A hypocalcaemic crisis can be managed by administering intravenous calcium supplementation in the immediate postoperative period if required (see Chapter 15).

Hypomagnesaemia can be a contributory cause of hypocalcaemia, especially in postoperative and hospitalized cases. Serum magnesium concentrations may be within the reference interval, since serum magnesium often does not accurately reflect intracellular stores. Assessment of the response to parenteral magnesium may be needed to infer magnesium deficiency. Oral magnesium (magnesium oxide, magnesium carbonate or magnesium sulphate) is used for mild, chronic magnesium deficiency (e.g. a daily dose of 200–300 mg). Intravenous magnesium (10% or 50% solution of magnesium sulphate) is used for severe hypomagnesaemia. A common regimen is 2–4 ml of a 50% solution given intravenously over 10–15 minutes, followed by similar amounts given daily. Several days of treatment are usually required to replenish magnesium stores.

Often, and particularly when postoperative hypocalcaemia has been severe and symptomatic, calcium supplementation will be used in the short term for stabilization of the case. For longer-term management, oral calcium supplementation is rarely necessary because most pet foods contain more than adequate amounts, provided sufficient vitamin D is present to allow absorption.

Prognosis

The short- to medium-term (<2 years) prognosis for primary hyperparathyroidism is excellent in all breeds. In all breeds other than the Keeshond, the long-term prognosis is also good. In the Keeshond, as in many human forms of primary hyperparathyroidism, recurrence is a distinct possibility. In humans with familial hyperparathyroidism, subtotal parathyroidectomy is commonly performed along with autologous transplantation of parathyroid tissue into the forearm due to the recognized risk of future tumour development in residual tissue. Keeshonds have a genetic drive to develop parathyroid adenomas; therefore, after one gland has been removed, more parathyroid tumours may develop if the individual lives long enough (Thompson and Skelly, 2020). Keeshonds that have been treated for primary hyperparathyroidism should be monitored throughout their remaining life for disease recurrence, particularly if the first surgery was performed at a relatively young age (<9 years old). It may be tempting to think that subtotal parathyroidectomy would be also be preferable in dogs, but this was shown to delay, but not prevent, recurrence in at least one dog (Thompson and Skelly, 2020). Although rare, it has also been shown that primary hyperparathyroidism can recur following successful treatment in dogs without a clear breed or familial predisposition (Thompson and Skelly, 2020). Clearly, this is an area that is poorly understood and requires further study.

Secondary hyperparathyroidism

Secondary hyperparathyroidism relates to non-endocrine causes of hypersecretion of PTH. Three forms of secondary hyperparathyroidism are described:

- Renal secondary hyperparathyroidism
- Nutritional secondary hyperparathyroidism
- Adrenal secondary hyperparathyroidism.

Renal secondary hyperparathyroidism

An animal with kidney disease and hypercalcaemia can be diagnostically challenging because primary kidney disease may be driving the hypercalcaemia, or another cause of hypercalcaemia may be leading to secondary kidney disease. The diagnostic dilemma is further complicated by the fact that, in many cases, PTH is the driving force for hypercalcaemia. The clinicopathological similarities between primary hyperparathyroidism and chronic kidney disease (CKD) with secondary hyperparathyroidism are covered in Chapter 14. If an animal with primary hyperparathyroidism has hypercalcaemia-induced kidney failure and phosphate concentrations increase, then another differentiating parameter is lost. Ionized calcium concentration is always increased in primary hyperparathyroidism, whereas less than 10% of dogs with CKD have increased ionized calcium concentrations. Therefore, most dogs with azotaemia and significantly increased ionized calcium concentrations in conjunction with high PTH concentrations will have primary hyperparathyroidism, but a careful diagnostic work-up is still required. The pathophysiological changes leading to renal secondary hyperparathyroidism are described in Figure 16.7.

The management of renal secondary hyperparathyroidism is summarized in Figure 16.8. The use of vitamin D is not recommended due to lack of evidence of any beneficial effect, particularly in cats. Both calcitriol and alfacalcidol have relatively short half-lives, so stopping therapy should rapidly result in resolution of any induced hypercalcaemia. Vitamin D preparations may be easier to use safely when dosing every other day as their activity depends on the length of time they are in contact with the intestinal wall. Phosphate restriction is pivotal, however, and has been shown to reduce the clinical features of renal secondary hyperparathyroidism. An evidence-based approach to the management of CKD is advised (International Renal Interest Society, 2023).

Phosphate retention
• Reduced capacity of the kidneys to excrete phosphate as glomerular filtration rate falls
Decreased concentration of calcitriol
• Increased phosphate concentrations in proximal tubular cells inhibit CYP27B1 (1-alpha-hydroxylase) activity and thus calcitriol synthesis • High phosphate concentrations stimulate FGF-23 synthesis and release from osteocytes, which further inhibits CYP27B1 • Damage to renal tubules further lowers the renal capacity to synthesize calcitriol
Ionized hypocalcaemia
• Relative calcitriol deficiency reduces calcium uptake from the intestine • Precipitation of calcium–phosphate complexes leads to soft tissue calcification • Skeletal resistance to the action of PTH
Abnormal parathyroid gland function
• PTH synthesis and secretion stimulated by low ionized calcium, the lack of negative feedback from calcitriol and hyperphosphataemia • Raised set-point for secretion of PTH leading to excessive PTH secretion even when extracellular ionized calcium concentrations are normal • Parathyroid gland hyperplasia (multiple)

16.7 Pathophysiology of renal secondary hyperparathyroidism. FGF-23 = fibroblast growth factor 23; PTH = parathyroid hormone.

Nutritional secondary hyperparathyroidism

Not all pets are fed a balanced diet. The rise of niche raw diets (also known as raw-meat-based diets or biologically appropriate raw food (BARF) diets) and boutique, exotic and grain-free (BEG) diets has led to an increase in diseases and syndromes related to dietary imbalances. This is coupled with the growing popularity of unusual breeds and owners' perceptions that their pets require specially formulated diets.

Nutritional secondary hyperparathyroidism is the consequence of an imbalance between calcium and phosphate that occurs when an animal is fed a predominantly meat diet. Such diets are low in calcium and high in phosphate; low vitamin D intake may also compound the problem. Raw diets may be associated with this condition (DeLay and Laing, 2002) and it is rare for pet owners feeding a complete dog or cat food that meets all dietary requirements to encounter this condition. The features of the condition usually manifest in young animals, where skeletal problems are present with low bone density and fibrous osteodystrophy. Nutritional secondary hyperparathyroidism tends to exert its effects on the long bones and pathological fractures can occur.

Adrenal secondary hyperparathyroidism

It has long been recognized that hypercortisolism can cause signs of dysregulation of calcium homeostasis and that affected animals can show soft tissue calcification (calcinosis cutis, bronchial tree calcification), but the reasons for this are still unclear. A syndrome of increased circulating concentrations of PTH has been identified in animals with hypercortisolism and this has been termed adrenal secondary hyperparathyroidism. Over 90% of 68 dogs with hypercortisolism had PTH concentrations above the reference interval, although total and ionized calcium concentrations were unaffected (Ramsey et al., 2005). The effects of hypercortisolism should be taken into account when reaching a diagnosis of primary hyperparathyroidism, particularly in dogs. Parathyroid hormone concentrations decrease to within the reference interval following successful treatment of hypercortisolism (Tebb et al., 2005). Recently, it has been suggested that adrenal secondary hyperparathyroidism is a physiological consequence of the increased serum phosphate and higher

Management	Side effects/limitations
Phosphate restriction	
Dietary phosphate restriction • Feeding phosphate-restricted commercial renal diets • Formulating home-made renal diets	• Palatability • Suitability for growing animal • Achieving nutritional balance
Oral intestinal phosphate-binding agents • Aluminium hydroxide 10–30 mg/kg q6–8h with meals • Calcium carbonate 30 mg/kg/day with meals • Chitosan and calcium carbonate 200 mg/kg q12h with meals • Sevelamer hydrochloride 30–40 mg/kg q8h with meals • Lanthanum carbonate, dogs 100 mg/kg/day, divided between meals, cats 400–800 mg/cat/day with meals	• Palatability • Nausea and anorexia • Constipation • Hypophosphataemia • Aluminium toxicity • Hypocalcaemia
Vitamin D therapy	
Directly inhibits parathyroid hormone secretion • Calcitriol 1.5–3.5 ng/kg/day • Alfacalcidol 1.5–3.5 ng/kg/day	• Beneficial effects still questioned • Calcium/phosphate need to be monitored regularly to prevent hypercalcaemia (at least weekly initially) • Hypercalcaemia will contribute to ongoing renal injury

16.8 Management of renal secondary hyperparathyroidism.

urinary calcium excretion rates in dogs with hypercortisolism (Corsini *et al.*, 2021). Although not widely studied, hyperparathyroidism is also likely with exogenous glucocorticoid administration.

References and further reading

Armstrong AJ, Hauptman JG, Stanley BJ *et al.* (2018) Effect of prophylactic calcitriol administration on serum ionized calcium concentrations after parathyroidectomy: 78 cases (2005–2015). *Journal of Veterinary Internal Medicine* **32**, 99–106

Burkhardt SJ, Sumner JP and Mann S (2021) Ambidirectional cohort study on the agreement of ultrasonography and surgery in the identification of parathyroid pathology, and predictors of postoperative hypocalcemia in 47 dogs undergoing parathyroidectomy due to primary hyperparathyroidism. *Veterinary Surgery* **50**, 1379–1388

Corsini A, Dondi F, Serio DG *et al.* (2021) Calcium and phosphate homeostasis in dogs with newly diagnosed naturally occurring hypercortisolism. *Journal of Veterinary Internal Medicine* **35**, 1265–1273

Dear JD, Kass PH, Della Maggiore AM and Feldman EC (2017) Association of hypercalcemia before treatment with hypocalcemia after treatment in dogs with primary hyperparathyroidism. *Journal of Veterinary Internal Medicine* **31**, 349–354

DeLay J and Laing J (2002) Nutritional osteodystrophy in puppies fed a BARF diet. *Animal Health Laboratory Newsletter* **6**, 23

Feldman EC, Hoar B, Pollard R and Nelson RW (2005) Pretreatment clinical and laboratory findings in dogs with primary hyperparathyroidism: 210 cases (1987–2004). *Journal of the American Veterinary Medical Association* **227**, 756–761

Gear RNA, Neiger R, Skelly BJS and Herrtage ME (2005) Primary hyperparathyroidism in 29 dogs: diagnosis, treatment, outcome and associated renal failure. *Journal of Small Animal Practice* **46**, 10–16

Goldstein RE, Atwater DZ, Cazolli DM *et al.* (2007) Inheritance, mode of inheritance, and candidate genes for primary hyperparathyroidism in Keeshonden. *Journal of Veterinary Internal Medicine* **21**, 199–203

Hostutler RA, Chew DJ, Jaeger JQ *et al.* (2005) Uses and effectiveness of pamidronate disodium for treatment of dogs and cats with hypercalcemia. *Journal of Veterinary Internal Medicine* **19**, 29–33

International Renal Interest Society (2023) IRIS treatment recommendations for CKD. Available from: www.iris-kidney.com/guidelines

Kallet AJ, Richter KP, Feldman EC and Brum DE (1991) Primary hyperparathyroidism in cats: seven cases (1984–1989). *Journal of the American Veterinary Medical Association* **199**, 1767–1771

Larson MJ, Oakes AB, Epperson E and Chew DJ (2019) Medication-related osteonecrosis of the jaw after long-term bisphosphonate treatment in a cat. *Journal of Veterinary Internal Medicine* **33**, 862–867

Lundberg AP, Roady PJ, Somrak AJ, Howes ME and Fan TM (2016) Zoledronate-associated osteonecrosis of the jaw in a dog with appendicular osteosarcoma. *Journal of Veterinary Internal Medicine* **30**, 1235–1240

Milovancev M and Schmiedt CW (2013) Preoperative factors associated with postoperative hypocalcemia in dogs with primary hyperparathyroidism that underwent parathyroidectomy: 62 cases (2004–2009). *Journal of the American Veterinary Medical Association* **242**, 507–515

Nelson RW and Elliott D (2003) Metabolic and electrolyte disorders. In: *Small Animal Internal Medicine, 3rd edn*, ed. RW Nelson and CG Couto, pp. 816–846. Mosby, St. Louis

Parker VJ, Gilor C and Chew DJ (2015) Feline hyperparathyroidism: pathophysiology, diagnosis and treatment of primary and secondary disease. *Journal of Feline Medicine and Surgery* **17**, 427–439

Pineda C, Aguilera-Tejero E, Raya AI *et al.* (2012) Feline parathyroid hormone: validation of hormonal assays and dynamics of secretion. *Domestic Animal Endocrinology* **42**, 256–264

Pollard RE, Long CD, Nelson RW, Hornof WJ and Feldman EC (2001) Percutaneous ultrasonographically guided radiofrequency heat ablation for treatment of primary hyperparathyroidism in dogs. *Journal of the American Veterinary Medical Association* **218**, 1106–1110

Ramsey IK, Tebb A, Harris E, Evans H and Herrtage ME (2005) Hyperparathyroidism in dogs with hyperadrenocorticism. *Journal of Small Animal Practice* **46**, 531–536

Rasor L, Pollard R and Feldman EC (2007) Retrospective evaluation of three treatment methods for primary hyperparathyroidism in dogs. *Journal of the American Animal Hospital Association* **43**, 70–77

Refsal KR, Provencher-Bolliger AL, Graham PA and Nachreiner RF (2001) Update on the diagnosis and treatment of disorders of calcium regulation. *Veterinary Clinics of North America: Small Animal Practice* **31**, 1043–1062

Riehl V, Hartmann A, Rohrberg A and Neiger R (2019) Percutaneous ultrasound-guided ethanol ablation for treatment of primary hyperparathyroidism in a cat. *Journal of Feline Medicine and Surgery Open Reports* **5**, 2055116919860276

Savary KCM, Price GS and Vaden SL (2000) Hypercalcemia in cats: a retrospective study of 71 cases (1991–1997). *Journal of Veterinary Internal Medicine* **14**, 184–189

Schaefer C and Goldstein RE (2009) Canine primary hyperparathyroidism. *Compendium: Continuing Education for Veterinarians* **31**, 382–389

Schenck PA, Chew DJ, Nagode LA and Rosol TJ (2006) Disorders of calcium: hypercalcemia and hypocalcemia. In: *Fluid, Electrolyte and Acid-Base Disorders in Small Animal Practice. 3rd edn*, ed. SP Dibartola, pp. 122–194. Saunders Elsevier, St. Louis

Simonds WF, Robbins CM, Agarwal SK *et al.* (2004) Familial isolated hyperparathyroidism is rarely caused by germline mutation in *HRPT2*, the gene for the hyperparathyroidism-jaw tumour syndrome. *Journal of Clinical Endocrinology and Metabolism* **89**, 96–102

Skelly BJ and Franklin RJM (2007) Mutations in genes causing human familial isolated hyperparathyroidism do not account for hyperparathyroidism in Keeshond dogs. *Veterinary Journal* **174**, 652–654

Tebb AJ, Arteaga A, Evans H and Ramsey IK (2005) Canine hyperadrenocorticism: effects of trilostane on parathyroid hormone, calcium and phosphate concentrations. *Journal of Small Animal Practice* **46**, 537–542

Thompson D and Skelly B (2020) Prevalence of canine primary hyperparathyroidism recurrence in Keeshond and non-Keeshond dogs after curative parathyroidectomy. *Veterinary Record* **187**, e93

Thompson KG, Jones LP, Smylie WA *et al.* (1984) Primary hyperparathyroidism in German shepherd dogs: a disorder of probable genetic origin. *Veterinary Pathology* **21**, 370–376

Warner J, Epstein M, Sweet A *et al.* (2004) Genetic testing in familial isolated hyperparathyroidism: unexpected results and their implications. *Journal of Medical Genetics* **41**, 155–160

Useful websites

Cornell University – Keeshonden PHPT Genetic Test
www.vet.cornell.edu/animal-health-diagnostic-center/testing/protocols/PHPT

Chapter 17

Disorders of vitamin D metabolism

Richard Mellanby

Introduction

Vitamin D plays an important role in regulating calcium metabolism and in the maintenance and development of skeletal health in companion animals. In addition, and paralleling human medicine, there is growing interest in understanding the role vitamin D has in non-skeletal health outcomes in dogs and cats. This chapter provides an overview of vitamin D metabolism and discusses both congenital and acquired vitamin D disorders in dogs and cats. It concludes with an overview of current understanding of the role vitamin D plays in non-skeletal health.

Role of vitamin D in skeletal health

The importance of vitamin D in skeletal health has been known for almost a century. The classic experiments of Sir Edward Mellanby, which involved supplementing dogs fed a restricted diet with either linseed or cod liver oil, demonstrated that cod liver oil, but not linseed oil, could protect dogs from developing rickets. The anti-rachitic factor in cod liver oil was later discovered to be vitamin D. Dogs and cats, unlike other mammals such as humans, cattle and sheep, cannot produce vitamin D cutaneously and are therefore reliant on their dietary intake. Vitamin D is available in two forms, namely vitamin D2 (ergocalciferol) and D3 (cholecalciferol), and most pet foods are supplemented with vitamin D3. Following intestinal absorption, vitamin D is rapidly metabolized to 25-hydroxycholecalciferol (calcifediol) in the liver, mainly by the CYP2R1 enzyme (25-hydroxylase). Nearly all circulating 25-hydroxycholecalciferol is protein bound, mostly to vitamin D-binding protein, leaving only a small amount readily available for cellular utilization. 25-hydroxycholecalciferol is subsequently converted by the CYP27B1 enzyme (1-alpha-hydroxylase) to the most active vitamin D metabolite, 1,25-dihydroxycholecalciferol (calcitriol), in the kidney. 25-hydroxycholecalciferol serves as a reservoir for the generation of 1,25-dihydroxycholecalciferol. Both 25-hydroxycholecalciferol and 1,25-dihydroxycholecalciferol are degraded by the CYP24A1 enzyme to 24,25-dihydroxycholecalciferol and 1,24,25-trihydroxycholecalciferol, respectively. The principal actions of 1,25-dihydroxycholecalciferol occur following binding to the vitamin D receptor (VDR), which is widely expressed on most canine tissues. The VDR–1,25-dihydroxycholecalciferol complex heterodimerizes with the retinoic acid receptor, which can influence numerous physiological processes by altering the expression of a wide range of genes.

The principal role of 1,25-dihydroxycholecalciferol, acting alongside parathyroid hormone (PTH) and calcitonin, is to maintain circulating calcium concentrations within a tight range (see Chapter 14). This is achieved mainly by the ability of 1,25-dihydroxycholecalciferol to increase the intestinal absorption of calcium. 1,25-dihydroxycholecalciferol also increases calcium resorption in the distal renal tubule and mobilizes the release of calcium from the skeleton in conjunction with PTH during periods of hypocalcaemia. When circulating concentrations of calcium decline, higher plasma PTH concentrations lead to an increase in renal CYP27B1 activity, which increases circulating 1,25-dihydroxycholecalciferol concentrations.

Measurement of vitamin D metabolites

A wide range of vitamin D metabolites can be measured using a variety of techniques. The main vitamin D metabolites measured in clinical cases are 25-hydroxycholecalciferol and 1,25-dihydroxycholecalciferol. 25-hydroxycholecalciferol has a half-life of 2–3 weeks, and its measurement is widely regarded as the most objective approach to assess vitamin D status. 25-hydroxycholecalciferol can be measured by a wide range of immunoassays, high-performance liquid chromatography (HPLC) and the widely considered gold standard technique of liquid chromatography–tandem mass spectrometry (LC–MS/MS) assay. 25-hydroxycholecalciferol can also be metabolized through a 3-epimerization pathway leading to the generation of C3-epimers of 25-hydroxycholecalciferol (3-epi-25-hydroxycholecalciferol). This can complicate the biochemical assessment of vitamin D status as the biological activity of 3-epi-25-hydroxycholecalciferol may not be equivalent to 25-hydroxycholecalciferol and some assays may not be able to distinguish between these two metabolites. However, a recent study found that serum 3-epi-25-hydroxycholecalciferol concentrations were very low in dogs (Hurst et al., 2020). In cats, 3-epi-25-hydroxycholecalciferol concentrations are higher relative to 25-hydroxycholecalciferol concentrations (Sprinkle et al., 2018). Free 25-hydroxycholecalciferol concentrations can also be quantified, and a reference interval derived using a quantitative immunoassay has recently been reported in the dog (Hurst *et al.*, 2020). Further studies are required to ascertain whether total or free 25-hydroxycholecalciferol measurement is the best assessment of vitamin D status in companion animals.

Since 1,25-dihydroxycholecalciferol is the vitamin D metabolite with the most impact on calcium homeostasis, there are also clinical indications for its measurement, notably in dogs with hypercalcaemia suspected to be caused by 1,25-dihydroxycholecalciferol exposure. As for 25-hydroxycholecalciferol, a range of assays have been reported, including immunoassays and LC–MS/MS methodologies. The Vitamin D External Quality Assessment Scheme (DEQAS), a global quality assurance scheme for laboratories measuring vitamin D metabolites, enables laboratories to benchmark their assay performance and accuracy against international standards. The measurement of both 25-hydroxycholecalciferol and 1,25-dihydroxycholecalciferol offers a comprehensive approach to assessing vitamin D homeostasis in dogs and cats.

Congenital vitamin D disorders

Congenital disorders of vitamin D homeostasis are rare in dogs and cats. They can be classified into three main types (Figure 17.1) (Dittmer and Thompson, 2011):

- Vitamin D-dependent rickets type 1A, caused by CYP27B1 deficiencies
- Vitamin D-dependent rickets type 1B, caused by mutations in the *CYP2R1* gene
- Vitamin D-dependent rickets type 2A, due to mutations in the *VDR* gene.

The main consequences of type 1A and type 1B disease are hypocalcaemia and skeletal abnormalities, which can be managed, with varying degrees of success, through calcitriol supplementation. In the rare type 2A disease, hypocalcaemia, secondary hyperparathyroidism and an increased concentration of 1,25-dihydroxycholecalciferol are typical biochemical changes seen alongside skeletal changes consistent with rickets. Alopecia may also be a feature of *VDR* gene mutations. Treatment is challenging and based around high-dose calcium and calcitriol supplementation.

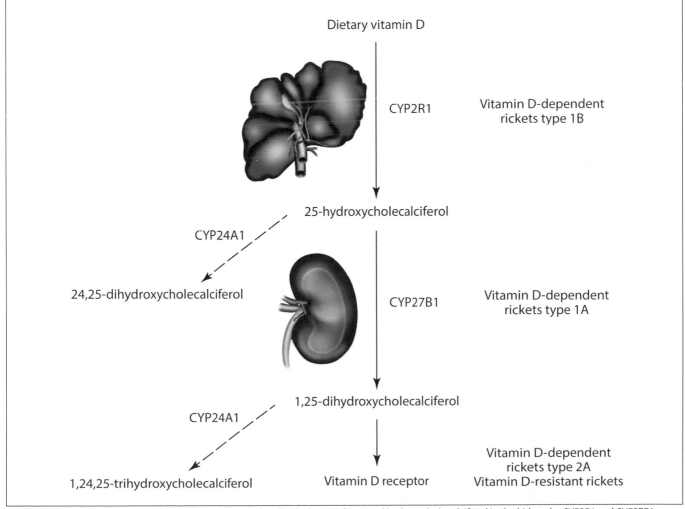

17.1 Vitamin D is converted to 25-hydroxycholecalciferol in the liver and to 1,25-dihydroxycholecalciferol in the kidney by CYP2R1 and CYP27B1 enzymes, respectively. 1,25-dihydroxycholecalciferol exerts its metabolic effects mainly through signalling via the vitamin D receptor. CYP24A1 plays an important role in the regulation of vitamin D status by degrading both 25-hydroxycholecalciferol and 1,25-dihydroxycholecalciferol. Mutations in *CYP2R1*, *CYP27B1* and *VDR* can lead to vitamin D-dependent rickets type 1B, type 1A and type 2A, respectively.

Acquired vitamin D disorders

Vitamin D deficiency

Figure 17.2 outlines key causes of vitamin D deficiency. An important cause of vitamin D deficiency in companion animals is the consumption of a deficient diet. This is rarely observed in dogs fed a commercially manufactured dog food, as indicated by a recent study that found that most proprietary dog foods contain vitamin D concentrations within the manufacturers' stated range (Kritikos *et al.*, 2018). Consequently, most cases of hypovitaminosis D occur in dogs and cats fed improperly prepared homemade diets. The hypovitaminosis D state may result in hypocalcaemia, which typically causes disturbances in neuromuscular function and secondary hyperparathyroidism. This can result in skeletal abnormalities, typically rickets in young animals and osteomalacia in older animals. In rickets, the classical skeletal change is impaired mineralization of physeal and epiphyseal cartilage, with lesions typically involving the fastest-growing bones such as the radius, tibia, metacarpals and metatarsals, leading to a stiff, lame gait and deformed limbs. On radiographic and post-mortem examinations, classical changes include widening of the physeal growth plates, metaphyseal flaring, poor skeletal mineralization and, potentially, pathological fractures (Figure 17.3).

Low vitamin D status can also occur with gastrointestinal disorders, especially in dogs with protein-losing enteropathy (PLE). Historically, it was considered that low total calcium concentrations observed in dogs with PLE were mainly due to a reduction in the amount of protein-bound calcium. However, wider availability of ionized calcium assays has resulted in a greater awareness that many dogs with PLE have reductions in both the ionized and protein-bound calcium concentrations. Whilst a blunted PTH response due to concurrent hypomagnesaemia has been postulated to be an important driver of hypocalcaemia in some cases of PLE, there is a growing consensus that very low concentrations of 25-hydroxycholecalciferol play an important role in the development of a hypocalcaemic state. Serum 25-hydroxycholecalciferol concentrations correlate inversely with the canine inflammatory bowel disease activity index (Gow *et al.*, 2011). Similarly, dogs with a chronic inflammatory enteropathy (CIE) and low serum 25-hydroxycholecalciferol concentrations had higher canine chronic enteropathy clinical activity index scores compared with dogs with CIE and reference interval serum 25-hydroxycholecalciferol concentrations (Wennogle *et al.*, 2019). In some dogs with PLE, the lack of vitamin D and secondary hypocalcaemia are so severe that neurological signs, including seizures, can be a significant clinical complication of the intestinal disease. The severity of the hypovitaminosis D state has been shown to correlate with adverse clinical outcomes in dogs with PLE (Allenspach *et al.*, 2010; Titmarsh *et al.*, 2015a).

The cause of hypovitaminosis D in PLE is likely to be multifactorial, with malabsorption of fat-soluble vitamin D, especially in dogs with lymphangiectasia, widely considered to be the most important cause. Ongoing systemic inflammation, reduced dietary intake of vitamin D and increased vitamin D metabolism may also be important in driving a vitamin D-depleted state. Protocols for the correction of chronic enteropathy-associated hypovitaminosis D have not been well established but parenteral administration of 1,25-dihydroxycholecalciferol is advisable in light of concerns about impaired gastrointestinal absorption of fat-soluble vitamins in dogs with PLE.

Dogs with pancreatic and hepatic disorders may also have low serum concentrations of 25-hydroxycholecalciferol. Dogs with weight loss and exocrine pancreatic insufficiency (EPI) have significantly lower serum 25-hydroxycholecalciferol concentrations than dogs with EPI and stable weight (Barko and Williams, 2018). Dogs with acute pancreatitis had lower vitamin D status than healthy dogs, and those that died had significantly lower serum 25-hydroxycholecalciferol concentrations compared with those that survived (Kim *et al.*, 2017). Vitamin D deficiency and rickets have also been occasionally reported in dogs with liver diseases, likely as consequences of impaired intestinal absorption of vitamin D. Treatment of the underlying cause may result in normalization of vitamin D status and circulating calcium concentrations. Acute or chronic management of hypocalcaemia may be required in severe cases, as detailed in Chapter 15.

- Congenital (see Figure 17.1)
- Dietary (improperly prepared homemade diets)
- Gastrointestinal disorders (protein-losing enteropathy)
- Pancreatic disorders
- Hepatic disorders

17.2 Causes of vitamin D deficiency.

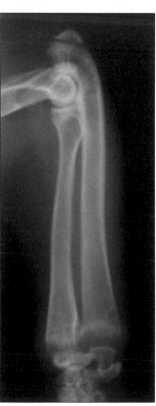

17.3 Radiograph of the forelimb of a 9-month-old male Domestic Shorthaired cat with high 25-hydroxycholecalciferol but low 1,25-dihydroxycholecalciferol values that was responsive to vitamin D supplementation, indicative of vitamin D-dependent rickets type 1A. There is widening of the distal radial and ulnar physes and flaring of the adjacent bone.
(Courtesy of Robert E. Shiel)

Vitamin D excess

Aetiology

Figure 17.4 outlines key causes of vitamin D excess. Disorders involving the excessive consumption of vitamin D typically occur as a result of the feeding of diets containing excessively high concentrations of vitamin D or as a consequence of inadvertent consumption of vitamin D-containing rodenticides or medications. The administration of inappropriate doses of vitamin D for therapeutic purposes in conditions such as primary hypoparathyroidism can also cause hypervitaminosis D. Hypervitaminosis D

- Dietary
  - Over-fortified food
    - Excessive vitamin D supplementation
    - Excessive vitamin D-rich ingredients (e.g. oily fish)
  - Consumption of vitamin D-containing medicines (e.g. oral supplements for human consumption, psoriasis creams)
- Rodenticide toxicity
- Endogenous overproduction of active vitamin D metabolites

17.4 Causes of vitamin D excess.

secondary to rodenticide consumption is well recognized and is likely to be an increasing problem as some rodenticide manufacturers switch to vitamin D-containing products. Although dogs can tolerate oral vitamin D doses at above recommended allowances without major ill effect (Young and Backus, 2016), marked hypervitaminosis D can lead to debilitating hypercalcaemia in both dogs and cats. This can occur due to the over-fortification of diets with supplementary vitamin D or through the addition of excessive amounts of vitamin D-rich ingredients. Historically, high concentrations of vitamin D have been observed in cat foods, which is considered to be most likely due to the high content of oily fish.

Consumption of vitamin D-containing medication is also an increasingly well recognized problem in companion animals. This may occur following the ingestion of oral vitamin D supplements or through the consumption of vitamin D analogue ointments that are widely prescribed for the treatment of psoriasis in humans. There have been reported cases of dogs developing hypervitaminosis D as a consequence of licking their owner's skin, which was covered in topical ointments containing 1,25-dihydroxycholecalciferol or vitamin D analogues, or through the consumption of detached 1,25-dihydroxycholecalciferol-containing skin plaques (Nakamura *et al.*, 2016; Fujita *et al.*, 2017).

Hypervitaminosis D can also occur from the endogenous overproduction of active vitamin D metabolites. This typically occurs in animals with granulomatous diseases where a dysregulated immune response results in the excessive production of 1,25-dihydroxycholecalciferol, typically by macrophages. This syndrome has been reported in dogs with sterile granulomatous lymphadenitis, granulomatous inflammation following placement of a biological implant, and infection with *Angiostrongylus vasorum* and *Mycobacterium avium* subspecies *hominissuis*. It has also been described in a cat with blastomycosis. Excessive production of 1,25-dihydroxycholecalciferol has also been postulated to be important in driving hypercalcaemia in dogs with autoimmune diseases such as immune-mediated polyarthritis. Successful treatment of the underlying condition typically decreases systemic 1,25-dihydroxycholecalciferol concentrations and resolves the associated hypercalcaemic state.

Clinical signs, diagnosis and management

If hypervitaminosis D is of sufficient magnitude to cause hypercalcaemia, clinical signs such as polydipsia, polyuria, lethargy and inappetence may occur. In severe cases, hypercalcaemia can lead to acute kidney injury and long-term complications such as widespread soft tissue mineralization. Routine clinicopathological tests show total and ionized hypercalcaemia. Phosphate concentrations are often within the upper reference interval or increased due to the increased renal and gastrointestinal absorption of phosphate, in contrast to the lower concentration of phosphate typically seen in animals with hypercalcaemia mediated by PTH or PTH-related protein. In animals with azotaemia secondary to kidney injury, interpretation of phosphate values becomes more complex, as detailed in Chapter 14. In most cases, vitamin D-mediated causes of hypercalcaemia are explored only once other more common causes of hypercalcaemia have been excluded, unless a clear source of vitamin D is apparent from the history.

Confirmation of toxicity is possible by measurement of the relevant vitamin D concentration. Two dogs diagnosed with dietary-induced hypervitaminosis D had serum 25-hydroxycholecalciferol concentrations of approximately 400 nmol/l (reference interval 17–140 nmol/l) when measured in a DEQAS-accredited laboratory (Mellanby *et al.*, 2005). Increased concentrations of 1,25-dihydroxycholecalciferol alone would be expected in cases of 1,25-dihydroxycholecalciferol toxicity or granulomatous disease. Assays for the measurement of some vitamin D analogues are not available commercially, and in such cases the diagnosis is confirmed by a history of exposure and exclusion of other causes of hypercalcaemia.

In cases of known exposure to vitamin D, immediate care is focused on induction of emesis and administration of activated charcoal alongside supportive care, typically involving the administration of intravenous fluids. The administration of an intravenous lipid emulsion lowered the serum 25-hydroxycholecalciferol concentrations in a dog that had consumed a large quantity of vitamin D (Perry *et al.*, 2016). Bisphosphonates have been used experimentally and clinically to treat hypervitaminosis D successfully, with intravenous administration of pamidronate or zoledronic acid most widely reported. Whilst bisphosphonates are effective and generally well tolerated in companion animals, complications such as osteonecrosis are increasingly recognized. As vitamin D is lipid soluble and may be sequestered in fat deposits, serum 25-hydroxycholecalciferol may take several months to return to within the reference interval.

Role of vitamin D in non-skeletal health

Following the discovery of vitamin D nearly a century ago, the main role of vitamin D was considered to be the regulation of calcium homeostasis and the development and maintenance of skeletal health. However, the discovery of the VDR on tissues other than the intestines, kidney and bone has resulted in intensive investigations into the non-skeletal health benefits of vitamin D in both humans and animals (Mellanby, 2016; Cartwright *et al.*, 2018).

Infectious diseases

Vitamin D status has been found to be lower in a wide variety of infectious diseases. Dogs with clinically active leishmaniosis, blastomycosis, babesiosis and spirocercosis had lower 25-hydroxycholecalciferol concentrations compared with healthy dogs. Similarly, cats with mycobacterial and feline immunodeficiency virus infections had lower vitamin D status than healthy cats. A negative relationship between 25-hydroxycholecalciferol concentrations and disease severity has also been reported in dogs with babesiosis and *Spirocerca lupi* infections (Rosa *et al.*, 2013; Dvir *et al.*, 2019).

Immune-mediated diseases

Dogs with a range of immune-mediated diseases have been found to have altered vitamin D homeostasis, and low serum 25-hydroxycholecalciferol concentrations are predictive of a poorer clinical outcome (Mick et al., 2019). Interest in the relationship between autoimmune diseases and vitamin D has been fuelled by the growing evidence that vitamin D metabolites can influence canine immune cell function and phenotype ex vivo, typically switching innate immune cells from a proinflammatory to a more anti-inflammatory response (Jaffey et al., 2018a).

Cardiovascular diseases

Circulating 25-hydroxycholecalciferol concentrations were significantly lower in dogs with congestive heart failure compared with unaffected dogs, even though the two groups had a similar dietary vitamin D intake (Kraus et al., 2014). 25-hydroxycholecalciferol concentrations were also found to be lower in dogs with stage B2 or C/D chronic valvular disease than in dogs with stage B1 disease (Osuga et al., 2015).

Oncology

Several studies have shown that vitamin D metabolites have anti-proliferative effects on canine tumour cell lines in vitro. In addition, the vitamin D status has frequently been reported to be lower in dogs with cancer than in control populations. For example, dogs with mast cell tumours had lower 25-hydroxycholecalciferol concentrations than healthy dogs despite having no significant differences in oral vitamin D consumption (Wakshlag et al., 2011). Another study found that the relative risk of cancer in dogs increased with decreasing 25-hydroxycholecalciferol concentrations (Selting et al., 2016). However, other studies have failed to find a difference in vitamin D homeostasis between dogs with and without cancer.

Kidney disease

Plasma 25-hydroxycholecalciferol concentrations have been found to be lower in dogs with chronic kidney disease (CKD). Lower 25-hydroxycholecalciferol concentrations and reduced CYP27B1 activity due to renal damage can cause circulating 1,25-dihydroxycholecalciferol concentrations to be lower in cats and dogs with CKD (Cortadellas et al., 2010; Parker et al., 2017). The decline in 1,25-dihydroxy-cholecalciferol concentrations is considered important in the development of secondary hyperparathyroidism, leading to interest in the potential therapeutic merits of 1,25-dihydroxycholecalciferol supplementation in companion animals with CKD. However, such supplementation is no longer recommended because of lack of supportive evidence that it confers any benefit. Disorders of vitamin D homeostasis may increase the risk of other renal disorders; a recent study suggested that altered vitamin D catabolism may predispose some dogs to the development of calcium oxalate urolithiasis (Groth et al., 2019).

Inflammation

Several studies have shown an inverse relationship between biomarkers of inflammation and vitamin D status in companion animals. For example, serum 25-hydroxycholecalciferol concentrations in dogs diagnosed with a chronic enteropathy have been shown to negatively correlate with circulating neutrophil and monocyte numbers and serum proinflammatory cytokine concentrations (Titmarsh et al., 2015c). Furthermore, two studies have observed that vitamin D status in dogs with a chronic enteropathy negatively correlated with the severity of intestinal inflammation (Titmarsh et al., 2015c; Wennogle et al., 2019). Hospitalized ill cats with neutrophil counts above the reference interval had lower serum 25-hydroxycholecalciferol concentrations (Titmarsh et al., 2017). Dogs with blastomycosis also had a negative relationship between vitamin D status and markers of inflammation. However, the widely reported negative association between vitamin D status and inflammation is not an absolute consensus finding, with one study reporting a positive association between C-reactive protein and 25-hydroxycholecalciferol concentrations in racing sled dogs (Spoo et al., 2015).

Dermatology

Serum 25-hydroxycholecalciferol concentrations in dogs with atopic dermatitis were found not to be significantly different from those in healthy dogs (Kovalik et al., 2012). However, atopic dogs that responded well to prednisolone had higher serum 25-hydroxycholecalciferol concentrations. Oral vitamin D treatment has been shown to improve clinical outcomes in an atopic dermatitis treatment trial, with an increase in serum 25-hydroxycholecalciferol correlating with a reduction in pruritus (Klinger et al., 2018).

Critical care

Several studies have identified a relationship between low vitamin D status and adverse clinical outcomes in hospitalized cats and dogs. A study of hospitalized ill cats found significantly lower 25-hydroxycholecalciferol concentrations in animals that died within 30 days of admission compared with those that survived (Titmarsh et al., 2015b). Similarly, significantly lower 25-hydroxycholecalciferol concentrations have been described in critically ill dogs that died compared with survivors (Cazzolli et al., 2019). Critically ill dogs and dogs with sepsis had significantly lower serum 25-hydroxycholecalciferol concentrations compared with healthy control dogs, and 25-hydroxy-cholecalciferol concentrations were an independent predictor of in-hospital and 30-day survival (Jaffey et al., 2018b). Low vitamin D status has also been associated with anaemia in hospitalized cats (Titmarsh et al., 2020).

Future directions

Whilst numerous studies have linked low vitamin D status to adverse non-skeletal health outcomes in cats and dogs, there is still significant uncertainty over the relationship between the two. In particular, it can be difficult to determine the direction of cause and effect. For example, serial measurements of circulating 25-hydroxycholecalciferol concentrations in experimental studies and in humans have shown that inflammation and infections can result in lower vitamin D status. A recent study revealed that 25-hydroxycholecalciferol concentrations declined significantly in the immediate postoperative period in dogs undergoing elective surgery to treat a ruptured cranial cruciate ligament but returned to baseline concentrations several weeks after surgery (Clements et al., 2020). To disentangle the relationship between vitamin D and non-skeletal health outcomes, human-focused studies have embraced Mendelian randomization approaches as well as examining the non-skeletal health benefits of long-term vitamin D supplementation in large-scale clinical trials. Recent large vitamin D supplementation trials have not shown any clear benefit in reducing the incidence of cardiovascular disease or cancer. However, human trials suggest that vitamin D supplementation can be helpful in respiratory tract disorders, notably in patients with low 25-hydroxycholecalciferol concentrations, and in improving survival times in patients diagnosed with cancer. Whilst these approaches may be challenging to undertake in the veterinary sector, long-term studies of healthy animals of known vitamin D status are necessary to further define the relationship between 25-hydroxycholecalciferol concentrations and non-skeletal health outcomes in dogs and cats.

References and further reading

Allenspach K, House A, Smith K et al. (2010) Evaluation of mucosal bacteria and histopathology, clinical disease activity and expression of Toll-like receptors in German shepherd dogs with chronic enteropathies. Veterinary Microbiology 146, 326–335

Barko PC and Williams DA (2018) Serum concentrations of lipid-soluble vitamins in dogs with exocrine pancreatic insufficiency treated with pancreatic enzymes. Journal of Veterinary Internal Medicine 32, 1600–1608

Cartwright JA, Gow AG, Milne E et al. (2018) Vitamin D receptor expression in dogs. Journal of Veterinary Internal Medicine 32, 764–774

Cazzolli DM, Prittie JE, Fox PR and Lamb K (2019) Evaluation of serum 25-hydroxyvitamin D concentrations in a heterogeneous canine ICU population. Journal of Veterinary Emergency and Critical Care 29, 605–610

Clements DN, Bruce G, Ryan JM et al. (2020) Effects of surgery on free and total 25 hydroxyvitamin D concentrations in dogs. Journal of Veterinary Internal Medicine 34, 2617–2621

Cortadellas O, Fernandez del Palacio MJ, Talavera J and Bayón A (2010) Calcium and phosphorus homeostasis in dogs with spontaneous chronic kidney disease at different stages of severity. Journal of Veterinary Internal Medicine 24, 73–79

Dittmer KE and Thompson KG (2011) Vitamin D metabolism and rickets in domestic animals: a review. Veterinary Pathology 48, 389–407

Dvir E, Rosa C, Handel I, Mellanby RJ and Schoeman JP (2019) Vitamin D status in dogs with babesiosis. Onderstepoort Journal of Veterinary Research 86, 1644

Fujita Y, Hanazono K, Uchida E et al. (2017) Renal failure in dogs kept by a man with severe psoriasis. Journal of the European Academy of Dermatology and Venereology 31, e184–e185

Gow AG, Else R, Evans H et al. (2011) Hypovitaminosis D in dogs with inflammatory bowel disease and hypoalbuminaemia. Journal of Small Animal Practice 52, 411–418

Groth EM, Lulich JP, Chew DJ, Parker VJ and Furrow E (2019) Vitamin D metabolism in dogs with and without hypercalciuric calcium oxalate urolithiasis. Journal of Veterinary Internal Medicine 33, 758–763

Hurst EA, Homer NZ, Denham SG et al. (2020) Development and application of a LC-MS/MS assay for simultaneous analysis of 25-hydroxyvitamin-D and 3-epi-25-hydroxyvitamin-D metabolites in canine serum. Journal of Steroid Biochemistry and Molecular Biology 199, 105598

Jaffey JA, Amorim J and DeClue AE (2018a) Effect of calcitriol on in vitro whole blood cytokine production in critically ill dogs. The Veterinary Journal 236, 31–36

Jaffey JA, Backus RC, McDaniel KM and DeClue AE (2018b) Serum vitamin D concentrations in hospitalized critically ill dogs. PLoS ONE 13, e0194062

Kim DI, Kim H, Son P et al. (2017) Serum 25-hydroxyvitamin D concentrations in dogs with suspected acute pancreatitis. Journal of Veterinary Medical Science 79, 1366–1373

Klinger CJ, Hobi S, Johansen C et al. (2018) Vitamin D shows in vivo efficacy in a placebo-controlled, double-blinded, randomised clinical trial on canine atopic dermatitis. Veterinary Record 182, 406

Kovalik M, Thoday KL, Berry J, van den Broek AHM and Mellanby RJ (2012) Prednisolone therapy for atopic dermatitis is less effective in dogs with lower pretreatment serum 25-hydroxyvitamin D concentrations. Veterinary Dermatology 23, 125–130, e27–e28

Kraus MS, Rassnick KM, Wakshlag JJ et al. (2014) Relation of vitamin D status to congestive heart failure and cardiovascular events in dogs. Journal of Veterinary Internal Medicine 28, 109–115

Kritikos G, Weidner N, Atkinson JL et al. (2018) Quantification of vitamin D_3 in commercial dog foods and comparison with Association of American Feed Control Officials recommendations and manufacturer-reported concentrations. Journal of the American Veterinary Medical Association 252, 1521–1526

Mellanby RJ (2016) Beyond the skeleton: the role of vitamin D in companion animal health. Journal of Small Animal Practice 57, 175–180

Mellanby RJ, Mee AP, Berry JL and Herrtage ME (2005) Hypercalcaemia in two dogs caused by excessive dietary supplementation of vitamin D. Journal of Small Animal Practice 46, 334–338

Mick PJ, Peng SA and Loftus JP (2019) Serum vitamin D metabolites and CXCL10 concentrations associate with survival in dogs with immune mediated disease. Frontiers in Veterinary Science 6, 247

Nakamura K, Tohyama N, Yamasaki M et al. (2016) Hypercalcemia in a dog with chronic ingestion of maxacalcitol ointment. Journal of the American Animal Hospital Association 52, 256–258

Osuga T, Nakamura K, Morita T et al. (2015) Vitamin D status in different stages of disease severity in dogs with chronic valvular heart disease. Journal of Veterinary Internal Medicine 29, 1518–1523

Parker VJ, Harjes LM, Dembek K et al. (2017) Association of vitamin D metabolites with parathyroid hormone, fibroblast growth factor-23, calcium, and phosphorus in dogs with various stages of chronic kidney disease. Journal of Veterinary Internal Medicine 31, 791–798

Perry BH, McMichael M, Rick M and Jewell E (2016) Reduction of serum 25-hydroxyvitamin D concentrations with intravenous lipid emulsion in a dog. Canadian Veterinary Journal 57, 1284–1286

Rosa CT, Schoeman JP, Berry JL, Mellanby RJ and Dvir E (2013) Hypovitaminosis D in dogs with spirocercosis. Journal of Veterinary Internal Medicine 27, 1159–1164

Selting KA, Sharp CR, Ringold R, Thamm DH and Backus R (2016) Serum 25-hydroxyvitamin D concentrations in dogs – correlation with health and cancer risk. Veterinary and Comparative Oncology 14, 295–305

Spoo JW, Downey RL, Griffitts C et al. (2015) Plasma vitamin D metabolites and C-reactive protein in stage-stop racing endurance sled dogs. Journal of Veterinary Internal Medicine 29, 519–525

Sprinkle MC, Hooper SE and Backus RC (2018) Previously undescribed vitamin D C-3 epimer occurs in substantial amounts in the blood of cats. Journal of Feline Medicine and Surgery 20, 83–90

Titmarsh H, Gow AG, Kilpatrick S et al. (2015a) Association of vitamin D status and clinical outcome in dogs with a chronic enteropathy. Journal of Veterinary Internal Medicine 29, 1473–1478

Titmarsh H, Kilpatrick S, Sinclair J et al. (2015b) Vitamin D status predicts 30 day mortality in hospitalised cats. PLoS ONE 10, e0125997

Titmarsh HF, Cartwright JA, Kilpatrick S et al. (2017) Relationship between vitamin D status and leukocytes in hospitalised cats. Journal of Feline Medicine and Surgery 19, 364–369

Titmarsh HF, Gow AG, Kilpatrick S et al. (2015c) Low vitamin D status is associated with systemic and gastrointestinal inflammation in dogs with a chronic enteropathy. PLoS ONE 10, e0137377

Titmarsh HF, Woods GA, Cartwright JA et al. (2020) Low vitamin D status is associated with anaemia in hospitalised cats. Veterinary Record 187, e6

Wakshlag JJ, Rassnick KM, Malone EK et al. (2011) Cross-sectional study to investigate the association between vitamin D status and cutaneous mast cell tumours in Labrador retrievers. British Journal of Nutrition 106, S60–S63

Wennogle SA, Priestnall SL, Suárez-Bonnet A and Webb CB (2019) Comparison of clinical, clinicopathologic, and histologic variables in dogs with chronic inflammatory enteropathy and low or normal serum 25-hydroxycholecalciferol concentrations. Journal of Veterinary Internal Medicine 33, 1995–2004

Young LR and Backus RC (2016) Oral vitamin D supplementation at five times the recommended allowance marginally affects serum 25-hydroxyvitamin D concentrations in dogs. Journal of Nutritional Science 5, e31

Chapter 18

Canine hypothyroidism

Carmel T. Mooney

Introduction

Hypothyroidism is considered a common endocrine disorder of dogs, although whether it is the most common one remains speculative. Over the past few decades, significant advances have been made in recognizing the type of dog affected and the expected clinical and clinicopathological features, and in the performance and accuracy of endocrine tests for diagnosis. Despite this, hypothyroidism can be challenging to diagnose and many myths have persisted regarding its associations and consequences. On the other hand, if appropriately diagnosed, hypothyroidism is one of the most satisfying endocrine disorders to treat, with an excellent long-term prognosis. Naturally occurring hypothyroidism in cats is rare (see Chapter 21).

Thyroid physiology

Thyroid hormone production

In dogs, the thyroid gland is divided into two distinct lobes, each located lateral to the proximal tracheal rings. Thyroid tissue is responsible for the production of the two active thyroid hormones, thyroxine (T4) and triiodothyronine (T3). The principal product of the thyroid gland is T4, which is entirely derived from thyroidal synthesis. By contrast, only approximately half of all circulating T3 originates from thyroidal production, the remainder being produced by peripheral deiodination of T4 in the skin, liver, skeletal muscle and kidneys. Most T3 is located intracellularly, with only approximately 20% present in the circulation. Triiodothyronine is three to five times more metabolically active than T4; therefore, T4 can be considered to act essentially as a prohormone.

Transport of thyroid hormones

For transportation in the circulation, thyroid hormones are usually bound to the plasma proteins, T4-binding globulin, albumin and transthyretin. A minor fraction of T3 and T4 is also carried by circulating lipoproteins. The protein-bound fraction acts as a reservoir to maintain adequate free hormone concentrations. In dogs, the unbound (free) fraction of T4 accounts for approximately 0.1% of the total hormone, compared with the approximately 1% of T3 that circulates unbound. These values are higher than the corresponding human values due to lower binding affinities and lower concentrations of the major carrier proteins in dogs. As a consequence of reduced affinity of the thyroid hormones for their carrier proteins, hormone turnover is more rapid than in humans. The half-life of T4 is only 10–16 hours in dogs, compared with about 7 days in humans.

Control of thyroid hormone production

Circulating thyroid hormone concentrations are regulated through a classical negative feedback mechanism (Figure 18.1). The main stimulus for their synthesis and secretion is a rise in serum thyrotropin (thyroid-stimulating hormone (TSH)) concentrations. Thyroid-stimulating hormone is synthesized and secreted from the pars distalis of the pituitary gland under the tonic stimulation of thyrotropin-releasing hormone (TRH) from the hypothalamus. The secretion of TSH and TRH is mainly inhibited by the negative feedback effect of circulating free T4. A complicated network of neuropeptides and neurotransmitters, including dopamine and somatostatin, also modulate TSH release.

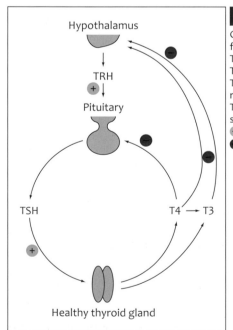

18.1 Control of thyroid function. T3 = triiodothyronine; T4 = thyroxine; TRH = thyrotropin-releasing hormone; TSH = thyroid-stimulating hormone; ⊕ = stimulation; ⊖ = inhibition.

Aetiology

Hypothyroidism results from a decrease in the production of T4 and T3, and potentially arises from a defect in any part of the hypothalamic–pituitary–thyroid axis. In dogs, spontaneous hypothyroidism usually develops because of irreversible loss of thyroid tissue, so-called primary disease, largely as a consequence of either lymphocytic thyroiditis or idiopathic atrophy. Only a small proportion of cases arise from disorders of the pituitary gland or hypothalamus – so-called central hypothyroidism.

Primary hypothyroidism

Lymphocytic thyroiditis

Canine lymphocytic thyroiditis (CLT), an autoimmune disorder, accounts for approximately 50% of cases of adult-onset hypothyroidism and has been likened to human Hashimoto's thyroiditis. Affected dogs experience either multifocal or diffuse infiltration of the thyroid tissue by lymphocytes, macrophages and plasma cells (Figure 18.2), along with the formation of lymphoid nodules, irreversible destruction of thyroid follicles and progressive replacement of normal glandular tissue by fibrous connective tissue. The associated clinical signs of hypothyroidism only develop after approximately 75% of the gland is destroyed. This process may take months to years, varying in progression from dog to dog, and may not result in hypothyroidism in all cases. There are variable periods of time during which significant thyroid pathology and, potentially, a suboptimal or failing gland are present but a clinical state of hypothyroidism has not yet become apparent.

Although the definitive diagnosis of lymphocytic thyroiditis requires thyroid biopsy, its existence can be inferred by demonstrating the presence of circulating autoantibodies against thyroid antigens. Commercially available tests include those for antibodies against T4, T3 and thyroglobulin (TgAAs): TgAAs are detected in approximately 50% of hypothyroid dogs while T4 and T3 autoantibodies are present in less than 10% and 30%, respectively. Anti-thyroid peroxidase antibodies, common in human hypothyroidism, have been demonstrated in only a small proportion of affected dogs, generally in the presence of other thyroid autoantibodies. Studies of thyroid autoimmunity in large numbers of dogs suggest a progression through the following stages (Figure 18.3):

- **Silent thyroiditis** – TgAA positive; euthyroid (all thyroid hormones within reference intervals)
- **Subclinical (compensating) hypothyroidism** – TgAA positive; euthyroid (T4 and T3 within reference intervals but with high endogenous TSH concentration)
- **Clinical disease** – TgAA positive or negative; overtly hypothyroid (T4 and T3 below reference intervals, TSH above or within reference interval).

Over time, antibody-positive dogs may become antibody negative. There is a presumed eventual decline in the inflammatory process as thyroid tissue is destroyed and, consequently, autoantibodies disappear from the circulation.

The recognition of these stages has significant implications, both for the progression of the disease and for choosing the most appropriate diagnostic tests. A recent study followed over 100 TgAA-positive euthyroid dogs for a median of 4 years (Egbert *et al.*, 2019). Approximately one third became overtly hypothyroid while approximately 15% became TgAA negative and euthyroid. The remaining dogs remained euthyroid and TgAA positive, although in some cases the autoantibody status changed to equivocal.

Idiopathic thyroid atrophy

Idiopathic thyroid atrophy accounts for most non-thyroiditis cases of hypothyroidism, and is characterized by the following:

- Degeneration of follicular cells
- Reduction in follicular size
- Replacement of the normal parenchymal tissue with adipose connective tissue, but without significant inflammatory infiltration (see Figure 18.2c).

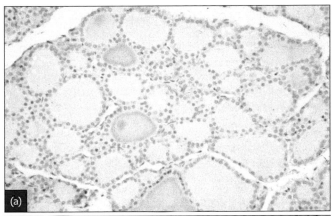
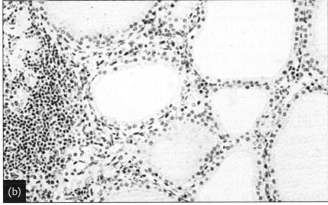
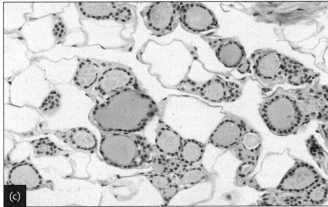

18.2 (a) Histological section of a healthy canine thyroid gland. (b) Histopathological section of a canine thyroid gland with lymphocytic thyroiditis. Note the inflammatory component replacing normal thyroid tissue. (c) Histopathological section of a canine thyroid gland with idiopathic thyroid atrophy. Note the loss of normal thyroid parenchyma without an inflammatory component. (Haematoxylin and eosin stain; original magnification X100)

Stage	Histopathological changes	Laboratory tests	Clinical signs
Silent thyroiditis	Evidence of mild inflammatory infiltration	Total T4, free T4 and cTSH within reference interval; TgAA positive	No overt clinical signs of thyroid dysfunction
Subclinical (compensating) hypothyroidism	More marked inflammatory infiltration with unaffected follicles exhibiting changes indicative of TSH stimulation	Total T4 and free T4 within reference interval; cTSH increased; TgAA positive	
Clinical hypothyroidism	Marked inflammatory response with associated destruction and replacement of >75% of the thyroid gland	Total T4 and free T4 decreased; cTSH increased; TgAA positive	Overt clinical signs of hypothyroidism
	Loss of active inflammation with destruction of most of the thyroid tissue	Total T4 and free T4 decreased; cTSH increased but may decline over time; TgAA negative	

18.3 The stages of canine lymphocytic thyroiditis. The disease does not always progress to overt hypothyroidism in all affected dogs. The rate of progression is variable. cTSH = canine thyroid-stimulating hormone; T4 = thyroxine; TgAA = thyroglobulin autoantibody; TSH = thyroid-stimulating hormone.

The underlying cause of this process is unknown. Histopathologically, it appears quite distinct from lymphocytic thyroiditis. However, it is unclear whether the two diseases are truly distinct or whether they represent different stages of the same disease process.

Theoretically, complete destruction of thyroid tissue due to CLT potentially leads to a reduction in immune stimulation and response, and eventual loss of thyroiditis and circulating autoantibodies with progression to thyroid atrophy. This theory is supported by the existence of both forms of hypothyroidism in certain breeds, but the tendency for lymphocytic thyroiditis to be diagnosed at an earlier age. In addition, the progression from lymphocytic thyroiditis to thyroid atrophy has been documented in some individual dogs. However, such a theory may be too simplistic, given that there appears to be a wide variation in the prevalence of TgAA-positive and TgAA-negative hypothyroidism across different breeds, suggesting a different rate of progression of CLT or a different aetiology for idiopathic atrophy.

Genetic associations

As in humans, canine hypothyroidism is likely to arise out of a combination of multiple genetic and environmental factors. It has long been recognized that hypothyroidism is more prevalent in pure breeds and particularly those of medium to large size. Numerous high-risk breeds are recognized, including the English Setter, Rhodesian Ridgeback, Giant Schnauzer, Hovawart, Old English Sheepdog, Boxer, Dobermann and Gordon Setter. Familial clustering has been shown in many breeds, such as Borzois, Great Danes and Beagles. Heritability is considered to be moderate to high in Hovawarts (Åhlgren and Uimari, 2016). Genetic risk factors for the development of autoimmune thyroid disease have been identified in humans, although none confers increased susceptibility in all cases. Susceptibility genes include those in the major histocompatibility complex, dog leucocyte antigen (DLA), as well as other regulators of immune and thyroid function. An association between DLA class II gene polymorphisms and hypothyroidism has been identified in certain breeds, including the Dobermann, Rhodesian Ridgeback, English Setter and Giant Schnauzer. However, such associations do not explain susceptibility in all dogs and only account for a proportion of the underlying genetic risk. Genome-wide association studies have identified a major hypothyroid risk locus on CFA12 shared by Gordon Setters, Hovawarts and Rhodesian Ridgebacks, and a protective locus on CFA11 in Giant Schnauzers (Bianchi et al., 2015, 2020). The former includes three genes that have not previously been linked with hypothyroidism but have functions that could potentially contribute to its development.

Whilst there is no doubt that a genetic component to the development of hypothyroidism exists in dogs, it is complex and can vary from breed to breed. Additionally, depending on local breeding practices, there may not be the same genetic contribution across any given breed from country to country. This complexity, and the paucity of data regarding the proportion of risk that is genetic, means that offering meaningful advice on breeding strategies is challenging.

Other causes of primary hypothyroidism

Other causes of primary hypothyroidism are uncommon in dogs, but include:

- Neoplastic destruction
- Antithyroid medication (particularly potentiated sulphonamides)
- Radiation therapy
- Congenital defects (see below).

Central hypothyroidism

Central hypothyroidism is caused by the failure of normal TSH secretion by the thyrotropic cells of the pituitary gland. The absence of such stimulation results in atrophic degeneration of the thyroid gland, characterized by follicular distension and flattening of the follicular epithelium, which is readily distinguishable from the changes typical of idiopathic thyroidal atrophy. It is commonly reported that central hypothyroidism accounts for approximately 5% of all spontaneous cases of hypothyroidism. However, it has rarely been reliably documented in dogs.

The most common cause of central hypothyroidism is suppression of pituitary TSH secretion by exogenous glucocorticoid administration or spontaneous hypercortisolism. This is usually a temporary and reversible condition for which treatment of the underlying cause is curative, and thyroid hormone supplementation is generally not indicated. Central hypothyroidism may also result from congenital TSH deficiency (see below) or be a consequence of pituitary neoplasia. Deficiency of TRH, although reported in humans, is rarely diagnosed in dogs and usually results from growth and extension of a pituitary tumour. Other rare cases of central hypothyroidism include lymphoplasmacytic adenohypophysitis, head trauma, non-traumatic intracranial haemorrhage and hypophysectomy usually carried out for the treatment of hypercortisolism.

Congenital hypothyroidism

Congenital hypothyroidism is reported, albeit uncommonly, both as single case reports and within particular breeds and families. It is possible that the true prevalence is higher than reported, as many affected puppies die early in life and may be misclassified as suffering from 'fading puppy' syndrome. Most cases are thought to be caused by thyroid hypoplasia, thyroid aplasia, dysgenesis or dyshormonogenesis that is associated with goitre. A defect in the *TPO* gene resulting in dyshormonogenesis has been described in Fox Terriers, Rat Terriers, Tenterfield Terriers, French Bulldogs and Spanish Water Dogs, for which breed-specific genetic tests are available. A defect in the sodium iodide symporter has been described in Shih Tzus (Soler Arias *et al.*, 2018). All recognized forms of congenital hypothyroidism with goitre appear to be inherited as autosomal recessive traits. A small number of dogs, including a family of Giant Schnauzers and related Miniature Schnauzers, have also been reported with congenital central hypothyroidism (Voorbij *et al.*, 2016).

Congenital hypothyroidism typically causes disproportionate dwarfism, helping to differentiate it from pituitary dwarfism caused by growth hormone deficiency (see Chapter 12). The abnormal physical appearance in congenital hypothyroidism develops as a consequence of epiphyseal dysgenesis and delayed epiphyseal maturation, one of the hallmarks of the condition. Affected puppies (Figure 18.4) have disproportionately wide skulls, macroglossia and delayed dental eruption. They may also exhibit some of the signs typical of the adult-onset disease. Chronic osteoarthritis is a common long-term complication in surviving dogs, due to developmental joint abnormalities. Impaired mental function is also common, particularly if instigation of treatment is delayed.

If congenital hypothyroidism is suspected, interpretation of thyroid hormone concentrations must take account of the higher values encountered in puppies compared with adult values. Healthy puppies up to 3 months of age typically have circulating total T4 values two to five times higher than those in adult dogs.

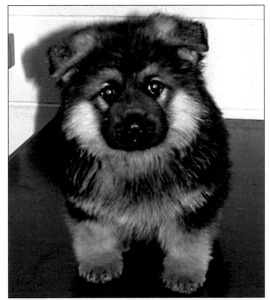

18.4 A 5-month-old male German Shepherd Dog with disproportionate dwarfism as a consequence of congenital hypothyroidism. Note the short legs, broad trunk and wide skull.

Prevalence and signalment

Adult-onset hypothyroidism is undoubtedly one of the most common endocrine disorders of dogs. However, estimates of prevalence are complicated by inconsistencies in the diagnostic criteria used to confirm the disease, particularly the use of tests in older studies that are now considered unreliable. It has been suggested that the true prevalence is 0.2–0.6% of the general canine population. However, a lower prevalence of 0.07% has been reported in an insured population of Swedish dogs, the majority of which are pedigree, which might be a more accurate reflection of true prevalence. The variable effect of breed is important; prevalence as high as approximately 15% has been recognized in Swedish Giant Schnauzers and Hovawarts (Ferm *et al.*, 2009).

Any breed can develop hypothyroidism. However, purebred medium to large dogs are most commonly affected overall, reflecting, at least in part, the genetic influence on the development of the condition (see above).

The disease is most common in middle-aged dogs and is only rarely recognized in animals younger than 2 years old. Overall, the mean age at the time of diagnosis is approximately 7 years old. Breeds at risk of CLT tend to develop the condition at an earlier age.

Reported effects of sex on the risk of hypothyroidism have been inconsistent. The largest study published to date, of over 90,000 dogs (including 1,700 hypothyroid cases), suggests that neutered animals are at greatest risk of developing hypothyroidism, with neutered females at greater risk than neutered males (Sundburg *et al.*, 2016).

Clinical features

Thyroid hormones influence the function of almost all organ systems within the body and a wide range of clinical signs can arise when they are deficient (Figure 18.5). Thyroid hormones act mainly as transcription factors to modify gene expression. At a cellular level, they influence multiple metabolic processes, from the regulation of mitochondrial oxygen demand to the control of protein synthesis. As a consequence, the onset of hypothyroidism is insidiously progressive and although the clinical signs can be varied and extensive, most are non-specific.

The most common clinical signs (approximately 70% of cases) relate to a decline in metabolic rate, together with a variety of dermatological changes. However, in some dogs only one abnormality is present, while in others clinical signs involving the neuromuscular, cardiovascular, reproductive, ophthalmic and gastrointestinal systems develop and may even predominate. Consequently, hypothyroidism is a differential for many presenting complaints in practice.

Metabolic features

Hypothyroidism is associated with a decline in metabolic rate. Related clinical signs, including weight gain, lethargy, exercise intolerance and weakness, occur in the majority of hypothyroid dogs. In hypothyroid humans, basal metabolic rate reduces by up to 40%; a decline in resting energy expenditure has also been demonstrated in hypothyroid dogs. The onset of metabolic signs in dogs is typically insidious and, consequently, often missed or dismissed by owners. However, the clinical response following appropriate therapy can be dramatic, retrospectively confirming the extent of the problem. At least one 'metabolic' sign is recognized in over 80% of hypothyroid dogs.

Metabolic
• **Lethargy** • **Weight gain** • **Exercise intolerance** • Cold intolerance

Dermatological
• **Poor quality, dry and brittle hair coat** • **Hair thinning** • **Endocrine alopecia** • **'Rat tail'** • **Hyperpigmentation** • Myxoedema and tragic facial expression • Secondary pyoderma • Seborrhoea • *Malassezia* infection • Otitis externa

Neurological
• Various neuropathies • Central vestibular disease • Myxoedema coma

Cardiovascular
• Bradycardia • Low-voltage R waves • Reduced myocardial contractility

Reproductive
• Galactorrhoea • Decreased fertility in bitch/dog • Prolonged parturition • Reduced puppy survival

Other
• Corneal lipidosis • Reduced tear production • Lipaemic uveitis • Small intestinal bacterial overgrowth • Gallbladder mucocoele

18.5 Clinical features associated with hypothyroidism in dogs. Those noted in bold are more common.

Lethargy

Lethargy is the most common metabolic change, affecting up to 80% of cases. The duration of the underlying illness appears to correspond with the severity of lethargy, which can be profound. Unusually, some affected dogs appear unperturbed by veterinary examination and may fall asleep during a consultation.

Exercise intolerance

Exercise intolerance affects just over 25% of all cases, although many owners confuse lethargy with exercise intolerance. Frequently, dogs appear to have a normal capacity for short-term exercise, or when excited will behave appropriately. However, this is relatively short-lived, and recovery is prolonged, as shown by a need for excessive rest or sleep thereafter.

Weight gain and obesity

There is no doubt that weight gain is a common finding in hypothyroidism, occurring in approximately 40% of cases during the few months prior to initial presentation. Weight gain occurs despite a normal or slightly reduced appetite and may be exacerbated by a concurrent unwillingness to exercise. In some affected dogs, weight gain can be marked, with recorded weights in excess of 75% above the expected breed average. Despite this, a large proportion of hypothyroid dogs do not gain significant weight, and hypothyroidism cannot be ruled out based on a lack of this finding alone. In addition, whilst obesity is extremely common in dogs, most cases relate to simple overfeeding and/or under exercising, with hypothyroidism accounting for only a small proportion of cases. Thus, the presence or absence of obesity is of little diagnostic consequence for hypothyroidism.

Cold intolerance

Cold intolerance or heat seeking is reported in approximately 10% of hypothyroid dogs; affected dogs may be noted as shivering excessively. However, the presence of heat seeking is non-specific as it is also a common feature in euthyroid dogs.

Dermatological features

Thyroid hormones play an important role in the maintenance of dermal health. Dermatological abnormalities can be extensive and more worrying to owners than the more subtle metabolic signs. They are reported in approximately 80% of affected dogs. Particular dermatological signs vary and reflect the severity and duration of the disease.

Scaling and scurfing

Hyperkeratosis causing scaling and scurfing of the skin, and poor hair coat quality, is common. Excessive dandruff or a dry dull coat is often noted in the early stages of the disorder. Otitis externa is reported in a number of hypothyroid dogs, and dryness and scaling of the external ear canal may be noted.

Alopecia

Thyroid hormones are necessary for the initiation of the anagen phase of hair growth. Absence of thyroid hormones results in persistence of the telogen phase; hairs become easily epilated, with resultant alopecia, and there is a failure of regrowth after clipping. Hair loss commonly begins in areas undergoing friction, such as on the neck in dogs that wear collars (Figure 18.6a) and on the tail, resulting in the typical 'rat tail' appearance of hypothyroidism (Figure 18.6b). Affected animals commonly develop a bilaterally symmetrical non-pruritic 'endocrine' alopecia, with progressive hair loss along the flanks and on the trunk, usually sparing the head and extremities (Figure 18.7). However, focal, multifocal and asymmetrical alopecia can also occur, and larger breeds may develop alopecia of the extremities (presumably as a result of friction) whilst the trunk remains relatively unaffected. Dorsal nasal alopecia (Figure 18.8) has been reported to be a particular feature of hypothyroidism but also occurs in other endocrine disorders.

Myxoedema

Accumulation of glycosaminoclycans in the skin occurs due to an imbalance in their thyroid-controlled production and degradation. It results in myxoedematous non-pitting thickening of the skin. This thickening is most pronounced over the head, where it can give rise to a 'tragic' facial expression with thickening of the lips, thickened skin over the forehead and drooping of the eyelids (Figure 18.9). In rare cases, myxoedema can progress to the more severe nodular cutaneous mucinosis.

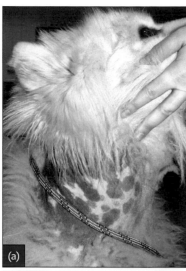

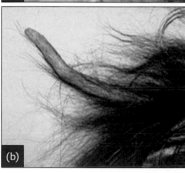

18.6 The hair loss of hypothyroidism typically begins in areas of friction such as (a) the neck in dogs that wear collars and (b) the tail ('rat tail').

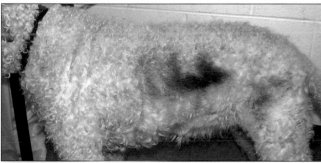

18.7 Truncal alopecia with hyperpigmentation in a hypothyroid dog.

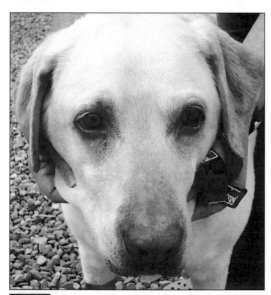

18.8 Nasal alopecia in a hypothyroid dog.

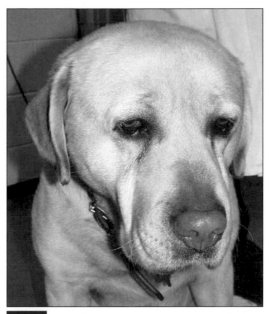

18.9 Tragic facial expression associated with hypothyroidism.

Secondary infection

Thyroid hormones assist the humoral and cellular immune responses, and consequently hypothyroidism reduces resistance to infection. Secondary recurrent, persistent superficial and deep bacterial and *Malassezia* infection is reported in 10–20% of hypothyroid dogs. Such disorders may be poorly responsive to standard therapy until the hypothyroidism is controlled. Pruritus may occur, resulting in self-excoriation and trauma, which can complicate the clinical and histopathological appearance. On the other hand, other causes of such diseases are more common and, at least for recurrent pyoderma, hypothyroidism is responsible for less than 10% of cases (Seckerdieck and Mueller, 2018).

Other changes

The remaining hair coat in affected dogs is usually dry and brittle and may become lighter in colour as a result of environmental bleaching. Hyperpigmentation of the skin is common and is particularly noticeable over alopecic regions. Comedones may also be noted, particularly on the ventrum, and seborrhoea (sicca or oleosa) affects up to 40% of hypothyroid dogs.

Breed-related differences in hair cycle and type may be responsible for some differences in clinical features. Arctic breeds typically lose primary hairs, giving the remaining hair coat a coarse woolly appearance. Hypertrichosis, rather than hair loss, is reported in Boxers and Irish Setters.

Histopathological appearance

The dermatohistopathological features of hypothyroidism are generally considered non-specific and are consistent with a number of endocrine diseases. These commonly include a predominance of telogen phase hair follicles (atrophic or hairless), dermal thickening and, more specifically, myxoedema and vacuolation of the arrector pili muscles. Inflammatory lesions may be present, with concurrent skin infection. Irritation associated with seborrhoea may also contribute to its development. Inflammatory changes generally consist of dermal and periadnexal accumulation of neutrophils, macrophages, lymphocytes and plasma cells. Folliculitis is generally the consequence of a secondary infection. If severe, these inflammatory changes have the ability to obscure some of the more subtle histopathological findings associated with hypothyroidism, and skin biopsy samples should preferably be collected from areas that are not obviously infected or inflamed.

Neuromuscular features

Hypothyroidism causes a variety of neurological and muscular disorders in humans, which are reported in as many as 75% of cases. However, while hypothyroidism has been implicated in canine myopathies, peripheral neuropathies and central nervous system (CNS) disorders, its influence has only been confirmed in some, and the causal relationship in others remains unproven or controversial.

The pathological basis for most central or generalized neuromuscular abnormalities is complex and probably multifactorial. Accumulation of glycosaminoglycans and decreased metabolism, and consequent impaired axonal transport, may contribute to peripheral neuropathies. CNS signs may occur because of atherosclerotic vascular disease or severe hyperlipidaemia, although a range of other metabolic derangements is possible.

Clinical manifestations

Clinical features of myopathy, peripheral polyneuropathy, megaoesophagus, laryngeal paralysis, peripheral and central vestibular disease, and myxoedema coma have all been reported in hypothyroid dogs, although none is common. They are rarely specifically cited in surveys of hypothyroid dogs, and hypothyroidism is uncommonly implicated as a cause in large case series of the specific abnormalities. Historically, seizures and isolated cranial nerve neuropathies were attributed to hypothyroidism, but it is now considered unlikely that they are causally related.

Myopathy: Myopathy as a distinct clinical entity is not well defined in hypothyroid dogs and clinically may be difficult to distinguish from neuropathies. However, experimentally, hypothyroid dogs develop electromyographic and morphological evidence of myopathy. These myopathic changes are consistent with altered muscle energy metabolism and carnitine depletion. The changes remain subclinical but may contribute to the non-specific signs of lethargy and exercise intolerance more commonly reported in hypothyroidism.

Peripheral polyneuropathy: This is probably the most well documented neurological abnormality attributed to hypothyroidism, although it remains uncommon. It may initially present as generalized weakness. Subsequent progression is variable, ranging from subtle gait alterations (often dragging or knuckling of the feet and excessive wear of the toenails (Figure 18.10)) and intermittent lameness to paraparesis and tetraparesis. Proprioceptive deficits are usually noted in the forelimbs, hindlimbs or both, and segmental reflexes may be diminished. Whilst there may be some response to thyroid hormone supplementation, often other therapies are concurrently used and spontaneous recovery cannot be ruled out.

Laryngeal paralysis and megaoesophagus: Both of these disorders have been associated with hypothyroidism, albeit rarely. However, based on the limited response to appropriate thyroid hormone supplementation in most cases, there is little evidence of a true causal relationship. Where response to thyroid hormone supplementation has

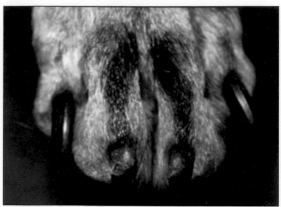

18.10 Excess wear of the middle digits in the forelimb of a dog with hypothyroidism, presumably as a consequence of a neuropathy or myopathy.

been reported for megaoesophagus, myasthenia gravis has not usually been specifically ruled out. Consequently, hypothyroidism should only be considered when other more common causes have been excluded and/or there are additional clinical and clinicopathological features suggestive of thyroid dysfunction.

Peripheral and central vestibular disease: In the past, peripheral vestibular disease has been associated with hypothyroidism. However, a recent large study suggested that less than 5% of dogs presenting with idiopathic vestibular disease, with or without concurrent facial nerve paralysis, were hypothyroid and, even when present, a complete response to thyroid hormone supplementation was not guaranteed (Chan *et al.*, 2020; Orlandi *et al.*, 2020). Thus, the relationship between hypothyroidism and peripheral vestibular disease remains speculative and potentially coincidental.

Central vestibular disease is better described in hypothyroidism, albeit rare. Affected dogs exhibit progressive central vestibular dysfunction that is rapidly and largely reversible with appropriate thyroid hormone supplementation. Other clinical signs of hypothyroidism appear to be uncommon in affected dogs, suggesting that it should be evaluated in all cases presenting for persistent or progressive central vestibular disease when other potential causes are not readily apparent.

Myxoedema coma: The most striking acute presentation of hypothyroidism is myxoedema coma, a rare complication of advanced hypothyroidism. Affected dogs are profoundly dull and present as stuporous or comatose, with hypothermia, bradycardia, hypotension and hypoventilation. Hypothyroidism is likely to have pre-existed for some time and other clinical features (e.g. skin thickening) may be readily apparent. In many cases, there is evidence of a precipitating disease, such as cardiac failure or overwhelming sepsis, that may or may not be related to the thyroid disease. Treatment consists of thyroid hormone supplementation (see 'Treatment and therapeutic monitoring', below) alongside appropriate medical supportive care. The prognosis is guarded but recovery can be expected with aggressive treatment.

Cardiovascular features

Thyroid hormones have direct positive chronotropic and inotropic effects on the heart. In addition, they stimulate myocardial hypertrophy and indirectly affect the cardiovascular system by increasing responsiveness to adrenergic stimulation. However, it is doubtful whether hypothyroidism truly causes significant cardiac disease. Mild and reversible electromechanical changes have been observed that respond to thyroid hormone supplementation, but these are unlikely to reflect clinically relevant cardiac dysfunction (Guglielmini et al., 2019).

Dilated cardiomyopathy

The most widely favoured link between cardiac disease and hypothyroidism in dogs is purportedly dilated cardiomyopathy (DCM). However, there is no clear evidence of a causal relationship, and the main link is likely to be similar breed predispositions for both diseases. At least for Dobermanns, where it has been most widely studied, hypothyroidism plays no role in the cause or progression of DCM (Beier et al., 2015). Reduced myocardial contractility has certainly been documented in isolated case reports of hypothyroid dogs, with improvement following appropriate treatment for the cardiac disease and/or hypothyroidism, but these remain rare. Overall, it is not considered necessary to test dogs with DCM for hypothyroidism unless other supportive clinical signs are present.

Other changes

Other cardiovascular abnormalities associated with hypothyroidism include bradycardia, a weak apex beat and arrhythmias. Electrocardiographic abnormalities include low-voltage R waves, inverted T waves and sinus bradycardia. These changes are usually reversible with appropriate therapy. A cholesterol-based pericardial effusion has been described in hypothyroidism, though this is rare.

Reproductive features

A wide range of reproductive abnormalities has been suggested to result from hypothyroidism, including persistent anoestrus, galactorrhoea, infertility, prolonged interoestrous interval, decreased male libido, abortion and stillbirth. Not all have been confirmed in experimentally induced or naturally occurring disease.

Experimentally, short-term hypothyroidism (median duration of 19 weeks) has no effect on interoestrous interval, litter size or gestation length. However, it is associated with prolonged parturition and reduced puppy survival in the periparturient period. More long-term disease is also associated with decreased fertility in the bitch but has no apparent deleterious effect on male reproduction. Naturally occurring hypothyroidism has been diagnosed in approximately 5% of male dogs with acquired infertility, representing a small proportion of possible causes (Domosławska and Zdunczyk, 2020). Reproductive abnormalities are expected to resolve on restoration of euthyroidism. Hypothyroidism is often blamed by dog breeders for poor reproductive performance, and the pressure to prescribe treatment without confirming a diagnosis may be considerable. However, whilst hypothyroidism may be one of the considerations in such cases, it is undoubtedly one of the more uncommon causes. Nevertheless, breeding animals may be of high value and hypothyroidism represents a cause that can be relatively easily ruled in or out.

Inappropriate galactorrhoea is a recognized but uncommon feature of hypothyroidism. Although previously presumed to be a consequence of increased circulating prolactin concentrations resulting from TRH stimulation, it is probably more complex. Prolactin secretion decreases in experimental hypothyroidism. In naturally occurring disease, prolactin concentrations do not decline, and are only significantly increased (potentially resulting in galactorrhoea) in the luteal phase of the oestrous cycle in the intact bitch.

Other clinical features

Corneal lipidosis (Figure 18.11) occurs in a small number of hypothyroid dogs as a consequence of alterations in the lipid profile of affected animals. Its response to appropriate therapy appears to be variable, despite the normalization of lipid values after successful thyroid hormone supplementation. Hypothyroidism has been described as a potential cause of lipaemic uveitis as a result of hyperlipidaemia (Violette and Ledbetter, 2019). However, the underlying reason for leakage of lipoproteins into the aqueous humour is unclear. Keratoconjunctivits sicca (KCS) has also been reported in association with hypothyroidism, although tenuously. Controversy arises because of similar breed predispositions for both disorders, problems with the diagnosis of hypothyroidism and the possibility of simply reflecting a wider autoimmune disorder. Tear production is reduced in hypothyroid dogs, although whether this progresses to overt clinical disease is unclear; it potentially exacerbates pre-existing KCS.

It has been suggested that hypothyroidism is a possible cause of behavioural abnormalities, particularly dominance and fear-related aggression. However, there is limited evidence to suggest that hypothyroidism is a cause of aggression in dogs and specific investigation is not warranted if a diagnosis of aggression has been made. It is possible that hypothyroidism could exacerbate the severity and frequency of aggressive episodes in dogs with pre-existing behavioural issues. Hypothyroidism could be considered as one of many differential diagnoses in such circumstances, particularly if there are supportive clinical and clinicopathological changes of reduced thyroid function. If dogs are diagnosed with hypothyroidism, thyroid hormone supplementation is recommended and may result in some improvement of behavioural issues, but a complete cure is unlikely.

Hypothyroidism has been reported in association with small intestinal bacterial overgrowth in a small number of dogs. This is presumed to be secondary to reduced gastrointestinal motility, a feature also recognized in human hypothyroid patients in whom constipation is a known complication.

Gall bladder mucocoele is becoming an increasingly recognized abnormality in dogs and is significantly associated with hyperlipidaemia (Kutsunai et al., 2014). Hypothyroidism is a recognized cause, although not all

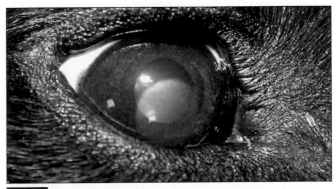

18.11 Corneal lipidosis associated with hypothyroidism.

affected cases have hyperlipidaemia. It is therefore unclear whether thyroid hormone deficiency could directly induce other contributing factors, such as gall bladder dysmotility, decreased bile flow or stasis and altered bile composition. In one study, approximately 25% of dogs with gall bladder mucocoele had thyroid hormone abnormalities supportive of primary hypothyroidism (Aicher et al., 2019). However, abnormalities suggestive of non-thyroidal illness (NTI) are widespread in dogs with gall bladder mucocoele even in those considered to have mild disease. Therefore, caution is advised in diagnosing hypothyroidism; other supportive clinical features should be present, and a comprehensive thyroid panel used for diagnosis. A prior diagnosis of hypothyroidism has limited impact on outcome following surgical cholecystectomy. Medical treatment of gall bladder mucocoele is possible but is associated with shorter long-term survival compared with surgical cholecystectomy (Parkanzky et al., 2019). However, whether a better response is possible in hypothyroid dogs adequately supplemented with levothyroxine together with standard medical management of gall bladder mucocoele is as yet unclear.

Hypothyroidism may be encountered in association with other immune-mediated disorders. The most common polyendocrinopathies reported include hypothyroidism in association with diabetes mellitus or hypoadrenocorticism (see Chapters 23, 28 and 36).

Commercial laboratories are frequently requested to perform thyroid function tests for dogs that exhibit polyuria and polydipsia (PU/PD); however, these signs are not true features of hypothyroidism unless caused by complications of concurrent glomerulonephritis, although this is rare.

Diagnosis

The following principles should be taken into consideration before diagnostic testing:

- The diagnosis of hypothyroidism is a clinical diagnosis and should not be based on laboratory tests alone
- None of the existing endocrine tests is 100% accurate. Performance frequently varies from being highly sensitive and poorly specific to highly specific and poorly sensitive
- The influence of commonly used medications and NTIs on thyroid function and test results can be significant and easily misinterpreted as indicating thyroid hormone deficiency.

Keeping these factors under consideration will undoubtedly help improve the ability to confirm or refute a diagnosis of hypothyroidism.

General approach

The recommended steps in investigating suspected hypothyroidism are depicted in Figure 18.12 and summarized as follows.

1. The dog should be of an appropriate age and breed.
2. Clinical signs of hypothyroidism must be present. If there are clinical signs unlikely to be associated with hypothyroidism (e.g. PU/PD, hepatomegaly), investigation for other disorders takes precedence.

3. There should be clinicopathological changes supportive of hypothyroidism. Routine clinicopathological analyses also serve to indicate the presence of NTI (see below).
4. Each case should be evaluated for previous and current drug therapy and testing postponed until a suitable withdrawal period has elapsed. The effect of drug therapy is of serious concern and some drugs can result in transient hypothyroidism.
5. Non-thyroidal illness should be excluded as far as is practical, by performing routine clinicopathological investigations and any additional appropriate diagnostic tests. Exclusion of NTI is the single most useful factor in reliably interpreting tests of thyroid function. If NTI is diagnosed, there may be no need to investigate thyroid function further. However, it is recognized that in some instances, hypothyroidism may be considered a complicating feature of another illness or an unrelated concurrent disorder, and in such cases interpretation of thyroid function tests should take the NTI into consideration. The effects of NTI on thyroid tests vary depending on the nature, severity and stage of the illness.
6. Once thyroid testing is considered feasible, first-line diagnostic thyroid tests should be performed (total T4 and endogenous canine TSH (cTSH)).
7. If results are equivocal, second-line diagnostic tests should be performed (free T4 by dialysis and/or TgAA).
8. If results remain equivocal, more advanced diagnostic tests should be considered, such as TSH/TRH response testing or thyroid imaging.

Routine clinicopathological features

The most common abnormalities associated with hypothyroidism include hyperlipidaemia and anaemia (Figure 18.13); their presence helps to provide supportive evidence of hypothyroidism.

However, due to the high prevalence of similar abnormalities in dogs with NTI, the predictive value of most routine parameters for hypothyroidism is relatively poor. Despite this, routine clinicopathological tests are of immense value in helping to exclude significant NTI.

Anaemia

A mild normocytic and normochromic anaemia affects approximately 40–50% of hypothyroid dogs. This is a consequence of reduced peripheral metabolic activity and a reduction in tissue oxygen demand. The severity of the anaemia generally reflects the chronicity of the hypothyroidism. Typically, it is mild (e.g. red blood cell (RBC) values 5.0–5.5 x 10^{12}/l) or RBC values are at the low end of the laboratory reference interval. Moderate to severe anaemia should prompt investigation for other causes. Hypothyroidism is one of several differentials for increased red cell distribution width, which occurs in approximately 25% of cases even in the absence of evidence of anaemia (Martinez et al., 2019).

Traditionally, hypothyroidism was thought to be associated with a variety of haemostatic abnormalities, in particular von Willebrand's disease. Isolated case reports suggesting an association between hypothyroidism and selected coagulation factor deficiencies are all questionable based on the methods used for diagnosing hypothyroidism or a failure to eliminate other potential causes. From experimental studies and evaluation of large case series of hypothyroidism, it is clear that coagulopathies are

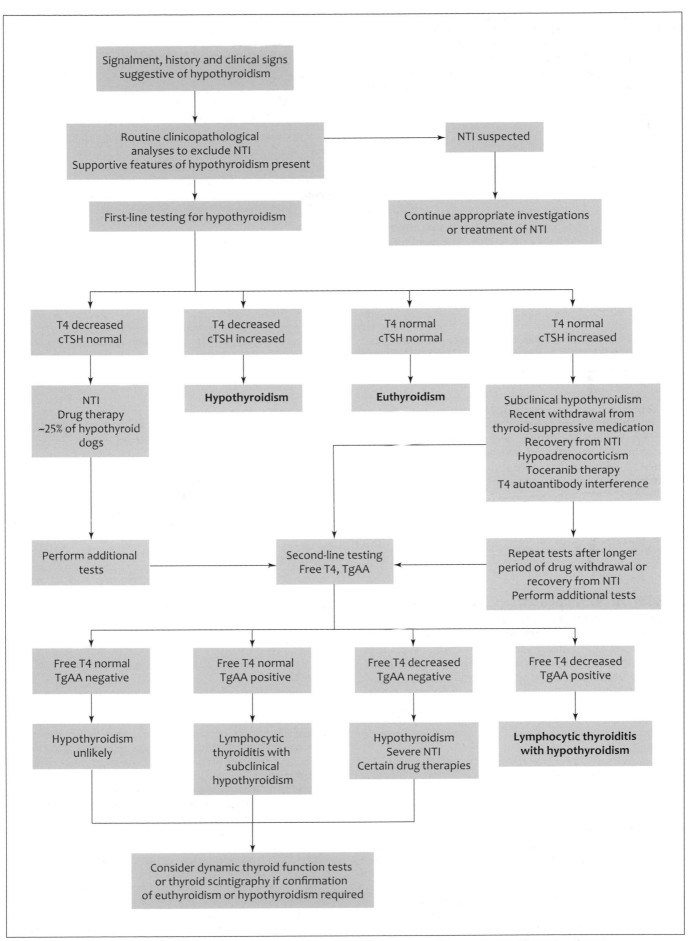

18.12 Diagnostic algorithm for hypothyroidism. cTSH = canine thyroid-stimulating hormone; NTI = non-thyroidal illness; T4 = thyroxine; TgAA = thyroglobulin autoantibody.

Abnormality	Prevalence (% of cases)	Severity	Pathophysiology
Hyperlipidaemia	80	Can be marked	Reduced lipid degradation
Anaemia	40–50	Usually mild, normochromic, normocytic	Reduced need for oxygen-carrying capacity
Increased creatine kinase activity	35	Rarely exceeds twice the reference interval	Decreased clearance, subclinical myopathy

18.13 Routine clinicopathological features of canine hypothyroidism.

not a feature of hypothyroidism *per se*, although undoubtedly certain breeds, notably Dobermanns, commonly suffer from both conditions. Moreover, thyroxine treatment has no effect on increasing production of von Willebrand factor or improving haemostatic function in affected dogs.

Hyperlipidaemia

Hypothyroidism is associated with both a reduction in the rate of lipid degradation and a reduction in lipid synthesis. The former is affected to a greater extent and thus there is an accumulation of lipids within the circulation. The principal changes are increases in high-density lipoproteins (HDLs), low-density lipoproteins (LDLs) and possibly very-low-density lipoproteins (VLDL) (see Chapter 7).

Hypercholesterolaemia is commonly reported, occurring in up to 80% of affected dogs. Hypertriglyceridaemia is additionally present in a similar proportion of cases. Whilst hyperlipidaemia is also a common feature of other endocrine disorders, notably diabetes mellitus and hypercortisolism, the magnitude of the cholesterol increase in hypothyroidism is typically greater and circulating cholesterol concentrations >15 mmol/l are not uncommon. Thus, whilst hypercholesterolaemia is not specific for hypothyroidism, an unusually severe increase should prompt its consideration.

Muscle enzyme activities

Increased creatine kinase (CK) activity is considered a feature of hypothyroidism attributable to decreased clearance from the circulation. However, the subclinical myopathy described in experimental cases (see above) may also play a role, as it is associated with modest increases in CK activity.

A mild increase in CK activity is reported in up to 35% of hypothyroid dogs. Severe increases are not a feature of hypothyroidism and are more likely to represent primary muscle disease.

Liver enzyme activities

Mild increases in liver enzyme activities, particularly alkaline phosphatase (ALP) and gamma glutamyl transferase (GGT), are present in approximately 30% of hypothyroid dogs. This is presumed to be a consequence of mild hepatic lipid deposition associated with hypothyroidism. The diagnostic utility of increased liver enzyme results is limited, as similar increases are a common finding in a wide range of NTIs. Marked increases in liver enzyme activities, particularly ALP, should prompt consideration of NTI, hypercortisolsm being an obvious example that could present with some similar, particularly dermatological, abnormalities (see Chapter 29).

Fructosamine

In human hypothyroid patients, circulating fructosamine concentrations increase when protein turnover is reduced, rather than as a result of any change in glycaemic control. Due to its widespread use as a monitoring tool for diabetic dogs, there has been much interest in the effect of other illnesses on the circulating concentration of fructosamine. Following exclusion of dogs with diabetes mellitus, increased fructosamine has a diagnostic specificity for hypothyroidism in excess of 80%. Given the relative ease with which diabetes mellitus can usually be excluded, fructosamine is therefore a useful additional screening test for suspected hypothyroidism. However, the magnitude of the increase is much less noticeable than in diabetes mellitus. Typical results from hypothyroid dogs are near the top end of the reference interval rather than markedly above it. In diabetic dogs with concurrent hypothyroidism, fructosamine concentration should be interpreted cautiously as an indicator of glycaemic control.

Other abnormalities

Decreased glomerular filtration rate is a possible sequela of hypothyroidism and is partially responsive to thyroid hormone supplementation (see Chapter 6). It is not surprising, therefore, that a proportion of dogs have increases in serum creatinine (approximately 30% of dogs) and symmetric dimethylarginine (SDMA) (4–50% of dogs depending on the cut-off used (14 or 18 μg/dl)) concentrations. However, such increases are mild and tend to normalize with successful therapy (Di Paola *et al.*, 2021).

Folic acid concentrations can be mildly decreased in hypothyroidism in association with increased homocysteine concentrations (Gołynski *et al.*, 2017). Circulating adiponectin concentrations are also increased in hypothyroidism, even allowing for such confounders as body condition score (Mazaki-Tovi *et al.*, 2015).

Endocrine tests

Knowledge of the normal production and control mechanisms of thyroid hormones (see 'Thyroid physiology', above) and the stages of thyroid disease (see 'Primary hypothyroidism', above) is essential in order to understand the performance of individual diagnostic tests. Additionally, NTI is capable of profoundly affecting thyroid function and must be taken into consideration for accurate interpretation.

The effect of non-thyroidal illness on thyroid function

Whilst the effects of NTI are varied, there is a continuum of change that progresses according to the severity of the particular disease. The first and most common effect is suppression of total T3 concentrations, which occurs even with mild illness. As disease severity progresses, there is a concomitant suppression of total T4 concentrations. There may then be a temporary increase in free T4 concentrations with eventual normalization and only rarely suppression in the most severe illnesses. In addition, over time there is an inappropriate or inadequate hypothalamic–pituitary response eventually manifesting as suppressed TSH concentrations. The cause of these disturbances is probably multifactorial and includes alterations in the set point of the hypothalamic–pituitary axis, changes in thyroid hormone receptor expression or function, reduced serum thyroid hormone protein binding, altered metabolism and reduced peripheral conversion of T4 to T3.

Glucocorticoids and circulating cytokines, including interleukins and tumour necrosis factor, may play a role in the development of some of these changes in NTI. During recovery from NTI, the abnormalities in thyroid hormone concentrations eventually resolve. However, TSH concentrations may transiently rise above the reference interval before T4 and T3 concentrations normalize. This is well described in humans, where high TSH concentrations are often found in hospitalized patients. It is suspected to occur in dogs, although this is less well described.

The changes described are considered to be a physiological adaptation to illness, and whilst some controversy and exceptions exist in humans, thyroid hormone supplementation is not required and may even have detrimental effects. The same is considered true in dogs, with studies of congestive cardiac failure demonstrating no difference in survival between dogs treated with T4 and placebo.

Total T4

Basal serum total T4 estimation has traditionally been the mainstay for the diagnosis of canine hypothyroidism and remains an excellent first-line diagnostic test for the disease. Its advantages and disadvantages are summarized in Figure 18.14.

Assay methods: Radioimmunoassay (RIA) is considered to be the gold standard technique for measuring circulating total T4 concentrations. However, due to constraints in using radioisotopes, non-isotopic and often fully automated methods have become routine (see Chapter 3). The lower binding affinity and concentration of T4-binding proteins in dogs compared with humans means that total T4 concentrations are considerably lower in dogs. Thus, it is well recognized that assays designed for human use must be modified to measure total T4 concentrations in dogs.

Diagnostic performance: There is universal agreement that circulating total T4 is usually decreased in hypothyroidism. In most studies, less than 5–10% of hypothyroid dogs have reference interval or, more rarely, increased values. With a few exceptions, finding a reference interval total T4 concentration is useful in helping to exclude a diagnosis of hypothyroidism. Unfortunately, whilst the diagnostic sensitivity (i.e. the percentage of affected dogs with subnormal values) is undoubtedly high, the specificity (i.e. the percentage of unaffected animals with normal results) is much lower, at approximately 75% (Figure 18.15). The specificity of total T4 is particularly poor because of the range of physiological (age, breed) and pathological (NTI, drug therapies) factors that are capable of suppressing circulating concentrations. Demonstrating a low total T4 concentration alone cannot be used to confirm a diagnosis of hypothyroidism.

Test	Sensitivity	Specificity
Total T4	95%	75%
Free T4	~80%	>90%
cTSH	75%	80%
Combined total T4 and cTSH	75%	>90%

18.15 Comparison of the test performance for different hormones for diagnosing hypothyroidism in the dog. All values are approximate. cTSH = canine thyroid-stimulating hormone; T4 = thyroxine.

Low total T4 values in euthyroid dogs: Several physiological mechanisms can result in decreased total T4 concentrations.

- **Daily variation** – healthy dogs exhibit fluctuation in total T4 concentrations on a daily basis and occasionally values fall below the reference interval. Unfortunately, there is no circadian pattern to this fluctuation and no recommendations on the timing of samples can be given.
- **Size** – healthy large and medium-sized dogs are often considered to have lower circulating total T4 values than small dogs. However, this is likely predicated on breed. Obese dogs have significantly higher total T4 values than non-obese members of the same breed.
- **Breed** – there is considerable evidence that total T4 concentrations vary between different breeds. This is most obvious in sighthounds, including Greyhounds, Whippets, Irish Wolfhounds, Scottish Deerhounds, Sloughis and Salukis, where total T4 values are often undetectable. Some other specific breeds, such as Basenjis and Dogues de Bordeaux, appear similar to sighthounds. Consequently, measurement of total T4 in these breeds cannot be used for investigating hypothyroidism and breed-specific reference intervals cannot be established. There may also be less obvious differences in other breeds that might benefit from a breed-specific reference interval. In their absence, breed effects should always be a consideration in interpretation.
- **Age** – total T4 concentrations progressively decline, from mid-normal values in middle-aged animals to low-normal values in elderly dogs. This is a physiological feature that is of importance because a high percentage of dogs evaluated for hypothyroidism are older.
- **Sex** – the influence of sex on thyroid hormone concentrations has been evaluated in several large studies, with conflicting results. Males and females show similar results, but total T4 values appear to increase during progesterone-dominated phases of the oestrous cycle and during pregnancy. Values may just exceed the upper reference limit and are therefore unlikely to have any clinical significance. Rapidly declining values, occasionally to below reference interval, have been demonstrated in non-infective abortion (Thuróczy et al., 2016).
- **Exercise** – training and endurance exercise in sled dogs are associated with a decline in total T4 values.

The specificity of total T4 concentration for diagnosing hypothyroidism is further confounded by the potentially profound suppressive effects of NTI and certain drug therapies.

Advantages
• Inexpensive, widely available and easily measured
• Highly sensitive marker for hypothyroidism
• Reference interval values suggest hypothyroidism is unlikely

Disadvantages
• Low values do not confirm hypothyroidism
• Decreased in certain breeds and in elderly dogs
• Decreased by most NTIs
• Decreased by a range of drugs

18.14 The advantages and disadvantages of total thyroxine measurements for the diagnosis of hypothyroidism in dogs. NTI = non-thyroidal illness.

- **Non-thyroidal illness** – the effect of NTI is widely recognized and is particularly common with hypercortisolism, neoplastic diseases, diabetes mellitus, hypoadrenocorticism, kidney disease, hepatic disease, pyoderma, infectious diseases and a variety of medical illnesses associated with systemic inflammation and/or requiring intensive care. As a general rule, the magnitude of suppression reflects the severity of illness, and less metabolically severe illnesses may in fact have little impact on thyroid function. Furthermore, the likelihood of recovery from NTI is inversely proportional to the degree of suppression of total T4 concentrations. As a general rule, any illness should be considered capable of suppressing total T4 concentrations and, when suppression is significant, total T4 values are indistinguishable from those that occur in hypothyroidism.
- **Drug therapies** – numerous categories of drugs interfere with thyroid hormone metabolism through a variety of mechanisms that can ultimately suppress total T4 values (Figure 18.16). These include glucocorticoids, clomipramine, anticonvulsants such as phenobarbital, non-steroidal anti-inflammatory drugs such as aspirin, carprofen and ketoprofen, and potentiated sulphonamides. Potentiated sulphonamides are capable of inducing hypothyroidism because of their effect on directly inhibiting thyroid hormone production. Some drugs even within the same categories have limited effect on total T4 concentrations, including imepitoin, potassium bromide, deracoxib and propranolol. If the effect of a drug has not been specifically evaluated in dogs, it should be considered as potentially capable of suppressing total T4 concentrations. Withdrawal of these drugs should be considered prior to testing for hypothyroidism. For many drugs, including thyroxine, a 6-week withdrawal period is often recommended. However, the time to normalization of thyroid function is variable and dependent on the specific drug, its dosage and duration of treatment. Ruling out hypothyroidism earlier than 6 weeks is possible if total T4 concentrations have returned to within the reference interval. Persistent thyroid hormone abnormalities dictate continued testing until at least 6 weeks have elapsed before a diagnosis is made.

Drugs	Effects
Glucocorticoids	Decrease total and free T4
Non-steroidal anti-inflammatory drugs	Decrease total T4
Potentiated sulphonamides	Decrease total and free T4 Increase cTSH
Barbiturates	Decrease total and free T4 Increase cTSH, but rarely above reference interval
Clomipramine	Decreases total and free T4 Decreases total T3
Toceranib	Increases cTSH
Thyroid hormone replacement therapy	Decreases cTSH through negative feedback and thus inhibits spontaneous thyroid function

18.16 Common drugs known to affect thyroid function tests in dogs. cTSH = canine thyroid-stimulating hormone; T3 = triiodothyronine; T4 = thyroxine.

Reference interval/high total T4 values in hypothyroid dogs: In a subset of dogs with CLT, autoantibodies can develop against specific epitopes on the thyroglobulin molecule corresponding to T4 (T4AAs) or T3 (T3AAs); T4AAs and T3AAs have no apparent clinical effect but are important because of their potential to interfere with the measurement of hormone concentrations. Their exact effect is variable and is dependent on autoantibody concentration and the assay binding affinities and separation methods employed. Falsely increased and falsely decreased values are possible and not always easy to predict. In general, T3AAs are more common, occurring in just over 5% of all samples submitted for investigation of hypothyroidism, compared with less than 2% for T4AAs. Although this prevalence appears relatively low, T4AAs occur in approximately 8% of hypothyroid dogs and 14% of those with CLT.

If T4AAs result in falsely increased total T4 values, markedly increased values may be found. These usually pose few diagnostic problems in a dog under investigation for hypothyroidism, as such results raise suspicion for the presence of T4AAs. However, their potential to artefactually increase low values to within the reference interval poses a greater diagnostic challenge; in many of these cases, a diagnosis of hypothyroidism may be ruled out erroneously. Thyroxine autoantibodies presumably account for the less-than-perfect sensitivity of total T4 for diagnosing hypothyroidism. Often the possibility of T4AAs is only considered because of other abnormal thyroid function test results (e.g. increased cTSH) or a persistent clinical suspicion. Some, but not all, commercial laboratories are capable of measuring actual T4AAs. An alternative is to measure TgAAs, as almost all dogs that are T4AA positive are also positive for TgAAs and such assays are more widely available. These antibodies have negligible effects in many dogs and total T4 values remain low and consistent with hypothyroidism in these cases.

Canine thyroid-stimulating hormone

Measurement of cTSH concentrations revolutionized the testing for canine hypothyroidism. In primary hypothyroidism, there is a loss of normal regulatory feedback on pituitary synthesis and secretion of cTSH. As the vast majority of hypothyroid dogs have primary hypothyroidism, an increased circulating cTSH concentration is expected. The advantage and disadvantages of this test are summarized in Figure 18.17.

When increased above the reference interval (up to approximately 0.6 ng/ml), values are typically between 1 and 3 ng/ml. Occasionally, marked increases in cTSH concentrations to values >10 ng/ml are identified. The reasons for such dramatic increases are unclear, but it has been suggested that they may be particularly prominent in the early stages of thyroid dysfunction. In accordance with this, there is a marked increase in cTSH

Advantage
• Helps differentiate hypothyroidism from other causes of low T4
Disadvantages
• Should not be interpreted alone
• Increased by certain drugs and recovery from NTI
• Within reference limits in a high proportion of hypothyroid dogs
• Increased in subclinical hypothyroidism

18.17 The advantage and disadvantages of canine thyroid-stimulating hormone measurements for the diagnosis of hypothyroidism in dogs. NTI = non-thyroidal illness; T4 = thyroxine.

concentration within 2–4 months of experimental induction of hypothyroidism, prior to a gradual decline over the next 2–3 years if left untreated.

Diagnostic performance: Measurement of circulating cTSH in isolation is not recommended, as it has a diagnostic sensitivity of only approximately 75% and a specificity of 80% (see Figure 18.15). It is usually recommended as a first-line test, together with total T4 estimation (Figure 18.18). The specificity of combined decreased total T4 and increased cTSH exceeds 90%. This combination of tests has therefore become the hallmark for the initial laboratory diagnosis of hypothyroidism. Together with the use of measurement of free T4 and TgAA as second-line diagnostic tests, the vast majority of dogs can reliably be categorized as either hypothyroid or euthyroid.

Reference interval cTSH values in hypothyroid dogs: Whilst circulating cTSH concentrations are increased above the reference interval in the majority of hypothyroid dogs, a significant proportion have reference interval values. A variety of possible explanations have been proposed.

- Although not documented in all studies, there is some evidence that concurrent NTI can decrease cTSH concentrations into the reference interval in hypothyroid dogs. To avoid any possible interference, any concurrent illness should be treated, or at least stabilized, prior to testing for hypothyroidism.
- Concurrent drug therapy, particularly with glucocorticoids, is known to suppress cTSH values, and may decrease concentrations into the reference interval in hypothyroid dogs. Drug withdrawal should be attempted before cTSH measurement.
- Some studies have suggested potential fluctuation of cTSH into the reference interval in some hypothyroid dogs with marginally increased cTSH values. This is supported by the demonstration of pulsatile ultradian secretion of cTSH in experimental hypothyroidism.
- Inappropriately low cTSH values are expected in central hypothyroidism. However, in contrast to the situation in humans, the current cTSH assays are incapable of distinguishing low values from reference interval values. Given that less than 5% of hypothyroid cases are centrally mediated, such a diagnosis could not account for the much higher proportion of dogs with decreased total T4 and concurrent reference interval cTSH values.

- The existence of varying isoforms of cTSH has been postulated to explain inappropriate reference interval cTSH values in hypothyroid dogs, although this is yet to be reliably documented in dogs.
- There is a reduction in pituitary cTSH secretion over time. Experimental induction of primary hypothyroidism results in an initial increase in cTSH concentration that wanes after 4 months, with cTSH values declining to within reference interval over 3 years. This is accompanied by pituitary enlargement and, histopathologically, emergence of cells that double immunostain for both growth hormone and TSH, indicative of transdifferentiation of somatotropes to thyrosomatotropes. Basal and TRH-stimulated growth hormone concentrations are increased while the cTSH response to TRH is blunted or absent. Similar endocrine changes are seen in naturally occurring primary hypothyroidism.

While the explanation for a reference interval value may be readily apparent in some dogs, in the majority it is not. Currently, the poor diagnostic sensitivity of cTSH measurement for hypothyroidism precludes its use as a screening test for the disease.

Increased cTSH values in euthyroid dogs: Increased cTSH values in euthyroid dogs are not such a concern as reference interval values in hypothyroid dogs. However, they can and do occur for a variety of reasons.

- cTSH may be increased in the early stages of thyroid disease for some time before total T4 values decline and clinical signs become apparent. This so-called subclinical or compensating hypothyroidism may explain increased cTSH in some euthyroid dogs. However, by definition such dogs should not be exhibiting clinical signs and are unlikely to undergo routine testing in practice. Despite this fact, these animals are being increasingly recognized during routine screening programmes such as those used by a number of breed clubs. Approximately one third of these dogs subsequently become hypothyroid (see above), and regular re-testing is therefore recommended.
- A variety of drugs potentially result in increased cTSH concentrations, particularly the potentiated sulphonamides. Sulphonamides interfere with thyroid hormone synthesis within the thyroid gland itself and potentially cause a temporary reversible state of

cTSH	Total T4	Interpretation	Suggested actions
Within reference interval	Decreased	NTI Drug therapy Approximately 25% of hypothyroid dogs	Treat NTI and retest Withdraw drugs and retest Perform second-line diagnostic tests such as free T4 and TgAA measurement
	Within reference interval	Euthyroid	Investigate other possible causes of clinical signs
Increased	Decreased	Hypothyroid Be aware similar results can be found in dogs treated with potentiated sulphonamides	Administer levothyroxine therapy
	Within reference interval	Recovery from NTI or various drug therapies Hypothyroidism with T4 autoantibody interference Subclinical hypothyroidism	Wait until recovery complete and retest Measure free T4 or TgAA to exclude antibody interference Assess TgAA and repeat thyroid function tests annually

18.18 Use and interpretation of total thyroxine (T4) and canine thyroid-stimulating hormone (cTSH) as 'first-line' endocrine tests. NTI = non-thyroidal illness; TgAA = thyroglobulin autoantibody.

thyroid hormone deficiency associated with increased circulating cTSH values. There appears to be some variation in effect depending on the specific preparation, and the dose and duration of therapy, but it is clear that total T4 values can decrease and cTSH values can increase within 1 and 2 weeks of starting therapy, respectively. The suppressive effect can be profound, and prolonged treatment may induce a clinical state of hypothyroidism. Withdrawal of the drug usually results in complete resolution within weeks. A transient rebound period, during which TSH is temporarily increased after cessation of glucocorticoid therapy, is recognized in humans and may occur in dogs. Certainly, increased cTSH concentrations have been reported in dogs with hypercortisolism treated with trilostane. Increased cTSH concentrations occur with toceranib treatment without a concurrent decrease in total T4 concentrations (Hume *et al.*, 2018; Harper *et al.*, 2020). A mild increase in cTSH concentration has also been reported as a consequence of phenobarbital-containing anticonvulsant treatment, but the increase has limited diagnostic significance as values do not generally exceed the upper limit of the reference interval.

- The recovery phase of NTI has also been associated with temporary increases in circulating TSH concentrations in both humans and dogs. This is presumed to reflect increased demand for thyroid hormone production with the progressive return to euthyroidism. Testing thyroid function during known recovery from NTI should therefore be avoided until the animal is clinically stable.
- Certain illnesses are associated with increased cTSH concentrations. Up to 40% of dogs with primary hypoadrenocorticism have increased cTSH concentrations but these are rarely associated with a decline in total T4 values (Reusch *et al.*, 2017). Values start to decrease within 2 weeks of glucocorticoid supplementation but can take up to 4 months to fully resolve. It is suggested that glucocorticoids have an inhibitory effect on the secretion of TSH and that this effect is lost in hypoadrenocorticism. However, this has not been proven and other, as yet unknown, mechanisms may play a role.

Free T4

Free T4 is the metabolically active portion of T4 and represents the hormone fraction that is available for tissue uptake. Theoretically, its measurement provides the most accurate assessment of cellular thyroid status. The advantages and disadvantages of this test are summarized in Figure 18.19.

Advantages
• Less affected by NTI and drug therapies than total T4
• Decreased values more specific for hypothyroidism than total T4

Disadvantages
• Must be measured by equilibrium dialysis
• More expensive than total T4 measurement
• More prone to sample handling effects
• Can be decreased in severe NTI or by certain drugs
• May be low-normal in early hypothyroidism

18.19 The advantages and disadvantages of free thyroxine (T4) measurements for the diagnosis of hypothyroidism in dogs. NTI = non-thyroidal illness.

Assay methods: The method used to measure free T4 concentrations is important. Only one method currently in routine use, free T4 by equilibrium dialysis (fT4d), is considered to be capable of measuring true free hormone concentrations. Using this technique, measurement of free T4 is a two-step procedure. The test takes longer to complete (24–48 hours) and is correspondingly more expensive than methods for total hormone analysis. The first step involves the dialysis of the test sample across a membrane impermeable to protein-bound T4 and T4AA. Only free hormone can cross the membrane into the dialysate, which is then subjected to an ultrasensitive T4 RIA.

The ability of most non-dialysis methods to truly measure free T4 concentrations is controversial. The most commonly used method is analogue based, where the analogue is designed to compete with free T4 in the sample without any anomalous interaction with the thyroid-hormone-binding proteins. These assays are designed for human use and are based upon the presence of high-affinity thyroid-hormone-binding proteins in the sample. Canine thyroid-hormone-binding proteins have lower affinity for T4 and are present at a lower concentration; these methods are therefore less reliable in dogs, particularly when additional factors (such as NTI) further decrease thyroid hormone affinity. A large laboratory-based study including concomitant measurement of total T4 and analogue-based free T4 concentrations in over 900 dogs demonstrated just over 5% disagreement, suggesting limited benefit to measuring both hormones simultaneously (Rasmussen *et al.*, 2014). Additionally, a more recent study demonstrated that free T4 concentrations are affected by severity of NTI in much the same way as total T4 and that values are often decreased when within reference interval as measured by equilibrium dialysis (Bennaïm *et al.*, 2022). Analogue assays are also affected by T4AAs in much the same way as total T4 methods (Randolph *et al.*, 2015).

Diagnostic performance: Measurement of fT4d is theoretically less affected by the variety of factors that affect total T4, including but not limited to NTI and T4AAs. The diagnostic specificity of fT4d is greater than 90%, which is significantly better than for total T4 (i.e. it is less likely to result in a false-positive diagnosis of hypothyroidism) (see Figure 18.15). The sensitivity of fT4d for hypothyroidism is approximately 80%, which is lower than the corresponding value for total T4. Overall, it is the most accurate single test for hypothyroidism. However, its expense, poorer availability, potential for sample handling errors (see Chapter 3) and poorer sensitivity preclude its widespread use as a first-line diagnostic test. If used as a second-line diagnostic test, its poorer sensitivity is relatively unimportant. It is particularly useful in cases in which total T4 concentration is decreased and cTSH concentration remains within the reference interval. In these cases, a free T4 concentration may help differentiate genuine hypothyroidism (low values) from NTI (reference interval values).

Reference interval free T4 values in hypothyroid dogs: A small proportion of hypothyroid dogs maintain free T4 values within the reference interval, albeit at the low end. This probably reflects an attempt to maintain adequate free T4 concentrations in the face of early hypothyroidism. There is some evidence that hypothyroid dogs with low-normal free T4 values have more thyroidal reserve than those with subnormal free T4 values.

Low free T4 values in euthyroid dogs: There is no doubt that free T4 is also affected by certain drug therapies and NTI, albeit to a lesser extent than total T4. Free T4 concentrations do decrease with NTI but are typically maintained within the reference interval in all but the most severe diseases. Certain drugs, including glucocorticoids, phenobarbital-containing anticonvulsant medications, clomipramine, aspirin, carprofen and potentiated sulphonamides, are also associated with decreased free T4 concentrations. Testing for hypothyroidism should be delayed until after such therapy is withdrawn. However, given the nature of the cases receiving such medications, complete withdrawal of these drugs is often unachievable. Efforts should be made to reduce the dose, but ultimately the results from dogs receiving such therapies should be interpreted with caution.

Thyroglobulin autoantibodies

Thyroglobulin is a large-molecular-weight glycoprotein and a normal component of the thyroid gland. The spontaneous development of antibodies to normal thyroid tissue, including thyroglobulin, is well recognized in CLT. Thyroglobulin autoantibodies are only one of several antibodies produced during the progression of CLT in dogs (see 'Lymphocytic thyroiditis', above). However, they are the most important because a reliable canine-specific method for their estimation is commercially available. The advantages and disadvantages of this test are summarized in Figure 18.20.

Diagnostic performance: The principal limitation of TgAA measurement is that not all dogs with hypothyroidism have lymphocytic thyroiditis, and even in those that do, TgAA-positive dogs may eventually become TgAA negative given time (see Figure 18.3). Therefore, whilst a positive TgAA result provides strong evidence of thyroid disease, a negative result does not rule it out.

Identification of TgAAs provides no information on thyroid function. The test is therefore not recommended for use alone but is of value when used alongside other tests such as measurement of total or free T4 and cTSH. Thyroglobulin autoantibody measurement is of particular value in cases with discordant T4 and cTSH results. Since the presence of TgAAs is highly specific for CLT, a positive result is of particular help in those cases with decreased total or free T4 values but unexpected reference interval cTSH results. Other advantages of TgAA estimation are that it is unaffected by concurrent drug therapy and that it can provide indirect evidence for the existence of T4AAs. The use of TgAA measurement as a second-line test is frequently recommended in these situations.

Positive TgAA results in hypothyroid dogs: Approximately half of all hypothyroid dogs have a positive TgAA result. However, epidemiological analysis of the prevalence of TgAA has shown considerable breed and age variation.

Advantages
• A positive result is suggestive of lymphocytic thyroiditis
• Postitive results occur before evidence of thyroid dysfunction
Disadvantages
• Provides no assessment of thyroid function
• A negative result does not rule out hypothyroidism

18.20 The advantages and disadvantages of thyroglobulin autoantibody measurements for the diagnosis of hypothyroidism in dogs.

Positive TgAA results peak in dogs between 4 and 6 years of age. This subsequently declines, presumably as thyroid tissue is destroyed. Elderly dogs (over 10 years of age) are much less likely to have positive TgAA results, making testing of less value in older animals. Certain breeds are overrepresented for CLT, and TgAA estimation is of particular value in these animals. The age at which the peak prevalence is observed also varies between breeds. The likelihood of identifying a positive result increases significantly when testing a predisposed breed of the appropriate age range, and this should be considered when selecting a second-line test and perhaps choosing between free T4 and TgAA. A positive TgAA result does not prove hypothyroidism but provides evidence of thyroid pathology that may be useful in supporting a diagnosis of hypothyroidism.

Positive TgAA results in euthyroid dogs: A positive TgAA result without thyroid hormone deficiency can occur in clinically healthy dogs in both the silent and subclinical or compensating stages of CLT. Not all of these dogs become hypothyroid. Assessment of TgAA status may be used by a section of the dog-breeding community to identify animals with CLT (see 'Genetic tests for hypothyroidism and lymphocytic thyroiditis', below).

Other diagnostic tests

Total T3: The diagnostic accuracy of total T3 is poorer than that of total T4 and as such it offers no real practical advantage. Consequently, total T3 measurement is not recommended. The poor diagnostic performance of total T3 reflects several factors:

- In early hypothyroidism, there may be increased peripheral conversion of T4 to the more metabolically active T3, thereby maintaining circulating concentrations within the reference interval
- T3AAs are more common than T4AAs, with the same potential for interfering with measured concentrations
- The effect of NTI is a progression from suppression of total T3 concentrations alone to lowering total T3 and total T4 concentrations concurrently. Thus, the overlap between total T3 values from hypothyroid dogs and those with NTI is more marked than is the case for total T4.

Free T3: Measurement of serum concentrations of free T3 is offered by a small number of commercial endocrine laboratories. The utility of this test for the diagnosis of hypothyroidism has not been evaluated. Therefore, measurement is of little value in the investigation of thyroid function.

Dynamic thyroid function tests: A number of dynamic thyroid function tests have been used in the past. However, the development of assays for cTSH, free T4 and TgAA has largely obviated the need for such tests in routine general veterinary practice. They tend to be reserved for specific circumstances in which a diagnosis cannot be confirmed in any other way.

The TSH response test was traditionally considered the 'gold standard' for diagnosing canine hypothyroidism. Intravenous administration of a supraphysiological dose of exogenous TSH results in maximal stimulation of the thyroid gland. Measurement of circulating total T4 values before and after administration provides an assessment of the functional reserve capacity of the thyroid, and minimal stimulation is expected in hypothyroidism. This test is considered to be more reliable than any other test for canine hypothyroidism. In early studies, TSH of bovine origin was used but this product is no longer available as a pharmaceutical preparation. Several studies have demonstrated comparable results using recombinant human TSH (rhTSH). Unlike bovine TSH, adverse reactions have not been reported following the administration of rhTSH to dogs. Samples for measurement of total T4 are taken before and 6 hours after the intravenous administration of 75 µg rhTSH/dog. This test is excellent at precluding a diagnosis of hypothyroidism but less good at definitively diagnosing the disease (Corsini et al., 2021). It can be prohibitively expensive.

The TRH response test, whereby total T4 is measured before and after TRH administration, was once recommended as a useful alternative to the TSH response test. Unfortunately, the TRH response test is considerably less reliable than the combined use of the currently available baseline tests and is therefore not recommended. At best, a good response to TRH can confidently exclude hypothyroidism. However, the lack of a T4 response to TRH is not confirmatory of hypothyroidism, being a common finding in both a wide variety of NTIs and dogs receiving certain medications.

Several investigators have evaluated the response of TSH to TRH administration (Pijnacker et al., 2018). A number of protocols have been used, but relatively low doses of TRH appear to be capable of causing significant pituitary TSH stimulation in euthyroidism whilst minimizing any side effects. Circulating cTSH concentrations are measured before and 30–45 minutes after intravenous administration of 10 µg/kg TRH. Humans with primary hypothyroidism exhibit an exaggerated and prolonged TSH response to TRH compared with healthy humans. However, the TSH response to TRH is blunted or absent in hypothyroid dogs compared with healthy dogs or those with NTI. Whilst capable of reliably distinguishing hypothyroidism from health and most NTIs, this test is not perfect.

Growth hormone, rather than cTSH, can also be measured during a TRH response test. In hypothyroid dogs there is usually an increased basal growth hormone concentration and an exaggerated response to TRH in samples taken 30–45 minutes after TRH administration. Whilst useful in distinguishing hypothyroidism from health and NTI, this test is of most value in diagnosing hypothyroidism in cases with low total T4 concentrations and reference interval cTSH concentrations (Pijnacker et al., 2018). Unfortunately, species-specific canine growth hormone assays are not commercially available.

Diagnostic imaging

Thyroid imaging has a well established role in the investigation of thyroid masses in humans, dogs and cats. In recent years, there has been growing interest in the use of imaging techniques for the diagnosis of canine hypothyroidism. In general, imaging findings are less affected by NTI and drug administration than are basal hormone concentrations. Although imaging techniques can be of value during the investigation of complex hypothyroidism cases, additional studies are warranted before their use can be recommended in a wider clinical setting.

Radiography

Radiography has no value in the investigation of acquired primary hypothyroidism. However, characteristic changes in the axial and appendicular skeleton are apparent in dogs with congenital hypothyroidism and disproportionate dwarfism. These changes include shortening of the long

bones, valgus deformities, epiphyseal dysgenesis and delayed ossification, shortening and broadening of the skull, and shortened vertebral bodies with scalloped ventral borders (Figure 18.21). Secondary degenerative joint disease can develop over time in affected animals. These changes can be particularly useful to differentiate this disorder from the proportionate dwarfism associated with growth hormone deficiency.

Thyroid ultrasonography

In euthyroid dogs, individual thyroid lobes are described as fusiform in longitudinal section and triangular in cross-section, with a smooth capsule. Echogenicity is homogeneous, and isoechoic or hyperechoic compared with the adjacent sternothyroid muscle (Figure 18.22). Thyroid volume can be calculated by applying the ellipsoid formula (volume (ml) = $\pi/6$ x length (cm) x width (cm) x height (cm)) to measured length, width and height, and summing the calculated volume for each lobe. Maximal cross-sectional area can also be calculated. There is no apparent difference in thyroid lobe measurements between healthy dogs and euthyroid dogs with NTI.

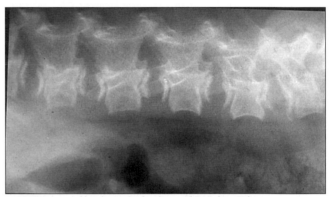

18.21 Lateral lumbar spinal radiograph in a dog with disproportionate dwarfism associated with congenital hypothyroidism. Note the shortened vertebral bodies with scalloped ventral borders.

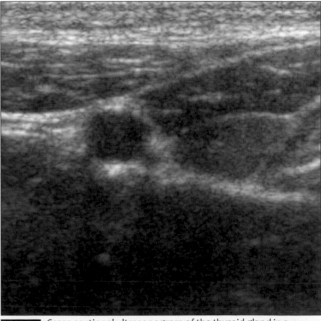

18.22 Cross-sectional ultrasonogram of the thyroid gland in a euthyroid dog. It is triangular in shape, homogeneous and hyperechoic compared with adjacent muscle.

By comparison, the thyroid lobes of TgAA-positive and TgAA-negative hypothyroid dogs display significantly decreased echogenicity and are typically heterogeneous in appearance in TgAA-negative cases but homogeneous in dogs with positive TgAA status. Thyroid lobes are often round or oval in shape, and have decreased length, width, height, volume and maximal cross-sectional area when compared with euthyroid dogs. Thyroidal volume has been suggested to be the most useful parameter to differentiate between hypothyroid and euthyroid individuals.

Although ultrasonographic results from hypothyroid dogs are statistically different from those obtained in euthyroid individuals, there is considerable overlap of all parameters between both groups. In addition, euthyroid dogs of different breeds display marked differences in thyroid lobe measurements. This has led to the suggestion of normalization of values to body surface area. However, this method has not been properly assessed, and studies of inter-breed variability independent of body size have not been performed. Thyroid ultrasonography has high inter-observer variability, even when performed by trained diagnostic imaging specialists, a factor that is likely amplified when performed by less skilled individuals with suboptimal equipment. Therefore, further studies are warranted to evaluate a larger range of NTIs and subclinical thyroid disease.

Computed tomography and magnetic resonance imaging

In theory, alterations in size and parenchymal features evident on computed tomography (CT) could allow differentiation between euthyroid and hypothyroid individuals, as has been described in human medicine. Enlargement of the pituitary gland, secondary to thyrotroph hyperplasia, has been detected by CT in dogs with experimental primary hypothyroidism, but this change is not specific for hypothyroidism. Given the high relative cost of these procedures and the requirement for deep sedation or general anaesthesia, it is unlikely that they will ever play a significant role in the assessment of primary hypothyroidism in dogs. However, they continue to play an important role in the investigation of central hypothyroidism associated with structural pituitary and/or hypothalamic lesions.

Thyroid scintigraphy

The use of nuclear medicine techniques for the assessment of thyroid function has been described for many years, predating the introduction of immunoassays. These procedures involve the administration of either technetium-99m as pertechnetate ($^{99m}TcO_4^-$) or radioactive iodine (^{123}I or ^{131}I) with subsequent quantification of thyroidal uptake using a scintillation counter or camera. The use of pertechnetate is preferred because of its shorter half-life, lower cost, more rapid uptake and lower radiation dose compared with radioactive iodine.

Whilst undoubtedly valuable for investigating thyroid masses in dogs, only a few studies have assessed the technique for the investigation of canine hypothyroidism and differentiation from NTI. The most common procedure involves the intravenous administration of between 110 and 160 MBq of $^{99m}TcO_4^-$. This is followed by thyroid imaging 40–60 minutes later. Calculation of $^{99m}TcO_4^-$ uptake has been shown to reliably differentiate hypothyroid dogs from euthyroid animals with low total T4 concentrations (Figure 18.23). Scintigraphy has also shown promise in confirming euthyroidism in specific breeds, such as Greyhounds,

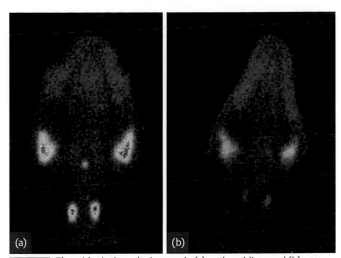

18.23 Thyroid scintigraphy images in (a) euthyroidism and (b) hypothyroidism. Thyroidal uptake measurements were 0.5% and 0.05% (reference interval 0.39–1.86%). Uptake is also noted in the salivary glands at the level of the ears.

where diagnosis of thyroid disease is complicated by decreased concentrations of multiple thyroid hormones in healthy animals.

In human medicine, however, altered radioisotope uptake has been described in association with several NTIs and different medications, and the scintigraphic appearance of inflammatory thyroid disease is variable. There is a dearth of information on the effect of a wide range of such factors on thyroid scintigraphy results in dogs. However, it is recognized that uptake values in dogs with hypercortisolism can mimic those found in dogs with hypothyroidism. In addition, values in the equivocal or non-diagnostic range do occur. The procedure requires specialist equipment and radiation isolation facilities. Therefore, although it is certainly a useful technique for the assessment of thyroid function, it is not a first-line test, and results should be interpreted in conjunction with clinical and clinicopathological findings.

Therapeutic trial as a diagnostic test

The use of a levothyroxine therapeutic trial as a diagnostic method has proved popular amongst some clinicians but should be avoided as much as possible. There are several disadvantages of a therapeutic trial. There may be diagnostic problems subsequent to thyroid hormone supplementation if the clinical response is suboptimal. Additionally, the pharmacological actions of levothyroxine may non-specifically improve some clinical signs in euthyroid dogs. Thyroid hormone supplementation suppresses thyroid function through negative feedback, with consequent normalization after cessation of treatment. In euthyroid levothyroxine-supplemented dogs, T4 and cTSH concentrations normalize within 1 week after 8–16 weeks of treatment (Ziglioli et al., 2017). However, more prolonged treatment could induce a state of functional hypothyroidism that potentially takes weeks or months to resolve after withdrawal of treatment. The use of a therapeutic trial is only appropriate when the index of suspicion for hypothyroidism remains high but diagnostic testing has repeatedly proven equivocal. Therapeutic trials should be considered a 'last resort' in these situations.

A true therapeutic trial for diagnostic purposes involves setting an objective, quantifiable target by which success or failure of therapy will be judged, starting treatment and then withdrawing therapy, subject to confirming adequate dosing and satisfying the predefined targets. This cessation is performed to ensure that any clinical resolution is genuinely a consequence of the treatment. Cessation of therapy should, of course, coincide with a return of clinical signs, which are then expected to resolve if therapy is reinstituted. A protocol for use of a therapeutic trial as a diagnostic test is shown in Figure 18.24.

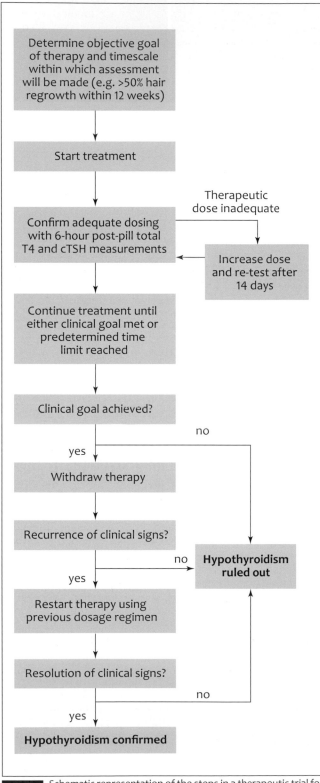

18.24 Schematic representation of the steps in a therapeutic trial for diagnosing hypothyroidism. cTSH = canine thyroid-stimulating hormone; T4 = thyroxine.

Genetic tests for hypothyroidism and lymphocytic thyroiditis

Given the hereditary nature of hypothyroidism in certain breeds, there is substantial interest in tests capable of identifying animals at increased risk for developing the disease. Measurement of TgAA may provide some useful information, as it is a marker of CLT, and its peak prevalence occurs at an earlier age than hypothyroidism. Samples are collected annually up to 4 years of age and every 2 years thereafter. There are no clear guidelines on how such information should be used for assisted breeding strategies as not all TgAA-positive dogs develop hypothyroidism. Genetic tests depicting certain DLA haplotypes and alleles known to increase risk of hypothyroidism are also available. However, it is difficult to recommend specific breeding practices based on such results. The development of hypothyroidism is complex and multifactorial. Not all recognized DLA haplotypes and alleles confer significant risk in all breeds. This complexity is highlighted by the finding of a DLA haplotype in Gordon Setters that is associated with protection against hypothyroidism but susceptibility to onychomadesis (Ziener *et al.*, 2015).

Effect of hypothyroidism on the diagnosis of other endocrine diseases

Primary hypothyroidism has significant effects on growth hormone secretion and concomitant increase in insulin-like growth factor-1 concentration has been noted. Hypothyroidism is also associated with significant increases in circulating leptin and insulin concentrations (neither of which is attributable to obesity alone), confirming the role of hypothyroidism in insulin resistance.

Treatment and therapeutic monitoring

Choice of preparation

All hypothyroid dogs require chronic thyroid hormone replacement therapy (THRT), and a variety of preparations are available. Crude thyroid products derived from desiccated porcine, ovine or bovine thyroid glands are obsolete, and synthetic products are preferable as they are more predictable and have a longer shelf life.

Both T3- and T4-containing products, as well as combination products, are available for the treatment of hypothyroidism. Synthetic sodium levothyroxine is the treatment of choice: as T4 is the principal secretory product of the thyroid gland and is the physiological prohormone for the more potent T3, re-establishment of reference interval circulating T4 and T3 concentrations is best achieved by administration of T4.

Triiodothyronine administration circumvents the normal physiological process of T4 deiodination to T3. Consequently, whilst circulating total and free T3 concentrations may be within the therapeutic range after T3 administration, total and free T4 concentrations remain subnormal. Administration of purely T3-containing products may result in adequate concentrations in organs such as the liver, kidneys and heart that derive their T3 from the circulation. However, the brain and pituitary gland may be deficient in T3 if the circulating concentration of free T4 is subnormal.

Conversely, it has been suggested that administration of sufficient T3 to provide adequate brain and pituitary concentrations may result in excessive concentrations in other organs.

Combination products containing both T4 and T3 are available for human use. These are not recommended for dogs as they do not reflect the thyroid production ratio in this species and provide excess T3.

In Europe, there are several authorized products for the treatment of hypothyroidism. They all contain levothyroxine alone, as either tablets or liquid for oral administration (see *BSAVA Small Animal Formulary*) and are the drugs of choice for canine hypothyroidism. They come in a range of dose sizes (0.1, 0.2, 0.3, 0.5 and 0.8 mg tablets and 1 mg/ml solution).

Levothyroxine pharmacokinetics

The pharmacokinetic profile of administered levothyroxine is similar in healthy and hypothyroid dogs. Bioavailability is variable and estimated to be between 10% and 50% of the orally administered dose. Whilst bioavailability is governed by the individual receiving the medication, it is also influenced by other factors. It varies depending on the product used and therefore not all products can be used interchangeably. In addition, administration with food significantly delays and inhibits levothyroxine absorption by approximately 45%, irrespective of food type (Iemura *et al.*, 2013). This does not mean that administration in food should be avoided; instead, the time between feeding and drug administration must be standardized in each individual dog, to avoid marked variations in levothyroxine absorption from day to day. Time to maximal T4 concentration is approximately 5–6 hours; the half-life is between 12 and 14 hours but is slightly lower if multiple daily doses are used.

Choice of dosing regime

Numerous therapeutic strategies have been recommended for the treatment of hypothyroid dogs, with dosages ranging from 10 µg/kg q8–12h to 44 µg/kg q12h. Today there is almost general agreement that a dose of approximately 20 µg/kg q24h suffices in most cases, at least initially (Lewis *et al.*, 2018). The clinical response to once-daily therapy is usually excellent, as long as adequate peak circulating hormone concentrations are achieved. This approach significantly improves owner compliance and is less expensive in the long term. Whilst the use of divided dosing certainly results in less fluctuation of circulating T4 concentrations compared with administration of the same total dose as a single daily bolus, the duration of biological action of thyroid hormones far exceeds their plasma half-life. There appears to be no difference in efficacy between administration of the drug once or twice daily (Lewis *et al.*, 2018).

Although the time of treatment is irrelevant, as there is no circadian release of T4 in dogs, morning dosing is recommended. This is to assist with the subsequent collection of monitoring samples, which are required approximately 6 hours after treatment.

Clinical monitoring

Adequately treated hypothyroid dogs should be clinically indistinguishable from healthy euthyroid animals. However, the time taken before all signs resolve varies based on the body system affected and the adequacy of therapy.

Clinical signs

Generally, metabolic signs such as mental dullness and lethargy are among the first to improve, usually appearing dramatically better within days of starting treatment. Often, it is only after treatment commences that the extent of the clinical problem is retrospectively noted by owners. Improvements in cardiovascular function and electrocardiographic changes should occur during the first 8 weeks of treatment, although some cases will take longer. Weight loss is a consistent feature of successful treatment, and a 10% weight reduction can be expected within 3 months of starting therapy. Treated dogs can also be expected to become more active and athletic, presumably as a consequence of the combination of improved mental alertness and weight loss.

Dermatological improvements (Figure 18.25) are expected to occur within a month of starting treatment, although it is common for a period of increased hair loss to precede regrowth. This apparent worsening may concern some owners, but it reflects increased follicular turnover and hair shedding in advance of normal hair replacement and should be considered as a positive sign during the early phase of treatment. Significant hair regrowth should be obvious within 3 months of starting treatment, although complete resolution may take a further 2–3 months.

The response of neurological signs to adequate THRT is more variable, and sometimes poorer, than that of other affected systems. In human hypothyroid patients, some neurological abnormalities take several years to resolve completely, and the same may be true for dogs. However, peripheral neuropathies typically improve within 1–3 months of starting treatment, if they are to respond at all.

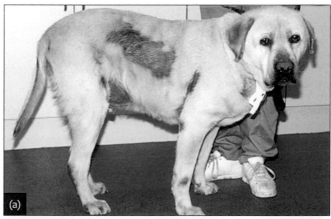

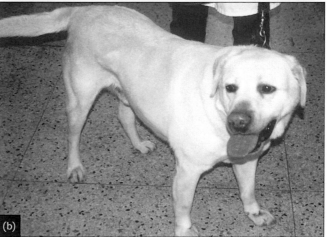

18.25 Appearance of a hypothyroid dog (a) before and (b) after thyroid hormone replacement therapy.

Central nervous system signs are expected to take longer to resolve, and although some improvement can be expected within 6 months, residual signs may persist in some dogs. There is limited evidence of improvement in laryngeal paralysis and megaoesophagus in most affected dogs, but this probably reflects the dubious causal links between these conditions and hypothyroidism.

Laboratory monitoring

The ultimate goal of therapy is the complete resolution of clinical abnormalities. However, there are now also well defined laboratory goals that can be expected to correspond to good clinical resolution. These are important given the wide inter-individual variation in absorption of levothyroxine. Therapeutic monitoring can be performed within 2 weeks of starting therapy or after making subsequent dosage alterations, allowing fairly rapid progress towards identification of a final maintenance dose of THRT. Once this is achieved, monitoring every 6 months thereafter is probably adequate. It is estimated that at least one dose adjustment is required in up to 20% of cases. Generally, an increased rather than a decreased dose is required. Only a small number of dogs require two or more dose adjustments. Fewer dose adjustments will be required if drug administration and feeding are standardized.

Total T4

Laboratory monitoring is aimed primarily at identification of peak circulating total T4 concentration. Total T4 measurements are currently preferred over free T4 measurements for monitoring purposes, for the simple reason that clinical resolution has been correlated with specific therapeutic ranges for total T4 but not free T4 values. Whilst it is probable that free T4 fluctuation is less marked following treatment than the total hormone concentration, peak circulating total T4 measurement is satisfactory. Total T4 determinations also have the advantage of being less expensive and more widely available.

Hypothyroid dogs receiving once-daily treatment have a marked increase in circulating total T4 values, which peak approximately 6 hours after treatment and then progressively decline until the next dose. In order to identify peak total T4 values, it is therefore recommended that samples are collected approximately 6 hours after pill administration. Adjustment of T4 to peak values using an estimated half-life can be made if samples are taken at a different time point but this is less reliable.

Optimal peak circulating total T4 concentrations should be in the region of 50–60 nmol/l in dogs receiving once-daily therapy. Values below approximately 35 nmol/l are usually associated with an inadequate clinical response, and an increase in dosage is indicated. Marked increases in peak total T4 to 90–100 nmol/l or higher are unnecessary and such values should probably prompt a decrease in the dose used. The magnitude of dose alterations is usually dictated by the next available tablet size when tablets are used. However, more accurate dose adjustment may be possible using the liquid formulation. Any dose adjustment required must take the low bioavailability (10–50%) of orally administered levothyroxine into account. A reasonable starting estimation is that doubling the dose will increase circulating total T4 concentrations by approximately 50%.

The measurement of pre-pill or 'trough' total T4 concentrations remains common practice. The rationale for this is to ensure that T4 values do not fall substantially below the reference interval. However, maintenance of reference interval total T4 concentrations over 24 hours is not essential, due to the prolonged biological action of T4 compared with its circulating half-life. In addition, dose adjustments based on trough values may give rise to significant under- or overtreatment in individual cases. Given the clinical studies which have correlated clinical resolution with peak T4 values alone, there appears to be no real value in performing trough T4 measurements.

Canine TSH

Measurement of cTSH alongside total T4 inevitably increases the expense of therapeutic monitoring. However, its measurement is usually recommended, as cTSH provides a longer-term assessment of the adequacy of treatment, unlike total T4, which only provides information concerning treatment on that particular day. Measurement of cTSH can therefore assist in identification of poor owner compliance where a particular effort to administer the medication is made on days corresponding to the monitoring visit. Unfortunately, in the proportion of hypothyroid dogs that do not have increased pre-treatment cTSH values, measurement during THRT is not of any additional value.

Circulating cTSH values usually decrease quickly to the reference interval after the institution of THRT. Circulating cTSH appears to be highly sensitive to the suppressive effects of THRT, such that suppression of cTSH may be achieved without also achieving optimal clinical control. Therefore, whilst maintenance of an increased or high-normal cTSH value is strong evidence of suboptimal therapy, suppression of cTSH does not necessarily confirm adequate treatment.

Clinicopathological tests

Improvements in the routine clinicopathological abnormalities associated with hypothyroidism following the instigation of THRT can be expected to occur broadly in parallel with the clinical response. Circulating cholesterol and triglyceride values decrease dramatically, and within just 2 weeks of starting therapy may be within or approaching the reference intervals. Whilst RBC values also start to improve quickly, this change is ongoing, and RBC values continue to increase during at least the first 3 months of THRT. Fructosamine concentration decreases significantly following the start of THRT as protein turnover increases. Mild reductions in ALP activity are also reported. It is presumed that this reflects the progressive normalization of hepatic metabolism, including the mobilization of hepatic lipid deposits once THRT starts and weight loss begins.

Therapeutic failure

Failure to achieve therapeutic circulating hormone concentrations, or absence of the expected clinical improvement, should prompt consideration of an underlying cause, and an increase in drug dose if appropriate, followed by monitoring after 2 weeks. This process should be repeated until hormone concentrations and/or clinical improvements are acceptable. Dogs with underlying gastrointestinal disease may demonstrate an increased THRT dose requirement to achieve adequate circulating hormone concentrations. Similarly, dogs receiving concurrent glucocorticoid therapy may require a slight increase in dose to achieve optimal control.

However, there is normally wide variation in individual dose requirements between individual hypothyroid dogs in any case, and there is no alternative to appropriate clinical and laboratory monitoring followed by review of the THRT dosage regime.

Potential complications of therapy

Dogs appear relatively resistant to levothyroxine over-dosing, presumably because of an ability to control the conversion of T4 to T3 and having virtually unsaturable thyroid-hormone-binding proteins. Doses up to 10 times that recommended administered over 6 months were well tolerated in dogs (Hare et al., 2018). Nevertheless, thyro-toxicosis can sporadically occur and is best avoided if possible. When it does occur, the clinical signs include PU/PD, polyphagia, panting, weight loss, hyperactivity, tachycardia and hyperthermia. Most signs should resolve within a few days of withdrawing therapy.

A gradual introduction of THRT has been recommended in dogs that have decreased ability to metabolize levothy-roxine and may be at increased risk of thyrotoxicosis, such as those that are elderly or suffer from hypoadrenocorticism or cardiac disease. However, such guidelines usually apply when the THRT dose being used is considerably higher than the standard dose. Overall, there is little published evidence of complications associated with THRT in dogs with concurrent illness. Nevertheless, care is advised in dogs with hypoadrenocorticism, and it should first be ensured that glucocorticoid replacement therapy has been established and life-threatening complications resolved. The treatment of hypothyroid dogs with concurrent insulin-dependent diabetes mellitus may result in a reduction in the animal's insulin requirement, and alterations in the insulin dose should be anticipated as THRT is started.

Anecdotal reports of hypersensitivity or allergies to levo-thyroxine are common. These are likely the result of a reaction to the dye or inactive ingredients in the formulation. There is one case report of a dog that had a delayed hyper-sensitivity, manifesting as skin disease, to two different levothyroxine formulations that shared two common inactive ingredients (Lavergne et al., 2016). Switching formulations, ensuring no shared ingredients, is recommended.

Thyroid hormone supplementation in myxoedema coma

In addition to the necessary symptomatic treatment (intra-venous fluids, electrolyte replacement, warming, etc.) in cases of myxoedema coma, thyroid hormone supplementation is also required. Due to the decreased metabolic rate and potential hypovolaemia/dehydration, oral, subcutaneous and intramuscular routes of administration are inadequate, at least initially. Sodium levothyroxine should therefore be administered intravenously, at a dose of 5 μg/kg q12h. Once stabilized, oral administration can be substituted. Resolution of abnormal mentation, ambulation and systolic hypotension should be expected within 30 hours.

References and further reading

Åhlgren J and Uimari P (2016) Heritability of hypothyroidism in the Finnish hovawart population. Acta Vetrerinaria Scandinavica 58, 39–43

Aicher KM, Cullen JM, Seiler GS et al. (2019) Investigation of adrenal and thyroid gland dysfunction in dogs with ultrasonographic diagnosis of gallbladder mucocele formation. PLoS ONE 14, e0212638

Allerton F (2023) BSAVA Small Animal Formulary, 11th edition – Part A: Canine and Feline, BSAVA Publications, Gloucester

Beier P, Reese S, Holler PJ et al. (2015) The role of hypothyroidism in the etiology and progression of dilated cardiomyopathy in Doberman pinschers. Journal of Veterinary Internal Medicine 29, 141–149

Bennaïm M, Shiel RE, Evans H and Mooney CT (2022) Free thyroxine measurement by analogue immunoassay and equilibrium dialysis in dogs with non-thyroidal illness. Research in Veterinary Science 147, 37–43

Bianchi M, Dahlgren S, Massey J et al. (2015) A multi-breed genome-wide association analysis for canine hypothyroidism identifies a shared major risk locus on CFA12. PLoS ONE 10, e0134720

Bianchi M, Rafati N and Karlsson Å (2020) Whole-genome genotyping and resequencing reveal the association of a deletion in the complex interferon alpha gene cluster with hypothyroidism in dogs. BMC Genomics 21, 307–324

Chan MK, Toribio J-ALML, Podadera JM and Child G (2020) Incidence, cause, outcome and possible risk factors associated with facial nerve paralysis in dogs in a Sydney population (2001–2016): a retrospective study. Australian Veterinary Journal 98, 140–147

Corsini A, Faroni E, Lunetta F and Fracassi F (2021) Recombinant human thyrotropin stimulation test in 114 dogs with suspected hypothyroidism: a cross-sectional study. Journal of Small Animal Practice 62, 257–264

Di Paola A, Carotenuto G and Dondi F (2021) Symmetric dimethylarginine concentrations in dogs with hypothyroidism before and after treatment with levothyroxine. Journal of Small Animal Practice 62, 89–96

Domosławska A and Zdunczyk S (2020) Clinical and spermatological findings in male dogs with acquired infertility: a retrospective analysis. Andrologia 52, e13802

Egbert RJ, Sist MD, Basu P et al. (2019) Temporal changes in thyroid status in euthyroid dogs with positive thyroglobulin autoantibodies. Journal of Veterinary Internal Medicine 33, 1041–1042

Ferm K, Bjornerfeldt S, Karlsson A et al. (2009) Prevalence of diagnostic characteristics indicating canine autoimmune lymphocytic thyroiditis in giant schnauzer and hovawart dogs. Journal of Small Animal Practice 50, 176–179

Gołynski M, Lutnicki K, Krumrych W et al. (2017) Relationship between total homocysteine, folic acid, and thyroid hormones in hypothyroid dogs. Journal of Veterinary Internal Medicine 31, 1403–1405

Guglielmini G, Berlanda M, Fracassi F et al. (2019) Electrocardiographic and echocardiographic evaluation in dogs with hypothyroidism before and after levothyroxine supplementation: a prospective controlled study. Journal of Veterinary Internal Medicine 33, 1935–1942

Hare JE, Morrow CMK and Caldwell J (2018) Safety of orally administered, USP-compliant levothyroxine sodium tablets in dogs. Veterinary Pharmacology and Therapeutics 41, 254–265

Harper A, Blackwood L and Mason S (2020) Investigation of thyroid function in dogs treated with the tyrosine kinase inhibitor toceranib. Veterinary Comparative Oncology 18, 433–437

Hume KR, Rizzo VL and Cawley JR (2018) Effects of toceranib phosphate on the hypothalamic-pituitary-thyroid axis in tumor-bearing dogs. Journal of Veterinary Internal Medicine 32, 377–383

Iemura R, Toyota M and Micallef MJ (2013) Effects of type of diet on pharmacokinetics of levothyroxine sodium oral solution. Research in Veterinary Science 94, 695–697

Kutsunai M, Kanemoto H, Fukushima K et al. (2014) The association between gall bladder mucoceles and hyperlipidaemia in dogs: a retrospective case control study. The Veterinary Journal 199, 76–79

Lavergne SN, Fosset FTJ, Kennedy P and Refsal KR (2016) Potential cutaneous hypersensitivity reaction to an inactive ingredient of thyroid hormone supplements in a dog. Veterinary Dermatology 27, 53–e16

Lewis VA, Morrow CMK, Jacobsen JA and Lloyd WE (2018) A pivotal field study to support the registration of levothyroxine sodium tablets for canine hypothyroidism. Journal of the American Animal Hospital Association 54, 201–208

Martinez C, Mooney CRT, Shiel RE et al. (2019) Evaluation of red blood cell distribution width in dogs with various illnesses. Canadian Veterinary Journal 60, 964–971

Mazaki-Tovi M, Abood S, Kol A, Farkas A and Schenck PA (2015) Increased serum concentrations of adiponectin in canine hypothyroidism. The Veterinary Journal 203, 253–255

Orlandi R, Gutierrez-Quintana R, Carletti B et al. (2020) Clinical signs, MRI findings and outcome in dogs with peripheral vestibular disease: a retrospective study. BMC Veterinary Research 16, 159–168

Parkanzky M, Grimes J, Schmiedt C, Secrest S and Bugbee A (2019) Long-term survival of dogs treated for gallbladder mucocele by cholecystectomy, medical management or both. Journal of Veterinary Internal Medicine 33, 2057–2066

Pijnacker T, Kooistra HS and Vermeulen CF (2018) Use of basal and TRH-stimulated plasma growth hormone concentrations to differentiate between primary hypothyroidism and nonthyroidal illness in dogs. Journal of Veterinary Internal Medicine 32, 1319–1324

Randolph JF, Lamb SV, Cheraskin JL et al. (2015) Free thyroxine concentrations by equilibrium dialysis and chemiluminescent immunoassays in 13 hypothyroid dogs positive for thyroglobulin antibody. Journal of Veterinary Internal Medicine 29, 877–881

Rasmussen SH, Andersen HH and Kjelgaard-Hansen M (2014) Combined assessment of serum free and total T4 in a general clinical setting seemingly has limited potential in improving diagnostic accuracy of thyroid dysfunction in dogs and cats. Veterinary Clinical Pathology 43, 1–3

Reusch CE, Fracassi F, Sieber-Ruckstuhl NS *et al.* (2017) Altered serum thyrotropin concentrations in dogs with primary hypoadrenocorticism before and during treatment. *Journal of Veterinary Internal Medicine* **31**, 1643–1648

Seckerdieck F and Mueller RS (2018) Recurrent pyoderma and its underlying primary diseases: a retrospective evaluation of 157 cases. *Veterinary Record* **182**, 434

Soler Arias EA, Castilo VA, Garcia JD and Fyfe JC (2018) Congenital dyshormonogenic hypothyroidism with goiter caused by a sodium/iodide symporter (*SLC5A5*) mutation in a family of Shih-Tzu dogs. *Domestic Animal Endocrinology* **65**, 1–8

Sundburg CR, Belanger JM and Bannasch DL (2016) Gonadectomy effects on the risk of immune disorders in the dog: a retrospective study. *BMC Veterinary Research* **12**, 278

Thuróczy J, Müller L, Kollár E and Balogh L (2016) Thyroxin and progesterone concentrations in pregnant, nonpregnant bitches, and bitches during abortion. *Theriogeniology* **85**, 1186–1191

Violette NP and Ledbetter EC (2019) Lipemic uveitis and its etiologies in dogs: 75 cases. *Veterinary Ophthalmology* **22**, 577–583

Voorbij AMWY, Leegwater PAJ, Buijtels JJCWM, Daminet S and Kooistra HS (2016) Central hypothyroidism in miniature schnauzers. *Journal of Veterinary Internal Medicine* **30**, 85–91

Ziener ML, Dahlgren S, Thoresen SI and Lingaas F (2015) Genetics and epidemiology of hypothyroidism and symmetrical onychomadesis in the Gordon setter and the English setter. *Canine Genetics and Epidemiology* **2**, 12

Ziglioli V, Panciera DL and Troy GC (2017) Effects of levothyroxine administration and withdrawal on the hypothalamic-pituitary-thyroid axis in euthyroid dogs. *Journal of Veterinary Internal Medicine* **31**, 705–710

Chapter 19

Feline hyperthyroidism

Carmel T. Mooney and Mark E. Peterson

Introduction

Hyperthyroidism (a form of thyrotoxicosis) is a disorder resulting from excessive circulating concentrations of the active thyroid hormones triiodothyronine (T3) and/or thyroxine (T4). First described in cats in 1979, hyperthyroidism has become not just the most common endocrine disorder of this species but a frequent diagnosis in small animal practice. It is unclear why such a phenomenon has occurred. Undoubtedly, increased awareness of the condition by veterinary surgeons (veterinarians) and their clients, easier availability of diagnostic tests, and a growing and ageing pet cat population may have all played a role. However, these factors, alone or together, cannot fully explain the trend.

The prevalence of hyperthyroidism varies nationally, although evidence for regional variation is lacking. It is considered reasonably common in many European countries, North America, South Africa, Australasia and Japan, but appears to be less common in Hong Kong. It is difficult to compare incidence rates and prevalence estimates accurately, due to differences in study design and populations tested. However, in the largest study of over 95,000 UK cats, an overall prevalence of 2.4% was reported, equating to 8.7% in cats aged 10 years of age or older (Stephens et al., 2014). A prevalence of up to 20% in older cats has also been reported from Ireland (Bree et al., 2018).

Aetiology

Benign adenomatous hyperplasia (adenoma) of one (<45% of cases) or, more commonly, both (>55% of cases) thyroid lobes is the most common pathological abnormality associated with hyperthyroidism in cats, occurring in approximately 98% of cases. Microscopically, the normal thyroid follicular architecture is replaced by one or more readily discernible foci of hyperplastic tissue, forming nodules ranging from smaller than 1 mm to larger than 2 cm in diameter. By contrast, thyroid carcinoma is a rare cause of hyperthyroidism in cats, accounting for approximately 2% of cases. There is some evidence that there is progression of benign to malignant disease over time, especially if not definitively treated (Peterson et al., 2016a). These cats usually have severe hyperthyroidism, large tumour volume, intrathoracic location and multifocal distribution, and are refractory to antithyroid drugs (so-called severe, huge, intrathoracic, multifocal disease, refractory to antithyroid drugs (SHIM-RAD) cases).

To date, the underlying aetiology remains obscure and, irrespective of the study, it is difficult to discern the cause of hyperthyroidism from its effects in diseased cats. Graves' disease is the most common form of hyperthyroidism encountered in humans. In this disease, autoantibodies are produced which bind to the thyrotropin (thyroid-stimulating hormone (TSH)) receptor, mimicking its activity. However, similar stimulating antibodies have not been identified in hyperthyroid cats and there is agreement that the feline condition is distinct from Graves' disease. Histopathologically, the feline disorder most closely resembles toxic nodular goitre (Plummer's disease), the second most common cause of hyperthyroidism in humans. Indeed, the feline condition offers a unique animal model for the study of toxic nodular goitre in humans. Similar to affected human tissue, adenomatous thyroid tissue from hyperthyroid cats retains its histopathological appearance and continues to grow and function in host mice and when cultured in TSH-free media. There are a variety of known and suggested causes of toxic nodular goitre in humans, including mutations of the TSH receptor and its G-protein alpha subunit leading to constitutive activation and excess thyroid hormone production. None has been convincingly documented in hyperthyroid cats.

Several epidemiological studies have identified potential risk factors for the disease, but a single dominant factor has not yet been detected. Several breeds, including Siamese, Himalayan, Persian and Burmese, and purebred cats overall have been reported to be at decreased risk of developing hyperthyroidism. Although there have been some inconsistencies across studies, sex and neutering are not associated with the development of hyperthyroidism.

Numerous environmental factors have been associated with an increased risk of hyperthyroidism, such as the use of cat litter and regular use of parasiticides, but the most commonly identified factor is the consumption of a diet composed entirely, or almost entirely, of canned cat food. In addition, certain varieties of canned cat food (fish or liver and giblet flavour) and cans with plastic linings and easy-open 'pop-top' lids have been implicated. Due to this dietary association, iodine intake has been linked to the pathogenesis of the disease. The iodine content of commercial cat food has been reported as being extremely variable and can be excessive or potentially deficient compared with recommended allowances. It has been postulated that wide swings in daily iodine intake may contribute to the development of thyroid disease. Selenium also plays an important role in the regulation of thyroid function in many species and, although the significance is unclear, circulating values appear to be high in cats, possibly through increased intake. There are many other agents (goitrogens and endocrine disrupters) that cats may be exposed to through food and its packaging or in the environment. These may be of particular importance in cats because of differences in metabolism, particularly in light of their inherently slower glucuronidation pathway. The potentially goitrogenic soy isoflavones, genistein and daidzein, are common constituents of commercially available cat foods and may be present in concentrations sufficiently high to exert some biological effect. The polyphenolic compound bisphenol A, which is used as a plasticizer in can linings, can act as a thyroid disruptor. High concentrations of polybrominated diphenyl ethers (PBDEs), also known as thyroid disruptors, have been demonstrated in cats. These are used as fire retardants and are potentially released as house dust that cats could consume during their normal grooming behaviour.

Given the variety of abnormalities and associations described, it is likely that hyperthyroidism is a multifactorial disease. Significantly, the same risk factors appear to exist in areas where hyperthyroidism is considered relatively uncommon, emphasizing the complexity of the pathogenesis of hyperthyroidism.

Clinical features

Signalment

Hyperthyroidism is a disease of middle-aged and older cats, with an average age at onset of 12–13 years. Virtually all affected cats are over 6 years of age, but only 5% are younger than 10 years old at the time of diagnosis. There has been one report of hyperthyroidism in a kitten but, given that the histopathological appearance was different, it likely represents a distinct disease entity. Hyperthyroidism can affect any sex and breed, although some purebred cats are less likely to develop the condition (see 'Aetiology', above).

Clinical signs

Thyroid hormones are responsible for a variety of actions, including the regulation of heat production and the metabolism of carbohydrates, proteins and lipids. They interact with the central nervous system by increasing overall sympathetic drive. Thyroid hormones also alter cardiovascular function both directly and indirectly. Consequently, when thyroid hormones are in excess, virtually every organ system is affected. Most cats present with a variety of clinical signs, reflecting multiple organ dysfunction, although in some cats one clinical sign may predominate. The signs vary from mild to severe, depending on the duration of the condition, the magnitude of increase in thyroid hormone production, the ability of the cat to cope with thyroid hormone excess, and the presence or absence of concomitant abnormalities in other organ systems. The disease is insidiously progressive and the signs, when mild, may be considered by owners as part of the generalized ageing process. For this reason, several months may elapse before veterinary attention is sought.

Overall, there are a number of clinical signs that are associated with hyperthyroidism, including: weight loss despite a normal or increased appetite, hyperactivity,

intermittent gastrointestinal signs such as vomiting or diarrhoea, tachycardia, cardiac murmur, palpable goitre, polyuria and polydipsia, and even congestive cardiac failure. However, the presence or absence of any one particular sign cannot confirm or exclude the disorder. In addition, because of the variety of signs that are potentially caused by hyperthyroidism, it is an important differential for many presenting complaints in older cats.

Increased awareness of the condition and earlier diagnosis have meant that, although any of the above clinical signs are possible, affected cats show fewer clinical signs than previously, and those shown are of lesser severity. Occasionally, a diagnosis is made before owners fully realize that their pet is ill. Up to 25% of cases are diagnosed incidentally either during a routine check or in the investigation of another disorder (Watson et al., 2018). The possible historical and clinical features are outlined in Figure 19.1.

Common features
• Weight loss
• Polyphagia
• Tachycardia
• Systolic heart murmurs
• Hyperactivity/irritability
• Intermittent gastrointestinal signs (vomiting or diarrhoea)
• Palpable goitre

Other features
• Polyuria and polydipsia
• Respiratory abnormalities (tachypnoea, panting)
• Other cardiac abnormalities (gallop rhythm, arrhythmias)
• Skin lesions (patchy or regional alopecia, unkempt coat)
• Moderate increase in temperature

Uncommon features
• Decreased activity
• Decreased appetite
• Congestive cardiac failure
• Hypertension
• Ventral neck flexion

19.1 Historical and clinical features of hyperthyroidism in cats.

General features

Almost all affected cats exhibit signs of mild to severe weight loss (Figure 19.2a) despite a normal or increased appetite, reflecting an overall increase in the metabolic rate. This increase in metabolic rate may be accompanied by a mild increase in body temperature or occasionally heat intolerance. The weight loss is reflective of both muscle and fat loss. The former appears to be more profound than the latter and it is not unusual now to diagnose hyperthyroidism in cats with a normal or increased body condition score (Peterson et al., 2016b). Routine recording of weight in older cats is advantageous, as subtle weight loss without any other obvious signs may be the first overt indication of the development of hyperthyroidism. In many cats, weight loss is the only clinical sign noted by owners.

If hyperthyroidism is allowed to progress untreated, more pronounced muscle wasting, fatigability, emaciation and cachexia will ultimately result, although this can take months to years. Severe muscle weakness, as demonstrated by ventroflexion of the neck, has been described, albeit rarely, and presumably relates to hyperthyroidism-induced hypokalaemia (see 'Biochemistry', below). A few affected cats exhibit intermittent periods of anorexia alternating with periods of normal or increased appetite, but this is often associated with concurrent non-thyroidal

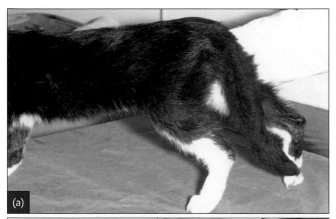

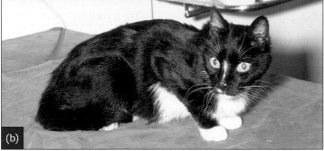

19.2 A hyperthyroid 11-year-old Domestic Shorthaired cat showing evidence of (a) weight loss and muscle atrophy and (b) an anxious facial expression.
(Reproduced with permission from Thoday and Mooney, 1992)

illness (NTI) rather than hyperthyroidism *per se*. In the absence of concurrent illness, the mechanism is unclear.

Hyperactivity, exhibited particularly as nervousness, restlessness, irritability and aggressive behaviour, may be apparent. These signs may be more obvious when attempts are made to restrain the animal and are therefore often more noticeable to veterinary surgeons than to owners themselves.

In extreme cases, tremor may be apparent and affected cats are often described as having an anxious or frantic facial expression (Figure 19.2b). There is impaired tolerance to stress, and even moderately stressful events (e.g. physical examination) can result in a so-called hyperthyroid crisis that can be life-threatening. The signs include overt respiratory distress, severe tachycardia, cardiac arrhythmias, dyspnoea and eventually extreme weakness. Hyperthyroid cats should therefore be handled appropriately in the practice environment.

Aimless pacing, vocalization and easily interrupted sleep patterns have been described, and this presumably reflects a state of confusion, anxiety and nervousness. Focal or generalized seizures characteristic of epilepsy have been described, albeit rarely. In such cases, there is a reduction in the severity of the seizures, or complete resolution, after treatment of the hyperthyroidism.

Polyuria and polydipsia

Polyuria and polydipsia occur in approximately one third of affected cases and can be marked in individual cats. Various mechanisms may be responsible, including concurrent chronic kidney disease (CKD) (not unexpected in a group of aged cats), decreased renal medullary solute concentration due to increased renal blood flow, electrolyte abnormalities (e.g. hypokalaemia), and primary polydipsia due to a hypothalamic disturbance associated with thyroid hormone excess.

Skin and coat changes

In older case series, skin and coat changes were common but were usually less of an owner concern than the metabolic changes described. Some cats presented with unkempt matted hair (Figure 19.3a), presumably because of a failure to groom. Longhaired cats particularly presented with alopecia (Figure 19.3b) (either bilaterally symmetrical or patchy), presumably resulting from excessive grooming. The latter has been suggested to reflect heat intolerance. Excessive nail growth with increased fragility has been described but is seen less frequently today.

Gastrointestinal features

Gastrointestinal signs are not uncommon and usually include intermittent vomiting and, less commonly, diarrhoea. Vomiting may result from a direct action of thyroid hormones on the chemoreceptor trigger zone or from gastric stasis. It appears to be more common in cats from multi-cat households and usually occurs shortly after feeding, indicating that it may simply be related to rapid overeating. In humans, rapid gastrointestinal transit contributes to the increased frequency of defecation and diarrhoea. In addition, malabsorption and steatorrhoea may result from excess fat intake associated with polyphagia, rapid gastric emptying and intestinal transit and/or a reversible reduction in pancreatic trypsin secretion. In cats, many of these mechanisms have not been fully investigated. However, orocaecal transit time appears to be accelerated in hyperthyroid cats compared with both healthy cats and those successfully treated for hyperthyroidism.

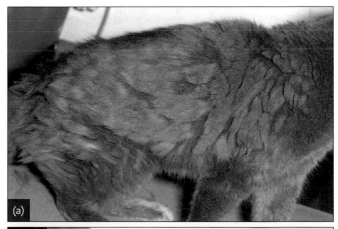

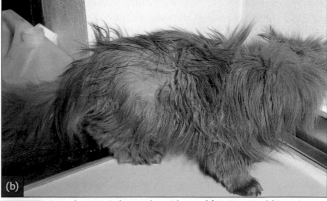

19.3 Coat changes in hyperthyroid cats. (a) A 13-year-old Russian Blue cat with extensive matting. (b) A 14-year-old pedigree cat with evidence of alopecia.

Cardiorespiratory features

Cardiovascular signs are common and are frequently the most significant findings on initial physical examination. Tachycardia (often with a heart rate >240 beats per minute) is documented in up to 50% of cases. A powerful apex beat and systolic murmurs are also commonly encountered. Such murmurs are generally grade I–III (of VI) and vary in intensity with the heart rate. They are frequently associated with dynamic right and left ventricular outflow obstruction, rather than primary mitral or tricuspid regurgitation as previously thought. Hyperthyroidism is probably the single most important factor for the development of murmurs in older cats. Gallop rhythms attributed to rapid ventricular filling can also occur. Arrhythmias, particularly ectopic atrial and ventricular arrhythmias, have also been noted on occasion.

These cardiac abnormalities are related to direct effects of thyroid hormones on cardiac muscle, indirect effects mediated through the interaction of thyroid hormones with the adrenergic nervous system, and cardiac changes that attempt to compensate for altered peripheral tissue perfusion. These effects result in a high cardiac output state and, consequently, cardiac hypertrophy and chamber dilatation. Congestive cardiac failure associated with pleural effusion and/or pulmonary oedema (coughing, dyspnoea, muffled heart sounds, ascites) can develop, although this is uncommon and generally only associated with severe hyperthyroidism. Usually, the cardiomyopathy associated with hyperthyroidism is reversible. Almost 50% of hyperthyroid cats have detectable circulating troponin I concentrations, which reduce after induction of euthyroidism, consistent with hyperthyroid-induced but reversible myocyte damage. However, in some cats, cardiomyopathy persists or worsens after treatment, suggesting a pre-existing cardiac defect or, more rarely, irreversible thyroid-hormone-related structural damage. Certainly, in cats that develop congestive cardiac failure, maintenance of treatment for their cardiac disease is required even with successful resolution of the hyperthyroidism.

Mild to moderate hypertension, reversible upon induction of euthyroidism, was originally considered important in hyperthyroid cats. However, it is now clear that hyperthyroid cats are typically only mildly hypertensive, if at all, and it may simply reflect the reduced tolerance of hyperthyroid cats to stressful situations such as veterinary examination ('white-coat syndrome' or situational hypertension). In accordance with this, hypertension-associated blindness and obvious ocular abnormalities are uncommon in hyperthyroid cats, even in the presence of documented hypertension. Although hyperthyroidism is associated with increased cardiac output, there is a decrease in systemic vascular resistance that mitigates against the development of significant hypertension. If moderate to severe hypertension and its target organ effects are demonstrated in a hyperthyroid cat, other potential causes such as CKD should be considered. Interestingly, some cats appear to develop hypertension after successful treatment of hyperthyroidism and this may result, at least in part, from the increase in systemic vascular resistance as thyroid hormone concentrations decrease, or from the associated decline in kidney function (see Chapter 6).

Respiratory abnormalities, chiefly tachypnoea, panting and dyspnoea at rest, are also common but tend to occur most frequently during periods of stress. In the absence of cardiac failure, respiratory muscle weakness due to chronic thyrotoxic myopathy (or even hypokalaemia) and decreased compliance of the lungs are the most likely explanations.

Apathetic hyperthyroidism

Cats may present with apathy or depression and anorexia rather than hyperactivity and polyphagia. Similarly affected human patients usually have severe cardiac complications induced by thyroid hormone excess. In cats, apathetic hyperthyroidism has also been associated with congestive cardiac failure. However, concurrent severe NTIs such as CKD or neoplasia may also be complicating factors. In cats presenting as apathetic, it is important that other illnesses are investigated as they may alter the therapeutic choice or eventual prognosis. While apathetic hyperthyroidism was previously recorded in approximately 10% of cases, this is less commonly seen today, presumably as hyperthyroidism is diagnosed earlier.

Palpable goitre

In healthy cats, the thyroid gland is divided into two distinct lobes positioned on either side just below the cricoid cartilage and extending ventrally for the first five or six tracheal rings. Thyroid lobes are not normally palpable. In hyperthyroid cats, either unilateral or bilateral thyroid enlargement (goitre) is almost always present (>90% of cases). Thyroid lobes are loosely attached to the surrounding tissues and tend to migrate ventrally as they enlarge, occasionally moving through the thoracic inlet into the anterior mediastinum. Ectopic thyroid tissue located anywhere from the base of the tongue to the base of the heart is occasionally (<4% of cases) involved in the pathogenesis of the condition. However, very few of these cases (<1%) have ectopic involvement alone (Peterson and Broome, 2015).

Sometimes goitre is visible, but more commonly palpation is required. Traditionally, to palpate for goitre the cat is placed in a sitting position with its head and neck facing the clinician:

- With the neck gently extended, the thumb and forefinger are placed on either side of the trachea and swept carefully downwards from the larynx to the manubrium
- It is important to avoid hyperextension of the neck as the thyroid lobes may become embedded in muscle or deviated retrotracheally, and therefore become more difficult to palpate
- Goitre is usually felt as a mobile subcutaneous nodule or 'slip' that slides under the fingertips
- When there are difficulties in palpation, visualization of small nodules may be aided by clipping the ventro-cervical area and moistening the skin with alcohol.

An alternative thyroid palpation technique (often called the Norsworthy technique) has also been described:

- The clinician is positioned behind the standing cat and the cat's head is raised and turned (45 degrees from the horizontal and vertical) to the right or left, depending on which side is being assessed
- The tip of the clinician's index finger is placed in the groove formed by the trachea and the sternothyroideus muscle just below the larynx, and then moved ventrally down to the thoracic inlet, evaluating each side in turn
- Palpation of a mobile subcutaneous nodule or 'slip' that slides under the fingertips indicates the presence of goitre.

Which of the two techniques is used is dependent on clinician preference. The traditional technique probably has greater agreement within and between examiners and has the added advantage, in some cases, of being able to visualize the goitre and its movement when palpation is equivocal. Some cats may interpret the face-to-face contact of the traditional technique as threatening or intimidating, and this is avoided using the Norsworthy technique. The Norsworthy technique also has the advantage of depicting the side of involvement, especially in cats with large goitres crossing the midline. Whichever technique is chosen, experience is probably the most critical factor for success.

Increasing enlargement of the thyroid lobes is usually synonymous with greater production of thyroid hormones and a clinically more severely affected case. However, this is not always the case, and extreme thyroid enlargement can occur in cats with thyroid cysts and thyroid carcinomas that are not associated with severe hyperthyroidism. Large cysts may be fluctuant and carcinomas irregularly shaped and less mobile.

A failure to find goitre is possible in hyperthyroid cats. The goitre may be barely palpable or in some cases there may be migration of the enlarged thyroid lobes through the thoracic inlet or involvement of ectopic thyroid tissue.

Although the likelihood of hyperthyroidism increases if goitre is present, thyroid hyperfunction is not synonymous with its presence. A palpable mass in this area could potentially represent lymph node enlargement, parathyroid neoplasia/hyperplasia or, more rarely, non-functional thyroid carcinoma. In addition, goitre may also be palpable in an as yet euthyroid individual, with eventual development of hyperthyroidism possible as the thyroid nodule continues to grow and secrete excessive thyroid hormone. It is not known how many cats with an evident thyroid slip eventually go on to develop hyperthyroidism. However, they require regular re-examinations to assess thyroid function, at 6-monthly intervals, or sooner if clinical signs dictate.

Diagnosis

A variety of procedures have been recommended for investigation of hyperthyroidism. Often these simply lend support to the diagnosis, but they may be particularly useful if concurrent disorders are suspected and an accurate prognosis is required. Detailed diagnostic imaging techniques are usually only required in cats in which compromised cardiac function is suspected. Specific thyroid function tests are necessary to confirm a diagnosis.

Diagnostic imaging

Hyperthyroidism is associated with a largely reversible hypertrophic cardiomyopathy. In approximately 50% of cats, there is evidence of mild to severe cardiac enlargement on thoracic radiography. This is accompanied by evidence of pleural effusion and pulmonary oedema in rare cases with congestive cardiac failure; such cases usually have severe hyperthyroidism. The most common echocardiographic abnormalities described include left ventricular hypertrophy, left atrial and ventricular dilatation, interventricular septum hypertrophy and dynamic outflow tract obstruction. However, currently, most of these changes are subtle if present at all in hyperthyroid cats and are of questionable clinical relevance. Increased fractional shortening remains common and invariably decreases upon successful treatment of the hyperthyroidism.

Rarely, hyperthyroidism is associated with a dilated form of cardiomyopathy with echocardiographic evidence of reduced myocardial contractility and marked ventricular dilatation. This is usually accompanied by evidence of severe congestive cardiac failure and probably represents end-stage cardiac disease.

Other changes are not uncommon in hyperthyroid cats. There is a high prevalence of pulmonary abnormalities (bronchial and bronchointerstitial patterns) and skeletal changes (intervertebral disc disease and spondylosis). However, these are not clinically relevant and presumably relate to the more advanced age of the cat (Kormpou et al., 2020). Abdominal ultrasonography is generally unremarkable in hyperthyroid cats. However, given the age of affected cases, up to 25% may have evident change in their kidneys (Nussbaum et al., 2015). Other abnormalities usually indicate distinct concurrent disorders.

Electrocardiography

Sinus tachycardia and increased R-wave amplitude in lead II are considered the most frequent electrocardiographic abnormalities recorded in hyperthyroid cats. Less common abnormalities include prolonged QRS duration, shortened Q–T interval, right bundle branch block, intraventricular conduction disturbances and a variety of atrial and ventricular arrhythmias. The likelihood of these changes usually increases with severity of disease and they may not be present in mildly affected cases.

Routine clinicopathological features

A variety of haematological, biochemical and urinalysis abnormalities are possible in hyperthyroid cats. None is specific and some are clinically insignificant. Their presence may lend support to a diagnosis of hyperthyroidism. More importantly, routine clinicopathological assessment is used to investigate other potential differentials for the presenting complaints or to identify comorbidities that may have an impact on treatment decisions and prognosis.

Haematology

Haematological changes are of limited diagnostic value or clinical impact. Mild to moderate erythrocytosis (increased packed cell volume, red blood cell count and haemoglobin concentration) and macrocytosis have been described (Figure 19.4). These changes presumably reflect thyroid-hormone-mediated stimulation of erythroid marrow, as well as the increased production of erythropoietin resulting from increased oxygen consumption. These features have not been confirmed in all studies.

Anaemia is a rare complication of hyperthyroidism in humans and is related to either bone marrow exhaustion or deficiencies in iron or other micronutrients. It has not been well described in hyperthyroid cats and, if anaemia is present, concurrent NTI is likely. Although overt anaemia is rarely encountered, increased Heinz body formation does occur in hyperthyroid cats, and platelet size may be increased. Clinically, these abnormalities appear to have minimal effect.

Not surprisingly, a stress leucogram, as evidenced by mature neutrophilia usually accompanied by lymphopenia and eosinopenia, is common. Occasionally, lymphocytosis and eosinophilia are present; this is thought to relate to a relative lack of cortisol induced by thyroid hormone excess.

Abnormality	Prevalence	Relevance
Erythrocytosis and macrocytosis	0–50%	Usually mild and clinically insignificant
Leucocytosis, neutrophilia, lymphopenia, eosinopenia	Common	Stress response
Lymphocytosis and eosinophilia	Uncommon	May reflect a relative cortisol deficiency induced by hyperthyroidism
Increased liver enzyme activities	>90%	Severity of increase reflects that of total T4. May not be increased in early or mild hyperthyroidism
Hyperphosphataemia	Up to 40%	May occur with or without concurrent azotaemia
Ionized hypocalcaemia	Up to 50%	Mild and clinically insignificant
Mild to moderate azotaemia	2–10%	Pre-existing chronic kidney disease not unexpected in older cats
Increased SDMA concentration	10%	May be a better predictor of post-treatment chronic kidney disease
Hyperglycaemia	Occasional	Stress response, rarely exceeds renal threshold
Hypokalaemia	Rare	May be severe enough to cause clinical signs
Hypocobalaminaemia	10–40%	Not significant as methylmalonic acid concentrations not increased
Increased beta-hydroxybutyrate concentrations	20%	Reflects the catabolism associated with hyperthyroidism
Urine specific gravity	Variable	Urine specific gravity <1.035 may be associated with an increased risk of developing post-treatment chronic kidney disease
Proteinuria	Common	Usually mild

19.4 Common haematological, biochemical and urinalysis abnormalities associated with hyperthyroidism.
SDMA = symmetric dimethylarginine; T4 = thyroxine.

Biochemistry

Liver enzymes: Mild to marked increases in the serum activities of alanine aminotransferase (ALT), aspartate aminotransferase (AST), alkaline phosphatase (ALP), gamma glutamyl transferase (GGT) and lactate dehydrogenase (LDH) are the most common and striking biochemical abnormalities of feline hyperthyroidism (see Figure 19.4). It has been suggested that these abnormalities are caused by malnutrition, congestive heart failure, hepatic hypoxia, infections and direct toxic effects of thyroid hormones on the liver. However, histopathological examination of the liver usually reveals only modest and non-specific changes. In addition, there are no significant abnormalities found on hepatic ultrasonography, and tests of liver function (bile acid stimulation) remain within the reference interval. Circulating ammonia concentration may be mildly increased in hyperthyroid cats. However, this is without clinical consequence and presumably reflects increased metabolism, and protein catabolism and deamination.

Not all of the liver enzymes are liver specific. Both liver and bone contribute to the increase in serum ALP activity. The bone isoenzyme usually contributes 20–30% towards total ALP activity, but its contribution can be as high as 80% in some cases.

Approximately 90% of affected cats have an increase in at least one of the above liver enzyme activities. The degree of increase is correlated with serum thyroid hormone concentrations and can be dramatic in severely thyrotoxic cats. However, the increase tends to be subtle, if present at all, in early or mild cases of hyperthyroidism. Concurrent and distinct hepatobiliary disease should be suspected if there are marked increases in ALT, ALP, AST, GGT or LDH activities with only mildly increased serum thyroid hormone concentrations. Nevertheless, hyperthyroidism is the most common reason for the development of increased liver enzyme activities in older cats.

Urea and creatinine: Undoubtedly, the effect of hyperthyroidism and its treatment on kidney function in cats is of particular clinical concern, as treatment of hyperthyroidism is associated with a decline in kidney function. Before treatment, mild to moderate increases in serum concentrations of urea, creatinine and symmetric dimethylarginine (SDMA) may be found in up to 10% of hyperthyroid cats and likely represent pre-existing and concurrent CKD. However, the abnormalities, at least in urea concentration, could be exacerbated by the increased protein intake and protein catabolism of hyperthyroidism. On the other hand, in hyperthyroid cats without azotaemia, the circulating creatinine concentration is significantly lower than in age-matched controls. This may be related in part to a loss of muscle mass and increased glomerular filtration rate. These effects have implications in assessing the existence of CKD in hyperthyroid cats (see Chapter 6).

Phosphate and calcium: Increased phosphate concentration without evidence of azotaemia occurs in up to 40% of hyperthyroid cats. In hyperthyroid humans, there is increased bone metabolism attributed to the direct effects of thyroid hormones on bone, which can lead to osteopenia and pathological fractures. This is associated with increased serum activity of the bone isoenzyme of ALP, increased concentrations of osteocalcin and phosphate, and a tendency towards increased serum calcium and decreased parathyroid hormone (PTH) and 1,25-dihydroxycholecalciferol (calcitriol, active vitamin D) concentrations.

In hyperthyroid cats, serum total calcium concentration is largely unaffected, but ionized calcium is mildly decreased in approximately 50% of cases and circulating PTH concentration is increased in 75% of cases. In addition, increased markers of bone turnover (osteocalcin, deoxypyridinoline, carboxyterminal propeptide of type 1 collagen, cross-linked carboxyterminal collagen telopeptide) and non-suppressed 1,25-dihydroxycholecalciferol concentrations have been found in a small number of hyperthyroid cats. The reasons for the differences between humans and cats, and the exact aetiology of the changes, are unclear. The combination of ionized hypocalcaemia and hyperphosphataemia can occur in CKD, but not all hyperthyroid cats with these changes have evidence of CKD or go on to develop CKD after induction of euthyroidism. Increased bone turnover could be responsible for hyperphosphataemia but would also likely result in hypercalcaemia. There may be a direct effect of thyroid hormones on increasing renal resorption of phosphate, inducing hypocalcaemia and stimulating PTH secretion.

The clinical consequences of hyperphosphataemia, ionized hypocalcaemia and hyperparathyroidism are unknown. There may be implications for skeletal integrity and kidney function. The increased secretion of PTH necessary to maintain ionized calcium at the low end of or below the reference interval might contribute to or exacerbate the hypocalcaemia often encountered after surgical thyroidectomy (see 'Postoperative complications', below). However, the ionized hypocalcaemia noted with hyperthyroidism is not severe enough to cause overt clinical signs.

Other biochemical changes: A number of other clinicopathological changes have been described in hyperthyroid cats but are either clinically insignificant or rarely encountered. Blood glucose concentrations are rarely affected, but nevertheless can be increased, reflecting a stress response. In cases with pre-existing diabetes mellitus, accelerated insulin catabolism increases requirements for exogenous insulin. In addition, the circulating fructosamine concentration is significantly lower in hyperthyroid cats compared with healthy cats, probably as a result of increased protein turnover. Caution is advised when using fructosamine as a means of monitoring diabetic cats with concurrent hyperthyroidism, especially when assessing for diabetic remission. Serum beta-hydroxybutyrate concentration is increased in approximately 20% of hyperthyroid cats. Thus, its increase cannot be used to support a diagnosis of diabetes mellitus in a hyperthyroid cat with hyperglycaemia. Hypokalaemia has occasionally been associated with hyperthyroidism and should be suspected in any cat with evidence of severe muscle weakness. Although once considered an important cause of hypocobalaminaemia, methylmalonic acid concentrations are not usually high in hyperthyroid cats and cobalamin supplementation is therefore not required (Geesaman *et al.*, 2016). Nevertheless, persistent hypocobalaminaemia in a euthyroid individual may require intervention as it may represent concurrent gastrointestinal disease. Other biochemical parameters such as cholesterol, sodium, chloride, bilirubin, ionized and total magnesium, albumin and globulin tend to remain within their respective reference intervals in hyperthyroid cats.

Urinalysis

Urinalysis is generally unremarkable but is useful in differentiating hyperthyroidism from other diseases with similar clinical signs, such as diabetes mellitus. Urine specific gravity is variable, ranging from dilute to concentrated. A urine specific gravity below 1.035 may help predict the development of CKD after induction of euthyroidism with reasonable sensitivity but poor specificity. Mild proteinuria is commonly observed and may reflect glomerular hypertension and hyperfiltration or differences in tubular handling of protein. Traces of ketones in the absence of glucosuria may be found. Urinary tract infections were once thought to occur in at least 12% of non-azotaemic hyperthyroid cats, with no recognizable risk factors and often without classic signs of lower urinary tract disease or urinalysis changes indicating infection. As a consequence, urine culture was considered to be indicated in hyperthyroid cats. More recently, it has been shown that hyperthyroid cats show a low prevalence of subclinical bacteriuria (<5%) that is no higher than in the general cat population. Urine culture should therefore only be performed in cats with lower urinary tract signs (Peterson *et al.*, 2020b).

Thyroid function tests

The diagnosis of hyperthyroidism is confirmed by demonstrating increased thyroidal radioisotope uptake or increased production of the thyroid hormones.

In cats, as in dogs (see Chapter 18), T4 is the main secretory product of the thyroid gland. Triiodothyronine is three to five times more potent than T4, but approximately 60% of circulating T3 is produced by extrathyroidal 5'-deiodination of T4. Over 99% of circulating T4 is protein bound, while approximately 0.1% is free and metabolically active. Overall, control of thyroid hormone production is provided by a negative feedback mechanism of circulating T4 and T3 on thyrotropin-releasing hormone (TRH) from the hypothalamus and TSH from the anterior pituitary. In hyperthyroid cats, there is autonomous and excessive secretion of thyroid hormones from the abnormally functioning thyroid gland.

Thyroidal radioisotope uptake

Hyperthyroid cats usually exhibit increased thyroidal uptake of both radioactive iodine (^{123}I or ^{131}I) and technetium-99m as pertechnetate ($^{99m}TcO_4^-$). Usually, the latter is preferred because of its short half-life and imaging time, relative inexpense, low radiation dose and consistent image quality. Percentage uptake, thyroid–background ratio or thyroid–salivary ratio may be calculated. Increased values are found in over 98% of hyperthyroid cats and are strongly correlated with circulating thyroid hormone concentration. Overall, calculation of the thyroid–salivary ratio is considered to be the most accurate diagnostic test, although quantitative percentage uptake better predicts functional volume and metabolic activity (Peterson *et al.*, 2016c).

Thyroid scintigraphy is considered to be the most sensitive and specific diagnostic test for hyperthyroidism. However, apart from the expense and difficulties in dealing with radioisotopes, few clinicians have access to such equipment. In addition, caution is advised in interpreting results from cats previously treated with antithyroid drugs, as radioisotope uptake can be enhanced for several weeks after drug withdrawal. Qualitative thyroid imaging may be useful in assessment of thyroid involvement prior to surgical thyroidectomy (see 'Surgical thyroidectomy', below).

Thyroid hormone concentrations

Total and free T4 concentrations, with or without measurements of TSH, are most commonly used for diagnosing hyperthyroidism in cats. A summary of how these hormones are interpreted in different situations is provided in Figure 19.5. A flow diagram outlining their use is provided in Figure 19.6.

Thyroid status	Total T4	Free T4	TSH
Euthyroidism			
Healthy	↔	↔	D/U
NTI	↔↓	↔↓↑	D/U
Hyperthyroidism			
Subclinical	↔	↔	D/U
Mild	↔↑	↔↑	D/U
Mild to moderate with NTI	↔↑	↑	U
Moderate to severe	↑	↑	U
Moderate to severe with NTI	↑	↑	U

19.5 Thyroid hormone concentrations in healthy cats, those with non-thyroidal illness (NTI) and those with hyperthyroidism stratified by severity of disease and presence or absence of concurrent NTI. D = detectable; T4 = thyroxine; TSH = thyroid-stimulating hormone; U = undetectable; ↔ = within reference interval; ↓ = decreased; ↑ = increased.

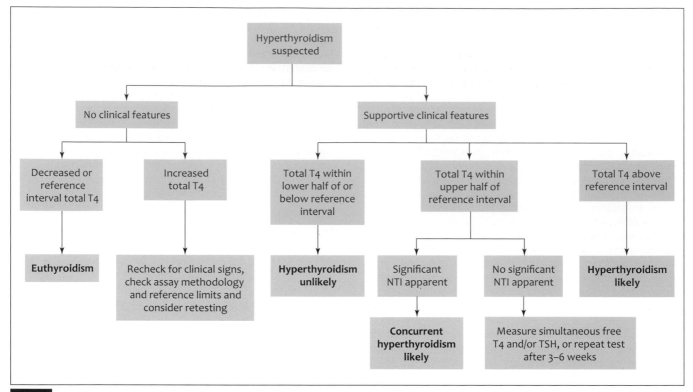

19.6 Diagnostic algorithm for investigating hyperthyroidism in cats. NTI = non-thyroidal illness; T4 = thyroxine; TSH = thyroid-stimulating hormone.

Total T4 concentration: Increased circulating total T4 concentration is considered to be the biochemical hallmark of hyperthyroidism and highly specific for its diagnosis, with few false-positive results reported. Methods for its measurement are readily accessible, relatively cheap and do not involve specific sample-handling requirements. Total T3 measurement is a less sensitive diagnostic test and is not routinely used in the investigation of hyperthyroidism.

There are several different methodologies that can be used to measure total T4 concentrations. Liquid chromatography–tandem mass spectrometry (LC–MS/MS) is rarely available commercially. Of the other methods, radioimmunoassay (RIA) is considered the gold standard method for measuring total T4 but is increasingly being replaced by non-isotopic automated and in-house techniques. Anecdotally at least, non-isotopic and especially in-house methods are responsible for the less-than-perfect specificity of total T4 measurements for diagnosing hyperthyroidism. Assays intended for measurement of total T4 in human serum are acceptable but must be fully validated for use with cat serum and, as for dogs, modified to allow for measurement of the lower circulating concentrations of hormone in this species. With few exceptions, total T4 is relatively constant across assay methodologies but under- and overestimation can occur in comparison studies. To account for any potential differences, technique- and laboratory-specific reference intervals should always be used. Reference intervals generally vary between 10 and 20 nmol/l at the lower limit and 45 and 60 nmol/l at the upper limit.

Most hyperthyroid cats (approximately 90%) exhibit an increased circulating total T4 concentration. While values up to approximately 20 times the upper limit of the reference interval have been reported, less dramatic increases are more common in the less affected hyperthyroid cats seen today. Over 50% of cases have total T4 values less than approximately 100 nmol/l and approximately 10% have reference interval total T4 concentrations. This corresponds to 20–40% of cases classified as having mild disease (Peterson *et al*., 2015). When within the reference interval, concentrations are usually within the mid to high end.

In mildly affected cases, serum total T4 concentrations can randomly fluctuate from above to within the reference interval. Non-specific fluctuation of thyroid hormones occurs in all hyperthyroid cats, but the degree of fluctuation is of little diagnostic significance in cats with pre-existing markedly increased hormone concentrations. Fluctuation and mild disease account for the majority (>80%) of cases with reference interval total T4 concentrations.

Moderate to severe NTI is also capable of significantly suppressing serum total T4 concentrations to the low end or below the reference interval in euthyroid cats and can be used as a prognostic indicator (Peterson *et al*., 2020a). Similarly, marginally increased serum total T4 concentrations may be suppressed to within the mid to high end of the reference interval in cats with concurrent mild hyperthyroidism and moderate to severe NTI. Occasionally, serum total T4 concentrations are suppressed to the lower half of the reference interval in hyperthyroid cats that are extremely ill. In such cases, the concurrent illness dictates the prognosis, and the existence of hyperthyroidism is of lesser clinical significance. Approximately 20% of hyperthyroid cats with reference interval circulating total T4 concentrations have an identifiable concurrent NTI.

In conclusion, while an increased total T4 value is usually indicative of hyperthyroidism, finding a single reference interval value does not preclude such a diagnosis. In older cats particularly, high-end reference interval values are highly suspicious for hyperthyroidism and such cases require regular re-evaluation (Lottati *et al*., 2019). In early or mild hyperthyroidism, serum total T4 concentrations will eventually increase into the diagnostic thyrotoxic range upon retesting 3–6 weeks later. However, in some cats a longer time is required, and it may be justifiable to wait until more overt clinical signs develop. Alternatively, other diagnostic tests may provide a means of diagnosing hyperthyroidism in these cats. Concurrent hyperthyroidism should always be suspected in severely ill cats with mid to high reference interval serum total T4 concentrations.

Finding an increased total T4 concentration in a euthyroid cat is unusual but occasionally occurs. Anecdotally, such results are more a feature of non-isotopic and particularly in-house methodologies (Peterson, 2013). A small number of healthy cats may consistently have total T4 concentrations that hover around the upper limit of the reference interval, representing normal population variation. Many commercial laboratories have decreased the upper limit of the total T4 reference interval to account for the lower total T4 values associated with ageing. Whilst this increases the sensitivity of total T4 measurement for diagnosing hyperthyroidism, it adversely affects specificity and potentially increases the number of false-positive diagnoses. Given that treatment is not without side effects and has a significant cost, loss of diagnostic specificity is undesirable. If an unexpected high total T4 value is found in a cat with few supportive signs of hyperthyroidism, it may be worthwhile repeating the test using a different assay methodology or diagnostic test (see below). If a repeat total T4 is persistently increased, the cat should be carefully re-examined for clinical features of hyperthyroidism, particularly the presence of goitre.

Free T4 concentration: In humans, measurement of free T4 is considered a more sensitive diagnostic test than total T4. Absolute free T4 concentrations are similar in humans and cats; therefore, when used, human assays do not require modification for cats. However, apart from LC–MS/MS, free T4 concentrations are only truly measured by techniques that involve the separation of free from bound hormone using equilibrium dialysis or ultrafiltration followed by ultrasensitive RIA. Controversy surrounds the validity of other non-isotopic methods that do not involve a separation step, particularly those involving analogues, for accurately measuring free T4 concentrations. If analogue free T4 concentrations are measured they rarely (approximately 5% of the time) provide any additional diagnostic information over total T4 concentrations alone (Rasmussen et al., 2014). The requirement for a separation step followed by RIA means that free T4 measurement is expensive and is not offered by all commercial laboratories. Free T4 is less stable than total T4 and inappropriate sample handling could falsely increase measured values (see Chapter 3). Reference intervals generally vary between 7.5 and 10.0 pmol/l at the lower limit and 40 and 50 pmol/l at the upper limit.

Free T4 concentrations are more consistently increased than total T4 in hyperthyroid cats (>98% of cases; Peterson et al., 2015). Importantly, free T4 concentrations are increased in the majority (>95%) of hyperthyroid cats that have reference interval total T4 values resulting from mild disease or the suppressive effect of concurrent NTI.

Although measurement of free T4 concentration is the most sensitive diagnostic test for hyperthyroidism, it is not recommended as a routine replacement for total T4 estimation. Apart from the limitations mentioned above, it has a considerably lower diagnostic specificity compared with total T4. Between 10% and 30% of euthyroid cats with NTI have increased circulating free T4 concentrations; these cats generally have corresponding total T4 values in the lower half of or below the reference interval. Caution is therefore advised in using serum free T4 measurements by equilibrium dialysis as the sole diagnostic test for

hyperthyroidism. Free T4 is more reliable if interpreted with a corresponding total T4 measurement. A mid to high reference interval total T4 with increased free T4 concentration is consistent with hyperthyroidism, whereas a low total and increased free T4 concentration is usually associated with NTI.

In hyperthyroid cats with an increased serum total T4 concentration, the free T4 concentration is concurrently high and its measurement adds no further diagnostic information. Given the high prevalence of increased total T4 values in hyperthyroid cats, it is more cost effective to initially measure total T4 concentration alone. If a diagnosis is not confirmed, consideration can be given to measurement of the corresponding free T4 concentration.

TSH concentration: In humans, measurement of circulating TSH concentration is usually used as a first-line discriminatory test of thyroid function. Hyperthyroidism can be indirectly assessed by detecting suppression of circulating TSH concentrations. However, TSH is species specific. There is greater similarity between feline and canine TSH than between feline and human TSH. Thus, there has been increasing interest in using the canine TSH (cTSH) assay for supporting a diagnosis of hyperthyroidism in cats. The limitations of this assay for cats should be recognized. Firstly, the canine assay only measures approximately 35% of recombinant feline TSH compared with 75% for cTSH (Rayalam et al., 2006). There is a much lower upper limit for the reference interval (approximately 0.30–0.32 ng/ml) in cats compared with dogs. Secondly, it is already well known that the canine assay is incapable of distinguishing low from normal values and there is no lower limit for the canine reference interval. This is problematic for a disease such as hyperthyroidism where suppressed values are expected. The lowest concentration that can be reliably measured is usually 0.03 ng/ml; results are therefore usually reported as detectable (≥0.03 ng/ml) or undetectable (<0.03 ng/ml).

The vast majority of hyperthyroid cats have undetectable TSH concentrations and diagnostic sensitivity is approximately 98% (Peterson et al., 2015). However, diagnostic specificity is poor at approximately 70%. Suppression of TSH is a known consequence of NTI in humans, and suppressed values in cats are more commonly seen with greater disease severity (Peterson et al., 2020a). Indeed, finding undetectable TSH together with low total T4 concentrations is predictive of poor short-term survival in cats with NTI. However, undetectable values also occur in approximately 25% of healthy cats, and this presumably reflects that the true lower limit of the reference interval is somewhere below 0.03 ng/ml but not accurately quantifiable using the current assays. Alone, an undetectable TSH concentration cannot be used to confirm a diagnosis of hyperthyroidism. However, such a value in combination with a high-end reference interval total T4 or increased free T4 concentration lends weight to a diagnosis of hyperthyroidism, particularly if there are compatible clinical signs present.

For the most part, finding a detectable TSH concentration is more indicative of euthyroidism and helps rule out hyperthyroidism in the majority of cats in which it is demonstrated. The reason why a small proportion (<2%) of hyperthyroid cats maintain detectable TSH concentrations is unclear. It is more commonly associated with mild hyperthyroidism, suggesting that the disease has not yet completely suppressed TSH. Recent thiamazole therapy may also play a role, particularly if it was associated with oversuppression of thyroid hormone production.

In humans, measurement of TSH can provide evidence for the existence of subclinical hyperthyroidism long before overt disease develops. In such cases, TSH suppression is demonstrable but total and free T4 concentrations remain within their respective reference intervals. It has been suggested that euthyroid cats with undetectable TSH concentrations are more likely to have histopathological evidence of thyroid nodular hyperplasia or to develop hyperthyroidism in the short term than those with detectable TSH values. However, any need to detect subclinical hyperthyroidism in cats is unclear, as its treatment may lead to a greater prevalence of iatrogenic hypothyroidism. On balance, finding a detectable TSH concentration is more likely indicative of euthyroidism and that hyperthyroidism will not develop in the short term.

An assay optimized for measuring feline TSH has recently been developed but is not yet widely available or clearly evaluated (Wood *et al.*, 2020). This new assay purports to have a lower limit of quantification of 0.008 ng/ml, which could potentially aid in differentiating the low values expected in hyperthyroidism and significantly improve diagnostic specificity. Further studies are required to assess its diagnostic performance for hyperthyroidism in cats.

Further diagnostic tests

In the majority of hyperthyroid cats with reference interval total T4 concentrations, identification of concurrent disease, repeat total T4 analysis or simultaneous measurement of free T4 or TSH allows confirmation of the diagnosis. Further diagnostic tests are rarely required. However, dynamic thyroid function tests have been recommended in the past as helpful in confirming a diagnosis of hyperthyroidism. They should only be considered for cats with clinical signs suggestive of hyperthyroidism when repeated measurements of total T4 concentration remain within the reference interval or free T4 or TSH analysis is unavailable or diagnostically unhelpful. More detailed information on these tests is available elsewhere in most standard textbooks.

T3 suppression test: In healthy individuals, T3 has a suppressive effect on pituitary TSH secretion and subsequently on T4 production by the thyroid gland. In hyperthyroidism, because of autonomous production of thyroid hormones and chronic suppression of TSH, this suppressive effect is lost. Thus, serum total T4 concentrations show minimal or no decrease in hyperthyroid cats following exogenous T3 administration. Simultaneous measurement of serum total T3 concentrations is required to ensure compliant administration and adequate absorption of the drug, and thus avoid false-positive results. Generally, the test is most useful in ruling out hyperthyroidism rather than confirming its existence.

TSH response test: Due to its poor diagnostic performance, this test is considered by many as obsolete. Exogenous TSH is a potent stimulator of thyroid hormone secretion. However, serum total T4 concentration shows little or no increase following exogenous TSH administration in hyperthyroid cats. This is presumably because the thyroid gland of affected cats secretes thyroid hormones independently of TSH control or because T4 is already being produced at or near the maximal rate with limited reserve capacity. Cats with equivocally increased serum total T4 concentrations tend to exhibit results which are indistinguishable from those of healthy animals, and the test is no longer recommended for evaluating hyperthyroidism. In addition, bovine TSH is no longer available for parenteral administration and the use of recombinant human TSH is limited by its cost.

TRH response test: Thyrotropin-releasing hormone is less expensive and easier to obtain than TSH. Serum total T4 concentrations increase minimally after TRH administration in mildly hyperthyroid cats. Compared with the T3 suppression test, this test is quicker and avoids tablet administration. However, TRH is associated with transient adverse reactions such as salivation, vomiting, tachypnoea and defecation. In addition, results of the test are indistinguishable in euthyroid and hyperthyroid cats with concurrent NTI and total T4 concentrations within or below the reference interval.

Treatment

The treatment of hyperthyroidism is aimed at removing or destroying abnormally functioning thyroid tissue, inhibiting thyroid hormone synthesis and release, or ameliorating the effects of excess thyroid hormones on peripheral tissue. Surgical thyroidectomy or thyroid ablation using radioactive iodine remain the only reasonable curative options available. Intrathyroidal infusion of ethanol, whilst somewhat efficacious in inducing euthyroidism, is rather crude in comparison and is associated with a high prevalence of adverse reactions, such as transient dysphonia, Horner's syndrome, gagging and laryngeal paralysis. Medical management, using antithyroid drugs or dietary iodine restriction, is non-curative and because of this cannot be recommended as sole therapy for the rare cases of hyperfunctioning thyroid carcinoma. The major advantages and disadvantages of the main forms of therapy are outlined in Figure 19.7. Treatment is tailored to each individual cat considering the factors outlined in Figure 19.8.

Medical management

Chronic medical management is a practical treatment option for many cats and is often the initial choice for the majority of cats. It requires no special facilities and is readily available. There is a rapid return to euthyroidism, which may be desirable in severely affected cases. Anaesthesia is avoided, as are the peri- and postoperative complications associated with surgical thyroidectomy and the prolonged hospitalization often necessary after radioactive iodine administration. Potential development of iatrogenic hypothyroidism is easily addressed by decreasing the drug dose or dosing frequency. However, medical management is not curative, is highly dependent on adequate owner and cat compliance, and requires regular biochemical monitoring to ensure the efficacy of treatment. The underlying lesions within the thyroid gland are not addressed and thyroid tissue continues to grow and may become more resistant to medical management. Prolonged use of antithyroid drugs over a period of years increases the chances of suspected malignant transformation of thyroid tissue. Medical management is therefore optimal for cats of advanced age or for those with concurrent diseases that may alter prognosis, for when owners refuse either surgery or radioactive iodine, or when facilities for such treatments are not available.

Short-term medical management is necessary prior to surgical thyroidectomy to decrease the metabolic and cardiac complications associated with hyperthyroidism,

Therapy	Persistent/recurrent hyperthyroidism	Time to achieve euthyroidism	Hospitalization	Adverse reactions	Availability	Cost
Radioactive iodine therapy	Rare	Usually within 2 weeks	5 days to 4 weeks	Few	Limited	High, up front
Surgical thyroidectomy	Possible (especially if inappropriate technique used)	Prior treatment recommended	1–10 days (dependent on postoperative complications)	Hypoparathyroidism	Experienced surgeon required	Intermediate, up front
Long-term medical management	Common (dependent on owner/cat compliance)	3–15 days	Not required	Possible and include potential malignant transformation	Readily available	Can be significant if long term (cost of treatment and monitoring)

19.7 The advantages and disadvantages of the three different treatment modalities for hyperthyroidism in cats.

- Severity of clinical thyrotoxicosis
- Presence/absence of concurrent illness
- Age of cat
- Access to/waiting list for radioactive iodine therapy
- Availability of experienced surgeon
- Adequate post-thyroidectomy care facilities
- Owner/cat compliance for drug administration
- Potential complications
- Cost

19.8 Factors for consideration prior to selecting a treatment modality for hyperthyroidism in cats.

and may be desirable in providing symptomatic control if there is a prolonged wait for radioactive iodine therapy. Short-term medical management can be used as trial therapy to determine the effect of restoring euthyroidism on kidney function.

The commonly used drugs, their mode of action, formulation, dosage regimes, indications and contraindications are detailed in Figure 19.9.

Thiamazole and carbimazole

The two drugs thiamazole (methimazole) and carbimazole are recommended for both short- and long-term management of hyperthyroidism. They have a potent and consistently reliable effect in suppressing thyroid hormone production. A related drug, propylthiouracil, often used in human medicine, is not recommended for cats because of a high incidence of serious adverse reactions (immune-mediated haemolytic anaemia and thrombocytopenia).

Thiamazole is specifically authorized for treatment of feline hyperthyroidism, in both Europe and the USA, and is presented as 1.25, 2.5 and 5 mg tablets and a 5 mg/ml liquid formulation. It is available elsewhere as a drug for human use. After administration, thiamazole is actively concentrated by the thyroid gland, where it inhibits thyroid hormone synthesis but not iodide trapping or release of preformed hormone. Thiamazole has good oral bioavailability and a serum half-life of 4–6 hours. Despite this, the intrathyroidal residence time, where thiamazole exerts its effect, is likely to be up to 20 hours, as it is in humans.

Carbimazole is available for human use in many European countries and Japan. It exerts its antithyroid effect through immediate conversion to thiamazole when administered orally. Serum concentrations of thiamazole achieved after carbimazole administration are less than after a similar weight of thiamazole, such that a 5 mg dose of carbimazole is approximately equal to 3 mg of thiamazole. Carbimazole is often touted as having a lower prevalence of adverse reactions such as vomiting and anorexia. This may be because it is tasteless whereas thiamazole purportedly has a bitter taste. However, this is questionable given that the liquid thiamazole preparation is not known to have a greater prevalence of such adverse effects compared with tablets in cats.

Carbimazole, as a novel once-daily controlled-release formulation (10 or 15 mg tablets), is authorized for treatment of hyperthyroid cats in Europe. Pharmacokinetic studies of this controlled-release formulation have shown no pronounced concentration peak and a sustained presence of thiamazole in plasma (>24 hours) with a half-life of approximately 9 hours after oral administration. Based on relative bioavailability and conversion, it is estimated that 15 mg of this preparation is equivalent to approximately 7.5 mg of conventional thiamazole. It has been shown that administration of this drug with food significantly enhances its absorption. While it is not necessary to administer it in food, in order to avoid potential variation in doses absorbed, the time between feeding and treatment should be as constant as possible. The same can be applied to thiamazole.

The effect of prior thiamazole treatment on the eventual outcome of radioactive iodine therapy is controversial. It has been variably suggested to enhance, worsen or have

Drug	Mode of action	Formulation	Dosage per cat	Indications	Contraindications
Thiamazole	Inhibition of thyroid peroxidase-catalysed reactions	1.25, 2.5, 5 mg tablets 5 mg/ml solution	1.25–2.5 mg q12h decreasing to 1.25 mg q12h or 2.5–5 mg q24h	Prior to surgery Chronic management	Immediately prior to ^{131}I therapy Severe adverse reactions
Controlled-release carbimazole		10, 15 mg tablets	10–15 mg q24h decreasing to 10 mg q24h		
Propranolol*	Beta-1/beta-2 adrenoceptor blocking agent	10 mg tablets	2.5–5 mg q8h	Symptomatic control	Alone, prior to surgery Chronic management
Atenolol*	Beta-1 adrenoceptor blocking agent	25 mg tablets 5 mg/ml syrup	6.25–12.5 mg q12h or q24h		

19.9 Commonly used drugs for the medical management of feline hyperthyroidism. * = Can be used alone for short-term symptomatic control of hyperthyroidism.

no effect on radioiodine treatment. Although thiamazole does not inhibit thyroidal iodine uptake, concurrent administration adversely affects the effective half-life of radioactive iodine and is not recommended. Generally, drug withdrawal is suggested anywhere from 5 to 9 days prior to radioactive iodine therapy.

Dosage regimens: The initial recommended dose of thiamazole is 1.25, 2.5 or 5 mg administered orally every 12 hours depending on the severity of the thyrotoxicosis. Today, as the majority of cats have mild to moderate disease, 1.25 or 2.5 mg doses are most commonly used. Using the total dose once daily is possible but attainment of euthyroidism is less reliable and more prolonged. The starting dose for controlled-release carbimazole is 15 mg/cat q24h. In mild cases, a lower starting dose of 10 mg/cat q24h is recommended.

The length of time to achieve biochemical euthyroidism is relatively short – it usually occurs within a week of starting therapy. For practical purposes and in order to ensure a reasonable clinical effect, cats are usually reassessed after 10 days (controlled-release formulations) or 3 weeks (conventional tablets/liquid). A serum total T4 concentration is measured and, if it is within the low end or below the reference interval, thyroidectomy can be performed, with the last dose administered on the morning of surgery. For severely affected cats, even if biochemical euthyroidism is achieved, a longer course of preoperative therapy may be required before the animal is considered a reasonable surgical candidate. The dose is adjusted as for long-term maintenance. If euthyroidism has not been achieved, the dose of thiamazole or carbimazole can be altered in 1.25–5 mg increments, reassessing the cat as detailed below. Lack of owner or cat compliance should first be eliminated as a reason for a failure of therapy. Similarly, if hypothyroidism is noted, the drug dosage should be decreased.

For long-term management once euthyroidism has been achieved, the daily dosage is adjusted, aiming for the lowest possible dose that effectively maintains euthyroidism. Retesting after each dose adjustment is required as described below. Achieving the lowest possible dose is limited by the available tablet sizes if tablets are being used, as neither conventional nor controlled-release formulations should be broken or crushed. Although divided doses of thiamazole are most effective in rapidly inducing euthyroidism, long-term once-daily dosing is often efficacious. Most cats are maintained on 1.25 or 2.5 mg q12h, or 2.5 or 5 mg q24h. For controlled-release carbimazole, the majority (approximately 90%) of cats can be effectively maintained on doses of 10–20 mg/cat q24h. A few cases require lower doses (10 mg/cat every other day) and only rarely do cats require higher doses.

While antithyroid drugs are routinely administered orally, compliance can be problematic, particularly in fractious or inappetent cats or where owners feel daunted by administering oral medications to their animals. Drug absorption is also potentially affected by concurrent intestinal disease and there are obvious difficulties in cats that vomit. Carbimazole and thiamazole can be compounded in a pluronic lecithin organogel or lipophilic formulation for transdermal administration. This is a safe and effective method of controlling hyperthyroidism but there are some notable differences compared with oral administration. The bioavailability of thiamazole is significantly lower and the efficacy of 10 mg administered transdermally q24h is estimated as half that of 5 mg oral carbimazole q12h (Hill *et al.*, 2014). A failure to take this into account may delay

the time to attain euthyroidism, but both routes can be equally efficacious (Hill *et al.*, 2011). Whatever formulation is used, it is applied in a thin layer to the non-haired portion of the pinnae, using a concentration approximating 5 mg/0.1 ml, which prevents excess vehicle build-up. It remains unclear whether there is sustained dermal absorption, or gastrointestinal absorption after oral ingestion through licking and grooming, although this is largely irrelevant to the outcome. Whilst transdermal products are undoubtedly an option for treating hyperthyroidism, none is specifically authorized for use in cats in Europe. Custom formulation increases the expense of therapy, and stability of the product is not guaranteed. Most importantly, handlers and other cats in the household are at increased risk of exposure to thiamazole if it is administered via this route, and owners must be appropriately advised on and understand the necessary precautions to take. Thiamazole is a suspected human teratogen, and pregnant women should only handle this drug and the treated cat's litter when using gloves, whether using tablets or transdermal preparations.

Monitoring strategies: Cats should be re-examined 10 days to 3 weeks after commencing therapy or after each dose adjustment and, once stability has been attained, every 3–6 months thereafter or as indicated clinically. Assessment of clinical signs is important in monitoring response to therapy. Demonstrable weight gain, reduction in appetite, resolution of tachycardia and a decrease in the grade or intensity of cardiac murmurs (if present initially) are all expected with successful treatment. Measurement of a serum total T4 concentration is usually indicated. The time of sampling in relation to dosing is not important, irrespective of the frequency of dosing. The aim is to maintain total T4 concentrations within the lower half of the reference interval, ensuring that free T4 concentrations remain within their reference interval (Daminet *et al.*, 2014). Treatment of hyperthyroidism can result in unmasking of kidney disease and induction of both overt and subclinical hypothyroidism (see below and Chapters 6 and 21). As a consequence, measurement of corresponding TSH and kidney function is also indicated. Ongoing regular assessment of hyperthyroid cats is necessary. Antithyroid medication has no effect on the underlying lesion and the thyroid nodules continue to grow and can enlarge, necessitating an increased dosage in the long term.

Increased serum activities of ALT and ALP decline progressively as euthyroidism is achieved (Figure 19.10). Although their measurement can be used as a nonspecific indicator of therapeutic efficacy, caution is advised. In some cats with concurrent hepatopathies, serum activities of these enzymes may not decline and without simultaneous measurement of total T4, an erroneous diagnosis of poor therapeutic efficacy may be made.

Adverse reactions: Most clinical adverse reactions occur within the first 3 months of therapy. It is unclear whether all are dose-related but aiming for the lowest possible dose appears prudent. Mild clinical side effects of vomiting, with or without anorexia and depression, occur in up to 25% of cats, usually within the first few weeks of therapy. In most cases, these reactions are transient and do not require drug withdrawal. Transdermal medication has the advantage of a lower prevalence of gastrointestinal adverse effects (approximately 5%). However, some cats resent manipulation of the ear and crusting and erythema can occur, although this is rare and easily avoided with routine gentle cleaning. Early in the course of therapy, mild and transient

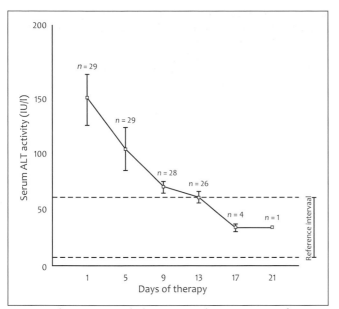

19.10 The progressive decline in serum alanine aminotransferase (ALT) activities in a series of hyperthyroid cats that became euthyroid with carbimazole at a dose of 5 mg q8h.
(Reproduced and modified with permission from Mooney et al., 1992).

haematological abnormalities including lymphocytosis, eosinophilia or leucopenia occur in up to approximately 15% of cases, without any apparent clinical effect. Self-induced excoriations of the head and neck have occasionally been described, usually within the first 6 weeks of therapy: permanent withdrawal of the drug together with symptomatic therapy is usually required, although there are anecdotal reports of recovery with symptomatic treatment but without drug withdrawal.

More serious haematological complications occur in <5% of cases and include agranulocytosis and thrombocytopenia, either alone or concurrently, or, more rarely, immune-mediated haemolytic anaemia. Fortnightly complete blood and platelet counts have been recommended, at least for the first 3 months of therapy, in order to detect such reactions. However, because of their rarity and unpredictability, assessment of a complete blood count, if clinical signs indicate, is a more cost-effective way of dealing with such reactions. A hepatopathy, characterized by marked increases in liver enzyme activities and bilirubin concentration, occurs in <2% of cats. Withdrawal of the medication and symptomatic therapy is required. If such reactions occur with thiamazole they will also occur with carbimazole, and an alternative treatment for hyperthyroidism is required. Other rarely reported side effects include a bleeding tendency without thrombocytopenia or prolongation of clotting times and acquired myasthenia gravis. Development of serum antinuclear antibodies without any clinical signs has been described in approximately 50% of hyperthyroid cats treated with thiamazole for >6 months, but only in cats receiving high-dose therapy ($\geq$15 mg/day).

The unmasking of kidney disease is also a recognized adverse effect of any of the possible treatment modalities for hyperthyroidism (see Chapter 6). It is exacerbated by the development of subclinical or overt hypothyroidism, with the latter known to adversely affect survival (see Chapter 21). The development of CKD is estimated to occur in between 15% and approximately 50% of treated hyperthyroid cats. The lowest prevalence occurs with antithyroid medication because it is less effective in consistently lowering thyroid hormone concentrations compared with more

curative treatment options such as surgery or radioactive iodine. Overt and subclinical hypothyroidism can develop in up to 50% of treated hyperthyroid cats but again is least likely with antithyroid medication. Both subclinical and overt hypothyroidism are easily managed by decreasing the antithyroid drug dose, and this has been shown to reverse increases in creatinine concentrations (Williams et al., 2014).

Lack of efficacy is considered to be an adverse effect, and it appears difficult to maintain serum total T4 concentrations within the reference interval with long-term medical management. Large laboratory surveys suggest that total T4 concentrations are frequently increased in cats undergoing long-term monitoring. This is also supported by approximately 70% of cats having one or more increased total T4 values when treated with long-term transdermal thiamazole (Boretti et al., 2014). This is exacerbated by the continued growth of thyroid tissue over time and the increasing need for higher dosages of antithyroid medication.

Over time, resistance to the effect of antithyroid drug medication may become apparent as thyroid volume and severity of disease increase. There is also evidence of malignant transformation of thyroid tissue. Over years of treatment there is development of large thyroid masses and increasing prevalence of both multifocal disease and intrathoracic masses suggestive of local and distant metastases (so-called SHIM-RAD cases) (Peterson et al., 2016a).

Alternative drugs

Occasionally, alternative medical therapies are required in cats because of adverse reactions to thiamazole or for other specific reasons. For the most part, these therapies are short-term and only recommended prior to a more permanent treatment option.

Propranolol and atenolol: These are the most frequently used beta-adrenoceptor-blocking agents in hyperthyroid cats. They are used to control tachycardia, tachypnoea, hypertension and hyperexcitability associated with hyperthyroidism. Although traditionally considered to have no discernible effect on serum thyroid hormone concentrations, propranolol may inhibit peripheral conversion of T4 to T3. These drugs are recommended when rapid control of clinical signs is desirable and may be used either alone or in combination with thiamazole. Alone, they are a useful treatment option for cats awaiting radioiodine therapy, or in those cases in which there is a delayed return to euthyroidism after treatment because neither has any direct effect on the thyroid gland. Propranolol is a non-selective beta-adrenoceptor blocker and is contraindicated in cats with pre-existing uncontrolled asthma. Atenolol is often preferred because it is a selective beta-1-adrenoceptor-blocking agent.

Stable iodine: High doses of stable iodine acutely decrease the rate of thyroid hormone synthesis (Wolff–Chaikoff effect) and release; these effects are erratic, inconsistent and short-lived, and escape from inhibition can occur. In addition, stable iodine is contraindicated prior to the administration of radioactive iodine and is associated with a high incidence of adverse reactions (excessive salivation and partial to complete anorexia), purportedly because of its 'brassy' taste. For these reasons it is not recommended for use in hyperthyroid cats. In many countries, stable iodine is specifically retained for human use, particularly in case of nuclear accidents.

Calcium ipodate and iopanoic acid: A number of oral cholecystographic agents (e.g. calcium ipodate and iopanoic acid) decrease T4 production, an effect presumably mediated by release of iodine as the drug is metabolized, although they can also acutely inhibit peripheral T4 to T3 conversion. However, they rarely normalize thyroid hormone concentrations and waning of effect is possible after short-term therapy. Neither drug is widely available and their use is not recommended in hyperthyroid cats.

Surgical thyroidectomy

Surgical thyroidectomy is an extremely effective treatment for hyperthyroidism; it is simple, quick, curative and cost-effective. In practice it is often considered the treatment of choice, particularly if radioactive iodine is unavailable.

Preoperative stabilization

Anaesthetizing hyperthyroid cats carries a significant risk of cardiac and metabolic complications serious enough to cause death, and it is therefore necessary to control the production or effects of excess thyroid hormone prior to surgery, as outlined above.

Anaesthetic management

Once the hyperthyroidism is well controlled, a variety of routine anaesthetic regimes can be used – with a few exceptions. Drugs that stimulate or potentiate adrenergic activity are capable of inducing tachycardia and arrhythmias so should be avoided, while drugs capable of preventing such arrhythmias are preferred. A balanced electrolyte solution should be administered intravenously during surgery and the immediate postoperative recovery period to help maintain renal perfusion in these older cats. Minimal anaesthetic time and continual monitoring are essential. Ventricular arrhythmia is a possible complication, particularly if the hyperthyroidism is not already adequately controlled. If such arrhythmias persist despite routine anaesthetic management, an intravenous beta-adrenoceptor blocker may restore normal sinus rhythm.

Surgical technique

The cat is placed in dorsal recumbency with the head extended, assisted by padding placed under the neck. Following aseptic preparation, a ventral skin incision is made from the larynx almost to the manubrium. The sternohyoideus and sternothyroideus muscles are separated by blunt dissection in the midline and gently retracted. Both thyroid lobes and the external parathyroid glands can then be visualized before excision (Figure 19.11). In addition, the right recurrent laryngeal nerve, which lies in close proximity to the right thyroid gland, can be identified and avoided. Following thyroidectomy, the surgical field is carefully examined for haemostasis before closing the incision routinely. Further details of techniques are given in the *BSAVA Manual of Canine and Feline Head, Neck and Thoracic Surgery.*

Unilateral versus bilateral removal: Bilateral lobe involvement occurs in over 50% of cases and thus the majority of cats require bilateral thyroidectomy. In many of these cases, lobe enlargement is not symmetrical, and the smaller lobe may not be clearly palpable. The decision whether to perform a unilateral or bilateral thyroidectomy is therefore often taken at the time of surgery. However, in

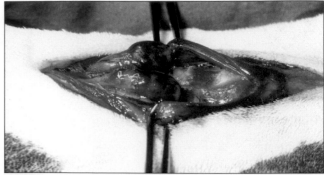

19.11 Appearance of bilateral thyroid lobe enlargement at the time of surgery. The external parathyroid glands are easily visualized as small spherical pale glands at the cranial pole of each thyroid lobe (cranial is to the right of the image).

some bilateral cases, one thyroid lobe may appear grossly normal and if left *in situ* will result in recurrence of the hyperthyroidism. In unilateral cases there is atrophy of the contralateral lobe, but the distinction between what is considered normal and atrophic is not clearly defined.

Thyroid scintigraphy, if available, is an extremely useful procedure to determine unilateral or bilateral lobe involvement and alterations in position or distant metastases from a functioning thyroid carcinoma (Peterson and Broome, 2015) (Figure 19.12). It is particularly useful in determining the site of hyperfunctioning ectopic/accessory tissue that may be present anywhere from the base of the tongue to the heart. High-resolution ultrasonography, in experienced hands, may be an alternative to thyroid scintigraphy, but there are few large studies investigating its use.

In the absence of thyroid imaging, both thyroid lobes should be carefully identified during surgery and, if abnormal in any way, removed. If a unilateral thyroidectomy is carried out, future monitoring for recurrence of the condition is required, although there may be an initial rapid decrease in total T4 concentrations before they slowly increase again. Routine bilateral thyroidectomy, whilst increasing the risk of postoperative complications, obviates the need for decision making at the time of surgery. However, ectopic thyroid tissue should be considered if hyperthyroidism persists after such a thyroidectomy.

Intracapsular versus extracapsular technique: Two techniques have been described for thyroidectomy, both of which attempt to preserve the cranial (external) parathyroid gland and maintain eucalcaemia (Figures 19.13 and 19.14).

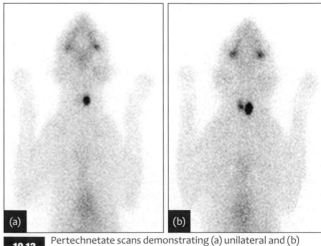

19.12 Pertechnetate scans demonstrating (a) unilateral and (b) bilateral thyroid lobe involvement.

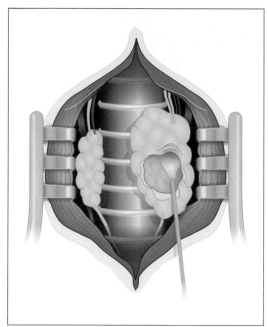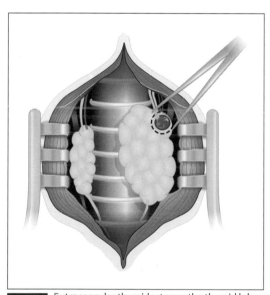

19.13 Intracapsular thyroidectomy: the thyroid capsule is incised and the thyroid lobe is removed. For the modified intracapsular technique, the capsule is subsequently excised.

19.14 Extracapsular thyroidectomy: the thyroid lobe and capsule are removed whilst preserving vascular supply to the external parathyroid glands. For the modified technique, the thyroid capsule deep to the cranial parathyroid gland is retained.

The choice of technique is less important if a unilateral thyroidectomy is being carried out, as only one parathyroid gland is necessary to maintain calcium homeostasis, but the decision requires careful consideration for bilateral thyroidectomy.

The original intracapsular technique involved incision through the thyroid capsule and blunt dissection of the thyroid lobe, leaving the capsule in situ, thereby preserving the blood supply to the cranial parathyroid gland. However, this technique is associated with a high rate of recurrence due to regrowth of tissue adherent to the capsule. The original extracapsular technique involved removal of the intact thyroid lobe with its capsule intact by dissecting away the cranial parathyroid gland and its blood supply. This technique significantly decreases the rate of recurrence but was associated with an unacceptably high rate of postoperative hypoparathyroidism. Both techniques have

therefore been successfully modified: the intracapsular technique by removal of the majority of the capsule after thyroid lobe removal; and the extracapsular technique by retaining the thyroid capsule deep to the parathyroid gland aided by the use of bipolar cautery, which minimizes blunt dissection around the cranial parathyroid gland. There is no significant difference in the rate of postoperative hypocalcaemia or recurrence between these two techniques and both are considered equally appropriate for bilateral thyroidectomy in cats. Haemorrhage obscuring the surgical field can be a problem with the modified intracapsular technique; for this reason, and because of its speed, the modified extracapsular technique may be preferred.

Postoperative complications

The most significant postoperative complication is hypocalcaemia. The tendency towards ionized hypocalcaemia and hyperparathyroidism in hyperthyroidism may play some role in the development of postoperative hypocalcaemia; however, it is generally agreed that it only occurs if the parathyroid glands are injured, devascularized or inadvertently removed during the course of surgery. Since only one parathyroid gland is required to maintain function, hypoparathyroidism only develops after bilateral thyroidectomy. If removal of the cranial parathyroid glands is noted at the time of surgery, small pieces can be transplanted into a muscular pouch in the neck, where revascularization and return of function may occur. There must be no possibility of thyroid carcinoma in such cases. Staged thyroidectomies (3–4 weeks apart) exploit the phenomenon of allowing time for the parathyroid gland on the side of the surgery to recover prior to the next thyroidectomy. However, any reduced risk of postoperative complications may not justify the risk and expense of two surgical procedures.

Hypocalcaemia occurs within 1–5 days of surgery. Biochemical hypocalcaemia alone does not warrant treatment, but treatment should be instituted if clinical signs develop or if the fall in calcium is rapid and precipitous. Clinical signs include anorexia, vocalization, irritability, muscle twitching, tetany and generalized convulsions. The treatment of postoperative hypocalcaemia is outlined in more detail in Chapter 15. Hypoparathyroidism is rarely permanent, and recovery of parathyroid tissue can occur days to months after surgery. This may be related to reversible parathyroid damage or activation of ectopic parathyroid tissue within the neck or mediastinum. However, it is also possible that calcium homeostasis is being maintained through a PTH-independent mechanism primarily relying on calcium absorption from the gastrointestinal tract. If this is the case, there is always the potential risk of developing signs of hypocalcaemia in the future, particularly if anorexia or gastrointestinal disease develops. Care should be taken to monitor these cats appropriately and implement supplementation again if and when necessary.

Monitoring of calcium concentrations should be performed within 12 hours of surgery and up to twice daily thereafter or as indicated by the change in calcium concentration. The risk of clinical signs of hypoparathyroidism appears to be greatest with early and significant changes in calcium. Whilst measurement of ionized calcium concentrations is preferred, there is usually no reason to suspect any abnormalities of calcium binding in hyperthyroidism and therefore measurement of total calcium usually suffices.

Recurrence must also be considered a potential complication. If a unilateral thyroidectomy was originally performed, development of lesions in the contralateral gland should pose no additional surgical risk providing parathyroid function is maintained. However, repeat thyroidectomies, following recurrence after bilateral thyroidectomy, are not recommended because of a higher incidence of severe life-threatening complications. Recurrence is also more likely following surgery on ectopic thyroid tissue. In both cases, an alternative form of therapy for hyperthyroidism is indicated.

It is difficult to assign accurately a risk for hypocalcaemia and recurrence in a cat undergoing bilateral thyroidectomy, as it is highly dependent on surgeon experience. In one study of the modified intracapsular technique performed by an experienced surgeon in a referral institute, a low rate of postoperative hypocalcaemia (<6%) and recurrence (5%) was found (Naan *et al.*, 2006). On the other hand, short- and long-term persistence/recurrence rates of over 20% and 40% were reported for bilateral thyroidectomies in primary care practice, where surgical technique was not recorded and variably experienced surgeons were used (Covey *et al.*, 2019).

Other rarer potential complications include haemorrhage, Horner's syndrome, laryngeal oedema or paralysis, and voice change. These can be avoided by a meticulous surgical technique. Serum total T4 concentrations are usually low for weeks to months after surgical thyroidectomy but eventually increase into the reference interval in many animals. Those that develop subclinical hypothyroidism require careful monitoring, whilst those with overt hypothyroidism require levothyroxine supplementation (see Chapter 21).

Radioactive iodine

Treatment with radioactive iodine is simple, safe and effective, and is the best treatment for most hyperthyroid cats. The radioisotope most commonly used is ^{131}I, which, like stable iodine, is concentrated by the thyroid gland. It has a half-life of approximately 8 days and emits both beta particles and gamma irradiation. The beta-particles, which cause 80% of the tissue damage, travel a maximum of 2 mm and have an average path length of 400 μm. They are therefore locally destructive but spare adjacent atrophic thyroid tissue, parathyroid tissue and other important cervical structures. [131]I can be administered intravenously or orally, but the subcutaneous route is preferred. It is equally effective, safer for personnel, is not associated with gastrointestinal side effects and can be performed under light sedation if necessary. However, whichever route of administration is used, the treatment requires special licensing and hospitalization facilities and an absolute requirement to satisfy local and national radiation safety regulations. As such, this treatment is generally confined to referral practices, and few are able to offer such facilities. Post-treatment hospitalization times for cats vary from 3–7 days up to 4 weeks, depending on local regulations. Due to the popularity of the treatment, waiting lists may be lengthy. This, and a possible delay in the return to euthyroidism of up to 6 months in a small number of cats (usually noted by a significant initial decrease in total T4 that just fails to reach the reference interval), may necessitate interim symptomatic control of the thyrotoxicosis. The use of radioactive iodine in animals is legally precluded in some countries.

The principal aim of treatment is to administer a dose of ^{131}I sufficient to restore euthyroidism and avoid both subclinical and overt hypothyroidism (see Chapter 21). There are several different methods used to calculate the optimal dose for individual cats. The preferred method is to calculate the dose using thyroid scintigraphy for assessment of thyroid volume and radioisotope uptake. Thyroid scintigraphy also confirms the diagnosis, and aids in depicting ectopic thyroid tissue or potential malignancy or resistance to treatment. Access to sophisticated nuclear medicine equipment is required. With this dosing regimen, mildly hyperthyroid cats typically receive 75–110 MBq, whilst those with severe disease and a large volume of thyroid tissue may require doses of 370–555 MBq. Such individualized dosing regimens are associated with an approximate 5% prevalence of overt hypothyroidism and 15% of subclinical disease, with high TSH concentrations decreasing over a period of months in over one third of these cases. Persistent hyperthyroidism is unusual.

The fixed-dose approach obviates the need for thyroid scintigraphy. In the past, presumably because of a more severe form of hyperthyroidism, fixed doses of 150–185 MBq were typically used. Whilst this may result in undertreatment of a number of animals (those with severe hyperthyroidism with large thyroid volume), its greatest problem is inducing hypothyroidism – particularly given the less severe form of hyperthyroidism seen today. In a recent study, the prevalence of subclinical and overt hypothyroidism was approximately three times higher (>60%) in cats treated with a fixed dose of 150 MBq compared with 75 MBq, with no difference in the prevalence of persistent hyperthyroidism (Lucy *et al.*, 2017). If fixed doses are used, lower doses should be considered for mild to moderate hyperthyroidism.

The third method of dose estimation is based on a scoring system, which includes the severity of the clinical thyrotoxicosis, increase in circulating total T4 concentration and the size of the goitre as estimated by palpation. Although variations between different scoring systems exist, typically doses of 75–180 MBq are used. Cats with low scores receive less than 120 MBq, intermediate scores between 120 and 150 MBq, and high scores 160 MBq or more. This is by no means an optimal method as it is reliant on some subjective factors (severity of signs and size of goitre) and does not take into account the possibility of ectopic tissue, or the need for even higher doses in severe cases with large thyroid volume or potential malignancy. It is also complicated if the total T4 assay does not quantify high values (e.g. many assays have an upper limit of approximately 200 nmol/l). Additionally, some sources only supply ^{131}I in a defined number of possible doses, and treatment before or after the known activity date may be required in order to administer the required dose, which is less than ideal. However, it is currently a commonly used method and presumably provides some benefits over a fixed (particularly high-dose) dose regimen. Using one such scoring system, overt hypothyroidism developed in approximately 40% of cats post treatment, although a relatively low upper limit of 0.2 ng/ml was used for TSH (as opposed to the more common use of between 0.3 and 0.32 ng/ml) (Fernandez *et al.*, 2019). Persistent hyperthyroidism occurs in approximately 10% of cases or less.

Complications

There are few complications of ^{131}I therapy, and the prognosis is excellent after successful therapy. Some cats develop self-limiting dysphagia and fever or voice change, presumably as a result of the radiation effects on the larynx, vocal cords and thyroid gland. Chronic kidney disease may develop as it does with other treatment options. This is discussed in greater detail in Chapter 6. There may be severe restrictions on handling cats in the immediate post-treatment isolation period. This can have implications with regard to any other complications that could arise unrelated to the administration of radioactive iodine. As a consequence, many centres offering this treatment only do so for relatively healthy hyperthyroid cats as opposed to those with clinically significant comorbidities.

Dietary iodine restriction

A diet with severely restricted iodine content (e.g. Hill's Prescription Diet y/d) has been available as an option for management of feline hyperthyroidism for several years. The rationale for its use is based on the fact that thyroid hormone production requires access to sufficient quantities of dietary iodine.

A dietary option has clear advantages for cats in which the more traditional curative options such as surgical thyroidectomy and radioiodine ablation are not suitable or available, where there are known or perceived complications with medical management or where owners simply refuse all other options. It is an attractive option given that oral or transdermal application of drugs is not required, anaesthesia or isolation are avoided, and feeding is a routine part of daily life. However, there are disadvantages that must also be considered before recommending this as a sole treatment option. Firstly, to achieve optimal success, the cat must eat the diet, and palatability can be a problem, particularly as thyroid hormone concentrations decline and the associated polyphagia decreases. Problems with palatability have been reported in over one third of cats (van der Kooij et al., 2014). The cat must not have access to other foods. This is difficult in cats that have outdoor access or that live in multi-cat households. However, exclusively feeding this diet for 2 years to healthy euthyroid adult cats had no significant effect on food intake, body condition or thyroid function compared with cats fed a similar diet without iodine restriction (Paetau-Robinson et al., 2018). Nevertheless, the consequences of longer-term feeding of such a diet are unknown and it is potentially a costly option for households of many cats. Additionally, this diet is relatively low in protein and so may not be ideal for all healthy or hyperthyroid cats.

The greatest disadvantage to dietary management is lack of predictable success and a more delayed onset of euthyroidism. Between 65% and 75% of cats attain euthyroidism, as defined by reference interval total T4 concentrations after 4–8 weeks of treatment (van der Kooij et al., 2014; Loftus et al., 2019). Success is most likely in hyperthyroid cats with mild to moderate disease. Maintenance of euthyroidism long-term is more difficult, with only approximately 40% of cases controlled at 6 months (Fritsch et al., 2014; Vaske et al., 2016). Over time, control of the clinical signs of hyperthyroidism is not often satisfactory (Hui et al., 2015). This may be because the total T4 concentration is not suppressed to anything less than the top end of the reference interval, it remains persistently high or there is a 'ping-pong' effect between high and reference interval values. As such, close monitoring of cats on such diets is required, at least monthly, to assess both the clinical signs and thyroid hormone concentrations. On the other hand, unmasking of CKD and its exacerbation through the development of overt or subclinical hypothyroidism is unlikely.

Combining antithyroid medication and dietary control is not recommended in the routine treatment of hyperthyroidism because of the increased risk of inducing hypothyroidism compared with using either treatment alone. In cats on long-term antithyroid medication with relapsing disease, severe hyperthyroidism and increasing thyroid volume, concurrent use of dietary control and increasing antithyroid dosage may be helpful. Dietary therapy can be used prior to surgical thyroidectomy but care must be taken to ensure that the cat is euthyroid prior to anaesthesia and alternative control methods should be used if this has not been attained. Stopping dietary therapy a few weeks prior to radioactive iodine therapy is often recommended. However, this is probably not strictly necessary. Iodine-restricted diets tend to increase radioactive iodine uptake (Scott-Moncrieff et al., 2015). Providing this is taken into account when calculating a dose of ^{131}I for treatment, there should be no issues. It may provide an additional way of increasing the dose delivered if warranted in an individual cat.

Thyroid carcinoma

Functional thyroid carcinoma accounts for approximately 2% of cases of feline hyperthyroidism (Peterson and Broome, 2015). However, not all thyroid carcinomas in cats are hyperfunctional. Affected cats present with similar clinical signs to those with benign adenomatous hyperplasia. Evidence for thyroid carcinoma includes palpable large multilobulated masses in the neck, signs of distant metastases (usually intrathoracic), supportive scintigraphic features (Figure 19.15), locally invasive appearance at the time of surgery, or persistence or rapid recurrence following either routine bilateral thyroidectomy or radioactive iodine therapy. Cats treated with antithyroid drugs over many years are more likely to show evidence of malignant transformation (Peterson et al., 2016a).

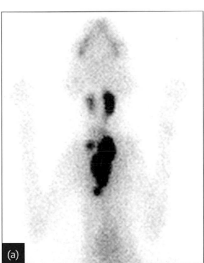

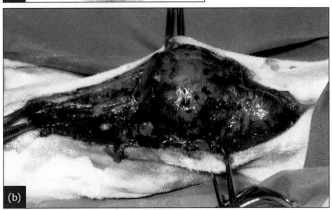

19.15 (a) Appearance of a pertechnetate scan in a case of thyroid carcinoma with multiple areas of uptake in the cervical and thoracic regions.
(b) Appearance of a large multilobulated thyroid carcinoma as visualized at the time of surgery.

References and further reading

Boretti FS, Sieber-Ruckstuhl NS, Schafer S *et al.* (2014) Transdermal application of methimazole in hyperthyroid cats: a long-term follow-up study. *Journal of Feline Medicine and Surgery* **16**, 453–459

Bree L, Gallagher BA, Shiel RE and Mooney CT (2018) Prevalence and risk factors for hyperthyroidism in Irish cats from the greater Dublin area. *Irish Veterinary Journal* **71**, 2

Brockman D, Holt D and ter Haar G (2018) *BSAVA Manual of Canine and Feline Head, Neck and Thoracic Surgery, 2nd edn.* BSAVA Publications, Gloucester

Covey HL, Chang YM, Elliott J and Syme HM (2019) Changes in thyroid and renal function after bilateral thyroidectomy in cats. *Journal of Veterinary Internal Medicine* **33**, 508–515

Daminet S, Kooistra HS, Fracassi F *et al.* (2014) Best practice for the pharmacological management of hyperthyroid cats with antithyroid drugs. *Journal of Small Animal Practice* **55**, 4–13

Fernandez Y, Puig J, Powell R and Seth M (2019) Prevalence of iatrogenic hypothyroidism in hyperthyroid cats treated with radioiodine using an individualised scoring system. *Journal of Feline Medicine and Surgery* **21**, 1149–1156

Fritsch DA, Allen TA, Dodd CE, Wedekind KJ and Sixby KA (2014) A restricted iodine food reduces circulating thyroxine concentrations in cats with hyperthyroidism. *International Journal of Applied Research in Veterinary Medicine* **12**, 24–32

Geesaman BM, Whitehouse WH and Viviano KR (2016) Serum cobalamin and methylmalonic acid concentrations in hyperthyroid cats before and after radioiodine treatment. *Journal of Veterinary Internal Medicine* **30**, 560–565

Hill KE, Gieseg MA, Bridges J and Chambers JP (2014) The pharmacokinetics of methimazole in a novel lipophilic formulation administered transdermally to healthy cats. *New Zealand Veterinary Journal* **62**, 208–213

Hill KE, Gieseg MA, Kingsbury D *et al.* (2011) The efficacy and safety of a novel lipophilic formulation of methimazole for the once daily transdermal treatment of cats with hyperthyroidism. *Journal of Veterinary Internal Medicine* **25**, 1357–1365

Hui TY, Bruyette DS, Moore GE and Scott-Moncrieff JC (2015) Effect of feeding an iodine-restricted diet in cats with spontaneous hyperthyroidism. *Journal of Veterinary Internal Medicine* **29**, 1063–1068

Kormpou F, Gil-Morales C, Warren-Smith C and Hibbert A (2020) Concurrent thoracic pathology identified with radiology in hyperthyroid cats referred for radioiodine therapy. *Journal of Feline Medicine and Surgery* **22**, 966–976

Loftus JP, DeRosa S, Struble AM, Randolph JF and Wakshlag JJ (2019) One-year study evaluating efficacy of an iodine-restricted diet for the treatment of moderate-to-severe hyperthyroidism in cats. *Veterinary Medicine: Research and Reports* **10**, 9–16

Lottati M, Aucoin D and Bruyette DS (2019) Expected total thyroxine (TT4) concentrations and outlier values in 531,765 cats in the United States (2014–2015). *PLoS ONE* **14**, e0213259

Lucy JM, Peterson ME, Randolph JF *et al.* (2017) Efficacy of low-dose (2 millicurie) *versus* standard-dose (4 millicurie) radioiodine treatment for cats with mild-to-moderate hyperthyroidism. *Journal of Veterinary Internal Medicine* **31**, 326–334

Mooney CT, Thoday KL and Doxey DL (1992) Carbimazole therapy of feline hyperthyroidism. *Journal of Small Animal Practice* **33**, 228–235

Naan EC, Kirpensteijn J, Kooistra HS and Peeters ME (2006) Results of thyroidectomy in 101 cats with hyperthyroidism. *Veterinary Surgery* **35**, 287–293

Nussbaum LK, Scavelli TD, Scavelli DM *et al.* (2015) Abdominal ultrasound examination findings in 534 hyperthyroid cats referred for radioiodine treatment between 2007–2010. *Journal of Veterinary Internal Medicine* **29**, 1069–1073

Paetau-Robinson I, Melendez LD, Forrester SD *et al.* (2018) Comparison of health parameters in normal cats fed a limited iodine prescription food vs a conventional diet. *Journal of Feline Medicine and Surgery* **20**, 142–148

Peterson ME (2013) More than just T4: diagnostic testing for hyperthyroidism in cats. *Journal of Feline Medicine and Surgery* **15**, 765–777

Peterson ME and Broome MR (2015) Thyroid scintigraphy findings in 2096 cats with hyperthyroidism. *Veterinary Radiology and Ultrasound* **56**, 84-95

Peterson ME, Broome MR and Rishniw M (2016a) Prevalence and degree of thyroid pathology in hyperthyroid cats increases with disease duration: a cross-sectional analysis of 2096 cats referred for radioiodine therapy. *Journal of Feline Medicine and Surgery* **18**, 92–103

Peterson ME, Castellano CA and Rishniw M (2016b) Evaluation of body weight, body condition, and muscle condition in cats with hyperthyroidism. *Journal of Veterinary Internal Medicine* **30**, 1780–1789

Peterson ME, Davignon DL, Shaw N *et al.* (2020a) Serum thyroxine and thyrotropin concentrations decrease with severity of nonthyroidal illness in cats and predict 30-day survival outcome. *Journal of Veterinary Internal Medicine* **34**, 2276–2286

Peterson ME, Guterl JN, Nichols R and Rishniw M (2015) Evaluation of serum thyroid-stimulating hormone concentration as a diagnostic test for hyperthyroidism in cats. *Journal of Veterinary Internal Medicine* **29**, 1327–1334

Peterson ME, Guterl JN, Rishniw M and Broome MR (2016c) Evaluation of quantitative thyroid scintigraphy for diagnosis and staging of disease severity in cats with hyperthyroidism: comparison of the percent thyroidal uptake of pertechnetate to thyroid-to-salivary ratio and thyroid-to-background ratios. *Veterinary Radiology and Ultrasound* **57**, 427–440

Peterson ME, Li A, Soboroff P, Bilbrough GE and Rishniw M (2020b) Hyperthyroidism is not a risk factor for subclinical bacteriuria in cats: a prospective cohort study. *Journal of Veterinary Internal Medicine* **34**, 1157–1165

Rasmussen SH, Andersen HH and Kjelgaard-Hansen M (2014) Combined assessment of serum free and total T4 in a general clinical setting seemingly has limited potential in improving diagnostic accuracy of thyroid dysfunction in dogs and cats. *Veterinary Clinical Pathology* **43**, 1–3

Rayalam S, Eizenstat LD, Davis RR, Hoenig M and Ferguson DC (2006) Expression and purification of feline thyrotropin (fTSH): immunological detection and bioactivity of heterodimeric and yoked glycoproteins. *Domestic Animal Endocrinology* **30**, 185–202

Scott-Moncrieff JC, Heng HG, Weng HY, Dimeo D and Jones MD (2015) Effect of a limited iodine diet on iodine uptake by thyroid glands in hyperthyroid cats. *Journal of Veterinary Internal Medicine* **29**, 1322–1326

Stephens MJ, O'Neill DG, Church DB *et al.* (2014) Feline hyperthyroidism reported in primary-care veterinary practices in England: prevalence, associated factors and spatial distribution. *Veterinary Record* **175**, 458

Thoday K and Mooney CT (1992) Historical, clinical and laboratory features of 126 hyperthyroid cats. *Veterinary Record* **131**, 257–264

van der Kooij M, Becvarova I, Meyer HP, Teske E and Kooistra HS (2014) Effects of an iodine-restricted food on client-owned cats with hyperthyroidism. *Journal of Feline Medicine and Surgery* **16**, 491–498

Vaske HH, Armbrust L, Zicker SC, Jewell DE and Grauer GF (2016) Assessment of renal function im hyperthyroid cats managed with a controlled iodine diet. *International Journal of Applied Research in Veterinary Medicine* **14**, 38–48

Watson N, Murray JK, Fontara S and Hibbert A (2018) Clinicopathological features and comorbidities of cats with mild, moderate or severe hyperthyroidism: a radioiodine referral population. *Journal of Feline Medicine and Surgery* **20**, 1130–1137

Williams TL, Elliott J and Syme HM (2014) Effect on renal function of restoration of euthyroidism in hyperthyroid cats with iatrogenic hypothyroidism. *Journal of Veterinary Internal Medicine* **28**, 1251–1255

Wood A, Ryder M and Harmon I (2020) White paper: *TRUFORMA® Point-of-Care Canine and Feline Thyroid-Stimulating Hormone (TSH) Assay.* Available from: zomedica.com/resource-center

Chapter 20

Canine hyperthyroidism and thyroid neoplasia

Miguel Campos

Introduction

Thyrotoxicosis refers to the clinical syndrome caused by excess circulating thyroid hormones, irrespective of the source. Hyperthyroidism refers specifically to increased thyroid hormone secretion from the thyroid gland. Hyperthyroidism in dogs is most frequently associated with functional thyroid neoplasia. Thyroid tumours represent 1.2–3.8% of all canine neoplasms and are almost always malignant (Brodey and Kelly, 1968; Harari et al., 1986).

Another important cause of thyrotoxicosis in dogs is the consumption of meat-based products (raw or commercial diets or treats) containing excessive amounts of thyroid tissue (Köhler et al., 2012; Broome et al., 2015). Rarely, thyrotoxicosis can also be caused by excessive administration or inadvertent ingestion of levothyroxine supplements (Shadwick et al., 2013). When suspicion of thyrotoxicosis arises due to the presence of typical clinical signs (e.g. weight loss, polyuria, polydipsia, polyphagia), a complete history (including dietary history) and a thorough physical examination (with cervical palpation) are helpful in identifying the underlying cause.

Clinicians can also be confronted with increased values for total thyroxine (T4) when investigating canine hypothyroidism (see Chapter 18). This can be attributed to the presence of T4 autoantibodies (T4AAs) in dogs with thyroiditis and their interference in the T4 immunoassay being used. Such cases are usually not too challenging, as the clinical signs are very different between hypo- and hyperthyroidism. It is also possible to measure T4AAs directly or surmise their presence by measurement of thyroglobulin autoantibodies (see Chapter 18).

Dietary thyrotoxicosis

Consumption of commercially available dog food, treats (e.g. dried gullet) or raw diets containing high concentrations of thyroid hormones can lead to clinical signs of hyperthyroidism, increased T4 and suppressed thyrotropin (thyroid-stimulating hormone (TSH)) concentrations (Köhler et al., 2012; Broome et al., 2015). This presumably occurs when meat-based products are erroneously contaminated with thyroid tissue or where neck parts are used in food production. In two separate studies of dogs with dietary thyrotoxicosis, after changing from a raw diet or a contaminated commercial diet to non-contaminated commercial food or pure muscle meat, or removing dried

gullet from the diet, all clinical signs resolved within a few days and circulating total T4 concentrations normalized upon re-examination 2 weeks to 2 months later (Köhler et al., 2012; Broome et al., 2015). Cervical scintigraphy in affected dogs demonstrates a diffuse, bilateral and symmetric reduction in uptake of technetium-99m as pertechnetate ($^{99m}TcO_4^-$) by the thyroid glands relative to salivary glands. A thorough dietary history is therefore essential when evaluating dogs with clinical signs of hyperthyroidism and increased T4 concentrations. This is particularly important when thyroid neoplasia is unlikely, such as in young dogs or when no cervical mass can be palpated.

Functional thyroid neoplasia

Classification of thyroid tumours

Approximately 90% of canine thyroid tumours detected clinically are carcinomas and are classified as either follicular thyroid carcinomas (FTCs), which arise from thyroid follicular cells, or medullary thyroid carcinomas (MTCs), which arise from the parafollicular cells (C-cells) (Wucherer and Wilke, 2005). Although thyroid adenomas account for 30–50% of thyroid masses reported in canine pathology studies, these benign tumours tend to be small, non-palpable and incidentally found during post-mortem examination rather than recognized during life (Brodey and Kelly, 1968; Leav et al., 1976).

Follicular thyroid carcinomas account for 64–71% of canine thyroid carcinomas while MTCs represent 29–36% (Carver et al., 1995; Campos et al., 2014a). According to the World Health Organization (WHO), FTCs can be classified histologically as well differentiated (follicular, compact, follicular-compact, papillary), poorly differentiated, undifferentiated or carcinosarcoma (Kiupel et al., 2008). In most veterinary studies, the prevalence of MTC is likely underestimated as these tumours may be difficult to distinguish from FTC of compact type by microscopic observation alone. In the absence of follicular architecture, follicular cell origin can be confirmed with immunohistochemistry for thyroglobulin, while C-cell origin can be confirmed with immunohistochemistry for calcitonin or for markers of neuroendocrine tissue (e.g. chromogranin A, synaptophysin).

Previously, MTCs were suggested to be more amenable to complete surgical resection and to have lower metastatic potential than FTCs (Carver et al., 1995). The lower prevalence of local invasiveness in MTCs has been observed in more recent studies but prognosis following thyroidectomy is comparable to that of FTCs (Campos *et al.*, 2014a).

Pathogenesis

The pathogenesis of canine thyroid neoplasia is largely unknown. In humans, studies have shown an association between thyroid neoplasia and iodine deficiency or excess, chronic stimulation by TSH, exposure to ionizing radiation and many different genetic alterations. Lymphocytic thyroiditis and exposure to ionizing radiation have both been reported as predisposing factors in dogs (Benjamin *et al.*, 1996, 1997). In a colony of 276 Beagles allowed to live their full lifespan without treatment, 16% of dogs developed hypothyroidism and 26% had evidence of lymphocytic thyroiditis at the time of death (Benjamin *et al.*, 1996). While 54% of hypothyroid dogs developed FTCs, only 23% of euthyroid dogs developed similar tumours. Chronic TSH stimulation of thyroid follicular cells may have been responsible for the strong association between lymphocytic thyroiditis, hypothyroidism and follicular thyroid neoplasia.

In agreement with human studies showing that mutations in the tumour suppressor gene *TP53* are uncommon in differentiated thyroid cancer, a somatic mutation in *TP53* has been identified in only one of 23 canine FTCs (Devilee *et al.*, 1994). It has also been shown that approximately 60% of canine thyroid tumours are DNA-aneuploid, which is comparable to what is observed in humans (Verschueren *et al.*, 1991). However, in dogs more than 80% of aneuploid thyroid tumours are hypodiploid, while in humans hypodiploidy is rare.

Common genetic events associated with human thyroid cancer include activating point mutations of *BRAF* (papillary carcinomas), *RAS* mutations (FTCs and MTCs without *RET* mutations), aberrant activation of the receptor tyrosine kinase *RET* (sporadic MTCs), activating mutations of *PIK3CA* (FTCs) and inactivating mutations of *PTEN* (follicular carcinoma). These genetic alterations lead to activation of the mitogen-activated protein kinase (MAPK) or the phosphoinositide 3-kinase/protein kinase B (PI3K/Akt) signalling pathways (or both), which play a predominant role in human thyroid gland oncogenesis. A study in 43 canine FTCs and 16 MTCs investigated known mutational hotspots and messenger RNA (mRNA) expression of genes commonly involved in human thyroid gland tumorigenesis: activating missense mutations in *K-RAS* also described in human thyroid cancer were found in one FTC and one MTC (Campos *et al.*, 2014b). No functional mutations were found in the sequenced regions of *BRAF*, *H-RAS*, *N-RAS*, *RET*, *PIK3CA* or *PTEN*, demonstrating that the mutations most frequently associated with human thyroid neoplasia are rare in dogs. Quantitative reverse transcription polymerase chain reaction (RT-PCR) for selected receptor tyrosine kinases and PI3K/Akt pathway members known to be commonly amplified in human thyroid cancer showed increased mRNA expression of vascular endothelial growth factor receptor-1 and -2 (VEGFR-1 and VEGFR-2), 3-phosphoinositide-dependent kinase-1, and v-akt murine thymoma viral oncogene homologues 1 and 2 in canine FTC, and of epidermal growth factor receptor (EGFR), VEGFR-1 and phosphatidylinositol-4,5-bisphosphate 3-kinase catalytic subunit alpha (PIK3CA) in canine MTC, when compared with healthy thyroid tissue (Campos *et al.*, 2014b). This suggests the involvement of the PI3K/Akt signalling pathway in the pathogenesis of canine thyroid cancer, particularly in FTC. Another study of canine FTCs also showed increased expression of VEGFR-2 and phosphorylation (activation) of EGFR and RET, which are known to signal through the PI3K/Akt and MAPK pathways (Urie *et al.*, 2012). In the only case report of canine familial MTC, no mutation was found after complete genomic sequencing of *RET* (Lee *et al.*, 2006).

In humans, thyroid tumours form part of the multiple endocrine neoplasia (MEN) syndrome type 2 (MEN-2), which is a genetic disorder caused by germline mutations in the *RET* proto-oncogene and is associated with a high lifetime risk of developing MTC. In dogs, large pathology studies have shown that MEN syndromes are rare (Beatrice *et al.*, 2018). Only two dogs have been described resembling MEN-2 and there is one case report of familial MTC (Peterson *et al.*, 1982; Lee *et al.*, 2006; Soler Arias *et al.*, 2016; see Chapter 35).

Clinical features

Signalment

Beagles, Golden Retrievers, Boxers and Siberian Huskies are at increased risk of developing thyroid neoplasia. There is no sex predilection and dogs over 7 years of age are more commonly affected (Leav *et al.*, 1976; Worth *et al.*, 2005; Wucherer and Wilke, 2005).

Clinical signs

Most dogs with thyroid tumours are presented due to the presence of a palpable cervical mass and are otherwise asymptomatic. In two studies including approximately 70 dogs with thyroid tumours, 62–83% of dogs had unilateral tumours, 11–22% had bilateral tumours and 6–16% had ectopic tumours (Campos *et al.*, 2014a; van den Berg *et al.*, 2020). There is no predilection for either the left or right thyroid lobe. Ectopic thyroid tumours are commonly located ventrally to the larynx (sublingual), invading the hyoid bone, but can potentially be located anywhere from the base of the tongue to the base of the heart (Broome *et al.*, 2014; Milovancev *et al.*, 2014; van den Berg *et al.*, 2020).

Weight loss is present in 26–33% of dogs, 20% present with cough, 19% present with polyuria/polydipsia (PU/PD) and 7–13% present with dyspnoea or stridor due to large or invasive tumours. In cases of advanced disease, dysphagia and dysphonia can also be observed.

Dogs with functional FTCs can present with clinical signs of hyperthyroidism such as PU/PD, weight loss, panting and aggressiveness. Rarely, dogs may also present with clinical signs of hypothyroidism, which could be present prior to the development of thyroid neoplasia (see 'Pathogenesis', above) or be due to extensive destruction of healthy thyroid tissue in cases of bilateral thyroid neoplasia.

Thyroid function

The majority of dogs (55–65%) with thyroid neoplasia are euthyroid. Approximately 20–30% of dogs are hyperthyroid and 30–40% have decreased circulating total T4 concentrations, mostly due to non-thyroidal illness and only occasionally due to hypothyroidism (Harari *et al.*, 1986; Marks *et al.*, 1994; Worth *et al.*, 2005; Campos *et al.*, 2014a; van den Berg *et al.*, 2020).

Diagnosis

Differential diagnosis

Causes for ventral cervical masses include thyroid neoplasia, carotid body tumours, and lymphadenomegaly of the submandibular, medial retropharyngeal or cervical lymph nodes.

Clinicopathological features

Although MTCs arise from calcitonin-producing C-cells, hypocalcaemia has not been reported to be associated with these tumours in dogs (Carver *et al.*, 1995; Campos *et al.*, 2014a). This may be related to the limited role of calcitonin in calcium balance compared with other hormones. On the other hand, paraneoplastic ionized hypercalcaemia has been reported in dogs with unclassified thyroid carcinoma, namely due to production of parathyroid hormone-related protein (PTHrP) (Lane and Wyatt, 2012; Scruggs *et al.*, 2015).

Cytology

When a thyroid tumour is suspected, cytology can provide important information regarding the thyroidal origin of the mass (Figure 20.1). However, cytology cannot be used to reliably distinguish benign from malignant disease, and thyroid tumours in dogs should be assumed to be malignant until proven otherwise. Given the high vascularization of these tumours, samples are often contaminated with blood and more than one aspirate may be needed to obtain a diagnostic sample. In a retrospective study, cytology correctly identified the thyroidal origin of the tumours in 10 of 11 dogs with thyroid carcinoma, while in another study diagnostic samples were obtained in only 8 of 17 cases (Thompson *et al.*, 1980; Harari *et al.*, 1986). If fluid is obtained after thyroid gland aspiration, demonstration of a markedly increased total T4 concentration confirms its thyroidal origin, but low values do not exclude such a diagnosis.

Biopsy

Definitive diagnosis of thyroid gland neoplasia requires histopathology. The safest way to obtain a definitive diagnosis is by excisional biopsy when possible. Thyroid tumours are highly vascularized and any biopsy procedure is commonly associated with haemorrhage. For tumours that are unresectable due to local invasiveness, a presumptive diagnosis based on cytology, scintigraphy or even computed tomography (CT) may be a preferable approach. Large-bore needle biopsies should be avoided, and even incisional biopsies carry a significant risk of haemorrhage.

Staging

It is crucial to thoroughly stage every dog with thyroid neoplasia in order to determine the best treatment modality. Dogs with tumours that are well encapsulated and have not metastasized have a good prognosis with surgery alone, while dogs with locally invasive tumours are better treated with radiation therapy or radioactive iodine. In the presence of distant metastases, treatment of the primary tumour can still be considered even if the long-term prognosis is less favourable. Staging is performed according to the WHO staging system and is based on the size (and mobility) of the primary tumour and presence of regional or distant metastases (Figure 20.2) (Owen, 1980).

Evaluation of local invasiveness

Up to 45% of canine thyroid tumours are unresectable due to local invasiveness (Carver *et al.*, 1995). Tumour palpation during physical examination can provide information as to whether the tumour is mobile or fixed in the neck. However, tumour size can greatly influence the impression during palpation and advanced imaging is recommended to better evaluate local invasiveness. In a retrospective study, although 17 of 38 FTCs and 5 of 19 MTCs were fixed at palpation, only 9 FTCs and no MTCs had macroscopic evidence of local invasiveness during surgery or post-mortem examination (Campos *et al.*, 2014a). These findings are corroborated by a study comparing clinical examination, ultrasonography, CT, magnetic resonance imaging (MRI) and pathology findings in 17 dogs with thyroid carcinoma (Taeymans *et al.*, 2013). Only 5 of 11 tumours considered fixed or partially fixed at palpation

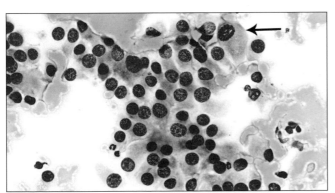

20.1 Fine-needle aspiration sample of a canine thyroid tumour interpreted as carcinoma, showing a sheet of neoplastic epithelial cells with indistinct cell borders and moderate anisocytosis and anisokaryosis. Note the mitotic prophase (arrowed). (Modified Wright's stain, X50 oil objective lens)
(Courtesy of Laureen Peters, Department of Clinical Veterinary Science, University of Bern)

Stage	Primary tumour (T)	Regional lymph nodes (N)	Distant metastases (M)
I	T1a,b	N0	M0
II	T0	N1a	M0
	T1a,b	N1a	M0
	T2a,b	N0 or N1a	M0
III	T3	Any N	M0
	Any T	N1b or N2b	M0
IV	Any T	Any N	M1
Key			
M0	No evidence of distant metastases		
M1	Distant metastases detected		
N0	No evidence of lymph node involvement		
N1	Ipsilateral lymph node involvement	N1a, movable	N1b, fixed
N2	Bilateral lymph node involvement	N2a, movable	N2b, fixed
T0	No evidence of tumour (microscopic residual disease)		
T1	Tumour maximum diameter <2 cm	T1a, movable	T1b, fixed
T2	Tumour maximum diameter 2–5 cm	T2a, movable	T2b, fixed
T3	Tumour maximum diameter >5 cm	T3a, movable	T3b, fixed

20.2 Clinical staging of canine thyroid tumours.
(Modified from Owen, 1980)

actually had imaging evidence of capsule disruption, while 5 of 6 masses considered mobile at palpation exhibited imaging signs of capsule disruption. In conclusion, palpation is not an accurate predictor of local invasiveness and advanced imaging (CT or MRI) should be performed to decide on the definitive treatment modality. Compared with CT and MRI, ultrasonography has a lower sensitivity and specificity for correctly identifying the thyroidal origin of a cervical mass and, most importantly, lower sensitivity for detecting tumour capsule disruption (Figure 20.3). Magnetic resonance imaging is the most sensitive imaging modality for detecting local invasiveness and may be crucial, in selected cases, to determine the best treatment option. However, in difficult cases with large cervical masses, a definitive assessment might only be possible during surgical exploration. Computed tomography likely offers the most cost-effective simultaneous evaluation of local invasiveness and metastatic spread in the preoperative evaluation of dogs with thyroid tumours.

Evaluation of regional and distant metastases

Thyroid tumours metastasize primarily to the lungs and regional lymph nodes (retropharyngeal, mandibular and cervical superficial) and up to 38% of dogs have evidence of pulmonary metastases at the time of diagnosis (Harari et al., 1986; Barber, 2007).

Thoracic radiographs provide a quick and relatively inexpensive evaluation for pulmonary metastases and may allow identification of ectopic thyroid neoplasia in the cranial mediastinum. However, CT is more sensitive for detection of pulmonary metastases and also allows a thorough evaluation of regional lymph nodes and local invasiveness, making it arguably the most complete imaging modality for treatment planning in these cases (Figure 20.4).

Another imaging modality that can be helpful in identifying regional and distant metastases is scintigraphy. The radioisotope most commonly used is $^{99m}TcO_4^-$, as it is trapped by cells that concentrate iodine (i.e. thyroid gland, salivary glands, gastric mucosa). Scintigraphy allows identification of cervical masses arising from the thyroid gland and it may also help to identify the presence of ectopic thyroid tissue (normal or neoplastic) and thyroid cancer metastases if the metastatic tumour cells take up the radioisotope (Figures 20.5 and 20.6) (Marks et al., 1994). Tumours with extensive capsular invasion have poorly circumscribed heterogeneous uptake, and most tumours causing hyperthyroidism have well circumscribed

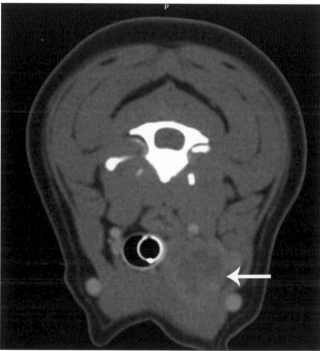

20.4 Computed tomographic image (transverse view) of a left-sided thyroid tumour in a dog (arrowed).
(Courtesy of the Department of Medical Imaging, University of Bern)

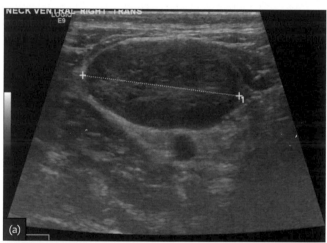

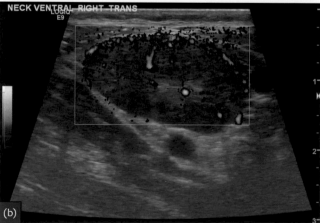

20.3 (a) Ultrasonographic image (transverse view) of a right-sided thyroid tumour in a 12-year-old male terrier cross. It measured 1.2 cm in width and 3.38 cm in length. (b) The tumour elicited significant Doppler signal.
(Courtesy of University College Dublin)

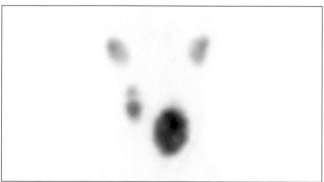

20.5 Ventrodorsal view of a thyroid pertechnetate scan of a dog with bilateral follicular thyroid carcinomas. The right-sided tumour presents a heterogeneous uptake pattern while the left-sided tumour exhibits a homogeneous uptake.
(Courtesy of the Department of Veterinary Medical Imaging and Small Animal Orthopaedics, University of Ghent)

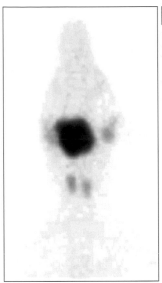

20.6 Ventrodorsal view of a thyroid planar pertechnetate scan of a dog with ectopic sublingual follicular cell thyroid neoplasia with a homogeneous uptake pattern.
(Courtesy of the Department of Veterinary Medical Imaging and Small Animal Orthopaedics, University of Ghent)

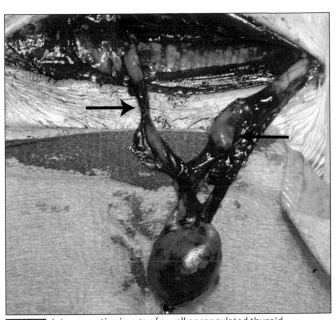

20.8 Intraoperative image of a well encapsulated thyroid carcinoma in a dog that had gross evidence of vascular invasion and tumour thrombi within the cranial and caudal thyroid veins (arrowed).
(Reproduced from Liptak (2007) with permission from the publisher)

and increased homogeneous uptake. Scintigraphy does not appear to offer additional benefit for detection of pulmonary metastases compared with thoracic radiographs. In a recent study, thoracic single-photon emission computed tomography (SPECT) provided higher sensitivity than radiographs for detecting thoracic metastases (Figure 20.7), but it is not yet widely available (van den Berg *et al.*, 2020).

Treatment

Thyroidectomy

Thyroidectomy is the preferred treatment modality for dogs with unilateral or bilateral thyroid tumours that are well encapsulated, with reported median survival times greater than 36 months in the absence of metastatic disease (Klein *et al.*, 1995; Tuohy *et al.*, 2012; Frederick *et al.*, 2020) (Figure 20.8). Dogs with metastases can also

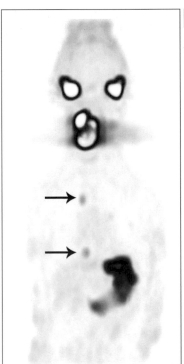

20.7 Pertechnetate single-photon emission computed tomography (SPECT) of a dog with a follicular thyroid tumour showing two thoracic metastases (arrowed).
(Courtesy of the Department of Veterinary Medical Imaging and Small Animal Orthopaedics, University of Ghent)

have prolonged survival after surgery. A median survival of 16.5 months in 15 dogs with metastases, 10 of which were lung metastases, variably treated with thyroidectomy and adjuvant chemotherapy, has been reported (Nadeau and Kitchell, 2011).

Advanced imaging of the neck and thorax prior to surgery is highly recommended to evaluate metastatic disease and local invasiveness, even if the tumour is freely mobile at palpation. Surgery typically allows marginal excision of the tumour. Wide resection of non-invasive tumours is not indicated because morbidity is unacceptably high and the rate of local recurrence following marginal resection is low (4–11%) (Liptak, 2007; Reagan *et al.*, 2019). Radical resection of deeply invasive tumours is not recommended due to high morbidity and because radiation therapy and radioactive iodine (^{131}I) are associated with prolonged survival and excellent quality of life in those cases. Cytoreductive surgery is also not recommended due to high vascularization and risk of haemorrhage. If cases are selected carefully, complications of unilateral thyroidectomy are uncommon and include haemorrhage (8%), aspiration pneumonia (3%) and laryngeal paralysis (2%) (Klein *et al.*, 1995; Nadeau & Kitchell 2011; Reagan *et al.*, 2019).

One important exception to the recommendation that invasive thyroid tumours should not be surgically removed is the existence of ectopic sublingual thyroid neoplasia invading the basis of the hyoid bone. Partial hyoidectomy appears to be well tolerated by dogs and allows *en bloc* removal of the entire tumour without major complications (Broome *et al.*, 2014; Milovancev *et al.*, 2014). Partial resection of the hyoid apparatus seems to be crucial to achieve a complete excision of the tumour in these dogs.

Dogs with well encapsulated bilateral thyroid tumours can also enjoy prolonged survival after bilateral thyroidectomy (Tuohy *et al.*, 2012). However, monitoring for iatrogenic primary hypoparathyroidism is critical after surgery. Over 70% of dogs undergoing bilateral thyroid lobectomy reportedly develop hypocalcaemia after surgery and calcitriol treatment may be required long-term.

Radiation therapy

Dogs with unresectable thyroid tumours can be adequately treated and enjoy a prolonged survival with radiation therapy (Théon *et al.*, 2000; Pack *et al.*, 2001). Typically, dogs receive 48 Gray (Gy) over 4 weeks on an alternate-day schedule of 4 Gy/fraction. A progression-free survival (PFS) rate of 80% at 1 year and 72% at 3 years has been described in dogs with locally advanced disease and no evidence of metastases (Théon *et al.*, 2000). Time to maximum tumour size reduction can be 8–22 months. Self-limiting acute radiation reactions include mild dysphagia, hoarseness and cough due to oesophageal, tracheal or laryngeal mucositis. Chronic radiation complications include skin fibrosis with permanent alopecia, dry cough due to chronic tracheitis, hypothyroidism and hypoparathyroidism (Théon *et al.*, 2000; Amores-Fuster *et al.*, 2017).

Palliative-intent hypofractionated radiation protocols have also been described for dogs with invasive thyroid tumours (Brearley *et al.*, 1999; Tsimbas *et al.*, 2019). A tumour response rate of just over 75% and a median survival of up to 29 months has been described in dogs without pulmonary metastases receiving 36 Gy divided in four weekly fractions of 9 Gy; the median survival for dogs with pulmonary metastases was 21 months (Brearley *et al.*, 1999). Advanced non-resectable thyroid carcinoma with tumour-related clinical signs, with or without distant metastases, is associated with a shorter survival time (Tsimbas *et al.*, 2019).

Radioactive iodine

^{131}I is an effective treatment modality for dogs with unresectable FTC (Adams *et al.*, 1995; Worth *et al.*, 2005; Turrel *et al.*, 2006). ^{131}I has the unique ability to target thyroid tumour tissue regardless of its location. However, treatment efficacy is highly dependent on sufficient uptake by the primary tumour and its metastases, so scintigraphy is mandatory prior to ^{131}I therapy for adequate case selection. Tumours causing hyperthyroidism are expected to have a high uptake of ^{131}I and many euthyroid dogs with FTC also constitute good candidates. Normal to increased scintigraphic uptake has been described in 69% of dogs with thyroid tumours and 79% of dogs with FTC (Campos *et al.*, 2014a; van den Berg *et al.*, 2020). Uptake is homogeneous in 16% of canine thyroid tumours while 84% have heterogeneous or variable uptake (van den Berg *et al.*, 2020). This could be related to loss of cellular differentiation in parts of the tumour, tumour necrosis or haemorrhage, and could limit treatment efficacy. In 13–28% of dogs, more than one ^{131}I treatment is necessary to achieve tumour control (Worth *et al.*, 2005; Turrel *et al.*, 2006). Other limitations of ^{131}I therapy include its limited availability and the need for high ^{131}I doses (410–7,100 MBq), which could necessitate a long hospitalization period depending on each country's regulations.

A study in 39 dogs treated with ^{131}I therapy reported a median survival time for dogs with stage II or III disease (28 months) that was significantly longer than for dogs with stage IV disease (12 months) (Turrel *et al.*, 2006). In 12 of the 39 dogs, the tumour became resectable 3–6 weeks after ^{131}I therapy and the dogs also underwent thyroidectomy. In another study, the median survival time reported for 32 dogs treated with ^{131}I as sole therapy (30 months) was similar to that for 11 dogs treated with ^{131}I as an adjunct to surgery (34 months) (Worth *et al.*, 2005). Thyroid function does not seem to be a prognostic factor.

Fatal myelosuppression is an important complication described in 3 of 39 (8%) dogs treated with ^{131}I (Turrel *et al.*, 2006). Although no specific factors could be associated with its development, all affected dogs had received higher doses of ^{131}I on a bodyweight basis (200, 210 and 220 MBq/kg) compared with the median dose (160 MBq/kg) (Turrel *et al.*, 2006).

Radiation therapy *versus* radioactive iodine

Although it is difficult to compare different studies, extrapolation from survival curves detailed by Worth *et al.* (2005) would indicate 70% 1-year and 34% 3-year survival rates for dogs treated by ^{131}I alone. This suggests that external beam radiation likely provides a longer progression-free interval and is superior to ^{131}I in the longer term (Théon *et al.*, 2000). External beam radiotherapy may provide a more uniform radiation dosage to the entire tumour compared with ^{131}I, which is limited in its distribution to functional FTC cells and those within 2 mm of functional cells (Worth *et al.*, 2005). With ^{131}I, tumour heterogeneity perhaps leads to areas of the tumour that may not be exposed to adequate radiation to ensure a more uniform cell death. Furthermore, ^{131}I therapy can only be expected to adequately treat dogs with FTC.

Chemotherapy

The role of chemotherapy in the treatment of canine thyroid carcinoma has not been fully elucidated (Barber, 2007). Partial responses are described in 44–54% of dogs undergoing chemotherapy and median survival times range from 3 to 8 months (Jeglum and Whereat, 1983; Fineman *et al.*, 1998). In 16 dogs with thyroid carcinoma, the use of doxorubicin, either as sole therapy or as an adjunct to surgery, was associated with a median survival time of 8 months (Jeglum and Whereat, 1983). Dogs presenting with distant metastases at the start of treatment (n = 5) had a median survival time of only 4 months. The effect of cisplatin has also been reported in 13 dogs with thyroid carcinoma, 8 of which had tumours larger than 5 cm (Fineman *et al.*, 1998). One dog went into complete remission, six dogs had partial remissions, three had stable disease and three had progressive disease. The uncensored median survival time was 3 months.

To date, no study has shown a clear benefit for the use of chemotherapy as an adjunct to surgery. In a retrospective study including 44 dogs with surgically excised thyroid carcinoma, the median survival time of dogs undergoing thyroidectomy alone (510 days; n = 28) was not significantly different than that of dogs also receiving adjuvant chemotherapy (518 days; n = 16) (Nadeau and Kitchell, 2011). Similar results have been reported in other studies (Castillo *et al.*, 2016). However, the effect of chemotherapy has only been evaluated in retrospective studies with relatively low numbers of dogs, and it seems reasonable to consider it in dogs at risk for metastatic disease after surgery, such as dogs with microscopic or macroscopic evidence of vascular invasion and dogs with bilateral disease (see 'Prognosis', below).

Other treatments

The use of toceranib phosphate, a receptor tyrosine kinase inhibitor that targets VEGFR, platelet-derived growth factor receptor (PDGFR), Kit, colony stimulating factor-1 receptor (CSF-1R) and FMS-like Tyrosine Kinase 3 (FLT-3), was initially reported in 15 dogs with thyroid carcinoma and showed clinical benefit in 12 cases (80%), with 4 experiencing partial remission and 8 stable disease (London *et al.*, 2012). These results were confirmed in a recent study including 42 dogs with thyroid carcinoma, 26 of which had naive disease and 16 of which had received prior therapy (Sheppard-Olivares *et al.*, 2020). The median starting dosage was 2.8 mg/kg. At the time of toceranib initiation, 18 of 26 dogs (69.2%) with naive disease and 10 of 16 dogs (62.5%) receiving prior therapy had presumed pulmonary metastases. Clinical benefit (complete remission, partial remission or stable disease) was observed in 23 of 26 dogs (88.5%) with naive disease and 12 of 16 dogs (75%) receiving prior therapy. Median progression-free interval and median survival time for treatment-naive dogs were 6.8 months and 18.5 months, respectively, and those for dogs previously treated were 33.4 months and 35.6 months, respectively. The objective response of thyroid tumours to toceranib phosphate suggests that specific receptor tyrosine kinases targeted by toceranib may be dysregulated. Adverse effects included primarily diarrhoea, anorexia, vomiting and neutropenia.

One study evaluated the use of retinoic acid for 6 months (n = 15) as an adjuvant treatment after thyroidectomy and compared it with adjuvant doxorubicin every 3 weeks for six complete cycles (n = 12) and thyroidectomy alone (n = 10) (Castillo *et al.*, 2016). In this study, time to recurrence was significantly longer in dogs receiving retinoic acid compared with dogs receiving chemotherapy or no adjuvant treatment.

In humans and dogs, FTC cells contain TSH receptors and endogenous TSH may stimulate the growth of neoplastic cells, contributing to tumour progression (Verschueren *et al.*, 1992). In humans with high-risk differentiated FTC, the benefit of TSH-suppressive therapy by supplementing thyroid hormones is well established, and many veterinary surgeons (veterinarians) recommend it routinely in the treatment of canine FTC. In one retrospective study, 13 of 28 dogs with differentiated FTC undergoing thyroidectomy also received levothyroxine supplementation lifelong after surgery but it did not appear to affect survival (Campos *et al.*, 2014a). For the moment, there is no clear evidence supporting the use of TSH-suppressive therapy in dogs with thyroid tumours. However, given the strong evidence in humans with differentiated FTC and the lack of large veterinary studies, its use should still be considered.

Anti thyroid drugs are not recommended as a first-line treatment for hyperthyroidism in dogs with thyroid tumours as this condition typically resolves after treatment of the underlying neoplasia. However, in selected cases, anti thyroid drugs may be indicated to specifically treat the hyperthyroid state. Examples include untreated dogs with clinical signs of hyperthyroidism and dogs with tumour recurrence/progression following thyroidectomy, radiation therapy or ^{131}I therapy. In such cases, thiamazole (methimazole) can be started at dosages similar to those used in hyperthyroid cats (2.5–5 mg q12h) with subsequent increases as needed to control clinical signs and T4 concentrations. If increasing doses of thiamazole or carbimazole are insufficient to control hyperthyroidism, adding an iodine-restricted diet has been shown to be successful (Looney and Wakshlag, 2017).

Prognosis

When considering factors associated with local invasiveness at the time of diagnosis, tumour size, tumour fixation at palpation, ectopic location, histological type (follicular

cell) and Ki-67 labelling index have all been implicated (Carver *et al.*, 1995; Campos *et al.*, 2014a). In dogs, MTC appears to be less locally invasive and more amenable to surgical resection than FTC (Carver *et al.*, 1995; Campos *et al.*, 2014a). However, following thyroidectomy, outcome is comparable. No factors have been specifically associated with local recurrence after complete thyroidectomy.

Increased tumour size has historically been associated with a higher prevalence of metastatic disease. However, an association between tumour size and prognosis following thyroidectomy has not been consistently found (Leav *et al.*, 1976; Klein *et al.*, 1995; Campos *et al.*, 2014a). Only recently, in a study including 156 dogs undergoing unilateral thyroidectomy for thyroid carcinoma, were tumour size and mitotic index associated with progression-free interval (Reagan *et al.*, 2019). In the same study, only mitotic index and perioperative complications were associated with survival time. Macroscopic and microscopic evidence of vascular invasion are independent predictors of disease-free survival (Figures 20.8 and 20.9) (Campos *et al.*, 2014a). Following thyroidectomy, dogs with macroscopic or microscopic evidence of vascular invasion had a significantly shorter disease-free survival (median 2.5 months and 12 months, respectively) compared with dogs without macroscopic or microscopic evidence of vascular invasion (median 23 months and 29 months, respectively) (Campos *et al.*, 2014a).

Survival in dogs undergoing bilateral thyroidectomy for discrete mobile thyroid carcinoma is comparable to what has been described for dogs with unilateral disease (Théon *et al.*, 2000; Nadeau and Kitchell, 2011; Tuohy *et al.*, 2012).

No prognostic factors for PFS have been demonstrated in dogs with unresectable differentiated thyroid carcinoma and no metastases treated with radiation therapy (Théon *et al.*, 2000). However, dogs with bilateral disease had a 16 times higher risk of developing metastases after radiation therapy and dogs with no evidence of tumour progression after treatment had a 15 times lower risk of developing metastases. Although the presence of metastatic disease very likely has an impact on prognosis, dogs with unresectable thyroid carcinoma and distant metastases can also enjoy prolonged survival when treated with palliative-intent hypofractionated radiation therapy (Brearley *et al.*, 1999). However, median survival is adversely affected if the dogs have advanced disease with tumour-related clinical signs (Tsimbas *et al.*, 2019). For dogs treated with ^{131}I, median

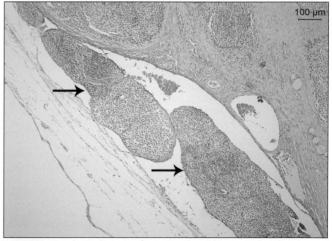

20.9 Histological image of a canine thyroid tumour showing vascular invasion (arrowed).

survival time with local or regional disease (stage II or III) is significantly longer than that of dogs with distant metastases at diagnosis (Turrel *et al.*, 2006). No other factors were found to be associated with survival. Survival times are similar in dogs with invasive thyroid carcinomas treated with ^{131}I alone or as an adjunct to surgery (Worth *et al.*, 2005). This suggests that radioiodine therapy is likely more important for longevity than surgery in this subset of dogs.

The median survival for dogs with thyroid tumours that remain untreated is approximately 3 months (Worth *et al.*, 2005; Campos, 2014).

References and further reading

Adams WH, Walker MA, Daniel GB, Petersen MG and Legendre AM (1995) Treatment of differentiated thyroid carcinoma in 7 dogs utilizing [131]I. *Veterinary Radiology & Ultrasound* **36**, 417–424

Amores-Fuster I, Cripps P and Blackwood L (2017) Post-radiotherapy hypothyroidism in dogs treated for thyroid carcinomas. *Veterinary and Comparative Oncology* **15**, 247–251

Barber LG (2007) Thyroid tumors in dogs and cats. *Veterinary Clinics of North America: Small Animal Practice* **37**, 755–773

Beatrice L, Boretti FS, Sieber-Ruckstuhl NS et al. (2018) Concurrent endocrine neoplasias in dogs and cats: a retrospective study (2004–2014). *Veterinary Record* **182**, 323

Benjamin SA, Saunders WJ, Lee AC et al. (1997) Non-neoplastic and neoplastic thyroid disease in beagles irradiated during prenatal and postnatal development. *Radiation Research* **147**, 422–430

Benjamin SA, Stephens LC, Hamilton BF et al. (1996) Associations between lymphocytic thyroiditis, hypothyroidism, and thyroid neoplasia in beagles. *Veterinary Pathology* **33**, 486–494

Brearley MJ, Hayes AM and Murphy S (1999) Hypofractionated radiation therapy for invasive thyroid carcinoma in dogs: a retrospective analysis of survival. *Journal of Small Animal Practice* **40**, 206–210

Brodey RS and Kelly DF (1968) Thyroid neoplasms in the dog. A clinicopathologic study of fifty-seven cases. *Cancer* **22**, 406–416

Broome MR, Peterson ME, Kemppainen RJ, Parker VJ and Richter KP (2015) Exogenous thyrotoxicosis in dogs attributable to consumption of all-meat commercial dog food or treats containing excessive thyroid hormone: 14 cases (2008–2013). *Journal of the American Veterinary Medical Association* **246**, 105–111

Broome MR, Peterson ME and Walker JR (2014) Clinical features and treatment outcomes of 41 dogs with sublingual ectopic thyroid neoplasia. *Journal of Veterinary Internal Medicine* **28**, 1560–1568

Campos M (2014) *Pathogenesis and treatment of canine thyroid tumors*. Thesis, Faculty of Veterinary Medicine, Ghent University

Campos M, Ducatelle R, Rutteman G et al. (2014a) Clinical, pathologic, and immunohistochemical prognostic factors in dogs with thyroid carcinoma. *Journal of Veterinary Internal Medicine* **28**, 1805–1813

Campos M, Kool MMJ, Daminet S et al. (2014b) Upregulation of the PI3K/Akt pathway in the tumorigenesis of canine thyroid carcinoma. *Journal of Veterinary Internal Medicine* **28**, 1814–1823

Carver JR, Kapatkin A and Patnaik AK (1995) A comparison of medullary thyroid carcinoma and thyroid adenocarcinoma in dogs: a retrospective study of 38 cases. *Veterinary Surgery* **24**, 315–319

Castillo V, Pessina P, Hall P et al. (2016) Post-surgical treatment of thyroid carcinoma in dogs with retinoic acid 9 cis improves patient outcome. *Open Veterinary Journal* **6**, 6–14

Devilee P, Van Leeuwen IS, Voesten A et al. (1994) The canine p53 gene is subject to somatic mutations in thyroid carcinoma. *Anticancer Research* **14**, 2039–2046

Fineman LS, Hamilton TA, de Gortari A and Bonney P (1998) Cisplatin chemotherapy for treatment of thyroid carcinoma in dogs: 13 cases. *Journal of the American Animal Hospital Association* **34**, 109–112

Frederick AN, Pardo AD, Schmiedt CW et al. (2020) Outcomes for dogs with functional thyroid tumors treated by surgical excision alone. *Journal of the American Veterinary Medical Association* **256**, 444–448

Harari J, Patterson JS and Rosenthal RC (1986) Clinical and pathologic features of thyroid tumors in 26 dogs. *Journal of the American Veterinary Medical Association* **188**, 1160–1164

Jeglum KA and Whereat A (1983) Chemotherapy of canine thyroid carcinoma. *Compendium on Continuing Education for the Practicing Veterinarian* **5**, 96–98

Kiupel M, Capen C, Miller M et al. (2008) *Histological Classification of Tumors of the Endocrine System of Domestic Animals*. Armed Forces Institute of Pathology, Washington, DC

Klein MK, Powers BE, Withrow SJ et al. (1995) Treatment of thyroid carcinoma in dogs by surgical resection alone: 20 cases (1981–1989). *Journal of the American Veterinary Medical Association* **206**, 1007–1009

Köhler B, Stengel C and Neiger R (2012) Dietary hyperthyroidism in dogs. *Journal of Small Animal Practice* **53**, 182–184

Lane AE and Wyatt KM (2012) Paraneoplastic hypercalcemia in a dog with thyroid carcinoma. *Canadian Veterinary Journal* **53**, 1101–1104

Leav I, Schiller AL, Rijnberk A, Legg MA and Kinderen PJ (1976) Adenomas and carcinomas of the canine and feline thyroid. *American Journal of Pathology* **83**, 61–122

Lee JJ, Larsson C, Lui WO, Höög A and Von Euler H (2006) A dog pedigree with familial medullary thyroid cancer. *International Journal of Oncology* **29**, 1173–1182

Liptak JM (2007) Canine thyroid carcinoma. *Clinical Techniques in Small Animal Practice* **22**, 75–81

London C, Mathie T, Stingle N et al. (2012) Preliminary evidence for biologic activity of toceranib phosphate (Palladia®) in solid tumours. *Veterinary and Comparative Oncology* **10**, 194–205

Looney A and Wakshlag J (2017) Dietary management of hyperthyroidism in a dog. *Journal of the American Animal Hospital Association* **53**, 111–118

Marks SL, Koblik PD, Hornof WJ and Feldman EC (1994) [99mTc]-pertechnetate imaging of thyroid tumors in dogs: 29 cases (1980–1992). *Journal of the American Veterinary Medical Association* **204**, 756–760

Milovancev M, Wilson DM, Monnet E and Seguin B (2014) Partial resection of the hyoid apparatus during surgical treatment of ectopic thyroid carcinomas in dogs: 5 cases (2011–2013). *Journal of the American Veterinary Medical Association* **245**, 1319–1324

Nadeau ME and Kitchell BE (2011) Evaluation of the use of chemotherapy and other prognostic variables for surgically excised canine thyroid carcinoma with and without metastasis. *Canadian Veterinary Journal* **52**, 994–998

Owen L (1980) *TNM Classification of Tumours in Domestic Animals*. World Health Organization, Geneva

Pack L, Roberts RE, Dawson SD and Dookwah HD (2001) Definitive radiation therapy for infiltrative thyroid carcinoma in dogs. *Veterinary Radiology & Ultrasound* **42**, 471–474

Peterson ME, Randolph JF, Zaki FA and Heath H 3rd (1982) Multiple endocrine neoplasia in a dog. *Journal of the American Veterinary Medical Association* **180**, 1476–1478

Reagan JK, Selmic LE, Fallon C et al. (2019) Complications and outcomes associated with unilateral thyroidectomy in dogs with naturally occurring thyroid tumors: 156 cases (2003–2015). *Journal of the American Veterinary Medical Association* **255**, 926–932

Scruggs JL, Nobrega-Lee M, Fry MM and Applegate R (2015) Hypercalcemia and parathyroid hormone-related peptide expression in a dog with thyroid carcinoma and histiocytic sarcoma. *Veterinary Clinical Pathology* **44**, 249–252

Shadwick SR, Ridgway MD and Kubier A (2013) Thyrotoxicosis in a dog induced by the consumption of feces from a levothyroxine-supplemented housemate. *Canadian Veterinary Journal* **54**, 987–989

Sheppard-Olivares S, Bello NM, Wood E et al. (2020) Toceranib phosphate in the treatment of canine thyroid carcinoma: 42 cases (2009-2018). *Veterinary and Comparative Oncology* **18**, 7–13

Soler Arias EAS, Castillo VA, Trigo RH and Aristarain MEC (2016) Multiple endocrine neoplasia similar to human subtype 2A in a dog: medullary thyroid carcinoma, bilateral pheochromocytoma and parathyroid adenoma. *Open Veterinary Journal* **6**, 165–171

Taeymans O, Penninck DG and Peters RM (2013) Comparison between clinical, ultrasound, CT, MRI, and pathology findings in dogs presented for suspected thyroid carcinoma. *Veterinary Radiology & Ultrasound* **54**, 61–70

Théon AP, Marks SL, Feldman ES and Griffey S (2000) Prognostic factors and patterns of treatment failure in dogs with unresectable differentiated thyroid carcinomas treated with megavoltage irradiation. *Journal of the American Veterinary Medical Association* **216**, 1775–1779

Thompson EJ, Stirtzinger T, Lumsden JH and Little PB (1980) Fine needle aspiration cytology in the diagnosis of canine thyroid carcinoma. *Canadian Veterinary Journal* **21**, 186–188

Tsimbas K, Turek M, Christensen N, Vail DM and Forrest L (2019) Short survival time following palliative-intent hypofractionated radiotherapy for non-resectable canine thyroid carcinoma: a retrospective analysis of 20 dogs. *Veterinary Radiology & Ultrasound* **60**, 93–99

Tuohy JL, Worley DR and Withrow SJ (2012) Outcome following simultaneous bilateral thyroid lobectomy for treatment of thyroid gland carcinoma in dogs: 15 cases (1994–2010). *Journal of the American Veterinary Medical Association* **241**, 95–103

Turrel JM, McEntee MC, Burke BP and Page RL (2006) Sodium iodide I 131 treatment of dogs with nonresectable thyroid tumors: 39 cases (1990–2003). *Journal of the American Veterinary Medical Association* **229**, 542–548

Urie BK, Russell DS, Kisseberth WC and London CA (2012) Evaluation of expression and function of vascular endothelial growth factor receptor 2, platelet derived growth factor receptors-alpha and -beta, KIT, and RET in canine apocrine gland anal sac adenocarcinoma and thyroid carcinoma. *BMC Veterinary Research* **8**, 67

van den Berg MF, Daminet S, Stock E et al. (2020) Planar and single-photon emission computed tomography imaging in dogs with thyroid tumors: 68 cases. *Journal of Veterinary Internal Medicine* **34**, 2651–2659

Verschueren CP, Rutteman GR, Kuipers-Dijkshoorn NJ et al. (1991) Flow-cytometric DNA ploidy analysis in primary and metastatic canine thyroid carcinomas. *Anticancer Research* **11**, 1755–1761

Verschueren CP, Rutteman GR, Vos JH, Van Dijk JE and de Bruin TWA (1992) Thyrotrophin receptors in normal and neoplastic (primary and metastatic) canine thyroid tissue. *Journal of Endocrinology* **132**, 461–468

Worth A, Zuber R and Hocking M (2005) Radioiodide ^{131}I therapy for the treatment of canine thyroid carcinoma. *Australian Veterinary Journal* **83**, 208–214

Wucherer KL and Wilke V (2005) Thyroid cancer in dogs: an update based on 638 cases (1995–2005). *Journal of the American Animal Hospital Association* **46**, 249–254

Chapter 21

Feline hypothyroidism

Sylvie Daminet and Mark E. Peterson

Introduction

Feline hypothyroidism is distinct from the canine condition and not directly comparable. Most commonly, clinicians are faced with iatrogenic hypothyroidism in cats resulting from overzealous treatment of hyperthyroidism. Naturally occurring spontaneous hypothyroidism (congenital or adult-onset) is also described and, although still considered rather uncommon, its true frequency remains unknown and is undoubtedly underestimated. Indeed, the lack of awareness amongst the veterinary profession, combined with greater familiarity with canine hypothyroidism and inappropriate extrapolation to cats, most likely contributes to this underestimation, especially of the naturally occurring disease.

Aetiology

The cause of hypothyroidism in cats is often suggested by signalment (e.g. young age in congenital hypothyroidism), medical history (e.g. treatment of hyperthyroidism or head trauma), and physical examination (e.g. palpable goitre, dwarfism).

Congenital hypothyroidism

In general, congenital primary hypothyroidism can be classified according to its pathogenesis, as thyroid dyshormonogenesis (a defect in the biosynthesis of thyroid hormones) or thyroid dysmorphogenesis (thyroid hypoplasia or aplasia). Both forms are well recognized in humans and usually inherited as autosomal recessive traits. There are several reports of congenital hypothyroidism in cats, mostly as single case reports or small case series. Most affected cats suffer from thyroid dyshormonogenesis (Sjollema *et al.*, 1991; Jones *et al.*, 1992; Mazrier *et al.*, 2003; Peterson, 2019; Iturriaga *et al.*, 2020). Dyshormonogenesis, due to defective thyroid peroxidase activity and impaired iodine organification, has been described in related Domestic Shorthaired and Abyssinian cats (Sjollema *et al.*, 1991; Jones *et al.*, 1992). Thyroid dysmorphogenesis has also been documented in related cats (Traas *et al.*, 2008). All of these reports suggest an autosomal recessive mode of inheritance.

In addition, hypothyroidism as a result of thyrotropin (thyroid-stimulating hormone (TSH)) resistance, which may have resulted from a gene mutation affecting the sodium–iodide symporter, has been suggested in a family of Japanese cats (Tanase *et al.*, 1991). Hypothalamic and pituitary forms of congenital hypothyroidism (central hypothyroidism) have not been well documented in cats.

Spontaneous adult-onset hypothyroidism

Spontaneous adult-onset hypothyroidism is currently considered extremely rare in cats. The relatively mild clinical signs combined with infrequent routine screening and a lack of awareness of this disease probably contribute to its low recognition. Reports of well documented cases are scarce. Lymphocytic thyroiditis similar to that observed in dogs (see Chapter 18), idiopathic atrophy and goitrous hypothyroidism have all been reported in cats (Rand *et al.*, 1993; Blois *et al.*, 2010; Peterson, 2015; Peterson *et al.*, 2018, 2019). More cats need to be diagnosed and studied extensively (including histopathology of the thyroid gland and scintigraphy) to clarify and understand the true pathophysiology of spontaneous adult-onset feline hypothyroidism.

Iatrogenic hypothyroidism

Iatrogenic hypothyroidism is a well recognized complication of all available treatment options for hyperthyroidism. It can result from an overdose of anti-thyroid medication, bilateral thyroidectomy or radioactive iodine (^{131}I) therapy.

The prevalence of drug-induced iatrogenic hypothyroidism in cats has probably been underestimated in the past as, in most cats, it is not associated with obvious clinical signs of hypothyroidism (Aldridge *et al.*, 2015; Peterson, 2019). Keeping the impact of hypothyroidism on kidney function in mind, detection of iatrogenic hypothyroidism, even if subclinical, is important.

After unilateral thyroidectomy, transient iatrogenic hypothyroidism is common as total thyroxine (T4) concentrations often decrease to below the reference interval within weeks to months. Most cats do not develop clinical signs of hypothyroidism and total T4 concentrations usually normalize spontaneously. Stimulation of the contralateral lobe serves to compensate for the thyroid tissue removed. With bilateral thyroidectomy, permanent iatrogenic hypothyroidism is expected, although in many cases remaining thyroid tissue might be sufficient to restore euthyroidism.

Iatrogenic hypothyroidism following ^{131}I therapy is relatively common, can be permanent or transient, overt or subclinical and, most importantly, may or may not require levothyroxine replacement therapy. Cats with bilateral disease and those treated with higher doses are predisposed to the development of hypothyroidism after treatment with [131]I. Over the last decade, there has been a tendency towards lower ^{131}I doses, which should lead to a decreased prevalence of iatrogenic hypothyroidism.

Iatrogenic central hypothyroidism is expected following hypophysectomy. Usually, cats undergoing such surgery are pre-emptively treated with levothyroxine prior to its overt development (see Chapter 13).

Clinical features

The most important clinical features observed with iatrogenic, congenital and spontaneous adult-onset hypothyroidism are outlined in Figure 21.1 and illustrated in Figures 21.2 and 21.3.

Although some signs are similar in hypothyroid dogs and cats, there are major differences that must be considered. Firstly, few hypothyroid cats, irrespective of underlying cause, develop obvious alopecia. Furthermore, inappetence is more likely, as is profound mental dullness. Kittens with congenital hypothyroidism can also develop severe constipation and, like dogs, have obvious dwarfism. In contrast, clinical signs can be rather discrete in adult-onset hypothyroidism.

Congenital hypothyroidism

In kittens, congenital hypothyroidism is likely greatly under-recognized, especially since routine screening is not done as it is in humans. Many of the signs observed in adult-onset hypothyroidism can also be present in affected kittens. However, thyroid hormones are essential for normal postnatal development of the skeletal and nervous systems; therefore, congenital hypothyroidism is characterized by disproportionate dwarfism and neurological abnormalities.

Typically, affected kittens appear normal at birth but a decrease in growth rate, compared with their littermates, becomes evident by 2 months of age. Disproportionate dwarfism can develop over the next few months. This is characterized by a large broad head, small ears, a round body and short neck and limbs. However, not all hypothyroid kittens exhibit disproportionate dwarfism. Most likely, the severity of the clinical signs (including the presence of dwarfism) is related to the completeness of the block in thyroid hormone secretion.

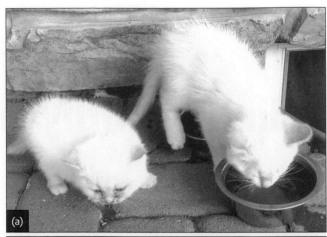

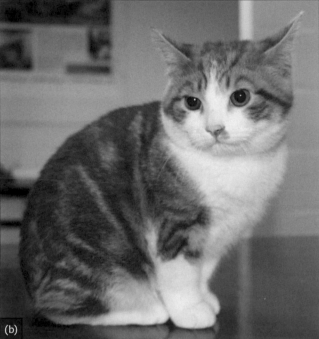

21.2 (a) Kitten (on the left) with congenital hypothyroidism with its normal-sized littermate (on the right). Note the disproportionate dwarfism (large head and short limbs) in the affected kitten. (b) Young adult cat with congenital hypothyroidism. In this case, the characteristics of disproportionate dwarfism are rather discrete (short limbs) and were not recognized by the owners. In some cats, partial block of thyroid hormone synthesis can lead to more discrete dwarfism and resulting delayed recognition.

(a, Reproduced from Feldman et al. (2019), Feline Endocrinology, Edra, with permission from the publisher)

Clinical sign	Iatrogenic hypothyroidism	Congenital hypothyroidism	Spontaneous adult-onset hypothyroidism
Lethargy	+	+ (even mental dullness)	+ (even mental dullness)
Weight gain or obesity	+	+	+
Inappetence	+	+	+*
Constipation	+	+* (even megacolon)	+
Goitre	– or +	possible	–
Disproportionate dwarfism	–	+*	–
Delayed closure of growth plates (on X-ray)	–	+*	–
Dermatological signs (especially seborrhoea and hairs that are easy to epilate)	+	+	+*

21.1 The most important clinical signs observed with iatrogenic, congenital and spontaneous adult-onset hypothyroidism. Clinical features can be mild or severe in all three forms of hypothyroidism or even absent, especially in spontaneous adult-onset cases. * = key feature; + = usually present; – = absent.

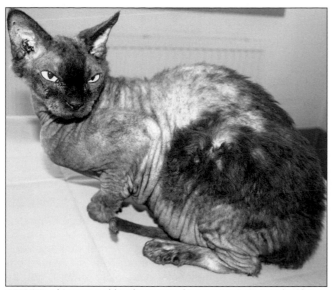

21.3 This 5-year-old male neutered Devon Rex presented with a history of lethargy, mental dullness and inappetence. The cat also had diabetes mellitus. This cat had very low circulating total thyroxine concentration, as well as an increased thyroid-stimulating hormone concentration, confirming primary hypothyroidism. The hair coat was seborrhoeic and easily epilated. Note the bilateral ceruminous otitis.
(Courtesy of E. Mercier and S. Daminet)

Additionally, affected kittens are generally mentally dull and may suffer from severe recurrent episodes of constipation. Occasionally, dullness and retarded growth may go unrecognized by the owners, who present their cat because of recurrent constipation. Seizures were reported as a major problem in two littermates affected by congenital hypothyroidism (Traas et al., 2008).

Although hair is usually present all over the body and obvious alopecia is not present, the hair coat consists mainly of undercoat with few guard hairs. The teeth are underdeveloped, and delayed tooth eruption and replacement of deciduous teeth is frequently observed. Hypothermia, bradycardia and palpable goitre (especially with organification defects) may be detected. With primary congenital hypothyroidism, the loss of normal negative feedback inhibition on the pituitary cells leads to increased TSH concentrations. In cats with thyroid dysmorphogenesis, little to no thyroid tissue is present to respond to this excessive TSH, and the thyroid gland will not be palpable. In contrast, in cats with thyroid dyshormonogenesis, the thyroid follicular cells remain intact despite their inability to produce adequate thyroid hormone concentrations. In these cats, the unrelenting stimulation of intact thyroid follicular cells by the high TSH concentrations results in thyroid hyperplasia, enlargement of the intact thyroid gland and clinically palpable goitre. Interestingly, the development of a palpable goitre takes time and may even be delayed in onset. In one family of affected kittens, goitre was not palpable in the first weeks of life but could be readily palpated at the age of 5–6 months (Jones et al., 1992).

Survival of untreated affected kittens depends largely on the aetiology of the congenital hypothyroidism. It is likely that many affected kittens die undiagnosed as part of 'fading kitten syndrome' or are euthanized because of suspected idiopathic megacolon or neurological disease before a definitive diagnosis is reached. Affected kittens can die within a few months. However, kittens suffering from a partial thyroid peroxidase activity defect can live to become adult cats without obvious clinical signs of disease. As clinicians become more aware that congenital hypothyroidism does occur in kittens and adolescent cats, its recognized prevalence will increase.

Spontaneous adult-onset hypothyroidism

Some cats are asymptomatic and therefore only diagnosed after a routine annual screening for hyperthyroidism is performed. Hair coat changes, lethargy and inappetence are the major clinical signs observed. Lethargy and inappetence can become severe over time. Dermatological signs are characterized by hypotrichosis, a dull, dry and unkempt hair coat (with possible matting), and seborrhoea sicca. Alopecia of the pinnae can develop in some cats. The hair coat is easily epilated and poor regrowth after clipping is possible. Hypothermia and bradycardia may be additional findings on physical examination. A palpable goitre is possible in cases of goitrous hypothyroidism. Obesity and weight gain are also important owner complaints. Many affected cats have concurrent chronic kidney disease (CKD).

Figure 21.4 summarizes the clinical signs and physical examination findings in 12 adult cats with naturally occurring primary hypothyroidism (Peterson, 2019).

Iatrogenic hypothyroidism

Although a recent or current treatment for hyperthyroidism is obvious, several factors can hamper diagnosis of iatrogenic hypothyroidism. Clinical signs are often mild or even absent. For example, half of the cats treated with ^{131}I do not have obvious clinical signs of hypothyroidism at the time of diagnosis. Weight gain and decreased activity can also easily be attributed to successful treatment of hyperthyroidism. Further, when present, clinical signs tend to develop gradually. Additionally, the most common owner complaints are polyuria and polydipsia due to development of post-treatment azotaemia, leading to a suspicion of CKD rather than iatrogenic hypothyroidism.

Clinical feature or finding	Number of cats	Prevalence
Primary reason for initial work-up by referring clinician		
Signs of hypothyroidism	7	58%
Routine monitoring for hyperthyroidism	3	25%
Palpable thyroid nodules (goitre)	2	17%
Historical, owner-reported signs		
Hair coat changes	9	75%
Lethargy/mental dullness	8	67%
Weight gain	6	50%
Polyuria and polydipsia	5	42%
Poor appetite	3	25%
Cold intolerance	2	17%
Physical examination findings		
Unkempt, dull coat	8	67%
Palpable goitre	7	58%
Overweight/obesity	6	50%
Dandruff, flaking dry skin	6	50%
Hair thinning/hypotrichosis	4	33%
Bradycardia (≤120 bpm)	1	8%

21.4 Clinical features of naturally occurring adult-onset primary hypothyroidism in 12 adult cats.
(Data from Peterson, 2019)

Diagnosis

The diagnosis of feline hypothyroidism can be challenging, regardless of the underlying cause. A presumptive diagnosis can be made based on a combination of compatible but often rather discrete clinical features and occasionally supportive abnormalities on routine clinicopathological analyses (anaemia and hypercholesterolaemia). Feline hypothyroidism should be confirmed by thyroid hormone testing and in some cases by thyroid scintigraphy. A number of thyroid function tests are available to aid in diagnosis. In most cats, the diagnosis of hypothyroidism relies largely on assessment of basal thyroid hormone analyses (i.e. serum total T4 and free T4), combined with serum TSH measurement.

As in dogs, total T4 can also be affected by many factors including assay technique, age, possibly certain drugs (although this is not evaluated as well in cats as in dogs) and, most importantly, non-thyroidal illness (NTI). For the latter, the more severe the systemic illness, the lower the total T4 concentration is expected to be. In conclusion, a decreased basal total T4 supports but does not equate to a definitive diagnosis of hypothyroidism.

The interpretation of free T4 concentration differs from that in dogs. In dogs, the use of free T4 by equilibrium dialysis (fT4d) has been shown to be of benefit as it has better specificity for the diagnosis of hypothyroidism compared with measurement of basal total T4 concentrations. However, a proportion of cats with non-thyroidal disease have increased, and a few have decreased, free T4 concentrations. This limits the use of free T4 in investigating hypothyroidism in cats. Non-equilibrium dialysis techniques for free T4 measurement are also available in cats; however, equilibrium dialysis is superior (Stammeleer et al., 2020).

In dogs with hypothyroidism, an increased serum TSH concentration confirms that the disease is primary (located within the thyroid gland). A specific assay for feline TSH measurement is not yet widely available. However, due to high homogeneity in TSH between the two species, the canine TSH (cTSH) assay can reliably be used in cats. The cTSH assay is useful in dogs but lacks diagnostic sensitivity, while in cats it is a much more sensitive diagnostic test. In cats, the upper limit of the reference interval is much lower than in dogs (typically 0.3–0.32 ng/ml (cats) versus 0.65–0.68 ng/ml (dogs)).

The use of the recombinant human TSH (rhTSH) stimulation test has been described in cats. Although it was evaluated in a limited number of cats, just as in dogs, it appears to be a valuable alternative to bovine TSH stimulation (Wakeling et al., 2020). This test is not for routine use but might offer added value in a research setting, or in practice when diagnosis remains unclear and scintigraphy is not readily available. The following protocol can be used to perform the rhTSH stimulation test in cats:

1. A blood sample is collected for basal total T4 measurement.
2. 25–50 µg rhTSH is administered intravenously.
3. A second blood sample is taken 6 hours later.

Recombinant human TSH vials can be aliquoted and stored frozen to make this test more affordable.

Thyroid scintigraphy using technetium-99m as pertechnetate ($^{99m}TcO_4^-$) has traditionally been used for the diagnosis of canine hypothyroidism and feline hyperthyroidism. As clinicians become more aware of feline hypothyroidism, it is likely to be used more as a tool for the diagnosis of feline hypothyroidism.

Congenital hypothyroidism
Routine laboratory features

Mild anaemia and/or hypercholesterolaemia can be observed in congenital hypothyroidism but are not consistently present. Due to of the limited number of reported cases, their exact prevalence remains unknown.

Thyroid hormone testing

In kittens and adolescent cats, a presumptive diagnosis of congenital hypothyroidism can be made on the basis of clinical features (e.g. dwarfism, mental dullness, epiphyseal dysgenesis) and low serum total T4 concentrations. However, a definitive diagnosis should not be based on a low total T4 alone, as many factors can also suppress serum total T4 concentrations, thus leading to a false-positive test result. In addition, the reference interval for serum total T4 may change as kittens age, and most laboratories have not established age-related reference intervals for thyroid hormone concentrations.

To confirm congenital hypothyroidism, serum total T4 (± fT4d) and TSH concentrations should be measured. The finding of low to low-normal total T4 concentrations (with or without low free T4) together with high concentrations of TSH confirms primary hypothyroidism. Demonstrating high TSH concentrations is the single most important endocrine test for diagnosis of feline hypothyroidism for two reasons: high TSH concentrations have been reported in all congenital hypothyroid cats in which TSH was measured, and increased values for TSH are not generally seen in cats with NTI (Peterson et al., 2020).

Diagnostic imaging

Radiography: As in dogs, radiography can be particularly useful to diagnose congenital hypothyroidism as the changes observed are pathognomonic. Radiographs demonstrate retarded skeletal development, particularly epiphyseal dysgenesis of vertebral bodies and long bones (Figure 21.5).

Thyroid scintigraphy: Thyroid scintigraphy using $^{99m}TcO_4^-$ is particularly useful to diagnose congenital hypothyroidism and can also help to differentiate dysmorphogenesis from dyshormonogenesis. In thyroid aplasia or hypoplasia, no thyroid tissue is visible on scintigraphy and thyroid uptake of the radioisotope is low or undetectable. In contrast, cats with dyshormonogenesis have an increased thyroidal uptake and both thyroid lobes are symmetrically enlarged. Scintigraphy with iodine-123 (^{123}I) can be a helpful diagnostic tool to further clarify the underlying mechanism in congenital hypothyroidism as it also allows assessment of the organification (incorporation of iodine) process, and not only the uptake of the tracer, as is the case with $^{99m}TcO_4^-$. In cases of dysmorphogenesis, an absence of uptake of ^{123}I is expected. Uptake of ^{123}I may be normal in cases with a thyroid peroxidase deficiency. However, organification is deficient and an abnormally rapid discharge of ^{123}I is observed after administration of perchlorate (perchlorate discharge test).

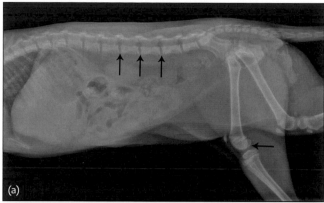

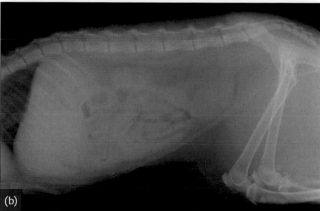

21.5 Radiographic changes in a cat with congenital hypothyroidism. (a) At the time of diagnosis (12 months of age), generalized delayed epiphyseal ossification (open physes) of the vertebrae and long bones was apparent (arrowed). Failure of fusion of the ischium, ilium and acetabulum, and poorly developed patellae were also noted. (b) After 1 year of treatment with levothyroxine, the ossification centres (physes) of all vertebrae, long bones and pelvis were closed and the patellae appeared normal.
(Reproduced from Feldman et al. (2019), Feline Endocrinology, Edra, with permission from the publisher.)

Spontaneous adult-onset hypothyroidism
Routine laboratory features

Besides a possible mild anaemia and occasionally hypercholesterolaemia, azotaemia appears to be the most striking abnormality observed in approximately half of the reported cases.

Many clinicians are aware of the complex interplay between thyroid and renal function that becomes apparent after treating hyperthyroidism. Decreased glomerular filtration rate and/or azotaemia is a well documented and potentially reversible complication of hypothyroidism in several species (see Chapter 6). Interestingly, some cats with primary spontaneous adult-onset hypothyroidism can also be presented with polyuria, polydipsia and other changes associated with CKD. With appropriate levothyroxine supplementation, the azotaemia can be reversible. It is important that clinicians recognize this essential relationship between renal and thyroid function and consider spontaneous hypothyroidism in the differential diagnosis of adult cats with CKD, especially in adolescent or middle-aged cats.

Thyroid hormone testing

Spontaneous primary hypothyroidism is extremely rare in cats and, by contrast, NTI is frequently observed. Hence, the diagnosis of spontaneous primary hypothyroidism should not be based solely on low to low-normal basal total I4 values but also on an increased serum TSH measurement (often >1.0 ng/ml). Indeed, all reported cats with spontaneous adult-onset hypothyroidism have extremely high serum TSH concentrations (7–40 times higher than the upper reference interval). Additionally, serum TSH concentration is the most specific diagnostic test for hypothyroidism: low serum total T4 and free T4 concentrations commonly develop in cats with NTI, including CKD, but high values for TSH have not been reported in these sick, euthyroid cats (Peterson et al., 2020).

In less straightforward cases, an rhTSH stimulation test might help distinguish true primary hypothyroidism from NTI, but its true added value has not yet been clearly documented in cats.

Thyroid scintigraphy

Thyroid scintigraphy is useful to both confirm the diagnosis of hypothyroidism and characterize the disease (atrophic *versus* goitrous subtypes) (Blois *et al.*, 2010; Peterson, 2015; Peterson *et al.*, 2018, 2019). Hypothyroid cats with thyroid atrophy have no detectable thyroid tissue on scintigraphy and minimal or absent thyroid uptake of the injected radionuclide, $^{99m}TcO_4^-$ (Figure 21.6). By contrast, high circulating TSH concentrations increase $^{99m}TcO_4^-$ uptake into the anatomically intact thyroid gland in untreated cats suffering from goitrous hypothyroidism,

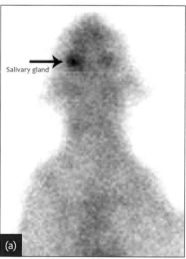

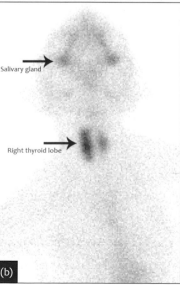

21.6 (a) Ventral view of a thyroid scintigraphic scan from the cat in Figure 21.3. Note the uptake of pertechnetate in the salivary glands and the absence of uptake in the cervical (thyroid) region. (b) This image shows the increased uptake of pertechnetate visible in the thyroid gland of a hyperthyroid cat.
(Courtesy of K. Peremans)

as evidenced by the intense ('hot') uptake of $^{99m}TcO_4^-$ into both thyroid lobes. Cats with goitrous hypothyroidism also have a marked increase in their measured thyroid mass or volume (2.5–8 times higher than the upper reference interval in one study; Peterson *et al.*, 2018).

Iatrogenic hypothyroidism

A few diagnostic pitfalls exist for iatrogenic hypothyroidism, despite the obvious history of previous or ongoing therapy for hyperthyroidism. Close monitoring using T4 and TSH measurements is recommended.

After therapy with ^{131}I, many cats develop a marked decrease in total T4 concentration, which is mostly transient, and a euthyroid state is usually expected after approximately 6 months. Up to 30% of cats may develop iatrogenic hypothyroidism following treatment with ^{131}I. Many of these cats do not show convincing clinical signs of hypothyroidism, but it can still adversely affect their kidney function. It is advisable to investigate iatrogenic hypothyroidism early in affected cats, particularly when there is evidence of impaired kidney function (Williams *et al.*, 2014). This underlines the importance of obtaining a definitive diagnosis in these cats, which is mainly achieved by monitoring total T4 or free T4 and TSH concentrations.

Routine laboratory features

Anaemia and hypercholesterolaemia are the classical haematological and serum biochemical markers of hypothyroidism, but these features are not common in cats with subclinical, or even overt, iatrogenic hypothyroidism (Peterson, 2019).

Thyroid hormone testing

In cats, a presumptive diagnosis of iatrogenic hypothyroidism can be made on the basis of a history of past or current treatment for hyperthyroidism (e.g. antithyroid drugs, surgical thyroidectomy or ^{131}I therapy) and low serum total T4 concentrations. However, the definitive diagnosis should not be based on a low total T4 concentration alone as it lacks diagnostic specificity and sensitivity; it is often low for other reasons and may be within the reference interval in some hypothyroid cats. A full thyroid hormone panel including total T4 and concurrent measurement of serum free T4 and TSH concentrations is recommended. The finding of decreased total (or free) T4 concentrations combined with high TSH concentrations confirms primary iatrogenic hypothyroidism (Peterson *et al.*, 2017). With a reported sensitivity for the diagnosis of iatrogenic hypothyroidism of 85–100% and a specificity of 57–98.5%, endogenous TSH measurement is a very useful test in cats (Peterson *et al.*, 2020; Stammeleer *et al.*, 2020; Wakeling *et al.*, 2020).

Thyroid scintigraphy

In cats treated with ^{131}I or surgery, follow-up thyroid scintigraphy can be helpful to determine the amount of residual functional thyroid tissue remaining after treatment.

Treatment

If obvious clinical signs of overt hypothyroidism are present, metabolic signs such as mental dullness and lethargy are the first to improve, generally within a few days of starting thyroid hormone replacement therapy. Weight loss and increased activity may also be noted within a few weeks, and an improvement in the hair coat (e.g. reduced shedding, dandruff, matted coat) should occur within 3–4 months of therapy.

With appropriate therapy, the prognosis is excellent for acquired hypothyroidism. For congenital hypothyroidism, the prognosis is somewhat more reserved, although many cats do well, and will largely depend on the underlying aetiology, severity of disease and age at diagnosis.

Many levothyroxine products (both brand name and generic) are available, although none are currently authorized for cats. Most of these are available as tablets, but an oral solution (Leventa 1 mg/ml) is marketed for use in dogs in many countries (not available in the USA). This liquid formulation is preferred over levothyroxine tablets by many owners since the small-volume formulation of the levothyroxine solution may be easier to administer or hide in the cat's food.

An initial levothyroxine dose of 20–40 µg/kg/day is recommended, with the goal of increasing serum total T4 concentrations and decreasing TSH concentrations back to their respective reference intervals.

Since the half-life of circulating T4 is very short in cats, it may be best to administer levothyroxine twice daily, but once-daily treatment works well in most cats. In addition, since food inhibits thyroid hormone absorption, levothyroxine is best given by mouth at least 1 hour before or 3 hours after feeding to ensure optimal absorption and consistent serum thyroid hormone concentrations. Since levothyroxine is best given on an empty stomach, bedtime dosing (at least 3 hours after the evening meal) works well for many owners. Depending on lifestyle, not all cat owners can easily follow these recommendations concerning the timing between the levothyroxine dose and feeding. If the levothyroxine dose must be given with food, it is important to standardize the time at which the levothyroxine dose is given in relation to feeding. Once a protocol is established, it should be used for each dosing period, especially on the day of thyroid hormone monitoring.

Other than food, many medications or supplements can also impair levothyroxine absorption, including calcium carbonate, aluminium hydroxide, sucralfate, and proton-pump inhibitors. If possible, a 4-hour separation time between administration of levothyroxine and other drugs is recommended. Reduced levothyroxine absorption has been reported in elderly human patients. Senior and geriatric cats may have a reduced ability to absorb nutrients from the gastrointestinal tract, which could play a role in levothyroxine malabsorption. Concurrent gastrointestinal disease can also impair levothyroxine absorption.

Further adjustment of therapy should be based on clinical response combined with total T4 and TSH therapeutic monitoring. Initial monitoring of post-pill serum total T4 and TSH concentrations is recommended 1 month after starting thyroid hormone therapy and then at 1- to 3-month intervals until the dose has stabilized. The levothyroxine dose is adjusted, as needed, to maintain near-normal concentrations of both serum T4 and TSH. Once the levothyroxine dose has been shown to be adequate, monitoring every 3–6 months thereafter is generally sufficient.

Congenital hypothyroidism

In congenital hypothyroidism, as the kitten grows and gains bodyweight, the dose of levothyroxine will have to be increased. Continued monitoring of post-pill serum total T4 and TSH concentrations is recommended at 2- to

3-month intervals during the first year of treatment, with dose adjustments made as needed to maintain near-normal concentrations of both serum total T4 and TSH.

Spontaneous hypothyroidism

In a recent study, serum TSH concentrations were used for long-term monitoring, with daily levothyroxine doses titrated to maintain TSH concentration within the reference interval while maintaining serum total T4 concentration within the reference interval. With that regime, cats needed a final daily levothyroxine dose of 100–200 μg/cat/day (16.7–55.6 μg/kg/day) (Peterson *et al.*, 2018). The median dose administered (31.3 μg/kg/day) was higher than that generally reported for thyroid hormone replacement in dogs (~20 μg/kg/day).

Treatment with levothyroxine improved or resolved clinical signs, when present, in all of the reported cats with spontaneous adult-onset hypothyroidism. Adequate thyroid hormone replacement also led to shrinkage of bilateral goitre when present; this is expected after lowering high serum TSH concentrations to within the reference interval, especially if TSH-induced diffuse thyroid hyperplasia was responsible for the goitre (Peterson, 2015; Peterson *et al.*, 2018.)

Iatrogenic hypothyroidism

If hypothyroidism is diagnosed in a hyperthyroid cat treated medically with an antithyroid drug, the daily dosage should be lowered to allow the serum total T4 concentration to increase back into the mid-normal range. On the other hand, if hypothyroidism has developed after treatment with ^{131}I or surgical thyroidectomy, then the clinician must decide whether to start treatment with thyroid hormone supplementation or to continue monitoring for remission of the hypothyroid state as the thyroid attempts to recover its normal function.

Most cats with confirmed overt hypothyroidism require lifelong thyroid hormone replacement therapy, whereas some treated cats, particularly those with subclinical hypothyroidism, will eventually go into remission.

Once thyroid hormone replacement therapy is initiated, cats need to be monitored to ensure that the daily levothyroxine dose is adequate and that overdosage does not develop. It is not possible to predict the final daily dose required in cats with iatrogenic hypothyroidism. Since most cats do not absorb levothyroxine well, overdosage is rare but when it does develop, the daily dose should be lowered. Many treated cats will require a slight increase in the initial daily levothyroxine dosage (e.g. from 150 μg to 200 μg), whereas a few may need a dramatic increase in daily levothyroxine dosage (up to 300–500 μg). As in the cats with naturally occurring hypothyroidism, cats with iatrogenic hypothyroidism tend to need a higher daily levothyroxine dose than generally required for hypothyroid dogs.

If hyperthyroid cats are closely monitored after treatment (i.e. by physical examination and serum total T4 and TSH concentrations), most cats with iatrogenic hypothyroidism will be diagnosed long before any obvious clinical features of hypothyroidism develop.

The most important routine serum biochemical parameter to follow after levothyroxine replacement for iatrogenic hypothyroidism is serum creatinine concentration. Many untreated older cats with iatrogenic hypothyroidism will develop mild to moderate azotaemia (IRIS stage 2 or 3 CKD). Of these, most will show improvement in their azotaemia as euthyroidism is restored (as documented by an increase in serum total T4 and a decrease in TSH concentrations) (Williams *et al.*, 2014; Peterson *et al.*, 2017). Even if the degree of azotaemia does not improve, adequate levothyroxine replacement tends to slow progression of the CKD and stabilize the azotaemia.

Since most hypothyroid cats will display few, if any, overt clinical signs, monitoring of serum total T4 and TSH concentrations is required to sufficiently judge the adequacy of thyroid hormone replacement therapy in these cats. Such laboratory monitoring is especially important given the wide variation in absorption of levothyroxine (and, therefore, the final daily dose) between individual cats.

Almost all cats treated on the basis of having severe (overt) persistent hypothyroidism, or new or worsening azotaemia, will need lifelong thyroid hormone replacement therapy. In some cats, it is possible for iatrogenic hypothyroidism to be transient, but most of those cats have mild, subclinical hypothyroidism and azotaemia is less common. If remission of hypothyroidism is suspected, levothyroxine therapy should be stopped for 1–2 weeks and serum total T4 and TSH measurements repeated; if reference interval concentrations are maintained without levothyroxine replacement, then the cat is euthyroid and does not require continued thyroid hormone supplementation.

Post-pill timing for levothyroxine monitoring

Hypothyroid cats receiving levothyroxine supplementation demonstrate an increase in circulating total T4 concentrations, which peaks only a few hours after treatment and then progressively declines until the next dose. If a regimen of twice-daily levothyroxine administration is used, then it is best to collect post-pill serum samples at the expected peak time (i.e. 4–6 hours after the morning dose of levothyroxine is given). Optimal peak serum total T4 concentrations are generally in the upper half of the reference interval (30–45 nmol/l); If peak post-pill serum T4 concentrations are adequate, high TSH concentrations should normalize. Peak serum T4 concentrations below 25 nmol/l are usually associated with very high serum TSH concentrations, indicating that an increase in dosage is needed or that levothyroxine administration should be changed to empty-stomach dosing, or both. Marked increases in peak total T4 concentrations into the hyperthyroid range are unnecessary, and the dose of levothyroxine should be lowered if they are observed, especially if the cat has lost bodyweight.

If using a once-daily treatment regimen, the same protocol as used for twice-daily dosing can be used. However, a later post-pill sampling time (e.g. 12 hours after levothyroxine) can also be used in order to get an estimate of the 'average' daily serum T4 concentration (between the peak and trough values). If bedtime dosing is used, this means that the cat is generally rechecked sometime in the morning. With 12-hour post-pill testing, the serum total T4 concentration will be lower than the expected peak value but should remain within the lower half of the reference interval. Again, if peak post-pill serum T4 concentrations are adequate, the serum TSH concentration should be normal.

No matter what monitoring protocol is chosen, owners should never modify the dosing schedule on the day before or the morning of thyroid testing in order to fit the correct timing for the predicted blood sampling time. Overall standardization and consistency of daily feeding and time of blood sampling over the years of monitoring is most important.

References and further reading

Aldridge C, Behrend EN, Martin LG *et al.* (2015) Evaluation of thyroid-stimulating hormone, total thyroxine, and free thyroxine concentrations in hyperthyroid cats receiving methimazole treatment. *Journal of Veterinary Internal Medicine* **29**, 862–868

Blois SL, Abrams-Ogg AC, Mitchell C *et al.* (2010) Use of thyroid scintigraphy and pituitary immunohistochemistry in the diagnosis of spontaneous hypothyroidism in a mature cat. *Journal of Feline Medicine and Surgery* **12**, 156–160

Feldman EC, Fracassi F and Peterson ME (2019) *Feline Endocrinology*. Edra, Milan

Iturriaga MP, Cocio JA and Barrs VR (2020) Cluster of cases of congenital feline goitrous hypothyroidism in a single hospital. *Journal of Small Animal Practice* **61**, 696–703

Jones BR, Gruffydd-Jones TJ, Sparkes AH and Lucke VM (1992) Preliminary studies on congenital hypothyroidism in a family of Abyssinian cats. *Veterinary Record* **131**, 145–148

Mazrier H, French A, Ellinwood NM *et al.* (2003) Goitrous congenital hypothyroidism caused by thyroid peroxidase deficiency in a family of domestic shorthair cats (abstract). *Journal of Veterinary Internal Medicine* **17**, 395–396

Peterson ME (2015) Primary goitrous hypothyroidism in a young adult domestic longhair cat: diagnosis and treatment monitoring. *Journal of Feline Medicine and Surgery Open Reports* **1**, 2055116915615153

Peterson ME (2019) Hypothyroidism. In: *Feline Endocrinology*, ed. EC Feldman, F Fracassi and ME Peterson, pp. 281–316. Edra, Milan

Peterson ME, Carothers MA, Gamble DA and Rishniw M (2018) Spontaneous primary hypothyroidism in 7 adult cats. *Journal of Veterinary Internal Medicine* **32**, 1864–1873

Peterson ME, Carothers MA, Gamble DA and Rishniw M (2019) ERRATUM: Spontaneous primary hypothyroidism in 7 adult cats. *Journal of Veterinary Internal Medicine* **33**, 1111–1111

Peterson ME, Davignon DL, Shaw N *et al.* (2020) Serum thyroxine and thyrotropin concentrations decrease with severity of nonthyroidal illness in cats and predict 30-day survival outcome. *Journal of Veterinary Internal Medicine* **34**, 2276–2286

Peterson ME, Nichols R and Rishniw M (2017) Serum thyroxine and thyroid-stimulating hormone concentration in hyperthyroid cats that develop azotaemia after radioiodine therapy. *Journal of Small Animal Practice* **58**, 519–530

Rand JS, Levine J, Best SJ and Parker W (1993) Spontaneous adult-onset hypothyroidism in a cat. *Journal of Veterinary Internal Medicine* **7**, 272–276

Sjollema BE, den Hartog MT, de Vijlder JJ, van Dijk JE and Rijnberk A (1991) Congenital hypothyroidism in two cats due to defective organification: data suggesting loosely anchored thyroperoxidase. *Acta Endocrinologica* **125**, 435–440

Stammeleer L, Buresova E, Stock E *et al.* (2020) Comparison of free thyroxine measurement by chemiluminescence and equilibrium dialysis following ^{131}I therapy in hyperthyroid cats. *Journal of Feline Medicine and Surgery* **22**, 1114–1120

Tanase H, Kudo K, Horikoshi H *et al.* (1991) Inherited primary hypothyroidism with thyrotrophin resistance in Japanese cats. *Journal of Endocrinology* **129**, 245–251

Traas AM, Abbott BL, French A and Giger U (2008) Congenital thyroid hypoplasia and seizures in 2 littermate kittens. *Journal of Veterinary Internal Medicine* **22**, 1427–1431

Wakeling J, Hall T and Williams TL (2020) Correlation of thyroid hormone measurements with thyroid stimulating hormone stimulation test results in radioiodine-treated cats. *Journal of Veterinary Internal Medicine* **34**, 2265–2275

Williams TL, Elliott J and Syme HM (2014) Effect on renal function of restoration of euthyroidism in hyperthyroid cats with iatrogenic hypothyroidism. *Journal of Veterinary Internal Medicine* **28**, 1251–1255

Chapter 22

Control of glucose homeostasis and investigation of hypo- and hyperglycaemia

Johan P. Schoeman

Glucose homeostasis

Glucose homeostasis is best understood if the metabolism is divided into an absorptive (fed) phase and a post-absorptive (fasting) phase.

Absorptive phase

The absorptive phase follows a typical meal in which carbohydrates, proteins and fats (in addition to minerals and vitamins) are ingested. These nutrients cross the gastro-intestinal tract and cause a rapid increase in circulating concentrations of monosaccharides and amino acids when carbohydrates and proteins, respectively, enter the blood. Fat, in turn, enters the lymph as triglycerides. In essence, the absorptive phase results in the storage of glucose as glycogen in liver and muscle tissue for later use.

The principal hormone involved in the coordination of events during the absorptive phase is insulin, which is secreted from the beta cells of the islets of Langerhans in the pancreas. Insulin promotes the expression of glucose transporter (GLUT)-4 proteins, which facilitate glucose uptake by muscle, adipose tissue and pancreatic alpha cells. As a consequence, when insulin concentrations are low, these tissues cannot remove glucose from the blood and hyperglycaemia ensues.

By contrast, insulin does not affect, and is not required for, the uptake of glucose through GLUT-2 transporters in the brain, liver, renal tubules, erythrocytes, leucocytes, pancreatic beta cells and gastrointestinal epithelium.

The primary stimulus for insulin release is an increase in blood glucose concentration, which typically occurs following the ingestion of a meal. Other factors, such as the concentrations of incretins, amino acids and potassium, which increase following a meal, also stimulate insulin secretion. Incretins are hormones secreted from the enteroendocrine cells and include glucose-dependent insulinotropic polypeptide (GIP) and glucagon-like peptide 1 (GLP-1), which stimulate insulin secretion from beta cells in a glucose-dependent manner.

Insulin, in turn, stimulates the uptake of amino acids and potassium by the tissues. Conversely, insulin secretion ceases once the blood glucose concentration decreases to within the reference interval, which heralds the commencement of the post-absorptive phase.

Post-absorptive phase

During the post-absorptive phase, no glucose is absorbed across the gastrointestinal tract, yet blood glucose concentrations need to be maintained, because nervous tissue is unable to oxidize other nutrients for energy – at least in the short to medium term. Cells of the central nervous system (CNS) are heavily dependent on glucose as an energy source, as are red blood cells. Indeed, although the brain constitutes only 2% of total body mass, it utilizes 25% of total body glucose. The brain relies on a large and sustained supply of glucose because it has three times the metabolic rate of peripheral tissues yet contains 10–30% less glucose. Maintenance of blood glucose concentration is accomplished through two major actions: the mobilization of stored sources of glucose and the utilization of other fuels to spare glucose for nervous tissue. The major counter-regulatory hormones coordinating these efforts and causing a degree of insulin resistance are glucagon, adrenaline (epinephrine), gluco-corticoids and growth hormone (GH). Glucagon and glucocorticoids are the primary stimulants of the gluco-neogenic pathways in the liver.

Glucagon

Glucagon is secreted from the alpha cells of the pancreas if blood glucose concentrations edge towards the lower limit of the reference interval. The glucose-sensing mechanism for the regulation of glucagon secretion resides within the interior of the alpha cell. Intriguingly, glucose entry through GLUT-4 transporters in the alpha cell is dependent on insulin. Consequently, in diabetic animals that lack insulin, glucose cannot enter the alpha cells to stop the release of glucagon, whose secretion therefore continues unabatedly, further fuelling high blood glucose concentrations (see Chapter 23).

Adrenaline

Adrenaline release from the adrenal medulla is primarily under the control of the hypothalamus and the sympathetic nervous system. Low blood glucose concentration is also sensed by the hypothalamic glucose receptors, stimulating the sympathetic nervous system and causing the release of adrenaline. Some sympathetic nerves are in direct contact with adipose tissue and release adrenaline directly into such tissue. Adrenaline promotes hepatic glycogenolysis and gluconeogenesis, and stimu-lates muscle glycogenolysis, lipolysis and ketogenesis; it also mobilizes gluconeogenic precursors (lactate, alanine and glycerol) and inhibits glucose utilization by insulin-sensitive tissues.

Growth hormone

Growth hormone release from the anterior pituitary is under complex control. Firstly, hypothalamic glucose receptors have a stimulatory effect on GH through the release of growth hormone-releasing hormone. Additionally, a rise in amino acid concentrations increases GH release. Growth hormone, among other functions, promotes gluconeogenesis, glycogenolysis, lipolysis and alanine release by muscle.

Glucocorticoids

Glucocorticoids are released from the adrenal cortex subsequent to stimulation by adrenocorticotropic hormone (ACTH) from the pituitary gland. In turn, ACTH release is primarily under the control of the nervous system and ACTH is secreted in response to a wide variety of stressors, which include cold, pain and hypoglycaemia.

Mobilization of glucose from body stores during fasting

During fasting, stored liver glycogen is rapidly broken down to glucose (glycogenolysis) and fulfils the energy needs of the body for a matter of hours. Conversely, glycogen stored in muscle tissue cannot be readily liberated as glucose. Muscle glycogen is broken down to glucose-6-phosphate, which is then catabolized via glycolysis to pyruvate and lactate. These two substances are then recovered by the liver, incorporated into the gluconeogenesis pathway and ultimately converted to glucose.

The catabolism of triglycerides within adipose tissue yields both fatty acids and glycerol. Fatty acids cannot be converted to glucose; however, glycerol can enter the gluconeogenesis pathway in the liver and be converted to glucose. Moreover, large portions of protein are stored in muscle tissue for the primary purpose of acting as a source of energy to be mobilized during fasting. The release of amino acids from muscle is stimulated by glucocorticoids and they too are converted to glucose in the liver.

The critical role the liver plays in ensuring a steady glucose supply partly explains why many forms of liver dysfunction are accompanied by hypoglycaemia. Whilst the liver is the main organ involved in gluconeogenic processes, the renal cortex also has limited gluconeogenic capabilities.

Glucose-sparing activities

The glycogenolytic and gluconeogenic capacities of the liver and kidneys are inadequate to provide enough metabolizable energy during the post-absorptive phase. It is thus necessary for the body to also oxidize other substances for energy. In this regard, muscle turns to oxidizing fat for energy, whilst adipose tissue catabolizes stored triglycerides to fatty acids and glycerol. Glycerol is converted to glucose as mentioned above, whilst fatty acids enter the tricarboxylic acid cycle in many tissues, where they are oxidized to carbon dioxide and water to yield energy. Fatty acids become the preferential energy source for the liver during the post-absorptive phase, rather than amino acids, which are preferred during the absorptive phase. This substitution spares amino acids for gluconeogenesis elsewhere. Some fatty acids are also converted to ketone bodies such as acetone, acetoacetic acid and beta-hydroxybutyrate. Ketone bodies are subsequently released into the blood and serve as an important fuel source for many tissues. Even nervous tissue can, several days after being deprived of glucose, begin to oxidize ketones for energy, yet it always prefers glucose.

Investigation of hypoglycaemia

Hypoglycaemia is defined as a circulating glucose concentration below the reference interval, typically less than 3.5 mmol/l. It is a common complication in the treatment of insulin-dependent diabetes mellitus and a frequent, but poorly recognized, cause of weakness and collapse. Occasionally, clinical signs are not obvious and hypoglycaemia is a serendipitous finding following measurement of circulating glucose concentration. In the critically ill or sedated animal, hypoglycaemia is a clinically silent, yet life-threatening, disorder that necessitates swift and decisive treatment to prevent lasting neuronal damage.

The following section presents an overview of the basic pathophysiology of hypoglycaemia and describes a rational, problem-oriented approach to the diagnosis of the potential underlying causes.

Pathophysiology of hypoglycaemia

Glucose represents the major source of energy for mammalian cells, particularly those in the CNS. Blood glucose concentrations are regulated by dietary intake, hormones and tissue utilization (see 'Glucose homeostasis', above).

When blood glucose concentrations decline, glucosensors (especially those in the glucagon-releasing alpha cells of the pancreas) are stimulated. These sensors initiate neuro-hormonal compensatory mechanisms that increase plasma glucose concentrations, increase glucose delivery to and uptake by the brain, and alter glucose metabolic pathways. This compensatory response involves the following:

- A decrease in insulin secretion and an increase in glucagon concentration
- Adrenaline and noradrenaline (norepinephrine) release at the onset of hypoglycaemia
- If hypoglycaemia persists for longer, a third mechanism, the secretion of cortisol and GH, is initiated (Cryer, 1997). This robust cortisol response to hypoglycaemia has also been shown in natural canine infection (Schoeman and Herrtage, 2007).

In certain circumstances, these physiological safeguards fail and hypoglycaemia develops.

Methods of circulating glucose measurement

A diagnosis of hypoglycaemia is made by documenting a low circulating glucose concentration. Misrepresentation of the animal's true glycaemic status because of a laboratory or processing error is a common occurrence in practice. The clinician should be aware of artefactual causes of hypoglycaemia, such as a poorly calibrated handheld glucometer, erythrocytosis, prolonged storage of blood, or lack of or delayed separation of plasma/serum from red blood cells.

Circulating glucose concentrations obtained with most portable glucometers are lower than those obtained by the reference hexokinase method. This difference is typically exacerbated as the true circulating glucose concentration decreases (Wess and Reusch, 2000). It is good practice to re-sample in order to verify hypoglycaemia, using a reference laboratory method, before embarking on an extensive diagnostic work-up. Blood should ideally be collected in fluoride oxalate tubes; serum or heparinized tubes may be used, but have to be centrifuged and the serum/plasma separated within 30 minutes of sample collection.

- The reference intervals for plasma glucose concentrations are approximately 3.5–6.5 mmol/l in dogs and 3.5–7.0 mmol/l in cats, with small variations depending on the laboratory and methodology used.
- When circulating glucose concentrations are reduced to below approximately 3.5 mmol/l, clinical signs indicative of sympathetic nervous system activation, such as nervousness, tremors and tachycardia, are observed.
- When circulating glucose concentrations fall below 1 mmol/l, seizure activity, severe brain damage, coma and death may occur due to marked neuronal dysfunction and cell death.

Differential diagnosis

Hypoglycaemia is typically a consequence of:

- Decreased glucose production, which may be caused by:
  - Inadequate dietary intake of glucose or other gluconeogenic substrates
  - Impaired hepatic gluconeogenesis
  - Deficiency of glucose counter-regulatory hormones
  - Impaired glycogenolysis
- Increased glucose utilization
- A combination of the above mechanisms (e.g. in sepsis, uraemia).

As causes of hypoglycaemia span the above mechanisms, the list of differential diagnoses is given according to the DAMNIT system and sub-categorized by the above-mentioned pathophysiological mechanisms where possible (Figure 22.1).

Decreased glucose production

Decreased glucose production may be the result of substrate, hormone or enzyme deficiencies.

Substrate deficiencies are most commonly caused by malnutrition and inadequate food intake, and usually occur in neonates and toy breeds. Insufficient functional hepatic mass (<75%), due to a portovascular anomaly or acute or chronic liver failure, is a common cause of hypoglycaemia. These hepatic disorders also result in impaired insulin catabolism, which further exacerbates the hypoglycaemia.

Inadequate production or release of insulin-antagonizing hormones, such as cortisol and GH, may result in hypoglycaemia. The circulating glucose concentrations in these disorders are usually only slightly decreased and other clinical and biochemical findings, such as dwarfism in panhypopituitarism and electrolyte abnormalities in primary hypoadrenocorticism, often predominate. Isolated glucocorticoid deficiency presents a diagnostic challenge unless the clinician retains a high index of suspicion for this disorder (see Chapters 28 and 31).

Hypoglycaemia insensitivity is a condition in human diabetic patients caused by impaired compensatory responses to hypoglycaemia. These patients develop decreased glucagon release and decreased hepatic responsiveness to adrenaline. Lower circulating glucose concentrations are thus endured without stimulation of normal compensatory mechanisms, and these patients become more prone to hypoglycaemic episodes (Korytkowski *et al.*, 1998; Ovalle *et al.*, 1998). Although poorly described, there is anecdotal evidence of hypoglycaemia insensitivity in some diabetic dogs and clinicians should maintain an awareness of these cases.

Dogs and cats with glycogen storage diseases due to specific glycogenolytic enzyme deficiencies are unable

Developmental
- Portovascular anomalies[a]
- Hepatic enzyme deficiencies[a]
• Von Gierke's disease (type 1 glycogen storage disease)
• Cori's disease (type 3 glycogen storage disease)
Artefactual
- Prolonged sample storage[b]
- Delayed separation of blood sample[b]
- Laboratory error
- Uncalibrated handheld glucometers
Miscellaneous
- Severe erythrocytosis[b]
- Prolonged starvation, malnutrition or chronic diarrhoea[a]
- Extreme exertion[b]
Metabolic
- Hepatic insufficiency[a, b]
• Acute liver failure
• Acquired portovascular anomaly
• Chronic liver fibrosis/cirrhosis
- Hypoadrenocorticism[a]
- Panhypopituitarism[a]
- Refeeding syndrome (cats)[b]
- Kidney disease[c]
- Puerperal eclampsia[b]
Neoplastic
- Pancreatic beta cell tumours (insulinoma)[b]
- Extra-pancreatic neoplasia[b]
• Hepatocellular carcinoma
• Hepatoma
• Haemangiosarcoma
• Leiomyoma/sarcoma
Idiopathic hypoglycaemia
- Hunting dog hypoglycaemia[b]
- Neonatal hypoglycaemia[c]
- Juvenile hypoglycaemia (especially in toy breeds)[c]
- Beta cell hyperplasia (nesidioblastosis)[b]
Iatrogenic
- Excess insulin therapy[b]
- Sulphonylurea therapy[b]
- Therapy with other oral hypoglycaemic drugs (e.g. acarbose, metformin)[a, b]
- Propranolol therapy[a]
Infectious
- Canine babesiosis[c]
- Canine parvovirus infection[c]
- Sepsis[c]
• Endocarditis
• Chemotherapy-associated neutropenia
• Severe pneumonia
• Peritonitis
Toxic
- Ethanol poisoning[a]
- Xylitol poisoning (dogs)[b]

22.1 Causes of hypoglycaemia arranged according to the DAMNIT system. [a] = decreased glucose production; [b] = increased glucose utilization; [c] = combination of decreased glucose production and increased glucose utilization.

to release glucose from the liver, resulting in glycogen accumulation, hepatomegaly and organ dysfunction. Nonetheless, enzyme deficiencies are the least common cause of decreased glucose production.

Increased glucose utilization

Hyperinsulinaemia drives glucose intracellularly whilst simultaneously inhibiting the mobilization of energy stored as amino acids, triglycerides or glycogen in muscle, fat and liver, respectively. Insulin's dual effect of increased utilization and decreased mobilization of glucose leads to profound hypoglycaemia.

Excessive administration of exogenous insulin to diabetic animals, in the form of overdosing or persistent dosing in the face of anorexia, is a common iatrogenic cause of hypoglycaemia (see Chapters 23 and 24). Previously well regulated diabetic cats can suddenly experience bouts of hypoglycaemia due to dramatically reduced insulin requirements as a consequence of diabetic remission.

The concomitant administration of oral hypoglycaemic drugs, such as glipizide or metformin, can also lead to increased insulin release and/or glucose utilization with resultant hypoglycaemia. Xylitol, a sweetener that is increasingly found in sugar-free confectionery and baked goods, is a documented cause of excessive insulin secretion and hepatic necrosis in dogs, with resultant profound hypoglycaemia (Dunayer, 2004).

Increased insulin production by hyperplastic (nesidioblastosis) or malignant (insulinoma) pancreatic beta cells causes excessive glucose utilization (see Chapter 27). A pancreatic beta cell tumour has been described that caused hypoglycaemia in a dog not by over-secretion of insulin, but by over-secretion of insulin-like growth factor-2 (Finotello et al., 2009).

In humans, severe malarial infection results in hypoglycaemia due to overproduction of insulin. Evidence of increased insulin concentrations has been found in hypoglycaemic dogs with babesiosis (Rees and Schoeman, 2008).

Diagnostic approach to hypoglycaemia

The most important diagnostic step is the recognition of hypoglycaemia as the cause of the clinical signs. This may seem obvious, but unfortunately many dogs with episodic collapse are treated for neurological or cardiac conditions for months prior to the demonstration of hypoglycaemia – occasionally for up to 3 years (see Chapter 27). If hypoglycaemia is strongly suspected yet not documented on the first occasion, 2-hourly circulating glucose measurements over a 12-hour (up to 24–72-hour) period of fasting should be performed. When a circulating glucose concentration of less than 3.5 mmol/l is confirmed, the sequence of diagnostic tests is mainly governed by the results obtained after a thorough review of the history, signalment, physical examination and clinicopathological data findings. The cause is frequently evident after interpretation of the above information, but a small proportion of cases need more advanced diagnostic investigation. Additional diagnostics such as measurement of serum insulin concentration, an ACTH response test, hepatic function tests, diagnostic imaging, blood culture and, occasionally, organ biopsy are then rationally employed based on these initial findings (Figure 22.2).

Signalment

Young animals are more prone to developing hypoglycaemia due to starvation, neonatal or juvenile hypoglycaemia, portovascular anomaly, parvovirus infection, babesiosis or glycogen storage disease. Middle-aged to older animals are more likely to be affected by insulinoma, other neoplastic conditions, acquired hepatic disease or hypoadrenocorticism. Bearded Collies and West Highland White Terriers may be predisposed to hypoadrenocorticism, whereas Yorkshire Terriers, Cairn Terriers, Irish Wolfhounds and Maltese are more likely to have portovascular

anomalies, and Boxers, Irish Setters and Siamese cats are more likely to develop insulinoma. Young Norwegian Forest Cats are prone to glycogen storage disease.

Historical features

Animals with hypoadrenocorticism and insulinoma usually have a more prolonged history (spanning a few months to years in the case of insulinoma) of intermittent weakness and collapse. In addition, peripheral neuropathies have been described in cases of insulinoma. Hunting dog hypoglycaemia cases have an obvious history of activity-associated clinical signs in lean individuals, whereas parvovirus-infected dogs have a classic history of vomiting or diarrhoea a few hours to days preceding weakness and collapse. Tick exposure and a short history of weakness, associated with marked anaemia, characterizes hypoglycaemia associated with virulent canine babesiosis (Keller et al., 2004). Sepsis should be suspected in those animals that have received immunosuppressive agents or undergone splenectomy, those with parvovirus infection, and those with hepatic dysfunction or endocarditis. A history of exposure to hypoglycaemic drugs, such as propranolol or insulin, or poisons such as ethanol, and especially the ingestion of xylitol, should be borne in mind in dogs with acute-onset weakness and collapse (Dunayer, 2004). Other appropriate areas of questioning include age of onset and whether siblings are affected (glycogen storage diseases), temporal relationship to meals (insulinoma, portovascular anomaly), vaccination history (parvovirus infection), and quality of the diet (malnutrition/starvation) or the presence of chronic diarrhoea (severe malassimilation).

Physical examination

Affected animals may show a variety of focal and generalized neurological signs. The most common clinical signs are intermittent, brief episodes (a few seconds to minutes) of altered consciousness (dullness, coma), weakness, ataxia, collapse and seizures. The severity of clinical signs is dependent on the rapidity of the fall in blood glucose concentration, the duration of hypoglycaemia and the absolute blood glucose concentration reached – some animals, especially hunting dogs, can tolerate quite low glucose concentrations without showing clinical signs. With a rapid fall in glucose concentration, additional signs such as muscle fasciculation, tachycardia and vomiting are observed, which are mainly attributable to sympathetic nervous system activation.

Clinical signs unrelated to hypoglycaemia, such as pyrexia, jaundice or bradycardia, are helpful in localizing the cause of the hypoglycaemia. However, there is evidence that severe hypoglycaemia may cause bradycardia of its own accord (Little, 2005).

Animals suffering from insulinoma may show signs of lower motor neuron dysfunction, such as decreased spinal reflexes related to the presence of peripheral neuropathy. They are generally in very good body condition because of the anabolic effects of insulin, whereas those with advanced kidney disease or prolonged starvation are clearly emaciated. Failure to identify abnormalities on physical examination in an older, large-breed dog is an important clue to the potential presence of an insulin-secreting tumour.

Animals with portovascular anomalies may have small stature and poor growth. Acquired or end-stage chronic liver disease cases are also generally in poor body condition with potential concomitant jaundice and ascites.

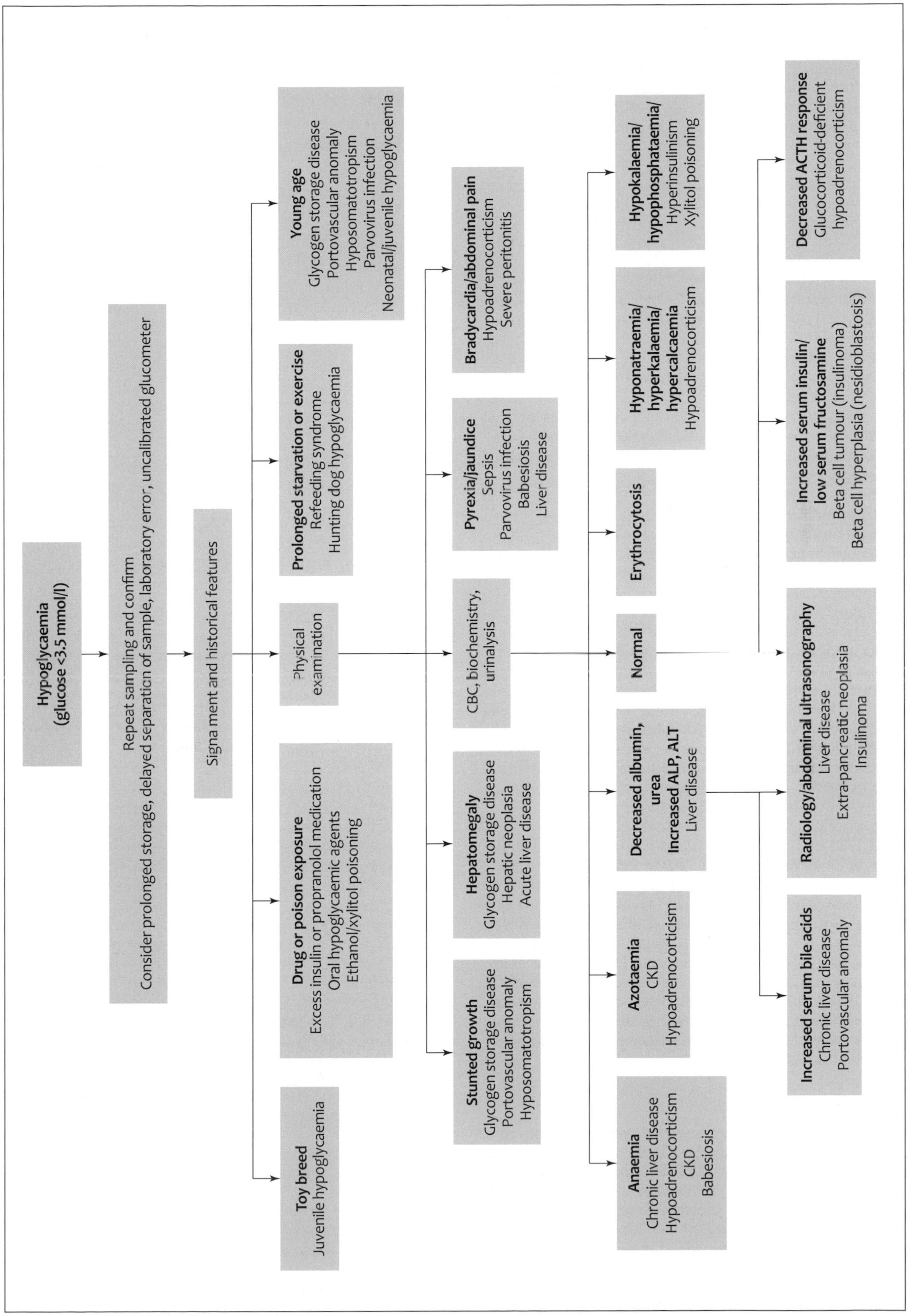

Hypoglycaemia (glucose <3.5 mmol/l)

Repeat sampling and confirm

Consider prolonged storage, delayed separation of sample, laboratory error, uncalibrated glucometer

Signalment and historical features

Physical examination

Toy breed
Juvenile hypoglycaemia

Drug or poison exposure
Excess insulin or propranolol medication
Oral hypoglycaemic agents
Ethanol/xylitol poisoning

Prolonged starvation or exercise
Refeeding syndrome
Hunting dog hypoglycaemia

Young age
Glycogen storage disease
Portovascular anomaly
Hyposomatotropism
Parvovirus infection
Neonatal/juvenile hypoglycaemia

Stunted growth
Glycogen storage disease
Portovascular anomaly
Hyposomatotropism

Hepatomegaly
Glycogen storage disease
Hepatic neoplasia
Acute liver disease

Pyrexia/jaundice
Sepsis
Parvovirus infection
Babesiosis
Liver disease

Bradycardia/abdominal pain
Hypoadrenocorticism
Severe peritonitis

CBC, biochemistry, urinalysis

Anaemia
Chronic liver disease
Hypoadrenocorticism
CKD
Babesiosis

Azotaemia
CKD
Hypoadrenocorticism

Decreased albumin, urea
Increased ALP, ALT
Liver disease

Normal

Erythrocytosis

Hyponatraemia/ hyperkalaemia/ hypercalcaemia
Hypoadrenocorticism

Hypokalaemia/ hypophosphataemia
Hyperinsulinism
Xylitol poisoning

Increased serum bile acids
Chronic liver disease
Portovascular anomaly

Radiology/abdominal ultrasonography
Liver disease
Extra-pancreatic neoplasia
Insulinoma

Increased serum insulin/ low serum fructosamine
Beta cell tumour (insulinoma)
Beta cell hyperplasia (nesidioblastosis)

Decreased ACTH response
Glucocorticoid-deficient hypoadrenocorticism

22.2   Diagnostic algorithm for hypoglycaemia. ACTH = adrenocorticotropic hormone; ALP = alkaline phosphatase; ALT = alanine aminotransferase; CBC = complete blood count; CKD = chronic kidney disease.

Animals with other extra-pancreatic neoplastic conditions are usually presented for clinical signs referable to these, such as hepatomegaly and other abdominal masses with or without ascites. Erythrocytosis may present as brick-red mucous membranes and seizures. Hypoglycaemia should always be suspected in any dog or cat presenting in status epilepticus, either as an inciting cause or as a complicating factor. The cardiovascular and neurological systems should be thoroughly evaluated during the physical examination because abnormalities in these systems are important differentials for weakness, collapse, syncope and seizure.

Minimum clinicopathological data

A complete haematological and biochemical profile will enable the confirmation of hypoglycaemia and help to rule out other causes of weakness and collapse, such as hypokalaemia and hypocalcaemia. Abnormalities that provide useful pointers as to which test might have to be employed next include:

- **Erythrocytosis** – acute haemorrhagic diarrhoea syndrome or erythropoietin-producing tumour
- **Non-regenerative anaemia** – kidney disease or neoplastic disease
- **Acute haemolytic anaemia** – babesiosis
- **Marked neutropenia** – parvovirus infection
- **A degenerative left shift** – sepsis
- **Lymphocytosis and/or eosinophilia** – hypoadrenocorticism
- **Increased liver enzyme activities and bile acid concentrations** – hepatic disease
- **Hyperkalaemia, hyponatraemia and hypercalcaemia** – hypoadrenocorticism
- **Azotaemia with inadequately concentrated urine** – chronic kidney disease or hypoadrenocorticism
- **Hypokalaemia and hypophosphataemia** – hyperinsulinism or xylitol poisoning
- **Low serum fructosamine concentration** – suggests a more chronic cause of hypoglycaemia.

Hepatic function tests

The bile acid stimulation test is the most practical and reliable way to assess liver function. It involves obtaining a serum sample when the animal is fasted, feeding a fatty meal and then re-sampling 2 hours later. Hypoalbuminaemia, low serum urea concentrations, hyperbilirubinaemia and prolonged bleeding times are additional indicators of hepatic dysfunction. Serum cholesterol concentrations in hepatobiliary disease are variable; hypercholesterolaemia is seen in cholestatic disease, whereas hypocholesterolaemia is observed in end-stage liver disease and portovascular anomalies.

Insulin concentration

Serum insulin concentrations should be below the reference interval in hypoglycaemic animals; it is abnormal for circulating insulin concentrations of hypoglycaemic animals to be within or above the reference interval and a diagnosis of insulinoma or nesidioblastosis is then very likely. Insulin should be measured with an assay that is validated for the species under investigation and always concurrent with a circulating glucose measurement. Guidelines for the interpretation of fasting insulin concentrations are detailed in Chapter 27.

Adrenocorticotropic hormone response test

This test is employed to assess adrenal reserve. Dogs and cats with hypoadrenocorticism will typically have low to undetectable cortisol concentrations both pre- and post-ACTH.

Diagnostic imaging

Abdominal radiography is generally of limited value in detecting insulinomas. Instead, it is used to identify other potential neoplastic conditions. Likewise, thoracic radiography may indicate pulmonary metastatic disease.

Abdominal ultrasonography, on the other hand, is the most useful test in hypoglycaemic dogs and cats if the underlying cause is not immediately apparent. It will reveal changes to the liver parenchyma in diseases such as chronic cirrhosis or may reveal anomalous blood vessels consistent with portovascular anomaly. Ultrasonography is also useful for the detection of extra-pancreatic neoplasms that may be associated with hypoglycaemia, such as hepatocellular carcinoma. In addition, small adrenal glands may be suggestive of hypoadrenocorticism in dogs and cats with consistent clinical signs.

Most insulinomas are quite small (<2 cm) and the ultrasonographic detection of insulinomas is not easy. The sensitivity of abdominal ultrasound is approximately 75% in dogs and unknown in cats, and a negative ultrasonographic examination does not rule the condition out. More advanced imaging may have to be considered in some cases.

Blood culture

Positive blood cultures are consistent with sepsis, but this is not a sensitive test. Sensitivity can be increased by taking at least three cultures over a 12-hour period and ensuring that blood samples are taken before the initiation of antibiotic therapy.

Organ biopsy

The method of biopsy is influenced by the organ size, the suspected diagnosis, the animal's clinical condition and the risk of haemorrhage. Ultrasound-guided biopsy can be a high-yielding procedure in diffuse disorders of the liver or in focal conditions in which suspicious lesions can be targeted. Fine-needle aspirates are preferred in animals with bleeding disorders, large cavitary lesions or abscesses, and may yield diagnostic samples and even reveal infectious agents that can be missed on histopathology. However, in animals that can tolerate the procedure, hepatic wedge biopsies (obtained through an exploratory laparotomy or, ideally, laparoscopy) give the most reliable results. Biopsy is often the only procedure to yield a definitive diagnosis in diseases with subtle or unevenly distributed lesions.

Investigation of hyperglycaemia

Increases in blood glucose concentration are primarily caused by the opposite processes to those that result in hypoglycaemia:

- Increased glucose production or release
- Decreased glucose utilization.

Figure 22.3 provides a full list of differential diagnoses for hyperglycaemia.

- Fear, excitement, extreme exercise, stress (especially cats)
- Severe trauma (especially bite wounds and head trauma)
- Postprandial
- Glucose infusion
- Diabetes mellitus
- Dioestrus (bitches)
- Conditions causing insulin resistance
  - Hypercortisolism (especially cats)
  - Hypersomatotropism (especially cats)
  - Hyperthyroidism (rarely)
  - Phaeochromocytoma
  - Glucagonoma
- Insulin overdose (counter-regulatory response)
- Acute pancreatitis
- Acute babesiosis
- Following surgical excision of an insulinoma
- Erroneous finding
  - Lipaemia
  - Haemolysis
  - Metronidazole administration (especially for the hexokinase method)
- Drugs that interfere with glucose regulation
  - Medetomidine
  - Butylscopolamine
  - Glucocorticoids
  - Progestins
  - Calcium channel blockers

22.3 Differential diagnoses for hyperglycaemia.

Most clinicians are familiar with stress hyperglycaemia in cats and tend to view more sustained hyperglycaemia in terms of the classic syndrome of diabetes mellitus caused by an absolute or relative lack of insulin. Yet, it is not always straightforward to distinguish incidental stress hyperglycaemia from diabetes mellitus. Clues in the history such as polyuria and polydipsia, weight loss despite polyphagia and laboratory findings such as glucosuria, ketonuria and high fructosamine concentration are helpful in diagnosing diabetes mellitus. However, historical clues may be overlooked or underappreciated by owners.

Additionally, although glucosuria is most commonly caused by diabetes mellitus, it can be caused by other conditions. Glucose undergoes filtration by the kidney but is almost entirely resorbed in the proximal tubules and is therefore not readily detectable in the urine of healthy dogs and cats. Importantly, any transient (acute kidney injury or inflammation) or permanent (primary renal glucosuria, Fanconi syndrome) impairment of proximal tubular resorption may lead to glucosuria. Glucosuria is also seen in conditions such as severe stress and following administration of glucose-containing fluids where the circulating glucose concentration exceeds the renal threshold (approximately 12–14 mmol/l in the dog and 14–16 mmol/l in the cat).

Whilst diabetes mellitus is indeed the most common and clinically relevant cause of overt and marked hyperglycaemia, there are many other causes of less severe hyperglycaemia. Recent research in critically ill human intensive care unit (ICU) patients has identified hyperglycaemia as an indicator of more severe disease and a poor prognosis. Moreover, its specific management confers a survival benefit. A negative impact of hyperglycaemia on morbidity and mortality has also been found in small animals (Torre *et al.*, 2007). Whilst in humans the worldwide epidemic proportions of obesity and diabetes mellitus contribute to the incidence of ICU hyperglycaemia, the situation is not quite the same in dogs. Yet, the increasing incidence of obesity and diabetes mellitus in the cat population means that hyperglycaemia is a likely comorbidity in many critically ill cats and may warrant specific intervention. A partial pancreatectomy for the treatment of insulinoma is yet another cause of hyperglycaemia, where the remaining insulin-secreting beta cells undergo atrophy in the presence of the tumour and the animal needs transient insulin treatment for a few days to weeks postoperatively (see Chapter 27).

A few studies on circulating glucose concentrations have been conducted in dogs and cats with various illnesses. Mild hyperglycaemia has been reported in association with traumatic brain injury, in dogs with babesiosis and in dogs with bite wounds (Syring *et al.*, 2001; Keller *et al.*, 2004; Schoeman *et al.*, 2011). However, there is no evidence yet that tight glycaemic control would confer any benefit in these populations.

Briefly, the approach to hyperglycaemia involves the following steps:

- Verify the glucose concentration and rule out stress hyperglycaemia, especially in cats
- Rule out obvious causes from the history, such as prior intravenous glucose administration, a recent high-carbohydrate meal or any drug administration such as anticholinergic agents, glucocorticoids, medetomidine, progestins or high-dose calcium channel blockers
- Rule out excessive secretion of counter-regulatory hormones:
  - Adrenaline in phaeochromocytoma (see Chapter 33)
  - Glucagon in glucagonoma (see Chapter 38)
  - Growth hormone in hypersomatotropism (see Chapter 13)
  - Glucocorticoids in hypercortisolism (see Chapter 29)
- Rule out systemic inflammatory response syndrome and sepsis or traumatic brain injury, which cause marked insulin resistance and subsequent hyperglycaemia.

References and further reading

Cryer PE (1997) Hierarchy of physiological responses to hypoglycemia: relevance to clinical hypoglycemia in type I (insulin dependent) diabetes mellitus. *Hormone and Metabolic Research* **29**, 92–96

Dunayer EK (2004) Hypoglycemia following canine ingestion of xylitol-containing gum. *Veterinary and Human Toxicology* **46**, 87–88

Finotello R, Marchetti V, Nesi G *et al.* (2009) Pancreatic islet cell tumor secreting insulin-like growth factor type-II in a dog. *Journal of Veterinary Internal Medicine* **23**, 1289–1292

Keller N, Jacobson LS, Nel M *et al.* (2004) Prevalence and risk factors of hypoglycemia in virulent canine babesiosis. *Journal of Veterinary Internal Medicine* **18**, 265–270

Korytkowski MT, Mokan M, Veneman TF *et al.* (1998) Reduced beta-adrenergic sensitivity in patients with type 1 diabetes and hypoglycemia unawareness. *Diabetes Care* **21**, 1939–1943

Lechner MJ and Hess RS (2019) Comparison of glucose concentrations in serum, plasma and blood measured by a point-of-care glucometer with serum glucose concentration measured by an automated biochemical analyzer for canine and feline blood samples. *American Journal of Veterinary Research* **80**, 1074–1081

Little CJL (2005) Hypoglycaemic bradycardia and circulatory collapse in a dog and a cat. *Journal of Small Animal Practice* **46**, 445–448

Ovalle F, Fanelli CG, Paramore DS *et al.* (1998) Brief twice-weekly episodes of hypoglycemia reduce detection of clinical hypoglycemia in type 1 diabetes mellitus. *Diabetes* **47**, 1472–1479

Rees P and Schoeman JP (2008) Plasma insulin concentrations in hypoglycaemic dogs with *Babesia canis rossi* infection. *Veterinary Parasitology* **152**, 60–66

Schoeman JP and Herrtage ME (2007) The response of the pituitary–adrenal and pituitary–thyroidal axes to the plasma glucose perturbations in *Babesia canis rossi* babesiosis. *Journal of the South African Veterinary Association* **78**, 215–220

Schoeman JP, Kitshoff AM, du Plessis CJ and Thompson PN (2011) Serial plasma glucose changes in dogs suffering from severe dog bite wounds. *Journal of the South African Veterinary Association* **82**, 41–46

Syring RS, Otto CM and Drobatz KJ (2001) Hyperglycemia in dogs and cats with head trauma: 122 cases (1997–1999). *Journal of the American Veterinary Medical Association* **218**, 1124–1129

Torre DM, deLaforcade AM and Chan DL (2007) Incidence and clinical relevance of hyperglycemia in critically ill dogs. *Journal of Veterinary Internal Medicine* **21**, 971–975

van Raalte DH, Kwa KAA, van Genugten RE *et al.* (2013) Islet-cell dysfunction induced by glucocorticoid treatment: potential role for altered sympathovagal balance? *Metabolism* **62**, 568–577

Wess G and Reusch C (2000) Evaluation of five portable blood glucose meters for use in dogs. *Journal of the American Veterinary Medical Association* **216**, 203–209

Chapter 23

Canine diabetes mellitus

Lucy Davison

Introduction

Canine diabetes mellitus is a common endocrinopathy characterized by relative or absolute deficiency of the hormone insulin. It is not a single disease, but rather can arise as the result of several different pathophysiological mechanisms converging on a similar set of clinical signs.

The past 10 years have seen an increase in knowledge of the factors underlying canine diabetes mellitus and its pathogenesis, although many questions remain unanswered. This chapter reviews current knowledge of the canine condition, including its pathogenesis and management, with a particular focus on recent findings that have a direct clinical impact. A general protocol for management of the newly diagnosed dog is also outlined. Investigation of the unstable diabetic dog is discussed in Chapter 25.

Prevalence and epidemiology

The most recent surveys of diabetes mellitus in the UK canine population reported a prevalence of 0.26–0.34% (Mattin *et al.*, 2014; Heeley *et al.*, 2020). However, an increasing incidence of diabetes mellitus in the global canine population is suggested by the fact that the proportion of diabetic dogs referred to second-opinion veterinary hospitals in the USA has increased from 19 per 10,000 cases to 64 per 10,000 cases over the past 30 years (Guptill *et al.*, 2003), as well as documentation of a rising number of cases in corporate veterinary practices (Aja, 2016). This, however, could also be related to improvements in diagnosis and management of diabetes mellitus by first-opinion veterinary surgeons (veterinarians), a greater willingness to refer problem diabetic cases and an increase in commitment by owners of diabetic dogs to pursue therapy. Owners of a dog with diabetes mellitus are more likely to develop type 2 diabetes mellitus than owners of non-diabetic dogs, although the reason for this is not clear (Delicano *et al.*, 2020).

Aetiology and classification of disease

Insulin is usually secreted in response to an increase in the circulating concentration of glucose (and amino acids) and is antagonized by several other hormones, including glucagon. As the presence of insulin allows glucose to be transported into cells from the blood, reduction in the amount or activity of this hormone results in an impaired ability to control blood glucose concentrations and hence hyperglycaemia ensues. In healthy animals, insulin is produced by the pancreas, an organ that contains both exocrine and endocrine tissue. The exocrine cells produce enzymes, such as trypsin, for digestion of food in the small intestine. The endocrine tissue, found in the islets of Langerhans scattered through the pancreas, produces hormones that are released into the circulation. Pancreatic beta cells constitute 60–80% of each islet, and it is these cells that are responsible for the synthesis of insulin, and whose destruction or dysfunction can lead to diabetes mellitus. Other endocrine cell types in the islets include delta cells, which secrete somatostatin, and alpha cells, which secrete glucagon. Islet cells can become exhausted in the face of persistent hyperglycaemia, although they have a capacity to recover once blood glucose has normalized. If islet damage is sustained, however, it becomes irreversible, since pancreatic islet cells have no capacity to regenerate.

In both humans and dogs, diabetes mellitus is a multifactorial disease, thought to involve genetic factors (Redondo and Eisenbarth, 2002; Denyer *et al.*, 2021, 2021b) and environmental factors, such as diet and infectious organisms (Fleeman and Rand, 2001; Hoenig, 2002; Catchpole *et al.*, 2005). Since multiple pathological processes can lead to canine diabetes mellitus, various classification systems have been proposed, but there is no universally accepted system in veterinary medicine. Human diabetes mellitus was initially classified into insulin-dependent diabetes mellitus (IDDM) and non-insulin-dependent diabetes mellitus (NIDDM), according to the patient's requirement for exogenous insulin therapy, although this system has now been replaced by classification based on pathophysiology. Classification by insulin dependency is not helpful in the dog, since almost all diabetic dogs are insulin dependent, with very few exceptions (Catchpole *et al.*, 2005). A more useful classification, therefore, is that which describes diabetes mellitus according to the underlying disease process (Gilor *et al.*, 2016). The most recent attempt to develop a classification system for canine diabetes mellitus was made by the European Society for Veterinary Endocrinology by an expert panel as part of Project ALIVE (Agreeing Language in Veterinary Endocrinology; see 'Useful websites', below) and is outlined in Figure 23.1. Such a classification also has practical relevance, as the underlying cause of the diabetes mellitus can impact significantly

Insulin-deficient diabetes mellitus (beta cell-related disorders)

- Reduced insulin secretion
  - Beta cell dysfunction
  - Beta cell destruction
    - Immune mediated
    - Loss associated with exocrine pancreatic disease
      - Pancreatitis
      - Neoplasia
      - Idiopathic
    - Toxicity (e.g. diazoxide)
    - Infection
    - Idiopathic
  - Beta cell death (apoptosis)
    - Glucotoxicity
    - Lipotoxicity
    - Idiopathic
  - Beta cell aplasia/abiotrophy/hypoplasia
- Production of defective insulin

Insulin-resistant diabetes mellitus (target organ disorders)

- Endocrine influence
  - Growth hormone
    - Endogenous hypersecretion
      - Pituitary origin
      - Mammary origin
    - Exogenous growth hormone
  - Steroids
    - Glucocorticoids
      - Endogenous hypersecretion
      - Exogenous glucocorticoids
    - Progesterone/progestins
      - Luteal phase
        - Pregnancy
        - Dioestrus
      - Exogenous progestins
    - Other
  - Catecholamines
  - Thyroid hormone
    - Hyperthyroidism
- Obesity
- Drugs
  - Thiazide diuretics
  - Beta adrenergic agonists
- Inflammatory mediators
- Disorders of receptor and intracellular signalling

23.1 Aetiological classification of diabetes mellitus disease complex in dogs as defined by Project ALIVE (see 'Useful websites', below). An individual can concurrently have more than one underlying cause.

on the glycaemic control that might be reasonably expected. Histopathologically, canine diabetes mellitus is generally characterized by extreme beta cell deficiency that can arise from multiple mechanisms (Shields et al., 2015).

Four of the most common categories of disease aetiology are discussed in more detail below.

Congenital or juvenile-onset canine diabetes mellitus

There are occasional reports of diabetes mellitus in dogs less than 6 months of age (Catchpole et al., 2005). Pancreatic histopathology is variable in these cases, but usually few islets are visible and those beta cells that are present are degenerate and vacuolated (Minkus et al., 1997). In a study of four dogs with juvenile-onset diabetes mellitus, the histopathology was consistent with congenital islet cell aplasia (Atkins et al., 1979). An inherited, early-onset form of diabetes mellitus characterized by abiotrophy of pancreatic beta cells has been reported in Keeshond dogs. Mating studies demonstrated that the condition was likely to result from an autosomal recessive mutation, although the precise genetic defect has not

been fully elucidated (Kramer et al., 1988). It is also possible that insulin receptor defects and other monogenic forms of diabetes exist in young diabetic dogs, although these have not yet been reported. Dogs with juvenile-onset diabetes mellitus can be successfully managed with insulin therapy, and although the establishment of good glycaemic control in the growing animal is challenging, it is not impossible. With the advent of genomic medicine, it is possible that monogenic forms of diabetes mellitus in dogs may be identified, which may be more appropriately managed with oral hypoglycaemic drugs than with injectable insulin, as has proven to be the case in humans.

Hormonal antagonism

Some dogs become clinically diabetic because of the presence of circulating hormones that are antagonistic to insulin, and comparisons with both type 2 and gestational diabetes mellitus in humans have been made. Gestational diabetes mellitus has been reported in dogs (Fall et al., 2008b) but another potentially more common example of hormonal antagonism is the progesterone-dominated phase of dioestrus in intact bitches. Dogs are non-seasonally mono-oestrous and, following a season (oestrus), all normal bitches enter a luteal phase (dioestrus) lasting approximately 60 days. As well as the potential diabetogenic effect of progesterone itself, growth hormone is synthesized in the mammary glands and released into the circulation during dioestrus, and this also counteracts the action of insulin. This results in glucose intolerance, which can progress to overt diabetes mellitus in a proportion of dogs. Although immediate ovariohysterectomy can result in a clinical cure in some cases, the beta cells may be irreversibly damaged, in which case ongoing therapy with exogenous insulin is required (Fall et al., 2010).

It also follows that glycaemic control is difficult to achieve with insulin therapy in intact bitches with diabetes, because of the varying degrees of insulin resistance during the oestrous cycle. It is therefore recommended that all bitches are neutered as soon as possible after diagnosis of diabetes mellitus. Notably, it has also been reported that pyometra in intact bitches (Poppl et al., 2013) and obesity in older dogs are associated with hyperinsulinaemia and glucose intolerance, although there are no reported cases of diabetes mellitus in dogs arising as a direct result of obesity (Mattheeuws et al., 1984).

Another hormone that antagonizes insulin is cortisol, a corticosteroid hormone produced by the adrenal cortex. Dogs with hypercortisolism, usually associated with a tumour of the pituitary gland or adrenal gland, have increased serum cortisol concentrations and are at risk of concurrent diabetes mellitus (Hoffman et al., 2018). Theoretically, diabetes mellitus caused by hypercortisolism can be transient and glucose homeostasis could return to normal when the primary disease has been adequately controlled (Hoenig, 2002). However, diabetic dogs with well controlled hypercortisolism typically still require insulin therapy, while poorly controlled hypercortisolism often necessitates an increase in insulin dose.

The proportion of diabetes mellitus in dogs caused by hormonal antagonism is uncertain, since many cases of hypercortisolism may be undiagnosed and the number of intact bitches in the UK is reducing as a result of elective neutering. One study reported that 34% of diabetic dogs referred to the University of Glasgow Veterinary School had hypercortisolism or dioestrus diabetes mellitus (Graham, 1995). In a cohort of 221 diabetic dogs from the University of Pennsylvania, USA, 50 dogs (22%) were reported to have evidence of concurrent adrenocortical dysfunction (abnormal low-dose dexamethasone suppression test and/or adrenocorticotropic hormone (ACTH) response test) (Hess *et al.*, 2000). In another study of 60 dogs with confirmed hypercortisolism, 23 dogs were hyperglycaemic with moderate to severe hyperinsulinaemia and five dogs were suffering from overt diabetes mellitus with a relative insulin deficiency (Peterson *et al.*, 1984). Exogenous steroid therapy can also have an impact on glucose metabolism and, therefore, it is not surprising that systemic glucocorticoid therapy has been associated with increased diabetes risk in dogs (Heeley *et al.*, 2020).

One way in which insulin resistance and hence pancreatic 'reserve' has been evaluated in newly diagnosed diabetic dogs with suspected hormonal antagonism is by intravenous glucagon stimulation testing (Montgomery *et al.*, 1996; Watson and Herrtage, 2004; Fall *et al.*, 2008a). This test evaluates serum insulin or insulin C-peptide (co-secreted with endogenous insulin and not cross-reactive with injected insulin in insulin assays) secreted in response to an intravenous dose of glucagon. A subnormal response indicates pancreatic exhaustion and insulin deficiency, whereas a supranormal response, particularly in a hyperglycaemic animal, implies insulin resistance due to hormonal antagonism.

Pancreatitis

It has become increasingly clear that inflammation of the pancreatic exocrine tissue can result in damage to the beta cells, leading to insulin-dependent diabetes mellitus (Davison, 2015). Canine pancreatitis exists in an acute form, characterized by vomiting and abdominal pain, and a chronic form, which can be more difficult to diagnose because of its more subtle clinical signs (Watson and Herrtage, 2004). When the pancreas becomes inflamed, digestive enzyme precursors (e.g. trypsinogen) are cleaved inside pancreatic acinar cells rather than in the small intestine, and active enzymes (e.g. trypsin) are released within the pancreas, causing local tissue damage. These enzymes are regulated by proteases such as alpha-2-macroglobulin that become depleted in pancreatitis.

Obese, older, female, small-breed dogs and spaniels are thought to be at increased risk of pancreatitis. However, the reason why some dogs suffer from acute disease whereas others suffer from chronic disease is not known (Watson *et al.*, 2007). Similarly, the reason why some dogs with pancreatitis develop diabetes mellitus whereas others maintain good glucose tolerance remains to be established. Preliminary findings indicate that some dogs suffering from chronic pancreatitis have reduced beta cell function on glucagon stimulation testing (Watson and Herrtage, 2004), and in some dogs it is possible that clinical signs of diabetes mellitus could be the first indication of a subclinical, low-grade pancreatitis.

A diagnosis of pancreatitis has an important clinical impact in a diabetic dog, as it can prove more difficult to achieve good glycaemic control. As early as 1971, one study reported that 6 of 10 diabetic dogs had histological evidence of pancreatitis on post-mortem examination (Cotton *et al.*, 1971), and that dogs with clinical or biochemical evidence of pancreatitis in addition to their diabetes mellitus had a poorer prognosis. A higher prevalence of acute and chronic pancreatitis in non-surviving diabetic dogs compared with diabetic dogs that had been well controlled and were euthanased for other reasons was demonstrated in a separate study (Ling *et al.*, 1977). Historically, serum biochemical or histopathological

evidence of pancreatitis has been reported to be present in 28–40% of diabetic dogs (Alejandro *et al.*, 1988) and post-mortem histopathological studies suggest that the prevalence of chronic pancreatitis in the canine population may be underestimated by clinicians (Watson *et al.*, 2007).

Another important potential clinical implication of chronic pancreatitis is the development of exocrine pancreatic insufficiency (EPI), in which poor digestion and absorption of food can make diabetes mellitus very difficult to control and lead to dramatic weight loss. This diagnosis can easily be missed if exocrine pancreatic disease has not previously been detected. In one study (Watson, 2003), two of four dogs with confirmed chronic pancreatitis had concurrent diabetes mellitus, which had occurred after the development of EPI in these cases. This progression is similar to that seen in humans, in whom the diagnosis of chronic pancreatitis typically predates the development of EPI by several years, with diabetes mellitus usually occurring even later in the disease process. The relationship between diabetes mellitus, pancreatitis and exocrine pancreatic disease is complex with a variable histopathological picture (Figure 23.2) (Watson, 2003).

One of the difficulties in establishing the prevalence of acute or chronic pancreatic inflammation in dogs with diabetes mellitus is the limited sensitivity and specificity of available diagnostic tests (Mansfield *et al.*, 2003). In addition, chronic pancreatitis can be almost asymptomatic, and many of the signs of acute pancreatitis (e.g. lethargy and vomiting) can be attributed to other conditions, including diabetic ketoacidosis. For this reason, despite its potential importance in prognosis, testing for exocrine pancreatic disease is rarely performed at the time of diagnosis of canine diabetes mellitus. Serum biochemical markers for pancreatitis include amylase and lipase activities, which are commonly, but not always, increased with pancreatic inflammation. Many other variables affect serum amylase and lipase activities, including renal function, so false-positive increases are also possible. Measurement of trypsin-like immunoreactivity (TLI), which is increased during pancreatic inflammation, can also be useful; however, serum concentration does not always correlate with the severity of disease (Mansfield *et al.*,

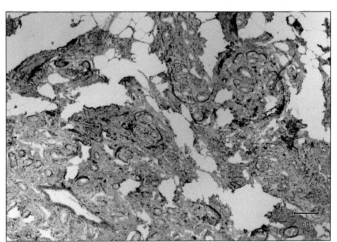

23.2 Histopathological section from the pancreas of a dog with concurrent chronic pancreatitis and diabetes mellitus. Grossly, there was very little pancreatic tissue remaining, and there is very little exocrine tissue visible histologically. A few remnants of islet tissue (dark brown) are present in this section immunostained for synaptophysin (monoclonal mouse anti-human clone SY38). This dog was totally insulin dependent despite the presence of some islet tissue, suggesting that the exocrine disease had also affected islet function. (Original magnification X40)
(Courtesy of Dr Penny Watson, University of Cambridge)

2003). In addition, the combination of EPI (decreased TLI) and acute pancreatic inflammation (increased TLI) has the potential to result in a TLI measurement within the reference interval (Hamilton *et al.*, 2021). Canine pancreas-specific lipase has been proposed as a more specific and sensitive marker for acute pancreatic inflammation (Steiner *et al.*, 2008), and its measurement should be considered in any newly diagnosed diabetic dog. In a small study of diabetic dogs with no clinical signs of pancreatitis at diagnosis, a quantitative pancreas-specific lipase concentration above the reference interval was detected in 5 of 30 cases, although none of these were above the diagnostic cut-off value for pancreatitis (Davison *et al.*, 2003a). More recently, a more pancreas-specific lipase, 1,2-o-dilauryl-raclglycero-3-glutaric acid-(6"-methylresorufin) ester (DGGR) lipase, has been suggested to provide similar evidence of pancreatitis as canine pancreas-specific lipase (Hope *et al.*, 2021). Ultrasound examination of the pancreas can also be valuable in some cases, but the sensitivity and specificity of this technique are variable, with a high degree of operator dependence. The gold standard for diagnosis of pancreatitis is pancreatic biopsy; however, this is an invasive procedure and difficult to justify, particularly as there is also a risk of missing a focus of inflammation confined to one area of the organ.

Autoimmunity

As diabetic dogs, almost without exception, are insulin dependent, it was historically thought that the canine disease had the same underlying autoimmune pathogenesis as human type 1 diabetes mellitus. As discussed above, chronic pancreatitis and hormonal antagonism are known to be responsible for the development of diabetes mellitus in some dogs, but it is possible that autoimmune destruction of beta cells is occurring in other cases, although the evidence for this is less convincing than in humans and rodents.

Human type 1 (usually insulin-dependent and juvenile-onset) diabetes mellitus is characterized by lymphocytic infiltration of the islets, known as 'insulitis', as well as the presence of serum autoantibodies to pancreatic proteins (including insulin, glutamic acid decarboxylase 65 (GAD65) and insulinoma antigen 2 (IA-2)) prior to the development of clinical signs (Taplin and Barker, 2008). In dogs, lymphocytic infiltration of pancreatic islets has been reported in a small proportion of cases (Alejandro *et al.*, 1988), but generally studies of canine pancreatic tissue in diabetes mellitus have demonstrated a more variable, heterogeneous pathology. There is some evidence of anti-beta cell antibodies in the serum of some diabetic dogs, suggesting that an immune-mediated mechanism might be responsible for beta cell destruction in a proportion of cases (Haines and Penhale, 1985). The antigen specificity of any autoimmune response in diabetic dogs is currently unknown. A small number of diabetic dogs may have autoantibodies to GAD65, IA-2 and insulin, similar to those seen in human type 1 disease (Davison *et al.*, 2008), but the majority of studies in dogs have not identified significant canine diabetes-associated autoimmunity (Ahlgren *et al.*, 2014). A recent study used a novel protein array platform for a range of autoantibodies; however, similar to previous work, results were variable and no consistent autoantibodies were identified (O'Kell *et al.*, 2022).

The potential increasing incidence of diabetes mellitus in dogs is another parallel with human type 1 disease. A seasonal pattern in the diagnosis of diabetes mellitus in dogs in the UK and the USA has been demonstrated, corresponding to the winter peak in diagnosis of type 1 diabetes mellitus in human patients (Atkins and MacDonald, 1987; Davison *et al.*, 2005; Qiu *et al.*, 2022). These similarities in disease onset between species have led to speculation that there may be similarities in environmental factors underlying the disease. It has been suggested that such environmental triggering events could be seasonal in nature (e.g. viral infections, which predominate in the winter months). Other factors that have been proposed as being involved in human diabetes mellitus and that could also play a role in the canine disease include dietary changes, obesity, inactivity and climatic change (Poppl *et al.*, 2017).

The age at onset of the disease in dogs, usually in 'middle age', is one of the features that contrasts with human type 1 diabetes mellitus, which is usually diagnosed in young children. It has therefore been suggested by some authors (Fleeman and Rand, 2001; Catchpole *et al.*, 2005) that canine diabetes mellitus is more comparable to the late-onset form of human type 1 disease known as latent autoimmune diabetes of the adult (LADA).

Clinical features

Signalment
Age
Diabetes mellitus is generally a disease of middle-aged and older dogs, usually diagnosed between the ages of 5 and 12 years, although there are some reports in dogs as young as 6 months of age (Davison *et al.*, 2005).

Breed
In the most recent UK survey of canine diabetes mellitus, crossbreed dogs and West Highland White, Yorkshire and Jack Russell Terriers predominated (Heeley *et al.*, 2020). However, as there is no compulsory dog registration scheme, it is difficult to estimate the proportions of each breed in the UK dog population. When databases such as the VetCompass database (see 'Useful websites', below) are used to compare prevalence in particular breeds to breed popularity, breeds such as Tibetan and Border Terriers, and the Samoyed emerge as being at particularly increased risk (Davison *et al.*, 2005, Heeley *et al.*, 2020). It is also interesting to note the relatively low numbers of some very popular breeds, such as German Shepherd Dogs, Boxers, Shih Tzus and Golden Retrievers, in the diabetic population, suggesting that such breeds might have a decreased risk of developing diabetes mellitus.

Breed associations with disease are likely to reflect underlying genetic risk factors. Human type 1 diabetes mellitus has a strong genetic association with the genes encoding the major histocompatibility complex (MHC) class II proteins, which are involved in antigen presentation to the immune system (Todd *et al.*, 1987). Recent genetic studies of canine diabetes mellitus have identified certain canine MHC alleles (encoding the dog leucocyte antigen (DLA) proteins) that are associated with increased risk of diabetes in some breeds (Denyer *et al.*, 2020). In addition, certain polymorphisms within other immune-response genes have been identified as contributing to risk of diabetes in certain breeds (Short *et al.*, 2009). Taken together, these findings implicate dysregulation of the immune response in some cases of canine diabetes mellitus, although many more susceptibility genes and mechanisms remain to be discovered.

Sex

Historically, a sex predisposition in bitches has been reported. In early surveys, approximately 70% of diabetic dogs were female (Marmor *et al.*, 1982); in more recent surveys, the female bias remains but is less obvious (Davison *et al.*, 2005; Heeley *et al.*, 2020). This relative reduction in the proportion of females being diagnosed is most likely related to an increased trend of neutering bitches, leading to a reduction in the proportion of cases resulting from insulin antagonism during the progesterone-dominated phase of dioestrus.

Additional risk factors

In a recent UK study, dogs documented as obese with a concurrent diagnosis of hypercortisolism or pancreatitis were at increased risk of diabetes mellitus (Heeley *et al.*, 2020).

Clinical signs

The majority of diabetic dogs are 'well' at the time of presentation, with the main complaints of the owner being polyuria, polydipsia and weight loss. Clinical signs of diabetes mellitus are summarized in Figure 23.3.

Polyuria and Polydipsia

Polydipsia is secondary to polyuria, which can also lead to signs of inappropriate urination, particularly if a secondary urinary tract infection is present. The polyuria arises as a result of the blood glucose concentration exceeding the renal threshold for resorption (12–14 mmol/l) and hence glucose escaping into the urine. This has a profound osmotic diuresis effect.

Polyphagia

A high proportion of diabetic dogs are also polyphagic as insulin is required for adequate activity of the hypothalamic satiety centre, which is involved in determining appetite.

Weight loss

Weight loss occurs partly as a result of glucosuria, but also because of metabolic changes resulting from cells being 'starved' of glucose (as insulin is not present to allow glucose into the cells). The body mobilizes fat and protein (muscle) stores for gluconeogenesis, which, as well as leading to weight loss, can result in hyperlipidaemia, hepatic lipidosis (hepatomegaly) and muscle wasting.

Generally, signs progress fairly rapidly but, in some rare cases, the disease has a gradual onset and the first sign noted by some owners may be the development of apparently 'acute' cataracts. A small proportion of dogs will present acutely unwell with ketosis or ketoacidosis, particularly if there are secondary complications such as pancreatitis or a urinary tract infection. Such dogs might be collapsed, tachypnoeic (acidosis) and smell of ketones, with a history of anorexia or vomiting. Ketoacidosis should be considered an emergency and requires immediate intensive treatment, which is discussed in detail in Chapter 26.

Diagnosis

A diagnosis of diabetes mellitus in dogs is usually made using a combination of clinical signs and documentation of a persistent fasting hyperglycaemia (>12–14 mmol/l) with glucosuria. Project ALIVE publishes guidance and criteria for diagnosing diabetes mellitus in dogs and cats (see 'Useful websites', below). Hyperglycaemia and glucosuria can be caused by several clinical syndromes; differential diagnoses are listed in Figure 23.4. A variety of other tests may be performed to aid in diagnosis and assist in determining any potential underlying cause.

Routine clinicopathological features

It can be helpful to perform routine haematology and serum biochemistry in dogs with suspected diabetes mellitus, to establish whether there are any other concurrent diseases and to confirm the diagnosis.

Common biochemical abnormalities in diabetes mellitus include hypercholesterolaemia and hypertriglyceridaemia, resulting from mobilization of fat stores and loss of inhibition of hormone-sensitive lipase in adipose tissue (see Chapter 7). Severe lipaemia can interfere with some biochemical assays, and consequently a fasting blood sample is preferred for biochemical analysis in diabetic dogs. Secondary fatty changes in the liver can also lead to persistent mild, moderate or severe increases in the activities of liver enzymes such as alkaline phosphatase and alanine aminotransferase.

Common
• Polyuria and polydipsia
• Weight loss
• Muscle wasting
• Polyphagia
Possible
• Cataracts
• Smell of ketones on breath
• Hepatomegaly
• Reduced exercise tolerance
• Recurrent bacterial infections

23.3 Clinical signs of diabetes mellitus.

Hyperglycaemia
• Diabetes mellitus
• Stress (usually <15 mmol/l)
• Iatrogenic
• Glucocorticoid treatment
• Progestin treatment
• Glucose-containing intravenous fluids
• Alpha-2 agonist sedatives
• Hormonal antagonism
• Hypercortisolism
• Dioestrus
• Phaeochromocytoma
• Hypersomatotropism (rare in dogs)
Glucosuria (renal threshold 12–14 mmol/l)
• Diabetes mellitus
• Stress
• Iatrogenic
• Glucose-containing intravenous fluids
• Renal tubular dysfunction
• Fanconi syndrome
• Primary renal glucosuria
• Acute or chronic kidney disease
• Nephrotoxins
• Interference with test
• Glucose in owner's collecting jar for urine (e.g. jam jar)
• Contamination with hydrogen peroxide or bacterial peroxidases

23.4 Differential diagnoses for hyperglycaemia and glucosuria.

It is uncommon to see marked haematological changes in diabetic dogs, although a stress leucogram (mature neutrophilia, lymphopenia, monocytosis, eosinopenia) can be detected in some cases. Occasionally, an increase in packed cell volume is noted, consistent with dehydration; however, in other cases a mild non-regenerative anaemia of chronic disease is seen.

Circulating glucose measurement

It is very important that any equipment used to assess circulating glucose concentrations in a diabetic dog is as accurate as possible. Historically, blood glucose meters designed and calibrated for human capillary blood have been employed to measure venous blood glucose concentrations in dogs. There are many such devices available, several of which have been tested for accuracy with canine blood, with variable results. The most accurate device is one that is well maintained, regularly calibrated against another machine or an external laboratory gold standard, and which draws up the correct volume of blood into a disposable chamber. Machines that are not well cared for, used infrequently or rely on blood being 'spotted' on to a test strip that is inserted into the machine tend to be less accurate. In addition, there are now specific veterinary glucometers available, including control calibrators for dog and cat blood, which may be more reliable (Figure 23.5). There can also be variability between individual glucometers of the same type so, when performing repeated measurements, it is advisable to use the same glucometer for each measurement to allow trends in blood glucose concentration to be more accurately assessed in individual animals.

Urinalysis

Urinalysis is important in the diabetic dog, primarily to confirm glucosuria but also to assess for evidence of concurrent urinary tract infection. In addition to assessment of haematuria, pH, proteinuria and ketonuria by dipstick, sediment analysis should always be performed for evidence of inflammation or bacterial infection. Diabetic dogs are particularly at risk of such infections as the high

glucose concentration in the urine favours bacterial growth. Clinical signs of urinary tract infection are very similar to those of diabetes mellitus, so a potential infection can easily be missed during history taking. Without adequate treatment, bacterial urinary tract infection will lead to insulin resistance and make it more difficult to achieve good glycaemic control, so culture and susceptibility testing of a cystocentesis urine sample is recommended both routinely and, particularly, where there is suspicion of infection.

Any evidence of proteinuria should be followed up with quantification of urinary protein by determination of urine protein:creatinine. Proteinuria should also prompt measurement of blood pressure and fundic examination if this has not already been performed as part of the general clinical examination.

Fructosamine and glycated haemoglobin

The long-term presence of hyperglycaemia can be confirmed by measuring concentrations of glycated blood proteins, such as fructosamine or glycated haemoglobin (HbA1c), which are increased in diabetic cases. As discussed below (see 'Monitoring glycaemic control'), these parameters are also used as a guide to glycaemic control once treatment has started, particularly in dogs that are resistant to repeated blood glucose sampling. Fructosamine is a term used to describe plasma proteins, mainly albumin, which have undergone non-enzymatic, irreversible glycosylation in proportion to their prevailing glucose concentration. In dogs, the serum fructosamine concentration is related to the average blood glucose concentration over the preceding 1–2 weeks but is also influenced by the rate of plasma protein turnover in the animal and may vary according to the breed and the individual (Momozawa et al., 2020). Glycated haemoglobin describes haemoglobin that has become irreversibly chemically bound to glucose, which occurs in proportion to the concentration of glucose in the plasma. In dogs, the HbA1c concentration reflects the average blood glucose concentration over the preceding 2–3 months. Most commercial veterinary laboratories now offer fructosamine assays and they are routinely used by most veterinary surgeons, but there is currently no widely available assay for HbA1c for dogs.

Further diagnostic tests for ketosis and ketoacidosis

In any 'unwell', inappetent or newly diagnosed diabetic dog, measurement of ketones in urine or preferably blood should always be performed. Further evidence for ketoacidosis can be gained from blood gas analysis, with demonstration of reduced blood pH and bicarbonate concentration in the ketoacidotic dog as a result of metabolic acidosis. The diagnosis and management of diabetic ketoacidosis are discussed in more detail in Chapter 26.

Functional testing and assessment of pancreatic inflammation

There are several other tests that can be performed at the time of diagnosis with the specific aim of categorizing the disease as being the result of insulin resistance, insulin deficiency and/or pancreatitis. These tests include the measurement of serum TLI and pancreas-specific lipase concentrations or DGGR lipase activity, increases of any or all of which can be indicative of exocrine pancreatic

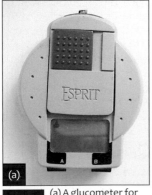
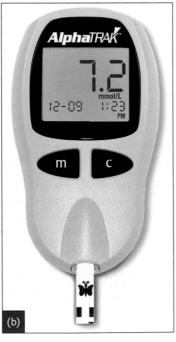

23.5 (a) A glucometer for human use, which draws up the correct volume of blood for testing into a disposable cartridge.
(b) Glucometers are available that are specifically designed to work with the blood of veterinary species.
(© Abbot Animal Health)

disease. As mentioned above, a diagnosis of concurrent pancreatitis can have an impact on the management and prognosis of the case, so it is important that the presence of pancreatic inflammation is not missed (Davison, 2015). Additionally, where insulin resistance is suspected, beta cell reserve can be assessed in untreated diabetic dogs by measurement of serum insulin or insulin C-peptide, and glucose concentrations before and after an intravenous injection of glucagon (see 'Hormonal antagonism', above).

Further endocrine testing (e.g. adrenal and thyroid function tests) is sometimes required if a concurrent endocrinopathy is suspected, although false-positive results can be obtained in stressed or sick animals. For this reason, it is often preferable to attempt diabetic stabilization prior to further endocrine testing.

Management

Once the diagnosis of diabetes mellitus has been made, it is important that treatment is instituted as soon as possible. The time and financial commitment required from the dog's owner should not be underestimated, and it is vital to make these details clear from the outset. Management of a diabetic pet requires daily administration of insulin, a fixed routine and enough financial support not only for insulin and consumables but also for monitoring, diagnostic tests and potential intermittent periods of hospitalization. Guidelines vary internationally because of variable insulin availability and licensing, but the key principles are the same (Behrend et al., 2018).

Many owners are anxious about how they and their dog will cope with treatment and may take several days to adjust to the idea of their pet being diabetic. However, even if the owner is undecided about their commitment initially, instigation of treatment should not be delayed by longer than a few hours as ketosis or ketoacidosis could develop and complicate the situation further. Once committed, even the most anxious owner can be taught to administer insulin to their pet and, in most cases, particularly after the first few months of stabilization are completed, the dog's quality of life should be very good. Although a wide variety of factors influence prognosis in individual cases (Gilor, 2019; Tardo et al., 2019), a study in Sweden demonstrated a median survival time of 2 years in diabetic dogs surviving more than 1 day beyond diagnosis (Fall et al., 2007), which is encouraging, given the advanced age of most dogs at the time of diagnosis. In a recent UK study, median survival time for all dogs was 15.6 months, rising to 20.2 months for those surviving at least 7 days post diagnosis (Heeley et al., 2020). However, it is also fair to warn owners that some dogs are more difficult to stabilize than others, and generally those dogs that have concurrent pancreatitis, ketoacidosis or hypercortisolism are more likely to fall into this more 'brittle' category with a poorer prognosis. Factors associated with reduced survival include being older than 10 years of age at diagnosis, having a circulating glucose concentration higher than 40 mmol/l at diagnosis and receiving prior glucocorticoid treatment (Heeley et al., 2020).

Diet and exercise

The key to achieving glycaemic control in diabetic dogs is a fixed daily routine. As the same dose of insulin is given each day, the type and amount of food should be the same, and ideally there should be no large variations in the amount of exercise the dog undertakes. Whilst ad libitum feeding can work well in some diabetic cats, it is not recommended in dogs. Similarly, between-meal 'snacks' are best avoided and if they must be used, for example, in training, the calories should be taken from the day's energy allowance and sugary or starchy treats avoided.

Type of diet

The most important factor when selecting a diet for a diabetic dog is whether the dog finds the food palatable and will eat it consistently. This is not usually a problem as diabetes mellitus tends to result in polyphagia. Dietary concerns relating to concurrent diseases (e.g. chronic kidney disease, urolithiasis, inflammatory bowel disease) must also be considered, and often take precedence over a specific 'diabetic' diet. Several very good commercial prescription diets are available for diabetic dogs. They are available in wet and dry formulations, broadly based on the principles that food should be palatable, nutritionally balanced and highly digestible. Additionally, to minimize postprandial hyperglycaemia, the diet should not contain large amounts of simple sugars. A diet lower in digestible carbohydrate results in lower postprandial glucose concentrations compared with standard maintenance diets in diabetic dogs (Elliott et al., 2012). Calories should be provided mainly by a combination of complex carbohydrates and protein, whilst fat should be particularly restricted in dogs with a history of pancreatitis. Various studies have been performed on the value of high-fibre diets in diabetic dogs, with some suggesting that higher-fibre diets are beneficial but may be less appropriate for diabetic dogs in poor body condition (Fleeman and Rand, 2001; Fleeman et al., 2009). Whilst weight remains an important guide to control of the disease, it can be difficult for a thin diabetic dog to regain weight. If weight loss continues despite satisfactory glycaemic control, measurement of TLI should be considered in case of underlying EPI.

Timing of feeding

Food should be divided into at least two meals a day; however, more frequent feeding is sometimes required in dogs receiving twice-daily insulin. The first meal should coincide with the first insulin injection, with some clinicians preferring the insulin to precede the meal by 30 minutes, some feeding 30 minutes prior to insulin and some recommending that insulin and food be given together. This is really a matter of personal preference, depending on the owner's routine and the dog's history or appetite. For example, it would be preferable to check that a dog with a history of episodes of inappetence is keen to eat its food before it receives insulin, to reduce the risk of hypoglycaemia occurring later in the day if it has been injected but does not eat. This is particularly important if the owner is not usually at home with the dog during the day. However, some dogs need the stimulus of the immediate fall in blood glucose concentration after injection (due to the soluble component of some lente insulins, e.g. Caninsulin) to stimulate their appetite and will only eat a full meal once the insulin has started to work. Such dogs are best injected as early as possible in the morning, particularly if the owner is out all day, to allow time for the insulin to work and for the owner to be able to check that the dog has eaten before they leave the house. In any circumstance, it is advisable to ask owners to contact the practice if their diabetic dog does not eat, since this can be a sign of more serious problems such as ketoacidosis or pancreatitis.

If the dog is being injected once daily and fed twice daily, each meal should contain 50% of the energy requirement for that dog and the second meal should be fed at the time of peak activity of insulin, 6–8 hours after injection. If dogs are receiving twice-daily insulin, then they should receive a meal with both injections, each containing 30–50% of the daily energy requirements. Often, dogs treated twice daily will also be hungry 6–8 hours after each injection, at the time of peak insulin activity. If this is the case, a smaller meal (10–20% of the daily energy requirements) can be provided at these times. Owners often prefer to use dry food for these smaller meals, and for good control they should be provided either every day or not at all, since variation in feeding can lead to glycaemic instability.

Exercise

Exercise need not be restricted in diabetic dogs, although it can take time to build up the muscle mass that is lost in the early phase of the disease. As with food and insulin, the most important factor is consistency; it is not ideal for a diabetic dog to have little or no exercise during the week and one or more very long walks at the weekend. Increasing exercise without increasing the amount of food runs the risk of hypoglycaemia but, conversely, increasing food too much without providing extra insulin can result in hyperglycaemia and osmotic diuresis. Hypoglycaemia is the most dangerous of these potential complications; it is therefore sensible to advise the owner of any diabetic dog to take a sugary snack or oral glucose gel with them when on a walk, in case their dog starts to show signs of hypoglycaemia.

Types of insulin

Diabetic dogs are insulin dependent, almost without exception. Owners familiar with treatment for human type 2 diabetes mellitus might enquire whether it is possible to control their dog's disease without injections, for example, using oral hypoglycaemic drugs, such as sulphonylureas. Many oral hypoglycaemic drugs act by stimulating insulin secretion; unfortunately, these are of no value in most diabetic dogs, since their pancreatic islets are usually irreversibly damaged by the time of diagnosis and are incapable of producing any insulin. The potential value of drugs such as alpha-glucosidase inhibitors, which delay absorption of dietary polysaccharides and could be used in combination with insulin, has yet to be determined in dogs. Ongoing research is also being performed into alternative insulin delivery routes such as mucosal or oral treatment, but problems with insulin degradation make these unacceptable for routine use at the present time, so injection remains the only effective method of insulin delivery. Future options may also include longer-acting depot insulin preparations and potentially islet or stem cell transplantation (Rhew et al., 2021), but neither of these options are currently in widespread use.

Species of origin

There are currently no recombinant canine insulin preparations available for veterinary use; the majority of dogs are treated with insulin purified from porcine pancreas or human recombinant insulin and insulin analogues (Figure 23.6).

There are two insulin preparations authorized for treatment of diabetes mellitus in dogs in the UK: Caninsulin, a

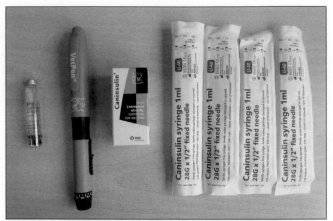

23.6 Caninsulin is one of the two types of insulin authorized for use in dogs. Caninsulin is available in two formulations: the VetPen and a suspension for injection with insulin syringes.

lente form of porcine insulin derived from pig pancreas, and ProZinc, a human recombinant insulin synthesized in a laboratory. Porcine insulin is homologous to canine insulin, whereas human insulin differs from canine insulin by two amino acids; however, both show similar clinical effects. Both preparations are formulated as 40 IU/ml, unlike most insulins for human use, which are typically formulated at 100 IU/ml. This relatively dilute formulation means that small dose adjustments are more accurate, but specific 40 IU/ml syringes must be used. However, where large doses are required for heavier dogs, the volume of insulin injected each day can become challenging for some owners.

Where no authorized preparation exists (e.g. a rapid-acting insulin suitable for intravenous or intramuscular use when treating diabetic ketoacidosis), human recombinant insulin in a 'neutral' or 'soluble' form at 100 IU/ml is usually used.

Duration of action

The duration of action of insulin depends not only on the preparation, but also on the route of delivery and the individual being injected. Soluble (neutral) insulin is the only preparation authorized in humans for intravenous and intramuscular injection, as well as the standard subcutaneous route. It also has the quickest onset (within 1 hour) and shortest duration (up to 4–6 hours) of activity, with the intravenous route providing the most immediate and shortest effect. Lente insulin, such as Caninsulin, has a more prolonged duration of action as it is insulin complexed with zinc to produce crystals of varying size, thereby delaying its absorption. It has a biphasic activity as 30–35% of the insulin is amorphous, with a more immediate effect. The remaining 65–70% of the insulin is in an ultralente or microcrystalline form, which peaks in activity at around 6–8 hours and lasts up to 12–24 hours. The longest-lasting insulins tend to be those in which the insulin is formulated with protamine and zinc (protamine zinc insulin (PZI)), such as ProZinc, which results in a suspension with a slower and more prolonged duration of activitiy. These insulins have a duration of activity of up to 24 hours in some dogs.

Other insulins

Where authorized preparations have not been successful in managing diabetes mellitus, recombinant insulin analogues have also been used successfully in dogs (Gilor and Fleeman, 2022). Figure 23.7 outlines the expected onset and duration of activity of several commonly used

Insulin type	Onset of activity	Peak of activity	Typical duration of activity	Type of insulin	Example
Soluble (neutral)	0–1 hours	0–2 hours	4–6 hours	Short acting	Actrapid 100 IU/ml human recombinant insulin
Lente	0–1 hours	4–8 hours	12 hours+	Intermediate acting	Caninsulin* 40 IU/ml porcine lente insulin
Protamine zinc	0–4 hours	5–20 hours	12–24 hours	Long acting	ProZinc* 40 IU/ml human recombinant insulin
Glargine	0–4 hours	'Peakless'	Up to 24 hours	Very long acting	Lantus 100 IU/ml and Toujeo 300 IU/ml human recombinant insulin analogue
Detemir	0–4 hours	8–10 hours	24 hours+	Very long acting	Levemir 100 IU/ml human recombinant insulin analogue. NB: this may be very potent in dogs
Degludec	0–4 hours	'Peakless'	24 hours+	Very long acting	Tresiba 100 IU/ml or 200 IU/ml human recombinant insulin analogue. NB: this may be very potent in dogs

23.7 Expected onset and duration of activity of several commonly used insulin preparations. * = UK veterinary-authorized preparations.

insulin preparations. Of particular interest is insulin glargine, a genetically engineered recombinant insulin analogue based on the human insulin amino acid sequence but with one asparagine in the insulin A chain replaced by glycine and two extra arginines on the C terminus of the B chain. This shifts the isoelectric point of the insulin, producing a solution that is completely soluble at a pH of 4 but forms subcutaneous microprecipitates when it is injected and exposed to the physiological pH of 7.4. This allows slow release of the insulin, which can last up to 24 hours in humans, with minimal peaks and troughs in activity. Other analogues include detemir, which is a genetically engineered human insulin analogue. The protein has been modified to allow it to bind albumin with high affinity in the subcutaneous and intravascular spaces. This prolongs the absorption of the insulin and minimizes peaks and troughs (Gilor and Graves, 2010; Fracassi et al., 2015). Detemir appears to be particularly potent in dogs and should be used with great caution, particularly in small dogs, to avoid hypoglycaemic episodes.

In addition to insulin analogues, other insulin therapies exist, including isophane insulin (neutral protamine Hagedorn) recombinant human lente insulin (some available in semi-automated insulin 'pens'), and mixed bovine/porcine insulin. These are in more widespread use in some countries, but are not authorized for dogs in the UK. The future of insulin therapy in dogs is likely to see increased use of, as yet unauthorized, longer acting 'basal' insulin preparations. These include a very highly concentrated preparation of glargine at 300 IU/ml, and another recombinant ultra-long-acting human insulin analogue called degludec. It may also include a once-weekly canine insulin preparation, but studies on its efficacy and safety are not yet available.

Stabilization protocol

Many protocols have been described for the initial management of diabetic dogs and each has its particular advantages and disadvantages. No single protocol is suitable for every dog, owner or veterinary practice, but a key feature common to every protocol is excellent communication between client and veterinary practice. The days immediately after diagnosis are also a vital period of education about diabetes for the client. Important factors to be discussed include the establishment of a daily routine of diet and exercise, the practicalities of insulin storage and injection technique, and monitoring of clinical signs and potential diabetic emergencies, such as hypoglycaemia. It is also important to arrange to neuter intact bitches that are diabetic as soon as some degree of glycaemic control has been achieved. If ovariohysterectomy

is performed expediently, there is some possibility that the beta cells might recover and the animal might not remain insulin dependent (Fall et al., 2008b, 2010). Much of this initial information can be provided in person by the veterinary surgeons and nurses within the practice; however, reinforcement by other available materials such as websites, literature and smartphone apps can be very valuable. It can also be very useful for the owner of a diabetic animal to keep a daily diary to record the general demeanour, appetite and thirst of their pet for monitoring purposes.

The importance of making sure the insulin is stored in the refrigerator to avoid extremes of light and temperature, not used past its expiry date, reconstituted before each injection and administered with the correct syringes or pen must be emphasized to the owner. Injection technique should be demonstrated to owners until they are comfortable with it, including drawing up the solution without air bubbles and safe sites for injection. Insulin is usually injected subcutaneously in the region of the dorsal neck, and the owner should be encouraged to rotate injection sites within this region every few days.

Most 'well' diabetic dogs are not ketoacidotic and have an excellent appetite, such that stabilization can be performed at home if preferred. This decision is primarily made depending on the clinical presentation of the dog, but also considers the lifestyle of the owner, their willingness/ability to travel to the practice and their confidence at giving insulin injections. It is even possible to stabilize 'well' dogs with ketonuria by this home method as long as they are eating well and making good clinical progress, but if they are inappetent or otherwise unwell, closer observation and more intensive treatment are recommended (see Chapter 26). Once the choice of insulin type has been made, a decision must be reached with regard to once-daily or twice-daily treatment, although twice-daily treatment is strongly recommended. Protamine zinc insulin, because of its longer duration of action, may be required only once daily in some dogs, whereas lente preparations are commonly injected every 12 hours. Although most owners would prefer to inject their dog only once daily, clinical evidence suggests that dogs are more stable (and the risk of hypoglycaemia is minimized) with twice-daily therapy (Hess and Ward, 2000; Fleeman and Rand, 2001). Another advantage of twice-daily treatment is that a 'missed' insulin injection, which can occur due to unexpected circumstances, is less likely to cause a problem as the dog will only go 24 hours, rather than 48 hours, between insulin doses.

As a guide, a starting dose of an authorized insulin preparation is usually in the region of 0.5 IU/kg, but can increase to 1 IU/kg with once-daily treatment; however, it is preferable to start with a low dose and work upwards than to risk hypoglycaemia. Adjustments to the initial dose are often made with respect to body condition score and weight, such that very large or obese dogs might receive a lower dose and very small dogs a slightly higher dose. Consideration must also be given to the presence of concurrent infection, inflammation or hormonal antagonism that might result in insulin resistance, although this should resolve with appropriate treatment of the underlying cause.

If the dog is being stabilized at home, it must return to the practice at least once daily, ideally at the time of expected peak activity of insulin (nadir glucose), for blood glucose measurement. If this is not possible, the dog can be stabilized on an in-practice basis. The main purpose of nadir blood glucose monitoring is not to assess glycaemic control in any detail but to establish that the blood glucose is not falling to a dangerously low concentration (<4 mmol/l) if the dog is more sensitive to insulin than expected. The disadvantage of this technique is that with single blood glucose measurements, the clinician can only estimate the time at which the blood glucose is likely to be at its lowest point. As a rough guide, somewhere between 4 and 8 hours post-injection is a useful starting point for blood glucose measurement when using a lente preparation, whereas 9–12 hours post-injection would be a more appropriate time to sample in PZI-treated dogs. The pharmacokinetics and pharmacodynamics of insulin will vary between individuals, hence the nadir might fall earlier or later than the blood glucose measurement, making the result potentially misleading. However, the in-home approach is still particularly useful for dogs that do not eat well in the practice and whose owners are at home most of the day and able to monitor for signs of hypoglycaemia. This approach can also be supported by teaching the owner to perform blood glucose measurements at home with a lancet device and glucometer, as long as results are regularly reported to the practice (see 'Monitoring glycaemic control', below). Alternatively, some owners will prefer that the dog receives its first few doses of insulin in hospital, perhaps visiting their pet to learn to administer the injections under veterinary or nursing supervision. The dog can then return home once it has been established by blood glucose measurement that the insulin dose is safe.

After 4–7 days of treatment, a 12–24-hour blood glucose curve to assess progress is recommended. Blood glucose curves can vary from day to day and can be influenced by many factors so must always be interpreted with caution (Fleeman and Rand, 2003). The main questions to be addressed by performing a curve include whether the insulin is working consistently, how long it is lasting and whether the nadir concentration of glucose is dangerously low (see 'Monitoring glycaemic control', below). It is likely that a dose adjustment will be made at this stage, or a recommendation to change to twice-daily treatment if the insulin is lasting less than 24 hours. Changes to management will also depend on other clinical parameters, such as the appetite, thirst and general demeanour of the dog, and it is preferable not to change more than one parameter (food, insulin, exercise regime) at a time during this phase. When changing a dog from once-daily insulin to twice-daily treatment, the dose used will depend on many factors, but it is preferable to make sure that the dose at each injection is the same and that the injections are given 12 hours apart. If a glucose curve has demonstrated that the once-daily insulin dose is safe but lasts less than 12 hours, then the same dose should be considered for twice-daily use. If the insulin appears to last slightly longer than 12 hours, but less than 24 hours, a guideline twice-daily dose would be 75% of the once-daily dose.

Once the frequency of insulin treatment has been determined, dose adjustments should be small (ideally maximum 1 IU at a time for smaller dogs and 2 IU for larger dogs). If larger dose adjustments are made because of consistently high blood glucose concentration, they should never be greater than 10% of the dose. The exception to this is dose reduction when profound hypoglycaemia has been detected, in which case a more dramatic reduction in dose (of up to 50%) can be undertaken. This phase of slow stabilization requires patience from the owner, dog and veterinary surgeon, with each dose change ideally being followed by a 3–5-day adjustment period at home and then, ideally, a 12–24-hour blood glucose curve. A steady and cautious approach in the weeks immediately following diagnosis increases the likelihood of a suitable dose of insulin being reached within 1–2 months, as the correct dose will not be 'overshot' by rapid and large dose adjustments. Depending on the dog and the owner, a combination of glucose curves and assessment of clinical parameters, such as 24-hour water intake and fructosamine measurement, is usually used to assess and achieve glycaemic control in the stabilization phase. If hospitalization is necessary, more frequent dose adjustments are often used; however, animals should be discharged only when dose adjustments are not required for at least 3 consecutive days.

Monitoring glycaemic control

Fructosamine

The introduction of diagnostic tests to measure fructosamine and HbA1c concentrations has helped improve monitoring of glycaemic control in dogs and prevent secondary complications. Changes in these parameters allow informed adjustments of insulin therapy to be made and decisions to be taken as to whether further investigations are required. In practical terms, this means that if the dog is not amenable to repeated glucose curves, an alternative, but often slower, method of adjusting the insulin dose is to use serum fructosamine measurement as a guide to glycaemic control. It is important, however, that this is performed alongside observation of clinical signs, such as weight change and measurement of water intake.

Fructosamine can be measured every 2–3 weeks using a single blood sample, with the advantage that this test can be performed at any time of day rather than at the specific timings needed for a blood glucose curve. Its most useful role is for monitoring a dog's progress longitudinally, that is, comparing a dog to itself over time and deciding whether glycaemic control is deteriorating or improving. In this situation, it is vital that the same laboratory is used for testing each time, as assays and reference intervals can vary substantially across laboratories. It is also recommended that a laboratory that participates in a hormone measurement quality assurance scheme is used. When the dog has reached a suitable dose of insulin, the fructosamine concentration will be steady, weight will be stable and the dog should not be drinking excessively. This route of stabilization is often more successful for dogs receiving twice-daily insulin as it is difficult to determine whether the duration of insulin activity is adequate in dogs treated once daily using fructosamine alone.

Although reference intervals can vary widely between laboratories, fructosamine values less than 400 µmol/l are generally accepted to represent very good glycaemic control whereas values above 550 μmol/l suggest very poor control. These values must be interpreted with caution, as fructosamine measurement is less accurate than blood glucose measurement for determining if a dog falls into 'poor', 'acceptable', 'good' or 'very good' glycaemic control compared with the general diabetic population. This is because the values representing these degrees of control can vary among cases; fructosamine concentration is not influenced exclusively by blood glucose but also by other factors, such as protein turnover. As a result, fructosamine should always be interpreted in light of clinical signs and previous measurements from the same dog. It is important to note that whilst it is desirable that fructosamine concentration is consistent with adequate glycaemic control (and blood glucose concentrations remain between 4 and 12 mmol/l in a blood glucose curve), this is not always completely achievable. It is more important to meet the clinical aims of therapy outlined in Figure 23.8.

A reassuring fructosamine result in a dog still showing clinical signs of instability does not suggest good glycaemic control, but instead might be the average result of a combination of hypo- and hyperglycaemic periods throughout the day. Conversely, an increased fructosamine value should not cause too much alarm in a dog that is doing well on assessment by clinical criteria (Figure 23.8). Rather than adjusting a regimen that is resolving clinical signs satisfactorily in such a case, it would be preferable to maintain the same regimen and repeat the fructosamine measurement and clinical assessment in 2–4 weeks' time. If fructosamine is continuing to increase, further investigation might be warranted, but if clinical signs and fructosamine are stable, then any adjustments should be considered very carefully as they might cause deterioration rather than improvement in a dog with an acceptable quality of life.

- Resolution of clinical signs such as polyuria and polydipsia
- Maintenance of a good appetite and stable bodyweight
- Owner perception that the dog has a good quality of life and is able to undertake a reasonable amount of daily exercise
- Minimal risk of complications, such as ketoacidosis, hypoglycaemia, infections or cataracts

23.8 Aims of diabetes mellitus therapy.

Urine glucose

If owners are able to collect urine easily from their dog, this offers a further method of assessing glycaemic control, since semi-quantitative dipsticks allow assessment of glucosuria and ketonuria. Approximately 44% of UK owners of diabetic dogs undertake urine monitoring of their pet (Heeley et al., 2020). Glucose will be present in the urine if the concentration in the blood exceeds the renal threshold (12–14 mmol/l), which is not unusual for at least some part of the day in many diabetic dogs, particularly just before an insulin injection. It is therefore important that urine glucose is assessed at the same time of day on each occasion, preferably in the morning, and that values are interpreted alongside other clinical data. A small amount of urine glucose in a morning sample is acceptable, but the owner should be instructed to seek veterinary advice if this amount increases in a consistent pattern or ketones are also present. Conversely, if no glucose is detected in a morning urine sample, then it is possible that the dog is at risk of hypoglycaemia and the insulin dose should be reviewed. Caution must be exercised in altering the insulin dose based on urine glucose alone, particularly

in dogs receiving once-daily therapy, as they almost always demonstrate morning glucosuria. Increasing the dose will not resolve glucosuria if the insulin is lasting less than 24 hours, and 'chasing' the urine glucose by gradual increase of the insulin dose is a common cause of insulin-induced hyperglycaemia (Somogyi response, see Chapter 25). In dogs at risk of ketoacidosis, intermittent urinalysis at home can also prove very useful in providing an early warning of ketonuria.

Blood glucose curve

Another potentially valuable method of evaluating the efficacy of insulin therapy in diabetic dogs is a serial blood glucose curve, involving repeated blood sampling every 1–2 hours over a 12–24-hour period. Veterinary glucometers, calibrated for canine and feline capillary blood, are generally preferable to those designed for use in humans (see Figure 23.5).

Blood glucose curves can be an important part of the assessment of glycaemic control in some dogs, but in others they provide very little useful diagnostic information, for example, if a dog will not eat during a hospital stay or is difficult to obtain repeat samples from. It is clear that even in stable dogs the blood glucose curve can vary dramatically from day to day, so care must be taken not to over-interpret findings (Fleeman and Rand, 2003). In the hours following a severe hypoglycaemic episode, for example, the presence of antagonistic hormones such as glucagon, adrenaline (epinephrine) and cortisol might prevent any further hypoglycaemic values from being obtained, despite the same dose of insulin being given. Stress can also contribute to increased blood glucose values in hospitalized dogs (although not to the same extent as in hospitalized cats), such that the blood glucose curve obtained in hospital might be very different from the curve that would be obtained at home. It is particularly important to avoid 'joining up' the various points on an hourly or two-hourly curve with lines, since this makes an assumption that no peaks or troughs are occurring in between samples and can be misleading. It is also important to wait for several days for a dog to 'equilibrate' to a new insulin dose before performing a curve by, for example, sending them home for a few days in between repeated curves if it is safe and practical to do so.

In an ideal diabetic dog, the blood glucose concentration would stay between 4 mmol/l and 12 mmol/l all day during a blood glucose curve. However, as blood glucose curves can be confusing and rarely look like textbook examples, it is useful for both owner and clinician to be realistic in the expectation of how much will be gained from the information generated. Methodical analysis of a blood glucose curve will usually allow a judgment to be made about glycaemic control and potential changes in treatment. Case selection is also important in gaining the most value from glucose curves, as they can be uncomfortable for the dog and require a lot of effort from practice staff. Unstable diabetic and newly diagnosed dogs being stabilized on insulin are most likely to benefit from a 12- or 24-hour curve, whereas performing a blood glucose curve simply to 'check' a dog that is already fulfilling all the aims of therapy described in Figure 23.8 is questionable as it is unlikely to alter clinical management.

There are several questions that can be asked when examining a blood glucose curve, although recommendations on management changes can vary between clinicians. As a guide, the following questions should be considered.

- **Is the insulin having any effect?** – This can be confirmed if the blood glucose concentration falls at any point in the 6–8 hours following an injection. It is also helpful to notice how long after food this effect is seen, and if the fall in glucose concentration had any associated effect on appetite.
- **How long is the effect lasting?** – This can be confirmed by noting the first time the blood glucose concentration starts to increase again, which can be as short as a few hours after injection.
- **Is the nadir (lowest blood glucose value) safe or potentially too low?** – If the blood glucose concentration falls below 4 mmol/l whilst the dog is being hospitalized for a blood glucose curve, it is at risk of clinically significant hypoglycaemia. This can occur because the dog is not eating the amount of food it would normally eat at home or because the insulin dose is too high. If there is any concern over hypoglycaemia as the curve is being performed, the dog should be fed and the blood glucose concentration checked again 30 minutes later, with monitoring continued and further insulin therapy withheld until the blood glucose concentration starts to increase.
- **Are there any factors that might also be contributing to the observations?** – A curve is unlikely to be representative of the dog's normal day-to-day glycaemic control if the dog is otherwise unwell (e.g. pancreatitis, urinary tract infection, ketoacidosis), will not eat its usual food or has very recently had a severe hypoglycaemic episode or a change in insulin dose. Similarly, stress during blood sampling, an inaccurate glucometer or haemolysed/lipaemic samples can also affect a blood glucose curve. These factors should always be considered as possible explanations of unexpected or erratic results.

Home glucose monitoring

In some cases, particularly where dogs are easy to handle but not suited to hospitalization, it may be possible for an owner to generate a blood glucose curve at home without performing venepuncture (Casella et al., 2003). This can be achieved using an automated lancet device in an area of hairless skin, such as the underside of the pinna (Figure 23.9).

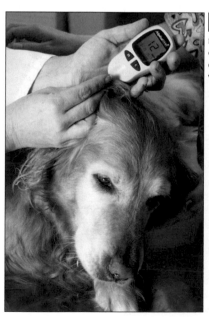

23.9 Use of a glucometer to measure glucose in a capillary blood sample obtained from the pinna with a lancet device.

Such devices use a spring-loaded disposable needle, which makes a pinprick incision through the skin and allows a small volume of capillary blood to escape, sometimes with the use of a vacuum. The glucose concentration can then be measured using a glucometer, which draws up the correct volume of blood. Care must be taken, however, to make sure that the welfare of the dog is not compromised by any such testing, since it can be painful if performed incorrectly. Problems can arise if testing is performed:

- Too frequently
- By a person without adequate training
- In a dog that does not tolerate the testing
- By an owner without direct veterinary supervision of the results generated.

Home glucose monitoring may be better reserved for more established diabetic cases rather than used in the initial stabilization phase, unless the owner is already experienced in diabetes mellitus management.

Continuous glucose monitoring

The generation of a blood glucose curve by repeated venepuncture, or even using a lancet device, can be stressful and painful for the dog, and there is also a risk that a significant blood glucose peak or nadir will fall between two sampling times and will not be recorded. An important technological advance in the management of human diabetes mellitus was the development of continuous glucose monitoring systems (CGMSs) such as the MiniMed, DexCom, GlucoDay and Freestyle Libre, which are increasingly being used successfully in diabetic dogs in a wide variety of settings (Davison et al., 2003b, Surman and Fleeman, 2013) (Figure 23.10).

Continuous glucose monitoring system devices require the subcutaneous implantation of a platinum glucose sensor (see Chapter 25). These can be left in place for periods ranging from 48 hours to 14 days and are usually very well tolerated in dogs. In some systems, the CGMS does not completely remove the need for blood sampling, as at least one blood glucose measurement must be taken in each 12-hour period in order to calibrate the machine and to check that the sensor is still active. The newer 'flash' glucose monitoring systems require minimal blood sampling and can give information in real time. Interstitial fluid glucose concentrations are measured every few seconds by the sensor and an average value is recorded every 5 minutes. Blood and interstitial fluid glucose concentrations are in equilibrium, and experimental studies have shown that differences are generally only seen when blood glucose concentration is changing rapidly, where a lag phase of between 3 and 14 minutes might be expected. The sensor communicates with a monitor (or in some cases a mobile phone app), so that when they are in close proximity a glucose reading can be obtained in 'real time'. The monitor can also store information regarding insulin injections and feeding, so that they can be superimposed on the glucose curve that is stored and generated by the associated software.

The main advantage of a CGMS is that a large amount of data can be collected and analysed without the need for repeated blood sampling, as well as the potential to identify subclinical hypoglycaemic episodes. Whilst such devices are increasingly accessible, the cost of the device and the disposable platinum sensors may be prohibitive for some owners. The working range of some devices precludes their use in dogs with blood glucose

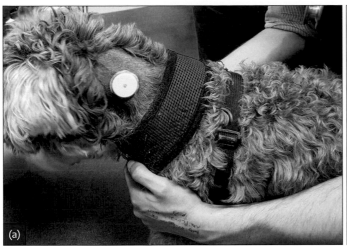
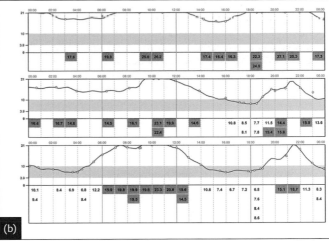

23.10 Use of a Freestyle Libre 'flash' Continuous Glucose Monitoring System (CGMS). (a) The disposable glucose monitoring sensor is inserted below the skin using a spring-loaded device and can remain in place for up to 14 days. Interstitial fluid glucose is measured every minute and the device stores readings every 15 minutes. The CGMS can be paired with a wireless electronic reader or a mobile phone app to provide information in real time and it is recommended that this pairing takes place at least every 8 hours. (b) The data can be downloaded periodically to generate a continuous interstitial fluid glucose trace using computer software, which helps to illustrate daily trends (data shown represent three consecutive days) and identify periods where interstitial glucose is outside the optimal range.

concentrations above the upper limit of detection (typically 22 mmol/l); however, CGMS devices can be particularly helpful in the investigation of unstable diabetic dogs, discussed in more detail in Chapter 25.

Long-term monitoring

Regular veterinary appointments are advisable, even in cases that are seemingly well controlled. Unlike cats, it is very rare for dogs to undergo a 'diabetic honeymoon' phase following insulin treatment, requiring dose reduction or discontinuation of insulin therapy. However, further insulin dose adjustments are sometimes necessary because of weight gain, concurrent disease or a change in management of the dog, such as increased exercise or a different diet. Regular planned assessment decreases the likelihood of diabetic emergencies, as changes in glycaemic control can be identified and treated early. The involvement of the nursing team in the regular assessment of diabetic dogs is also very valuable, sharing the responsibility of care so that several people, rather than one single veterinary surgeon, are familiar with each case.

Ideally, a routine clinical appointment should be scheduled approximately every 2 months for a well controlled diabetic dog, to address the factors listed in Figure 23.11. In dogs that are stable with an established routine, this type of appointment is an excellent opportunity for nursing staff to become involved in the care of diabetic dogs. If the owner reports any problems or any factors listed in Figure 23.12 become apparent, further investigations should be undertaken.

- Measure bodyweight (monthly)
- Review diary records with owner, looking for any changes in:
  - Appetite
  - Thirst
  - Behaviour
- Check urine sample for evidence of infection and/or ketones
- Monitor dental hygiene
- Discuss any concerns about diet/feeding
- Review insulin injection technique if required
- Check owners are prepared for potential diabetic emergencies
- Fructosamine measurement every 4–6 months or more regularly if any concerns

23.11 Assessments to be made at a regular diabetic appointment.

- Episodes of collapse or unusual behaviour (hypoglycaemia)
- Appetite or thirst have changed significantly (unstable diabetes mellitus or concurrent disease, e.g. exocrine pancreatic insufficiency, chronic kidney disease)
- Blood, protein or ketones are present in the urine (cytology and bacterial culture and susceptibility testing should be performed in any case of haematuria in a diabetic animal)
- Bodyweight has altered significantly
- There are signs of infection (e.g. periodontal disease)
- There has been a deterioration in vision (cataracts)
- There are lumps appearing at injection sites (injection reactions can result in erratic absorption of insulin)
- The animal is quiet or depressed (possibly hypoglycaemia or concurrent illness)
- There has been vomiting or diarrhoea (vomiting with no change in insulin dose might lead to dangerous hypoglycaemia)
- There has been a change in hair coat or body shape (might suggest another endocrinopathy, e.g. hypothyroidism, hypercortisolism)

23.12 Findings that should prompt further investigation at a diabetic assessment appointment.

Management of concurrent illness

Any concurrent illness in a diabetic dog should be managed as swiftly as possible. Diabetic dogs are particularly at risk of bacterial and fungal infection because the higher glucose concentration in their blood and interstitial fluid promotes growth of these organisms and because of inherent immunosuppression (Hess *et al.*, 2000). If not recognized and treated, infection and inflammation will lead to insulin resistance, more severe hyperglycaemia and exacerbation of infection. Antibiotic use in diabetic dogs should be based on the results of bacterial culture and susceptibility testing. In the case of fungal disease or more severe bacterial infection, prolonged treatment courses and intensive management of blood glucose concentration may be necessary for adequate control.

Any disease that reduces appetite or leads to vomiting will also have an impact on glycaemic control. Owners should always be advised to contact the practice if their diabetic dog does not eat or is vomiting. With reduced caloric intake for any reason, there is a risk of hypoglycaemia at the time of peak activity of insulin. In mild disease, such as vomiting related to dietary indiscretion, a reduction of insulin dose by 50% for 1 or 2 days until recovery of appetite is acceptable. Longer periods of inappetence, such as those associated with acute pancreatitis, require further diagnostic intervention and careful monitoring of blood glucose concentrations. Management of the diabetic dog with acute pancreatitis should follow the same principles as management in a non-diabetic dog, including analgesia, small low-fat meals if the dog is not vomiting and antiemetic treatment (e.g. maropitant) if necessary. In such cases, it can be useful to manage blood glucose concentrations with several small doses (0.1–0.3 IU/kg) of soluble (neutral) insulin given by the intramuscular route throughout the day (depending on the amount of food eaten and the blood glucose measurement), rather than the longer-acting preparation usually administered. Neutral (soluble) insulin has the advantage of having a rapid onset of action but also a short duration, meaning that the animal is less at risk of hypoglycaemia if it does not eat for several hours. Dogs with chronic pancreatitis may also benefit from intermittent oral antiemetic drugs such as maropitant if nausea and/or inappetence are features of their condition.

Another challenge in diabetic dogs is the use of drugs that antagonize insulin or contain sugar in the form of a syrup. In particular, corticosteroids such as prednisolone will have a detrimental effect on glycaemic control and an increase in insulin dose may be required to compensate for this. If possible, the use of such drugs should be avoided, but this is not always practical. For example, in severe cases of allergic or immune-mediated disease it might become necessary to use corticosteroids, but their use should be avoided in diabetic dogs for more minor indications and consideration should be given to alternative regimens where possible. Topical treatment is less likely to cause a problem, but in some cases even eye, ear or skin preparations can result in insulin resistance. If the use of corticosteroids is unavoidable, the minimum effective dose should be used, and the use of other appropriate 'steroid-sparing' drugs considered (e.g. ciclosporin or azathioprine in immune-mediated disease). Injectable depot preparations of corticosteroid have a more variable duration and activity, making it very difficult to predict changes in insulin requirements that might be required, so should be avoided in favour of shorter-acting once-daily oral preparations. Ciclosporin is known to affect blood glucose concentrations in humans by inhibiting insulin secretion. However, this is less likely to cause a problem in diabetic dogs as they usually have no functioning islets remaining and are entirely dependent on exogenous insulin for appropriate glycaemic control.

General anaesthesia

The period of starvation required for general anaesthesia in diabetic dogs can cause concern regarding glycaemic control. The most likely indications for general anaesthesia in a diabetic dog are ovariohysterectomy, cataract surgery or management of severe dental disease. Diabetic dogs are at risk of developing hypoglycaemia and cerebral damage during anaesthesia, and blood glucose concentrations can remain uncontrolled for many hours after a surgical procedure. It is advisable to perform anaesthesia on diabetic dogs as early as possible in the day to allow them to recover in time to eat before the onset of peak insulin activity. Following an overnight fast from midnight, a common regime is to give the dog half of its usual insulin

dose in the morning but no food. The dog should be placed on intravenous glucose fluid therapy throughout the anaesthetic, and blood glucose should be monitored regularly throughout the procedure, with an intravenous glucose bolus (of up to 1–2 ml/kg 25% glucose) administered if blood glucose falls below 5 mmol/l. On recovery, the dog should be encouraged to eat as soon as possible (preferably its usual diet) and blood glucose should be monitored every 1–2 hours. Once-daily insulin-treated dogs can return to their normal routine the following morning, whereas twice-daily treated dogs, if recovering well, can receive their insulin and food as normal in the evening.

Long-term complications

Although insulin therapy can be used successfully to manage the majority of diabetic dogs, suboptimal glycaemic control can lead to secondary complications, such as hypoglycaemic seizures, cataract formation, recurrent infections or diabetic ketoacidosis. Canine diabetes mellitus is also thought to be a risk factor for development of atherosclerosis, although this is usually only apparent at post-mortem examination and does not generally cause clinical signs (Hess et al., 2003). Unlike human diabetic patients, diabetic dogs do not commonly suffer from clinical signs associated with diabetic nephropathy or peripheral neuropathy. It is possible that this represents a difference in pathophysiology between the two species, but it may also be related to the difference in lifespan; secondary complications can take many decades to develop in humans, and diabetic dogs usually live for only a few years following diagnosis.

Ocular disease

Ocular complications occur with variable frequency, with cataracts being the most common (Figure 23.13). Cataracts are thought to occur as a result of osmotic disruption of the lens due to an accumulation of sorbitol (a metabolic product of excess glucose) and are more common in

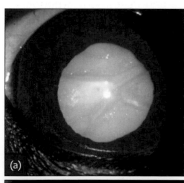
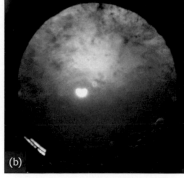

23.13 Diabetic cataracts. (a) Early diabetic cataract showing vacuoles, before the sudden onset of mature lens opacity. (b) Mature diabetic cataract – note the water clefts in the lens. The dark iris results from lens-induced uveitis, which can be associated with the hypermature cataracts seen in diabetes mellitus. (Courtesy of Dr David Williams)

poorly controlled dogs. High activity of the aldose reductase pathway within the canine lens compared with the feline lens has also been demonstrated, which is thought to play a role in cataract development (Richter *et al.*, 2002). Even most well controlled diabetic dogs are likely to develop cataracts within 2 years of diagnosis, which will eventually result in blindness. Although owners are often reluctant to allow a diabetic pet to undergo surgery, a great improvement in quality of life can be obtained by early surgical management of cataracts, even if only one eye is treated. Other ocular complications of diabetes mellitus can include keratoconjunctivitis sicca, lens rupture, bacterial conjunctivitis and uveitis, with the diabetic retinopathy seen in humans being very rare.

Dermatological complications

Ulcerative skin lesions and cutaneous xanthoma have occasionally been reported in unstable diabetic dogs. Hepatocutaneous syndrome is a rare complication of diabetes mellitus and some hepatic diseases. Severe crusting lesions of the feet and distal limbs, face and perineum are seen, and are thought to be related to an excess of glucagon. Diagnosis is confirmed by skin biopsy and this complication carries a poor prognosis.

Hypoglycaemia

Hypoglycaemia is rare in diabetic dogs but can be life-threatening if it occurs, so clients should be well educated about how to avoid and treat this condition. Dogs are usually protected from hypoglycaemia by hormones that are produced as blood glucose concentration falls, such as glucagon, adrenaline and cortisol. Hypoglycaemia is most likely to occur when an animal does not eat its usual amount of food, exercises more than usual or receives too high a dose of insulin (sometimes accidentally). Clinical signs of mild hypoglycaemia can include lethargy and behavioural changes such as aggression or restlessness, stumbling when walking and an increased appetite. If the animal is not fed and hypoglycaemia is allowed to progress, neurological status will deteriorate to convulsions or coma, eventually resulting in cerebral damage and death. Mild hypoglycaemia can be treated by feeding any food that is not high in fibre, particularly sugar-rich food such as sweets or biscuits. If the animal cannot eat voluntarily, glucose can be applied to the oral mucous membranes in the form of glucose gel or glucose solution, where it can be directly absorbed, until the animal has recovered well enough to be fed.

Clinical signs may become evident at a glucose concentration of <3.3 mmol/l, although some dogs cope well with much lower concentrations, particularly if the fall in blood glucose has not been rapid. In the home environment, the owner should apply honey or sugar syrup to the oral mucous membranes whilst arranging to bring the dog to the practice. In the collapsed hypoglycaemic animal, for example following an insulin overdose, intravenous glucose must be provided immediately to limit cerebral damage. An initial intravenous bolus dose of 2 ml/kg of 25% glucose is appropriate, followed by a 5% glucose infusion, which can be increased or decreased depending on clinical response. Glucagon has also been used to manage acute hypoglycaemia induced by insulin overdose, particularly if hypoglycaemia is difficult to control. A 1 mg vial of glucagon can be added to 1 litre of 0.9% sodium chloride, which is then administered as a 50 ng/kg bolus, followed by constant rate infusion of 10–40 ng/kg/min, depending on response.

References and further reading

Ahlgren KM, Fall T, Landegren N et al. (2014) Lack of evidence for a role of islet autoimmunity in the aetiology of canine diabetes mellitus. *PLoS ONE* 9, e105473

Aja D (2016) *Banfield State of Pet Health Report 2016*. Vancouver: Banfield Pet Hospital

Alejandro R, Feldman EC, Shienvold FL and Mintz DH (1988) Advances in canine diabetes mellitus research: etiopathology and results of islet transplantation. *Journal of the American Veterinary Medical Association* 193, 1050–1055

Atkins CE, Hill JR and Johnson RK (1979) Diabetes mellitus in the juvenile dog: a report of four cases. *Journal of the American Veterinary Medical Association* 175, 362–368

Atkins CE and MacDonald MJ (1987) Canine diabetes mellitus has a seasonal incidence: implications relevant to human diabetes. *Diabetes Research* 5, 83–87

Behrend E, Holford A, Lathan P, Rucinsky R and Schulman R (2018) 2018 AAHA Diabetes Management Guidelines for Dogs and Cats. *Journal of the American Animal Hospital Association* 54, 1–21

Casella M, Wess G, Hassig M and Reusch CE (2003) Home monitoring of blood glucose concentration by owners of diabetic dogs. *Journal of Small Animal Practice* 44, 298–305

Catchpole B, Ristic JM, Fleeman LM and Davison LJ (2005) Canine diabetes mellitus: can old dogs teach us new tricks? *Diabetologia* 48, 1948–1956

Cotton RB, Cornelius LM and Theran P (1971) Diabetes mellitus in the dog: a clinicopathologic study. *Journal of the American Veterinary Medical Association* 159, 863–870

Davison LJ (2015) Diabetes mellitus and pancreatitis – cause or effect? *Journal of Small Animal Practice* 56, 50–59

Davison LJ, Herrtage ME and Catchpole B (2005) Study of 253 dogs in the United Kingdom with diabetes mellitus. *Veterinary Record* 156, 467–471

Davison LJ, Herrtage ME, Steiner JM, Williams DA and Catchpole B (2003a) Evidence of anti-insulin autoreactivity and pancreatic inflammation in newly diagnosed diabetic dogs [abstract]. *Journal of Veterinary Internal Medicine* 17, 395

Davison LJ, Slater LA, Herrtage ME et al. (2003b) Evaluation of a continuous glucose monitoring system in diabetic dogs. *Journal of Small Animal Practice* 44, 435–442

Davison LJ, Weenink SM, Christie MR, Herrtage ME and Catchpole B (2008) Autoantibodies to GAD65 and IA-2 in canine diabetes mellitus. *Veterinary Immunology and Immunopathology* 126, 83–90

Delicano RA, Hammar U, Egenvall A et al. (2020) The shared risk of diabetes between dog and cat owners and their pets: register based cohort study. *BMJ* 371, m4337

Denyer AL, Massey JP, Davison LJ et al. (2020) Dog leucocyte antigen (DLA) class II haplotypes and risk of canine diabetes mellitus in specific dog breeds. *Canine Medicine and Genetics* 7, 15

Denyer AL, Catchpole B, Davison LJ and Canine Diabetes Genetics Partnership (2021a) Genetics of canine diabetes mellitus part 1: phenotypes of disease. *The Veterinary Journal* 270, 105611

Denyer AL, Catchpole B, Davison LJ and Canine Diabetes Genetics Partnership (2021b) Genetics of canine diabetes mellitus part 2: current understanding and future directions. *The Veterinary Journal* 270, 105612

Elliott KF, Rand JS, Fleeman LM et al. (2012) A diet lower in digestible carbohydrate results in lower postprandial glucose concentrations compared with a traditional canine diabetes diet and an adult maintenance diet in healthy dogs. *Research in Veterinary Science* 93, 288–295

Fall T, Hansson Hamlin H, Hedhammar A et al. (2007) Diabetes mellitus in a population of 180,000 insured dogs: incidence, survival, and breed distribution. *Journal of Veterinary Internal Medicine* 21, 1209–1216

Fall T, Hedhammar A, Wallberg A et al. (2010) Diabetes mellitus in elkhounds is associated with diestrus and pregnancy. *Journal of Veterinary Internal Medicine* 24, 1322–1328

Fall T, Holm B, Karlsson A et al. (2008a) Glucagon stimulation test for estimating endogenous insulin secretion in dogs. *Veterinary Record* 163, 266–270

Fall T, Johansson Kreuger S, Juberget A et al. (2008b) Gestational diabetes mellitus in 13 dogs. *Journal of Veterinary Internal Medicine* 22, 1296–1300

Fleeman LM and Rand JS (2001) Management of canine diabetes. *Veterinary Clinics of North America: Small Animal Practice* 31, 855–880

Fleeman LM and Rand JS (2003) Evaluation of day-to-day variability of serial blood glucose concentration curves in diabetic dogs. *Journal of the American Veterinary Medical Association* 222, 317–321

Fleeman LM, Rand JS and Markwell PJ (2009) Lack of advantage of high-fibre, moderate-carbohydrate diets in dogs with stabilised diabetes. *Journal of Small Animal Practice* 50, 604–614

Fracassi F, Corradini S, Hafner M et al. (2015) Detemir insulin for the treatment of diabetes mellitus in dogs. *Journal of the American Veterinary Medical Association* 247, 73–78

Gilor C (2019) Discussing prognosis for canine diabetes mellitus: do we have relevant data? *Veterinary Record* 185, 689–691

Gilor C and Fleeman LM (2022) One hundred years of insulin: Is it time for smart? *Journal of Small Animal Practice* 63, 645–660

Gilor C and Graves TK (2010) Synthetic insulin analogs and their use in dogs and cats. *Veterinary Clinics of North America: Small Animal Practice* 40, 297–307

Gilor C, Niessen S, Furrow E and DiBartola S (2016) What's in a name? Classification of diabetes mellitus in veterinary medicine and why it matters. *Journal of Veterinary Internal Medicine* 30, 927–940

Graham PA (1995) *Clinical and epidemiological studies on canine diabetes mellitus.* PhD thesis, University of Glasgow

Guptill L, Glickman L and Glickman N (2003) Time trends and risk factors for diabetes mellitus in dogs: analysis of veterinary medical data base records (1970–1999). *Veterinary Journal* **165**, 240–247

Haines DM and Penhale WJ (1985) Autoantibodies to pancreatic islet cells in canine diabetes mellitus. *Veterinary Immunology and Immunopathology* **8**, 149–156

Hamilton K, O'Kell AL and Gilor C (2021) Serum trypsin-like immunoreactivity in dogs with diabetes mellitus. *Journal of Veterinary Internal Medicine* **35**, 1713–1719

Heeley AM, O'Neill DG, Davison LJ *et al.* (2020) Diabetes mellitus in dogs attending UK primary-care practices: frequency, risk factors and survival. *Canine Medicine and Genetics* **7**, 6

Hess RS, Kass PH and Van Winkle TJ (2003) Association between diabetes mellitus, hypothyroidism or hyperadrenocorticism, and atherosclerosis in dogs. *Journal of Veterinary Internal Medicine* **17**, 489–494

Hess RS, Saunders HM, Van Winkle TJ and Ward CR (2000) Concurrent disorders in dogs with diabetes mellitus: 221 cases (1993–1998). *Journal of the American Veterinary Medical Association* **217**, 1166–1173

Hess RS and Ward CR (2000) Effect of insulin dosage on glycemic response in dogs with diabetes mellitus: 221 cases (1993–1998). *Journal of the American Veterinary Medical Association* **216**, 217–221

Hoenig M (2002) Comparative aspects of diabetes mellitus in dogs and cats. *Molecular and Cellular Endocrinology* **197**, 221–229

Hoffman J, Lourenço B, Promislow D and Creevy K (2018) Canine hyperadrenocorticism associations with signalment, selected comorbidities and mortality within North American veterinary teaching hospitals. *Journal of Small Animal Practice* **59**, 681–690

Hope A, Bailen EL, Shiel RE and Mooney CT (2021) Retrospective study evaluation of DGGR lipase for diagnosis, agreement with pancreatic lipase and prognosis in dogs with suspected acute pancreatitis. *Journal of Small Animal Practice* **62**, 1092–1100

Kramer JW, Klaassen JK, Baskin DG *et al.* (1988) Inheritance of diabetes mellitus in Keeshond dogs. *American Journal of Veterinary Research* **49**, 428–431

Ling GV, Lowenstine LJ, Pulley LT and Kaneko JJ (1977) Diabetes mellitus in dogs: a review of initial evaluation, immediate and long-term management, and outcome. *Journal of the American Veterinary Medical Association* **170**, 521–530

Mansfield CS, Jones BR and Spillman T (2003) Assessing the severity of canine pancreatitis. *Research in Veterinary Science* **74**, 137–144

Marmor M, Willeberg P, Glickman LT *et al.* (1982) Epizootiologic patterns of diabetes mellitus in dogs. *American Journal of Veterinary Research* **43**, 465–470

Mattheeuws D, Rottiers R, Kaneko JJ and Vermeulen A (1984) Diabetes mellitus in dogs: relationship of obesity to glucose tolerance and insulin response. *American Journal of Veterinary Research* **45**, 98–103

Mattin M, O'Neill D, Church D *et al.* (2014) An epidemiological study of diabetes mellitus in dogs attending first opinion practice in the UK. *Veterinary Record* **174**, 349

Minkus G, Breuer W, Arun S *et al.* (1997) Ductuloendocrine cell proliferation in the pancreas of two young dogs with diabetes mellitus. *Veterinary Pathology* **34**, 164–167

Momozawa Y, Merveille AC, Battaille G *et al.* (2020) Genome wide association study of 40 clinical measurements in eight dog breeds. *Scientific Reports* **10**, 6520

Montgomery TM, Nelson RW, Feldman EC, Robertson K and Polonsky KS (1996) Basal and glucagon-stimulated plasma C-peptide concentrations in healthy dogs, dogs with diabetes mellitus, and dogs with hyperadrenocorticism. *Journal of Veterinary Internal Medicine* **10**, 116–122

O'Kell AL, Shome M, Qiu J *et al.* (2022) Exploration of autoantibody responses in canine diabetes using protein arrays. *Scientific Reports* **12**, 2490

Peterson ME, Altszuler N and Nichols CE (1984) Decreased insulin sensitivity and glucose tolerance in spontaneous canine hyperadrenocorticism. *Research in Veterinary Science* **36**, 177–182

Poppl AG, de Carvalho GLC, Vivian IF, Corbellini LG and Gonzalez FHD (2017) Canine diabetes mellitus risk factors: a matched case-control study. *Research in Veterinary Science* **114**, 469–473

Poppl AG, Mottin TS and Gonzalez FHD (2013) Diabetes mellitus remission after resolution of inflammatory and progesterone-related conditions in bitches. *Research in Veterinary Science* **94**, 471–473

Qiu LNY, Cai SV, Chan D and Hess RS (2022) Seasonality and geography of diabetes mellitus in United States of America dogs. *PLoS ONE* **17**, e0272297

Redondo MJ and Eisenbarth GS (2002) Genetic control of autoimmunity in Type I diabetes and associated disorders. *Diabetologia* **45**, 605–622

Rhew SY, Park SM, Li Q *et al.* (2021) Efficacy and safety of allogenic canine adipose tissue-derived mesenchymal stem cell therapy for insulin-dependent diabetes mellitus in four dogs: a pilot study. *Journal of Veterinary Medicine and Science* **83**, 592–600

Richter M, Guscetti F and Spiess B (2002) Aldose reductase activity and glucose-related opacities in incubated lenses from dogs and cats. *American Journal of Veterinary Research* **63**, 1591–1597

Shields EJ, Lam CJ, Cox AR *et al.* (2015) Extreme beta-cell deficiency in pancreata of dogs with canine diabetes. *PLoS ONE* **10**, e0129809

Short AD, Catchpole B, Kennedy LJ *et al.* (2009) T cell cytokine gene polymorphisms in canine diabetes mellitus. *Veterinary Immunology and Immunopathology* **128**, 137–146

Steiner JM, Newman S, Xenoulis P *et al.* (2008) Sensitivity of serum markers for pancreatitis in dogs with macroscopic evidence of pancreatitis. *Veterinary Therapeutics* **9**, 263–273

Surman S and Fleeman L (2013) Continuous glucose monitoring in small animals. *Veterinary Clinics of North America: Small Animal Practice* **43**, 381–406

Taplin CE and Barker JM (2008) Autoantibodies in type 1 diabetes. *Autoimmunity* **41**, 11–18

Tardo AM, Del Baldo F, Dondi F *et al.* (2019) Survival estimates and outcome predictors in dogs with newly diagnosed diabetes mellitus treated in a veterinary teaching hospital. *Veterinary Record* **185**, 692

Todd JA, Bell JI and McDevitt HO (1987) HLA-DQ β gene contributes to susceptibility and resistance to insulin-dependent diabetes mellitus. *Nature* **329**, 599–604

Watson PJ (2003) Exocrine pancreatic insufficiency as an end stage of pancreatitis in four dogs. *Journal of Small Animal Practice* **44**, 306–312

Watson PJ and Herrtage ME (2004) Use of glucagon stimulation tests to assess beta-cell function in dogs with chronic pancreatitis. *Journal of Nutrition* **134**, 2081S–2083S

Watson PJ, Roulois AJA, Scase T *et al.* (2007) Prevalence and breed distribution of chronic pancreatitis at post-mortem examination in first-opinion dogs. *Journal of Small Animal Practice* **48**, 609–618

Useful websites

European Society of Veterinary Endocrinology – Project ALIVE
www.esve.org/alive/intro.aspx

European Society of Veterinary Endocrinology – Laboratory Quality Assurance Scheme
www.esve.org/esve/eve-qas

VetCompass
www.vetcompass.org

Chapter 24

Feline diabetes mellitus

Jacquie Rand and Susan Gottlieb

Introduction

Diabetes mellitus is defined as a disorder of persistent hyperglycaemia regardless of underlying cause. The typical clinical signs are polyuria and polydipsia (PU/PD) and weight loss. It is one of the most common endocrine disorders in cats, although the prevalence varies depending on the population studied. For example, the highest prevalence that has been reported is 1 in 100 cats from an Australian veterinary laboratory (Rand et al., 1997). The prevalence most commonly reported is approximately 1 in 200, as observed in an Australian primary-care, feline-only practice (Baral et al., 2003), in UK primary-care small animal practices (O'Neill et al., 2016), and in an insured population in the UK (McCann et al., 2007). The lowest prevalences reported are 1 in 400 using data from USA referral institutions (Panciera et al., 1990) and 1 in 830 in a population of insured cats in Sweden (Öhlund et al., 2015).

The majority of cats have a disorder similar to type 2 diabetes mellitus in humans, although a minority of cases are attributed to other specific types of diabetes. Risk factors include obesity, breed, age, physical inactivity, confinement indoors, prior administration of glucocorticoids or progestins, and underlying endocrinopathies such as hypersomatotropism and hypercortisolism. Most of these risk factors decrease insulin sensitivity, leading to increased demand on pancreatic beta cells to produce insulin. The incidence of feline diabetes mellitus observed in private practice increased between 1970 and 1999 (Prahl et al., 2007). This is presumably because of increased prevalence of predisposing factors, particularly obesity and physical inactivity, but might also reflect improved diagnosis. More recent changes in frequency have not been reported.

Treatment of diabetes mellitus should, where possible, initially be aimed at normalizing circulating blood glucose concentrations to maximize the probability of remission. This is achieved through administration of insulin, feeding a low-carbohydrate diet and appropriate adjustment of insulin dose based on close monitoring of glycaemic response. In some situations, the primary goal is to control clinical signs, with a lesser need for intense monitoring and stringent insulin dosing protocols. However, survival times are significantly longer in cats that achieve diabetic remission (Callegari et al., 2013). The implications for longevity should be carefully discussed with owners of diabetic cats before implementing a protocol based purely on controlling clinical signs, as such a protocol will likely achieve suboptimal glycaemic control and decrease the probability

of remission (Nack and DeClue, 2014). In most cats, adequate glycaemic control is readily achieved, whilst in some cats consistent glycaemic control is difficult.

Cats are prone to stress hyperglycaemia, which complicates the interpretation of blood glucose concentrations and may lead to inappropriate insulin dosage changes. Home monitoring of blood glucose concentrations helps to overcome this confounding effect. Although the majority of cats are initially insulin dependent, a substantial proportion of newly diagnosed cats undergo remission if good glycaemic control is achieved using insulin therapy with diligent monitoring of glycaemic response.

Aetiology and classification of disease

The causes of feline diabetes mellitus are varied. In primary-care practices in Western countries, the majority of diabetic cats have type 2 diabetes mellitus. The remainder have diabetes mellitus best classified as other specific types of diabetes (O'Brien et al., 1985; Goossens et al., 1998), which typically results from insulin resistance caused by hypersomatotropism or hypercortisolism (Niessen et al., 2013), or from conditions that destroy pancreatic beta cells (pancreatitis or neoplasia) (Nelson, 2000; Rand and Marshall, 2005; Caney, 2013; Gottlieb et al., 2020). Type 1 diabetes mellitus resulting from immune-mediated destruction of beta cells is rare in cats (Woods et al., 1994).

Type 2 diabetes mellitus

Based on clinical characteristics and islet pathology, and depending on the population studied, approximately 60–90% of diabetic cats appear to have type 2 diabetes mellitus, which results from a combination of impaired insulin secretion and insulin resistance (O'Brien et al., 1985; Lutz and Rand, 1996; Feldhahn et al., 1999; Marshall et al., 2009; Roomp and Rand, 2009; Gottlieb et al., 2015). Amyloid deposition in pancreatic islets is a common histopathological finding in diabetic cats and humans with type 2 diabetes (O'Brien et al., 1985; Panciera et al., 1990; Porte, 1991; Herndon et al., 2014).

Insulin resistance

Insulin resistance is a hallmark of type 2 diabetes mellitus. Diabetic cats are, on average, six times less sensitive to insulin than are healthy cats (Feldhahn *et al.*, 1999). This is of a similar magnitude to the insulin resistance in humans with type 2 diabetes mellitus. In humans, insulin resistance is predominantly the result of the sum of the underlying insulin resistance (insulin sensitivity), which is genetically determined, coupled with acquired insulin resistance, which is largely the result of obesity and physical inactivity.

Genetic and acquired factors contributing to insulin resistance are also present in cats. Risk factors for acquired insulin resistance associated with feline diabetes mellitus include obesity, physical inactivity and previous drug therapies (glucocorticoids and progestins). A range of insulin sensitivities are present in healthy, ideal-weight cats, and insulin sensitivity is likely genetically determined in cats, as in humans. Cats with insulin sensitivities below the population median have three times the risk of developing impaired glucose tolerance with weight gain (Appleton *et al.*, 2001). Higher insulin concentrations in non-diabetic Burmese cats compared with non-diabetic domestic cats suggest that genetically determined insulin resistance is a factor. Burmese cats are reported to be at increased risk of diabetes mellitus in Australia, New Zealand, Sweden and the UK (Rand *et al.*, 1997; Lederer *et al.*, 2009; Öhlund *et al.*, 2015).

Weight gain has a particularly profound effect on insulin resistance. In one study, insulin sensitivity was decreased by approximately 50% in cats that had increased their bodyweight by an average of 44% over 10 months (Appleton *et al.*, 2001). In humans and dogs, physical inactivity leads to insulin resistance independent of bodyweight. Although insulin sensitivity has not been compared in inactive and active cats, indoor cats and cats rated as less active by their owners are at increased risk of developing diabetes mellitus (Slingerland *et al.*, 2009).

Drugs, especially long-acting or repeatedly administered glucocorticoids, induce insulin resistance and are a frequent precipitator of clinical signs of diabetes mellitus in cats, especially when other risk factors are present. Hypersomatotropism and, to a lesser extent, hypercortisolism cause marked insulin resistance, with hypersomatotropism being reported as a frequent cause of other specific types of diabetes mellitus (Niessen *et al.*, 2007; Schaefer *et al.*, 2017).

Hyperglycaemia induces insulin resistance in dogs and humans that is reversible with improved glycaemic control (Vuorinen-Markkola *et al.*, 1992; Matsumoto *et al.*, 2001; Fleeman, 2007). Hyperglycaemia is also likely a cause of insulin resistance in cats, given the molecular mechanisms involved (Tomás *et al.*, 2002; Samuel and Shulman, 2012). Hyperlipidaemia may also contribute to insulin resistance (Nishii *et al.*, 2012; Samuel and Shulman, 2012).

Decreased insulin secretion

Loss of beta cell function is another hallmark of type 2 diabetes mellitus. While the exact mechanisms are unknown, especially in the early stages of failure, several mechanisms have been identified that result in reduced response to a glucose challenge and impaired insulin secretion (Alejandro *et al.*, 2015). Some of these include endoplasmic reticulum stress within beta cells as a result of increased glucose and lipid concentrations associated with nutrient overload and obesity, alterations in protein function and gene expression, proinflammatory cytokine induction in islets, and inflammation of islets (Tanaka *et al.*, 1999; Alejandro *et al.*, 2015; Galicia-Garcia *et al.*, 2020). Once glucose concentrations are persistently increased, glucose toxicity, compounded by increased lipid concentrations

(glucolipotoxicity), further suppresses beta cell function and damages beta cells. Ultimately, some of these mechanisms lead to beta cell apoptosis and loss. Another contributor reported to decrease beta cell function and mass in type 2 diabetes mellitus is formation of misfolded polymers of amylin (islet amyloid polypeptide). These include intracellular aggregates ranging from small soluble dimers and hexamers to large soluble oligomers and amyloid fibrils, as well as extracellular deposits of misfolded aggregates as islet amyloid (O'Brien *et al.*, 1985, 1995; Johnson *et al.*, 1992; Zini *et al.*, 2009; Link *et al.*, 2013; Mukherjee *et al.*, 2015). It is likely that both the soluble misfolded oligomers and the larger aggregates induce injury (Mukherjee *et al.*, 2015). Large amyloid deposits may serve as a reservoir for more toxic smaller oligomers. The soluble intracellular amylin oligomers mediate beta cell dysfunction and death (Mukherjee *et al.*, 2015). Several mechanisms have been proposed for the toxicity of amylin oligomers, including:

- Membrane permeabilization – the amylin oligomers form pore-like structures in the membrane, resulting in leakage, calcium dysregulation and cytotoxicity
- Mitochondrial damage
- Endoplasmic reticulum stress
- Induction of inflammation.

Overexpression of amylin, as occurs in obesity-induced insulin resistance and associated with a sustained increase in glucose concentration, increases formation of toxic aggregates (Mukherjee *et al.*, 2015; Galicia-Garcia *et al.*, 2020). Of note, the species that spontaneously develop type 2 diabetes mellitus (humans, non-human primates and cats) also express amyloid-prone sequences of amylin (Henson and O'Brien, 2006).

Some loss of function is reversible in type 2 diabetes mellitus, as occurs in the early stages of glucose toxicity (Link *et al.*, 2013). In humans, early intensive insulin therapy has been demonstrated to improve reversible components of glucose toxicity (Retnakaran, 2015). Loss of beta cells occurs in the later stages of glucose toxicity, resulting in irreversible loss of insulin secretion. Chronic hyperglycaemia creates a continuous cycle resulting in progressive loss of insulin secretion (Poitout and Robertson, 2008; Zini *et al.*, 2009; Link *et al.*, 2013). In some cats, pancreatitis may compound loss of beta cells (Goossens *et al.*, 1998).

Other specific types of diabetes

Other specific types of diabetes mellitus account for approximately 5–40% of cases, depending on the population studied. These types are more commonly seen in referral practice, especially tertiary referral practice, where most referred diabetic cats have disease that is difficult to control and are atypical of the majority of diabetic cats seen in primary-care practice (O'Brien *et al.*, 1985; Goossens *et al.*, 1998; Berg *et al.*, 2007).

Other specific types of diabetes mellitus result from an underlying condition causing decreased insulin secretion or impaired insulin action (insulin resistance), or both. After type 2 diabetes mellitus, hypersomatotropism, linked to marked insulin resistance, is the most commonly diagnosed underlying cause of diabetes mellitus, reported in up to 30% of cases in referral institutions in the UK and USA (Berg *et al.*, 2007; Niessen *et al.*, 2007, 2013). In cats referred with poor diabetic control and insulin doses exceeding 2 IU/kg per injection, the prevalence may be even higher. Diabetes mellitus is also linked to hypercortisolism, chronic end-stage pancreatitis and pancreatic adenocarcinoma (reported to account for 9–18% of cases in referral practice), although the reported frequencies are lower than for hypersomatotropism (O'Brien *et al.*, 1985). Pancreatitis might be underestimated as a cause of diabetes mellitus.

Glucose toxicity

Regardless of the cause of diabetes mellitus, endogenous insulin secretion at diagnosis is usually low because of the interaction between glucose toxicity and beta cell function. Glucose toxicity describes the suppression of insulin secretion from beta cells secondary to prolonged hyperglycaemia (Unger and Grundy, 1985; Zini *et al.*, 2009; Link *et al.*, 2013). Insulin secretion in healthy cats is suppressed to concentrations found in insulin-dependent diabetic cats within 3–7 days of maintenance of blood glucose concentrations of approximately 30 mmol/l (Link *et al.*, 2013). Glucose toxicity is dose dependent, and less suppression occurs at lower circulating glucose concentrations.

Glucose toxicity is particularly important when superimposed on hyperfunctioning beta cells that are already compromised as a result of loss of beta cell mass (Imamura *et al.*, 1988). In cats, formation of misfolded polymers of amylin, amyloid deposition and pancreatitis may result in loss of beta cell mass and increased demand on the remaining beta cells to secrete insulin. With hyperfunctioning and stressed beta cells, even mild hyperglycaemia can cause a further rapid deterioration of beta cell function, and worsening hyperglycaemia eventually contributes to signs of overt diabetes mellitus (Imamura *et al.*, 1988).

Suppression of insulin secretion by glucose toxicity is initially functional and reversible but later results in structural changes of beta cells. Over weeks and months such changes become irreversible and beta cells are irreversibly lost. This largely explains why cats with poorly controlled diabetes mellitus for more than 6 months have a significantly reduced probability of remission, even after good glycaemic control is achieved (Roomp and Rand, 2009).

Clinical features

Signalment

The typical diabetic cat is 10–13 years of age and male (ratio of 2:1 male:female). Domestic Shorthaired cats are the most commonly diagnosed breed. In the USA, Maine Coon, Domestic Longhaired, Russian Blue and Siamese cats are over-represented. In the UK, Sweden and Australasia, Burmese cats are at increased risk; their frequency in the diabetic population is approximately three times that in the overall population. In Australasia, 1 in 10 Burmese cats over 8 years of age has diabetes mellitus (Rand *et al.*, 1997; Lederer *et al.*, 2009). Norwegian Forest Cats, Tonkinese and Abyssinians have also been identified as predisposed in a Swedish population of cats (Öhlund *et al.*, 2015).

Clinical signs

The classical clinical signs of diabetes mellitus are:

- PU/PD (80% of cats)
- Weight loss (70% of cats)
- Increased appetite (reported by only 20% of owners).

At the time of diagnosis, some cats have a reduced rather than increased appetite. This is probably the result

of one or more factors including dehydration, electrolyte disturbances, ketonaemia and precipitating conditions such as infection or pancreatitis.

Clinical signs are usually present for weeks to months but may be missed by some owners. Cats are more often overweight than of normal weight or underweight (Scarlett *et al.*, 1994). Depression, anorexia and dehydration may be present in some cats, but others are apparently healthy at initial presentation. In those cats that present with other specific types of diabetes mellitus, clinical signs indicative of the underlying disorder may be present. Muscle wasting and diffuse peripheral neuropathy are commonly reported (50% of diabetic cats) and result in weakness, difficulty in jumping and unsteadiness of gait. A plantigrade stance is less common and is probably indicative of more longstanding diabetes mellitus (Figure 24.1). In one study of diabetic cats, all cats had evidence of widespread deficits in peripheral motor nerve function, especially in the pelvic limbs but also the thoracic limbs, based on nerve conduction tests, and half the cats had evidence of decreased sensory nerve function (Mizisin *et al.*, 2002). Severity was associated with increasing blood glucose concentration.

Because diabetic cats are typically over 8 years old, other concurrent diseases that may be masked by diabetes mellitus should be considered, including chronic kidney disease (CKD) and hyperthyroidism.

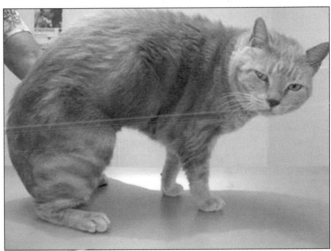

24.1 Cat with plantigrade stance.
(Reproduced from Rand, 2013, with permission from the publisher.)

Diagnosis

A diagnosis of uncomplicated diabetes mellitus is made based on the presence of appropriate clinical signs, persistent fasting hyperglycaemia and glucosuria. Other changes on routine clinicopathological analysis may include mild anaemia, a stress leucogram, hypercholesterolaemia, hypertriglyceridaemia and increased liver enzyme activities. Sick dehydrated diabetic cats may also have evidence of ketonaemia or ketonuria, acidosis, prerenal azotaemia and electrolyte disturbances including increased or decreased potassium and phosphate concentrations (see Chapter 26).

Additional diagnostic tests to identify other specific causes of diabetes, such as hypersomatotropism, hypercortisolism, pancreatitis and pancreatic neoplasia, are not usually performed initially unless pre-existing clinical signs are suggestive or there is a poor response to treatment and/or evidence of significant insulin resistance. Measurement of feline pancreas-specific lipase at the time of diagnosis is recommended if there are any signs consistent with pancreatitis. All cats in which poor glycaemic control is present at least 2–4 weeks after initiation of treatment, especially when the insulin dose exceeds 0.5 IU/kg/injection, should be screened for hypersomatotropism by measurement of insulin-like growth factor-1 (IGF-1). Earlier testing is not recommended because insulinopenia present at the time of diagnosis of diabetes mellitus may cause a falsely low concentration of IGF-1, as production is reliant on hepatic growth hormone receptors being stimulated by insulin (Niessen et al., 2013).

Blood glucose concentration

Feline diabetes mellitus is typically diagnosed when the blood glucose concentration exceeds the renal threshold, causing glucosuria and obligatory water loss and hence PU/PD. These signs are associated with a blood glucose concentration of at least 14–16 mmol/l (Kruth and Cowgill, 1982).

No epidemiological studies have been performed in cats to demonstrate whether there are adverse health effects associated with persistent mild to moderate hyperglycaemia (7–14 mmol/l). In humans, however, the cut-off blood glucose concentration for diabetes mellitus has been consistently lowered as more information has become available on the adverse effects of mild hyperglycaemia, including microvascular damage and retinopathy. The authors consider a persistent, non-stressed blood glucose concentration of >10 mmol/l to be diabetic. It is likely that if cats were classified as diabetic with a persistent fasting blood glucose concentration of 7–<10 mmol/l, a greater proportion would be non-insulin-dependent and could be controlled with weight loss and diet alone.

Humans with impaired glucose tolerance or impaired fasting glucose concentrations are considered prediabetic and are at greater risk of developing type 2 diabetes mellitus (American Diabetes Association, 2014). Cats in diabetic remission with impaired fasting glucose concentrations or impaired glucose tolerance are also at increased risk of relapse compared with cats with normal fasting glucose concentration and glucose tolerance. In one study, cats with impaired fasting glucose concentrations of 7.5–8.5 mmol/l had a 79% probability of relapse (Gottlieb et al., 2015). However, impaired fasting glucose concentration or glucose tolerance indicating a prediabetic state are rarely diagnosed in cats. In most cats, a mildly increased blood glucose concentration identified in the veterinary clinic is assumed to be stress hyperglycaemia, and truly prediabetic cats are therefore usually missed.

Stress hyperglycaemia

Acute stress, particularly if associated with struggling, can increase the blood glucose concentration by up to approximately 10 mmol/l, but this often resolves within 3–4 hours. Transient illness-associated hyperglycaemia may persist for several days. Stress hyperglycaemia rarely results in blood glucose concentrations that exceed 16 mmol/l; more often, glucose concentrations are in the 7–12 mmol/l range.

If blood glucose concentration is lower than 20 mmol/l with no, or minimal, glucosuria and typical clinical signs are absent, blood glucose concentration measurement should be repeated 4 or more hours later. Repeat glucose measurement should be made using a glucose meter validated for feline blood and with the sample obtained preferably from the ear while the cat remains quietly in its carrier or cage, to minimize stress. If the stress has largely resolved the blood glucose concentration should be within the reference interval. If the cat remains hyperglycaemic, it may be prudent to hospitalize it overnight and repeat blood glucose measurement the following morning to determine whether the hyperglycaemia is persistent.

If hyperglycaemia is marked (>20 mmol/l), treatment with insulin should be instituted within 24 hours if the glucose concentration has not normalized, because high blood glucose concentrations can rapidly (within 24 hours) suppress insulin secretion and predispose to diabetic ketoacidosis (Link et al., 2013).

Fructosamine concentration

Measurement of circulating fructosamine concentration is useful in some situations where the history is unreliable or unclear and stress hyperglycaemia cannot be ruled out. However, repeat measurement of the glucose concentration 4 hours later is usually more accurate and is recommended. In general, the serum fructosamine concentration is not a sensitive indicator of persistent mild to moderate hyperglycaemia (Link and Rand, 2008). In cats with circulating glucose concentrations <20 mmol/l, the fructosamine concentration does not reliably differentiate stress hyperglycaemia from diabetes mellitus. In healthy cats infused with glucose to maintain circulating glucose concentrations of 17 mmol/l for 6 weeks, the serum fructosamine concentration was not consistently above the upper limit of the reference interval (Link and Rand, 2008). Therefore, fructosamine measurement may significantly underdiagnose diabetes mellitus in cats with persistent hyperglycaemia and glucose concentrations <20 mmol/l. There can be wide variation in measured fructosamine concentrations between individual cats for a given concentration of circulating glucose, and false-positive and false-negative results can occur (Lutz et al., 1995; Crenshaw et al., 1996). Concurrent uncontrolled hyperthyroidism or hypoproteinaemia may also result in false-negative results, as serum protein concentrations and turnover will also affect fructosamine concentrations (Reusch and Haberer, 2001; Gal et al., 2017).

Glycated haemoglobin

Glycated haemoglobin (HbA1c) results from glucose binding to haemoglobin in circulating red blood cells; HbA1c may be used as a measure for diagnosis or to help monitor glucose control. It is an alternative to fructosamine measurements in cats to differentiate between stress hyperglycaemia and diabetes mellitus (Elliott et al., 1997; Bennett, 2002). However, its availability is limited and results are usually not available within 24 hours, limiting its usefulness. Because it reflects blood glucose concentration over approximately 70 days, it is of use only in monitoring glucose control in long-term diabetic cats, and not for adjustment of the insulin dose in the initial stabilization period.

Ketones and lipids

Ketosis and hyperlipidaemia are likely to occur in diabetic cats with circulating glucose concentrations over 20 mmol/l, especially if present for 2 or more weeks. Experimentally, as few as 14 days of marked hyperglycaemia (at approximately 30 mmol/l) are required for plasma beta-hydroxybutyrate concentrations to exceed the reference interval in healthy cats infused with glucose (Link, 2001).

Although 60–80% of diabetic cats are ketonaemic based on plasma beta-hydroxybutyrate measurements, ketonuria is present in a smaller percentage. Urine biochemistry test strips detect only acetoacetate and acetone, while beta-hydroxybutyrate is the major ketone present in diabetic ketosis. Awaiting a positive stick test result can delay the diagnosis of ketonuria in cats by approximately 5 days (Link, 2001). For an accurate diagnosis of ketosis and ketonuria, it is preferable to measure the plasma or urine beta-hydroxybutyrate concentration. Although its measurement is only offered as a routine test by some veterinary laboratories, portable meters are available for use with whole blood.

Diabetic cats with mild to moderate hyperglycaemia (<20 mmol/l) do not typically develop ketonaemia and ketonuria. Consequently, measurement of plasma beta-hydroxybutyrate is not useful for differentiating such cases from stress hyperglycaemia (Link, 2001). Healthy cats fasted for 24 hours and those on a low-carbohydrate energy-restricted diet for weight loss may also have mildly increased plasma beta-hydroxybutyrate concentrations (approximately 0.7 mmol/l and 1.4 mmol/l, respectively, with a reference interval upper limit of 0.6 mmol/l).

A diabetic ketoacidosis crisis can occur within days of demonstrating increased plasma beta-hydroxybutyrate concentrations, and prompt insulin therapy should be considered in all such cases (see Chapter 26).

Urinalysis

Glucosuria in the presence of persistent hyperglycaemia is considered to be diagnostic of diabetes mellitus. Many cats also have secondary urinary tract infections. The sediment should therefore be examined for evidence of bacteria. However, there may not be an active sediment in all cases and urine culture is recommended. Diabetes mellitus must be confirmed by documentation of hyperglycaemia and not just glucosuria, given that other causes of glucosuria are possible, including IRIS stage 4 CKD (Zeugswetter et al., 2019). Indeed, Fanconi syndrome, although very rare in cats, can result in both glucosuria and ketonuria, and in other species is associated with PU/PD.

Treatment

Goals of therapy

The principal goal for treatment of feline diabetes mellitus has changed over the past 10 years from ameliorating clinical signs to achieving euglycaemia without the need for insulin or other hypoglycaemic therapy, commonly called diabetic remission. Remission has enormous health and quality-of-life (QOL) benefits for diabetic cats, and cost and lifestyle benefits for their owners. Because remission is so advantageous, in general, the treatment protocol selected should maximize its probability if possible.

Knowledge of the likely aetiology of diabetes mellitus for each cat is important in determining the treatment goals for individual cases. In all newly diagnosed cats with type 2 diabetes mellitus and in cats with correctable or reversible causes of other specific types of diabetes, including some cats with hypersomatotropism, hypercortisolism, previous glucocorticoid therapy and pancreatitis, treatment should be primarily directed at achieving remission.

The primary goal of therapy in cats with long-term diabetes mellitus (>12–24 months) and causes of other specific types of diabetes mellitus that cannot be corrected (e.g. end-stage pancreatitis, pancreatic adenocarcinoma and untreatable hypersomatotropism) is control of clinical signs and avoidance of clinical hypoglycaemia. Attempts should be made to identify such cases if possible. However, these cats are not typically identified until months after diagnosis, when poor control associated with a high insulin dose becomes evident or remission does not occur despite excellent glycaemic control.

Diabetic remission

Diabetic remission is defined as occurring when a cat that was previously diagnosed as diabetic and treated with insulin is able to maintain a normal (<6.5 mmol/l) or pre-diabetic (<10 mmol/l) blood glucose concentration without insulin therapy for at least 2–4 weeks. Diabetic remission is possible only if there are functional beta cells remaining. Timely resolution of glucose toxicity is critically important for its achievement.

Three factors are crucial in achieving optimal remission rates in newly diagnosed diabetic cats (Bennett et al., 2006; Roomp and Rand, 2009):

- Early initiation of appropriate insulin therapy
- Diligent and frequent monitoring of circulating glucose concentrations with appropriate adjustment of insulin dose
- Feeding a suitable diet.

Several variables linked to a higher probability of remission emerged from one study involving 55 cats treated with glargine insulin (Roomp and Rand, 2009). This study highlights that achieving excellent glycaemic control as early as possible is imperative. Remission rates were 84% for cats that started intensive glycaemic control within 6 (median 4) months of diagnosis of diabetes mellitus. The rate of remission significantly decreased to 35% for cats in which the same protocol was instituted more than 6 months after diagnosis, even if they subsequently achieved excellent glycaemic control. Other variables associated with increased probability of remission included prior glucocorticoid treatment and the absence of clinical signs of overt peripheral neuropathy. Sex, weight at diagnosis, age at diagnosis, presence of diabetic ketoacidosis at diagnosis, existence of CKD or hyperthyroidism, and frequency of asymptomatic hypoglycaemia were not predictors of remission. Obesity was not shown to be negatively linked with achieving remission. In another study, older age and lower cholesterol concentrations were associated with increased probability of remission (Zini et al., 2010).

Treatment with glucocorticoids in the 6 months prior to diagnosis of diabetes mellitus was associated with an increased likelihood of diabetic remission. Sudden acquired marked insulin resistance associated with glucocorticoid treatment likely triggers a more acute onset of clinical signs, which presumably results in treatment being sought earlier, before extensive loss of beta cells occurs. Consequently, there is earlier resolution of glucose toxicity coupled with resolution of the acquired insulin resistance following withdrawal of steroids, facilitating diabetic remission.

A plantigrade stance or other milder signs of peripheral neuropathy, such as difficulty in climbing stairs, are associated with a significantly reduced probability of diabetic remission. It is likely that cats with signs of neuropathy have had uncontrolled hyperglycaemia for longer periods than those without neuropathy and, therefore, sustained greater destruction of beta cells arising from prolonged glucose toxicity, resulting in lower remission rates.

Although 'diabetic remission' is the term commonly used to describe previously diabetic cats that maintain euglycaemia without insulin or oral hypoglycaemic therapy, most cats in remission do not have normal glucose tolerance (Gottlieb *et al.*, 2015). The majority (80%) have a mildly impaired capacity to normalize blood glucose concentrations after a glucose challenge. Some (20–30%) have impaired fasting glucose concentrations as well as glucose intolerance. Impaired fasting glucose implies a blood glucose concentration above the reference interval but less than that considered diabetic (6.5–9 mmol/l) (Gottlieb *et al.*, 2015). Cats with impaired fasting glucose and/or impaired glucose tolerance should be considered prediabetic and should be managed with a low-carbohydrate diet and normalization of bodyweight. Cats with impaired fasting glucose concentrations should be very closely monitored for relapse of diabetes mellitus (glucose concentrations >10 mmol/l). Impaired fasting glucose concentration and impaired glucose tolerance are both predictors of relapse in cats (Gottlieb *et al.*, 2015).

Treatment protocols for 'healthy' diabetic cats

'Healthy' diabetic cats are those with minimal dehydration and no, or only mild, ketosis. Cats with marked depression and dehydration, with or without ketoacidosis, should initially be treated in the same way as cats with diabetic ketoacidosis until they are stable (see Chapter 26). The protocols described below can be instituted for healthy diabetic cats and sick diabetic cats once they are stable. Protocols that provide the greatest probability of achieving remission should initially be implemented, and all such protocols require insulin administration.

The aim of insulin therapy is to ensure blood glucose concentrations are above the lower limit of the reference interval (typically reported as 3–4.5 mmol/l for non-stressed cats) and less than 10 mmol/l throughout the day, thus maximizing the chance of diabetic remission. The type of insulin used has a major influence on the likelihood of achieving such rigorous glycaemic control. However, success is also dependent on the intensity of monitoring, appropriate dose adjustments and dietary control. Although remission is achievable with most commonly used regimes, the remission rates can vary from 20% to 90% depending on the protocol implemented and the population of cats studied (Marshall *et al.*, 2009; Roomp and Rand, 2009, 2012; Riederer *et al.*, 2016).

Insulin choice

In many countries, including those within the UK and the European Union, only insulins authorized for veterinary use can be prescribed as the first line of therapy (see Chapter 23 for examples of types of insulin). The only readily available insulin authorized for veterinary use globally is a porcine-derived lente insulin. Protamine zinc insulin (PZI), a 40 IU/ml human-recombinant insulin, is authorized for use in cats in the UK, the European Union and the USA. As both these insulins are 40 IU/ml, it is important that they are used only with the appropriate insulin syringes; using 100 IU/ml syringes can result in incorrect dosing, unless this is specified to owners. Older insulin types such as isophane (neutral protamine Hagedorn (NPH)) and ultralente are not authorized for use in cats and are rarely, if ever, used today. More recently, longer-acting human-use insulin analogues have been assessed in cats; these include glargine 100 IU/ml,

glargine 300 IU/ml, detemir 100 IU/ml, and degludec 100 IU/ml or 200 IU/ml. However, in those countries with veterinary-use-only constraints, these may be prescribed only if treatment with an insulin authorized for cats has failed to achieve adequate glycaemic control.

Data published so far indicate that the use of insulin analogues such as glargine may result in higher remission rates in newly diagnosed diabetic cats compared with PZI, and PZI remission rates may be higher than those for lente insulin, although large controlled studies are lacking (Marshall *et al.*, 2009; Roomp and Rand, 2013). A small study of recently diagnosed diabetic cats demonstrated that 2 out of 8 cats (25%) achieved remission with porcine lente insulin, 3 out of 8 (37.5%) with PZI, and 8 out of 8 (100%) with glargine (Marshall *et al.*, 2009). Remission rates for detemir are similar to those for glargine (Roomp and Rand, 2012). Further support for higher remission rates using long-acting insulins such as glargine compared with lente insulin comes from a study of 55 diabetic cats (Roomp and Rand, 2009). These cats had previously been treated for a median of 16 weeks with other insulins, principally porcine lente insulin, but failed to achieve remission. After changing to glargine within 6 months of diagnosis, remission rates of 84% were attained, although intensive glucose monitoring and dietary control were implemented concurrently. Similar results were obtained with detemir (Roomp and Rand, 2012).

Given these results, glargine and detemir are the preferred insulin choices. However, PZI or porcine lente insulin may have to be used initially because of legal obligation or availability issues. Remission rates for cats are appreciably lower if intensive glucose control is not introduced early. Consequently, if veterinary-authorized insulins are used and diabetic remission is not achieved within 4–8 weeks, it is recommended to change to glargine or detemir to assist remission.

Lente insulin

When given twice daily, intermediate-acting insulins such as lente insulin have too short a duration of action for effective glycaemic control in a high proportion of cats. Because of this short duration of activity, there is usually suboptimal exogenous circulating insulin for several hours before each insulin injection, resulting in minimal glucose-lowering effect for approximately 4–8 of every 24 hours (Martin and Rand, 2007). Therefore, pre-insulin blood glucose concentrations are usually high (sometimes exceeding 20 mmol/l) and the goal of achieving glucose concentrations between 3–4.5 and 10 mmol/l, which is important for diabetic remission, is not achieved throughout the day. Although clinical signs may be relatively well controlled, the potential marked hyperglycaemia twice daily will continue to suppress insulin secretion and damage beta cells, contributing to lower remission rates in comparison with results obtained using longer-acting insulins (Marshall *et al.*, 2009; Roomp and Rand, 2009).

Protamine zinc insulin

Protamine zinc insulin has a longer duration of action compared to lente insulin, and because of this it is often preferred for use in cats, especially as it is approved for use in cats in the UK, the European Union and the USA. However, in some studies it has been shown to be linked with lower remission rates in comparison to the new long-acting insulin analogues detemir and glargine (Marshall *et al.*, 2009; Roomp and Rand, 2009).

Glargine

Glargine is a synthetic insulin analogue. It is produced using recombinant DNA technology utilizing *Escherichia coli*. The insulin molecule is modified by replacing asparagine at position 21 of the A chain with glycine, and by adding two arginines at the terminal portion of the B chain. This is reflected in the name glargine. The modification shifts the isoelectric point, producing a molecule that is totally soluble at a pH of 4. In subcutaneous tissues, where the pH is 7.4, the acidic solution is neutralized, allowing the formation of microprecipitates that steadily break down. This slow release of glargine into the systemic circulation produces its sustained action. The formation of microprecipitates is dependent on the interaction of the acidic insulin and the relatively neutral subcutaneous tissues; it is therefore imperative that glargine is not mixed with other insulins or diluted before administration.

Glargine as a 100 IU/ml solution is designed for once-daily administration in humans and is marketed as a 'peakless' insulin with respect to its glucose-lowering effect. This lack of peak relates to the glucose utilization rate of glargine, a factor determined by the amount of intravenous glucose necessary to maintain a constant circulating glucose concentration after insulin is injected subcutaneously. However, when viewing the glucose and insulin concentration curves in diabetic and healthy cats, there are definite glucose nadirs and insulin peaks associated with glargine use. The blood-glucose-lowering effect and duration of action in cats are comparable to those in diabetic humans (Marshall *et al.*, 2008a).

Clinical experience demonstrates that glargine has a long duration of action in cats and, in stabilized cats, is not usually associated with marked hyperglycaemia at the time of the next insulin injection, as occurs with lente insulin.

Glargine is now also available as a 300 IU/ml formulation, which has different pharmacokinetics to the 100 IU/ml formulation. It has a more even distribution of metabolic effect and longer duration of action of over 24 hours in healthy cats compared with glargine 100 IU/ml, which may make it suitable for once-daily administration in some cats (Saini *et al.*, 2021). A study of eight diabetic cats (five newly diagnosed) reported that it was safe and effective to use, with two cats going into remission during the study period (8 weeks) and two cats achieving remission after the study completion (within 12 weeks) (Linari *et al.*, 2022).

Detemir

The synthetic insulin analogue detemir has an extended duration of action, which is achieved via a different mechanism from that of glargine. Detemir is produced using recombinant DNA technology in yeast (*Saccharomyces cerevisiae*), and the insulin molecule is modified by the addition of an acylated fatty acid chain. This modification facilitates reversible binding to plasma proteins, particularly albumin, from where detemir is slowly released into the plasma. The modification also prolongs self-association in the injection depot, which delays absorption from subcutaneous tissue at that site and contributes to the long duration of action (Kurtzhals, 2004).

Glargine *versus* detemir

No clinical differences were detected between cats treated with glargine (n = 55) and with detemir (n = 18), except that a 30% lower maximal dose was required in the detemir-treated cats (median maximum glargine dose was 2.5 IU (range = 1.0–9.0 IU) compared with a median maximum detemir dose of 1.75 IU (range = 0.5–4.0 IU)) (Roomp and Rand, 2009, 2012). Glargine is currently the insulin of choice in diabetic cats because it has been used more widely and its pharmacokinetics and dynamics are better known in this species in comparison with detemir, and because it can be used intramuscularly to treat diabetic ketoacidosis (Marshall *et al.*, 2013). However, data from healthy cats and humans suggest that detemir has a longer duration of action and less variability between and within individuals compared with glargine (Gilor *et al.*, 2010). Experimentally, detemir had a longer duration of action (median 800 minutes; range 525–915 minutes) than glargine (median 470 minutes; range 295–950 minutes) and showed less variation in duration of action in healthy cats (Gilor *et al.*, 2010). In humans, detemir has also been shown to be more consistent in its duration of action in comparison with glargine. In a retrospective study of 14 diabetic cats treated with detemir, 13 achieved control of clinical signs within 3 months and three of those achieved remission (Hoelmkjaer *et al.*, 2015). Detemir or glargine 300 IU/ml are particularly indicated in those cats for which glargine 100 IU/ml appears to have too short a duration of action with twice-daily administration.

Storage of glargine and detemir

Many questions arise because of the manufacturers' instructions regarding shelf life for glargine and detemir and the subsequent cost implications for owners managing diabetic cats. Glargine is marketed for human use with a shelf life at room temperature of 28 days after opening. It is reasonably fragile but is chemically stable in solution for 6 months if kept refrigerated. Detemir is marketed with a 6-week shelf life at room temperature after opening. Longer expiration periods are not usually recommended on multiple-use injectable medication vials for humans, even if a preservative is present, because of the risk of bacterial contamination. Glargine and detemir preparations contain the antimicrobial preservative meta-cresol, which is thought to be bacteriostatic rather than bactericidal. Authorization bodies believe that there is a reasonable probability of contamination with microbes through multiple daily punctures to withdraw medication past the arbitrary expiration date. However, in veterinary practice, owners of diabetic cats routinely use refrigerated glargine or detemir for up to 6 months, or more, with no evidence of problems. Owners should be instructed to immediately dispose of any insulin that appears cloudy or discoloured, because this may represent bacterial contamination or precipitation. For cats requiring small doses of insulin, detemir can be diluted using a special diluting medium available from the manufacturer, although this is not always available in veterinary practices. Diluting with sterile water or saline increases the risk of bacterial contamination, and the effects on stability and efficacy have not been reported (Barone *et al.*, 2011). Dilution of detemir is generally not recommended for cats.

Degludec

Insulin degludec is an ultra-long-acting insulin analogue and, in humans, has a longer duration of action than glargine 100 IU/ml and detemir. Degludec is insulin modified by deletion of one threonine residue and addition of a fatty acid that prolongs the duration of activity by increased self-association, precipitation at the injection site and albumin binding. In healthy cats, insulin degludec was shown to have a longer duration of action than PZI (Salesov *et al.*, 2018). However, insulin degludec had a shorter duration of action compared with glargine 300 IU/ml in healthy cats (Gilor *et al.*, 2019). In eight diabetic cats (five of them newly diagnosed) treated with insulin degludec and followed over a 12-month period, glycaemic control was achieved with a mean dose of 0.75 IU/kg/day (Oda *et al.*, 2020). Remission was not achieved in any of these cats during this period; however, full details of dosing protocols were not reported.

AKS-267c

A new ultra-long-acting insulin administered once weekly has been reported to successfully control clinical signs and blood glucose concentrations in five previously treated diabetic cats that had good glycaemic control following treatment with glargine for at least 2 months (Gilor *et al.*, 2021). AKS-267c is a recombinant fusion protein of a synthetic insulin and feline immunoglobulin fragment crystallizable (Fc) region. The dose of AKS-267c was titrated weekly for 7 weeks based on continuous glucose monitoring. There was no evidence of clinical hypoglycaemia or adverse events. Glycaemic control was no different between once-weekly AKS-267c and twice-daily glargine protocols, with the former offering QOL and other benefits to diabetic cats and their owners. This insulin is not yet commercially available.

Frequency of insulin administration

It is important to reduce the daily exposure of beta cells to marked hyperglycaemia to aid recovery of beta cell function and maximize the likelihood of successful diabetic remission (Robertson *et al.*, 2000; Link, 2001). This is more achievable if insulin is administered twice daily rather than once daily in diabetic cats.

Intermediate-acting insulins such as lente must be given twice daily in cats. However, in many cats, glycaemic control would be improved if administration were three times daily, because the duration of action is typically shorter than 8 hours. In dogs, once-daily insulin administration is associated with an increased risk of clinical hypoglycaemia and this is also likely in cats (Hess and Ward, 2000).

Although PZI is a long-acting insulin, improved glycaemic control occurs with twice-daily administration. Glargine and detemir are also considered to be long acting. The mean duration of action of 0.25 IU/kg glargine in healthy cats was at least 20 hours, although in some cats it was as short as 14 hours (Marshall *et al.*, 2009). Another study measuring glucose utilization rate in healthy cats found that the median duration of glargine action was 8 hours but could be as short as 5 hours after administration of 0.5 IU/kg (Gilor *et al.*, 2010). It is clear that the duration of action of glargine, and probably detemir, varies substantially between healthy and diabetic cats and within the same cat from day to day. Despite the variability and lack of well controlled pharmacodynamic studies in cats, clinical observations suggest that remission rates in recently diagnosed diabetic cats are higher when glargine or detemir are administered twice daily in comparison with once daily. Twice-daily dosing is recommended (Weaver *et al.*, 2006; Marshall *et al.*, 2009; Roomp and Rand, 2009, 2012).

Insulin dose

Dosing protocols can be successfully used for adjusting insulin dose with a range of insulins. However, it needs to be recognized that the dosing rules differ depending on whether the insulin used is intermediate acting and unlikely to have a carry-over effect at the next insulin injection, or is long acting with a high probability of carry-over effects.

For long-acting insulin, both the nadir and the pre-insulin blood glucose concentration (just prior to insulin injection) are used as a basis for increasing the dose. By contrast, with intermediate-acting insulin, only the nadir blood glucose concentration is used. This is because exogenous insulin is unlikely to be present immediately before the subsequent insulin injection, so the pre-insulin blood glucose concentration does not reflect the glucose-lowering effect of exogenous insulin, and reflects only the duration of insulin action or the presence of endogenous insulin.

Regardless of the type of insulin used, an initial dose of 0.25–0.5 IU/kg of the cat's ideal bodyweight is recommended for a newly diagnosed cat, at 12-hourly intervals depending on blood glucose concentrations. During the first 3 days of therapy, blood glucose concentrations should be carefully monitored every 2–4 hours during the day and the insulin dose reduced if the blood glucose concentration at any one time is low.

When changing cats to glargine from other types of insulin, they can typically be given the same dose, with the exception of cats receiving high doses (>3 IU/injection/cat) of insulin. Care should be exercised in these cats until it is known how they will respond, and a smaller dose should be used initially. For detemir, a 30% lower dose than previously used for other insulins is recommended as a starting dose, and the dose can be increased within a few days if inadequate control is achieved (Roomp and Rand, 2012).

Because blood glucose concentrations can ideally be measured every 2 hours (lente) or every 3–4 hours (glargine, detemir and PZI), portable glucose meters and continuous/flash glucose monitoring systems are useful tools, provided they are interpreted correctly (see 'Glucose meters', below). The protocols illustrated in Figures 24.2–24.4 have been developed for use with intermediate (lente) and long-acting (glargine 100 IU/ml, glargine 300 IU/ml, detemir and PZI) insulins.

Pre-insulin blood glucose concentration (mmol/l)	Dose adjustment
Newly diagnosed (<2 months insulin therapy)	
>13	Increase dose by 0.5 IU
7–13	Keep dose the same
4–<7	Decrease dose by 0.5 IU
<4	Do not give insulin and call the clinic to discuss
Longer term (>2 months insulin therapy)	
>25	Increase dose by 1 IU
15–25	Increase dose by 0.5 IU
7–<15	Keep dose the same
4–<7	Decrease dose by 0.5 IU
<4	Do not give insulin and call the clinic to discuss; check for remission depending on dose

24.2 Low-intensity home blood glucose monitoring protocol for glargine 100 IU/ml or detemir using only pre-insulin blood glucose concentration. Blood glucose cut-off points are based on measurement using a glucometer calibrated for feline blood. Remission rate is approximately 50% in newly diagnosed diabetic cats. If using glargine 300 IU/ml, increase only one insulin dose per day and wait at least 3 days before increasing the second dose per day if indicated. If using a glucometer calibrated for human blood, decrease the target glucose concentration by 20% (approximately 1 mmol/l).
(Adapted with permission from Rand and Gottlieb, 2017)

Parameter used for dose adjustment	Dose adjustment
Begin with 0.5 IU/kg q12h if blood glucose concentration >20 mmol/l **or** 0.25 IU/kg of ideal weight q12h If blood glucose concentration is lower. Monitor response to therapy for first 3 days. If no monitoring is occurring in first week, begin with 1 IU/cat q12h	Do not increase in first week unless minimal response to insulin occurs. Decrease if necessary
Pre-insulin blood glucose concentration >12 mmol/l, provided nadir is not in hypoglycaemic range **or** Nadir blood glucose concentration >10 mmol/l	Increase dose by 0.25–1 IU depending on the degree of hyperglycaemia and total insulin dose (greater or less than 3 IU/cat) and how close blood glucose concentration is to 10 mmol/l
Pre-insulin blood glucose concentration of 10–12 mmol/l **or** Nadir blood glucose concentration of 5–9 mmol/l	Keep the dose the same
Nadir blood glucose concentration of 3.5–<5 mmol/l	Use nadir glucose, water intake, urine glucose and next pre-insulin glucose concentration to determine whether the insulin dose should be decreased or maintained
Pre-insulin blood glucose concentration <10 mmol/l **or** Nadir blood glucose concentration <3.5 mmol/l	Reduce dose by 0.25–1.0 IU depending on the blood glucose concentration and total dose (greater or less than 3 IU/cat) and how close blood glucose concentration is to 10 mmol/l. If total dose is 0.5–1.0 IU q12h, change to q24h. If total dose is 0.5–1.0 IU q24h, stop insulin and check for diabetic remission
Observation of clinical signs of hypoglycaemia	Reduce dose by 50%

24.3 Semi-intensive protocol for glargine 100 IU/ml, detemir or protamine zinc insulin, based on monitoring glucose in hospital or at home initially weekly using a glucometer calibrated for cats. If using a glucometer calibrated for human blood, decrease the target blood glucose concentration by 20% (approximately 1 mmol/l). If using glargine 300 IU/ml, increase only one insulin dose per day and wait at least 3 days before increasing the second daily dose if indicated.

(Adapted with permission from Rand and Gottlieb, 2017)

Parameter used for dose adjustment	Dose adjustment
Phase 1: Initial dose and first 3 days on glargine	
Begin with 0.25 IU/kg of ideal weight q12h	If the cat received another insulin previously, increase or reduce the starting dose taking this information into account. Glargine has a lower potency than lente or protamine zinc insulin in most cats
Cats with a history of developing ketones that maintain blood glucose concentration >17 mmol/l after 24–48 hours of insulin treatment	Increase dose by 0.5 IU
Blood glucose concentration <4 mmol/l	Reduce dose by 0.25–0.5 IU depending on whether the cat is receiving a low or high dose of insulin (greater or less than 3 IU/cat) and how close blood glucose concentration is to 10 mmol/l
Phase 2: Increasing the dose	
Nadir blood glucose concentration >16.6 mmol/l	Increase dose by 0.5 IU every 3 days
Nadir blood glucose concentration of 11.1–16.6 mmol/l	Increase dose by 0.25–0.5 IU every 3 days depending on whether the cat is receiving a low or high dose of insulin
Nadir blood glucose concentration of 6.5–<11 mmol/l and peak >11 mmol/l	Increase dose by 0.25–0.5 IU every 5–7 days depending on whether the cat is receiving a low or high dose of insulin
Nadir blood glucose <3.5 or <4 mmol/l – actual cut-off depends on the frequency of monitoring and previous response to insulin dose changes when blood glucose is around the lower limit of the reference interval	Reduce dose by 0.25–0.5 IU depending on whether the cat is receiving a low or high dose of insulin; if clinical signs of hypoglycaemia occur, reduce dose by 0.5 to >1 IU depending on severity
Pre-insulin blood glucose of 4–6.5 mmol/l	Initially test which of the alternative methods is best suited to the individual cat: a. Feed cat and reduce the dose by 0.25–0.5 IU depending on whether the cat is receiving a low or high dose of insulin b. Feed cat, wait 1–2 hours and when the glucose concentration increases above 6.5 mmol/l, give the normal dose. If the glucose concentration does not increase within 1–2 hours, reduce the dose by 0.25 IU or 0.5 IU (as above). c. Split the dose: feed cat, give most of the dose immediately and then give the remainder 1–2 hours later, when the glucose concentration has increased above 6.5 mmol/l. If all these methods lead to an increased blood glucose concentration and pre-insulin blood glucose concentration is still 4–6.5 mmol/l, give the full dose and observe closely for signs of hypoglycaemia. For most cats, the best results in phase 2 occur when insulin is dosed as consistently as possible, giving the full normal dose at the regular injection time
Phase 3: Holding the dose. Aim to keep blood glucose concentration between 4 and 11 mmol/l throughout the day	
Nadir blood glucose <3.5 or <4 mmol/l	Reduce dose by 0.25–0.5 IU depending on whether the cat is receiving a low or high dose of insulin
Nadir or peak blood glucose concentration >11.0 mmol/l	Increase dose by 0.25–0.5 IU depending on whether the cat is receiving a low or high dose of insulin and on the degree of hyperglycaemia

24.4 Intensive protocol for glargine or detemir with home blood glucose monitoring a minimum of 3 times per day (average 5) during stabilization period (6–12 weeks) using a glucometer calibrated for cats (Roomp and Rand, 2009). If using glargine 300 IU/ml, increase only one daily insulin dose and wait at least 3 days before increasing the second daily dose if indicated. (continues) ▶

(Adapted with permission from Rand and Gottlieb, 2017)

Parameter used for dose adjustment	Dose adjustment
Phase 4: Reducing the dose. Phase out insulin slowly by 0.25–0.5 IU depending on dose	
The cat regularly (every day for at least 1 week) has a nadir blood glucose concentration 4–6.5 mmol/l, and stays under 6.5 mmol/l overall	Reduce dose by 0.25–0.5 IU depending on whether the cat is receiving a low or high dose of insulin
Nadir glucose concentration of 3–<4 mmol/l at least three times on separate days	Reduce dose by 0.25–0.5 IU depending on whether the cat is receiving a low or high dose of insulin
Blood glucose concentration drops below 3 mmol/l once	Immediately reduce dose by 0.25–0.5 IU depending on whether the cat is receiving a low or high dose of insulin
Peak blood glucose concentration >11 mmol/l	Immediately increase dose to last effective dose
Phase 5: Remission. Euglycaemia for a minimum of 14 days without insulin. Monitor blood glucose at least twice daily to ensure it remains ≤6.5 mmol/l. If blood glucose increases to 6.5–<10 mmol/l, institute other therapy such as insulin sensitizers or glucagon-like peptide 1 agonists to maintain blood glucose ≤6.5 mmol/l. If ≥10 mmol/l, reinstitute insulin once or twice a day depending on the severity of hyperglycaemia	

24.4 (continued) Intensive protocol for glargine or detemir with home blood glucose monitoring a minimum of 3 times per day (average 5) during stabilization period (6–12 weeks) using a glucometer calibrated for cats (Roomp and Rand, 2009). If using glargine 300 IU/ml, increase only one daily insulin dose and wait at least 3 days before increasing the second daily dose if indicated.
(Adapted with permission from Rand and Gottlieb, 2017)

Dose adjustments

After the initial 3 days of treatment there are two or three phases of treatment for diabetic cats. Initially, there is a phase of increasing dose followed by a phase of consistent dosing and finally, for cats going into remission, a phase of decreasing dose.

In the phase of increasing dose, depending on the insulin being used, either nadir alone or nadir and pre-insulin blood glucose concentrations are used as a basis for increasing the dose. If close monitoring is occurring, doses can be increased every 3–7 days by 0.25–0.5 IU/injection depending on whether a low (<3 IU/injection/cat) or high (>3 IU/injection/cat) dose of insulin is being used and the degree of hyperglycaemia (see Figure 24.3). For glargine 100 IU/ml or 300 IU/ml and detemir, the aim is to increase the dose until the blood glucose concentration is between 4–4.5 and 10 mmol/l (initially aiming for <12 mmol/l); that is, consistently within or just above the reference interval throughout the day. In lente-treated cats, this is not achievable, but the aim is for the nadir blood glucose concentration to be in the high end of the reference interval (5–9 mmol/l) until the cat is well controlled, because the risk of clinical hypoglycaemia with potent intermediate-acting insulins appears to be higher than with longer-acting insulins. Once the cat is well controlled, small insulin dose increases can be trialled to determine whether improved glycaemic control can be achieved without clinical signs of hypoglycaemia. Approximately 25% of cats treated with glargine or detemir will show an increase in glucose concentration in the first 2 or 3 days after a dose increase, which generally lasts for <24 hours. The dose should be maintained and the fluctuations disregarded.

In the phase of consistent dosing, the dose is held once the blood glucose concentrations throughout the day are between 4–4.5 and <11 mmol/l (detemir, glargine and PZI) or the nadir is between 5 and 9 mmol/l (lente). This phase of consistent dosing may last several months, although in some cats it lasts only weeks. In lente-treated cats, once it is known how an individual cat responds to insulin, a nadir closer (4–7 mmol/l) to the reference interval can be aimed for.

The final phase involves a reduction in the dose once the pre-insulin blood glucose is consistently <11 mmol/l or if the nadir glucose concentration is <4 mmol/l (see Figures 24.2–24.4). Decreasing the dose too rapidly may reduce the chance of remission by withdrawing insulin before beta cells have fully recovered from glucose toxicity. Instead, insulin should be reduced but not withheld until the total insulin dose is 0.5 IU/cat once a day. In this phase of decreasing dose, it is critical that the rate of decrease is slow and conservative, ideally adjusting only every 7–14 days. Insulin is phased out gradually in a step-by-step manner (in 0.25 IU or 0.5 IU decrements), which is dependent on the overall dose administered. Anecdotally, cats that are very slowly weaned off insulin are less likely to relapse soon after insulin is withdrawn. If the blood glucose concentration fails to remain within the reference interval after a dose reduction, the insulin dose is immediately increased to the last effective dose.

During the first weeks of insulin therapy, a frequent error is to cease insulin administration prematurely. This is often done when a pre-insulin blood glucose concentration is within the reference interval. To determine whether remission has occurred, the insulin is stopped if the pre-insulin blood glucose is <10 mmol/l or if the nadir blood glucose concentration is <4 mmol/l and the cat is receiving a minimal dose (e.g. 0.5 IU once a day). The cat is then reassessed 12 hours later and, if at that time the blood glucose concentration has not increased above 10 mmol/l, the cat is re-checked again in 1 week. Insulin is immediately reinstituted if the blood glucose concentration increases to 10 mmol/l or higher within 12 hours of withholding insulin. For cats that remain insulin dependent, a dose reduction may be required after the phase of consistent dosing, once the insulin resistance associated with hyperglycaemia resolves.

For a small number of cats, a small dose (e.g. 0.5–1 IU) of insulin administered every 24–48 hours is necessary when there is insufficient beta cell function to maintain euglycaemia without insulin, but daily dosing would result in hypoglycaemia. In a further few cats, blood glucose concentrations remain in the reference interval for a few days following a dose reduction but then begin to increase again, and the dose will need to be increased.

The average dose for cats that remain stable on glargine, detemir, lente or PZI is 0.4–0.6 IU/kg q12h. Occasionally, cats need high total doses of insulin (5–10 IU/cat) to control blood glucose concentrations. In many of these cats, the dose can be decreased once control is achieved. However, cats with hypersomatotropism often require high (>10 IU/cat) or, on occasion, extreme (>50 IU/cat) doses to control blood glucose concentrations.

Any cat that is still poorly controlled after 8 weeks of therapy and is receiving a dose of >0.5–1 IU/cat q12h should have IGF-1 concentration measured. If hypersomatotropism is confirmed, good glycaemic control will not be possible without specific treatment of the underlying disorder. In addition, the potential for remission will vary between the treatment options chosen (see Chapter 13). In the absence of specific treatment, palliative care with insulin can help manage blood glucose concentrations. If palliative care is chosen, it is strongly recommended that owners of cats with hypersomatotropism measure blood glucose concentration at home before each insulin dose, especially if very high insulin doses are being used, because growth hormone and, subsequently, blood glucose concentrations can vary widely from day to day.

Dose variations

There is a large variation in the glucose-lowering effect of a given dose of insulin between cats and within the same cat from day to day. This is also reported in humans and dogs. There are a variety of factors that contribute to this, including differences in the rates and percentage of insulin absorbed from the subcutaneous injection site, variation in insulin sensitivity between cats and variation in the actual dose received per kg of metabolic weight (Marshall et al., 2008b).

The very small volume of insulin used in cats makes dose errors likely. These errors are likely to be reduced by using 0.3 ml insulin syringes designed for 100 IU/ml insulin with 0.5 unit (and, if available, 0.25 unit) gradations. Many cats receive <2 IU at each injection. One study demonstrated that even trained paediatric nurses using 100 IU insulin and 0.3 ml syringes were unable to dose any amount under 2 IU accurately (Casella et al., 1993). Although 40 IU/ml syringes may make measuring small doses easier, these should be used only with the appropriate insulins (e.g. lente and PZI), as use with 100 IU/ml insulins can result in errors in dose if owners do not understand the difference in volume between the syringes with each gradation. Insulin dosage pens are able to administer more accurate doses; some allow dose adjustments of 0.5 IU, which can help with small adjustments in insulin dosing.

Adverse effects of insulin

Hypoglycaemia

Biochemical hypoglycaemia is common in insulin-treated cats. Clinical hypoglycaemia is infrequent in cats treated with glargine or detemir but appears to be more common in cats treated with lente insulin (Marshall et al., 2009; Roomp and Rand, 2009, 2013). In humans with type 1 and 2 diabetes treated with glargine, the prevalence of clinical hypoglycaemia is also considerably reduced compared with those using shorter-acting insulins such as NPH insulin (Fonseca et al., 2004; Fulcher et al., 2005). This is thought to be associated with glargine's consistent insulin action related to its slow release from the injection site over 24 hours, compared with a sharp peak of insulin action associated with the rapid release of intermediate-acting insulin from the injection site (Marshall et al., 2009). In one study of 55 cats treated with glargine using an intensive protocol designed to achieve euglycaemia, asymptomatic or biochemical hypoglycaemia was common, occurring at some point in up to 94% of cats (Roomp and Rand, 2009). However, there was only one associated mild episode of clinical hypoglycaemia. Detemir is associated with a similarly low rate of clinical hypoglycaemia.

Signs of clinical hypoglycaemia in cats can be severe and life-threatening, and are the reason why some owners elect to euthanase diabetic cats. Although concern about hypoglycaemia is a factor reducing the QOL for owners of diabetic cats and leads to decisions to euthanase, owners should be informed that biochemical hypoglycaemia is common with glargine and detemir and is an indicator to reduce the insulin dose, not to elect for euthanasia, because clinical hypoglycaemia is uncommon. It is also important for clients to understand that although insulin dosing protocols typically use 4–4.5 mmol/l as the lower limit of desired blood glucose concentration, the lower limit of normal blood glucose in an unstressed cat after an overnight fast is 3 mmol/l.

Somogyi effect (rebound hyperglycaemia)

Marked hyperglycaemia following an episode of hypoglycaemia is often referred to as the Somogyi effect and is usually attributed to an insulin overdose triggering a counter-regulatory hormone response. However, in human patients, several studies have shown that the Somogyi effect is uncommon and that most episodes of hyperglycaemia following hypoglycaemia are not due to a rebound effect but are the result of inadequate duration of insulin action (Bolli and Gerich, 1984; Carroll and Schade, 2005). A large-scale review of 10,767 blood glucose curves in 55 cats treated with an intensive glargine protocol found that only 0.42% of curves fitted the criteria of hypoglycaemia followed by marked hyperglycaemia, even though 93% of cats experienced at least one episode of biochemical hypoglycaemia (Roomp and Rand, 2016). Hypoglycaemia followed by marked hyperglycaemia occurred in approximately 25% of cats and occurred on a median of three (range 1–11) occasions. In 10% of curves showing hypoglycaemia followed by hyperglycaemia, there was no glucose-lowering effect following the next insulin dose, suggesting insulin resistance after the hypoglycaemic event. However, there was no difference in peak glucose concentration after a hypoglycaemic or euglycaemic nadir, suggesting that a rebound phenomenon was not involved in the subsequent hyperglycaemia. Similarly, in humans, there is no association between counter-regulatory hormone concentration and blood glucose concentrations following hypoglycaemia, but insulin concentration is lower when there is hyperglycaemia, which is consistent with inadequate insulin action (Gale et al., 1980). Anecdotally, hyperglycaemia following hypoglycaemia, occasionally followed by insulin resistance, appears to be more frequent with lente and other intermediate-acting insulins, which are more potent and lead to a more rapid reduction in blood glucose concentration following insulin injection. This hyperglycaemia with or without insulin resistance is usually attributed to a Somogyi effect but, based on current knowledge, this appears to be unlikely. A comparison of rebound hyperglycaemia in healthy and diabetic cats treated with either lente or degludec insulin found that 25% of diabetic cats with hypoglycaemia appeared to have rebound hyperglycaemia; the same prevalence has been reported in glargine-treated cats (Zini et al., 2018). However, without measurements of insulin or counter-regulatory hormones, it is not possible to know whether the hyperglycaemia was truly due to rebound hyperglycaemia or inadequate duration of action. The availability of continuous glucose monitoring (see below) provides the technology required to more accurately document the true prevalence of hyperglycaemia following hypoglycaemia associated with use of intermediate- and long-acting insulins. In most cats, marked hyperglycaemia within 24 hours of hypoglycaemia is more likely reflective of short duration of insulin action. Hypoglycaemia is indicative that the insulin dose needs to be reduced; when followed by hyperglycaemia, a longer-acting insulin is also indicated. It is recommended that cats receiving lente insulin are switched to glargine 100 IU/ml, and that cats receiving glargine 100 IU/ml are switched to 300 IU/ml or to detemir.

Glucose variability

Glucose variability refers to glycaemic excursions, including episodes of hypoglycaemia and hyperglycaemia, during the course of a day or on different days. In human diabetes mellitus, glucose variability is an indicator of glycaemic control, and high glucose variability is considered a risk factor for hypoglycaemia, other diabetic complications and mortality (Suh and Kim, 2015; Krämer et al., 2020). The j index is one measure of glucose variability that includes the mean and standard deviation in one score. In cats treated with lente insulin, the j index was shown to be strongly correlated with clinical signs, in particular water intake, and other measures of glycaemic control such as urine glucose concentration (Martin and Rand, 2007), and was the most sensitive index tested for differentiating between cats with and without clinical signs. However, both the standard deviation and the j index require more complex calculations for clinicians than just using maximum, minimum and mean blood glucose as indicators of glucose variability. The association of lower glucose variability with lower risk for hypoglycaemia, improved glycaemic control and, in humans, lower mortality is further evidence that long-acting insulins are a more appropriate choice for use in diabetic cats.

Oral hypoglycaemic agents

Oral hypoglycaemic drugs stimulate beta cells to secrete insulin (e.g. glipizide), decrease glucose absorption from the gastrointestinal tract (e.g. acarbose) or increase insulin sensitivity (e.g. metformin, roziglitazone). Sole use of oral hypoglycaemic agents that stimulate insulin secretion is associated with a reduced probability of remission (remission rate <20%) compared with treatment with a long-acting insulin, and is not recommended (Feldman et al., 1997; Roomp and Rand, 2009). Remission rates associated with most other oral hypoglycaemic drugs are likely similar, and so use of these drugs as sole agents is also not recommended. However, the use of oral hypoglycaemic agents can be life-saving for cats when the owner elects for euthanasia rather than insulin injections. They may also be valuable during periods of remission in cats with mild hyperglycaemia.

Sodium-glucose co-transporter (SGLT) 2 inhibitors were recently approved for use in cats in the USA and will likely become the first line of therapy in newly diagnosed diabetic cats. They reduce renal tubular glucose absorption, which increases urinary glucose excretion and lowers circulating glucose concentrations. Bexagliflozin is authorized in the USA for otherwise healthy cats not previously treated with insulin (Hadd et al., 2023) and velagliflozin is set to be approved in 2023 (Niessen et al., 2022; Behrend, 2023), with others likely to follow. The dose for bexagliflozin is 15 mg orally once daily to cats >3 kg bodyweight. Tablets can be crushed in food and have high acceptability in cats (98% of treatments consumed). Within 8 hours of the first treatment, blood glucose may decrease by 50% or more. Mean blood glucose is below the renal threshold from day 7, with 50% of cats having blood glucose in the

reference range by 30 days and more than 80% of cats by 180 days. Clinical hypoglycaemia is not a risk and biochemical hypoglycaemia is rare. Cats must have some endogenous insulin secretion (evidenced by lack of ketonuria at diagnosis) to prevent ketoacidosis, which can happen as soon as 48 hours after beginning therapy and mostly occurs within 2 weeks of starting therapy. Typically, diabetic ketoacidosis is associated with normal or near normal blood glucose concentrations (<13.9 mmol/l) and termed euglycaemic diabetic ketoacidosis. It occurred in 7% of newly diagnosed cats and can be fatal, requiring prompt treatment with insulin along with 7.5% dextrose to prevent hypoglycaemia and nutritional support to prevent rapid onset of hepatic lipidosis. Home blood monitoring of beta-hydroxybutyrate concentration is important, and lethargy or inappetence should be rapidly investigated because onset of euglycemic diabetic ketoacidosis can be rapid. Dehydration and corticosteroid administration are risk factors for diabetic ketoacidosis in humans. Other serious adverse events include pancreatitis and hepatic lipidosis, and cats with pre-existing evidence of pancreatitis and anorexic cats should be excluded. Diarrhoea was the most common adverse effect (50% of cats) followed by vomiting (33% of cats) and both were typically mild and transient, likely associated with inhibition of the SGLT2 transporters in the gastrointestinal tract. Other common mild adverse effects are anorexia, lethargy and dehydration (Hadd et al., 2023).

During treatment, home monitoring of blood glucose and beta-hydroxybutyrate concentrations, clinical signs and bodyweight, and periodic in-clinic monitoring of fructosamine, feline pancreas-specific lipase, liver parameters, cholesterol and triglyceride is advised. Glucosuria persists for 6–7 days after cessation of therapy. Although not approved for use in insulin-treated cats, bexagliflozin improved glycaemic control and reduced insulin dose in poorly controlled cats (Benedict et al., 2022), but concurrent use with insulin will carry a risk of clinical hypoglycaemia. To reduce the risk of hypoglycaemia, it is recommended that the insulin dose be reduced by 50% before the first dose of bexagliflozin is administered, and the dose of insulin should be subsequently adjusted based on at-home blood glucose and beta-hydroxybutyrate monitoring. Further studies are necessary to evaluate the long-term efficacy and safety of these drugs, including use in cats with hypersomatotropism where surgery or radiation is not an option. Guidelines need to be developed for withdrawing treatment to determine if a cat is in remission, and for concurrently treating cats with insulin to prevent ketoacidosis when there is insufficient endogenous insulin for SGLT2 inhibitors to be used as sole therapy. In humans, low carbohydrate diets are not recommended due to the increased risk of diabetic ketoacidosis; further research is required to determine dietary recommendations for cats.

Emerging therapies include incretins, gastrointestinal hormones that stimulate insulin release in response to food intake and include glucagon-like peptide 1 (GLP-1) agonists and dipeptidylpeptidase-4 (DDP-4) inhibitors (Reusch and Padrutt, 2013). Hypoglycaemia is rare, as the actions are glucose dependent. In newly diagnosed diabetic cats treated with glargine and a low-carbohydrate diet, those also treated with the GLP-1 agonist exenatide had improved glycaemic control and remission rates (Riederer et al., 2016). Exenatide has also been associated with improvement in glucose variability in diabetic cats treated with insulin (Krämer et al., 2020). Further studies are required before their widespread use.

Dietary management

Dietary management of feline diabetes mellitus using a low-carbohydrate diet (<15% metabolizable energy (ME) from carbohydrates) is one of the three key strategies for increasing the probability of remission. A complete and balanced low-carbohydrate diet should be fed, including in those diabetic cats requiring weight loss. Low-carbohydrate diets are associated with increased remission rates and minimize the need for beta cells to secrete insulin. Importantly, in a study comparing remission rates between a moderate-carbohydrate (26% ME) and low-carbohydrate (12% ME) diet with similar protein content (37% ME versus 40% ME), the low-carbohydrate diet was associated with significantly higher remission rates (68% versus 41%) (Bennett et al., 2006). In addition, decreasing the carbohydrate content (from 50% to 25% ME) significantly reduces blood glucose concentrations in healthy cats by 20–25% for 3–18 hours after eating, if fed once or twice daily or if fed ad libitum. For diabetic cats with reduced or no endogenous insulin secretion, the increase in blood glucose after eating is likely to be more pronounced than in healthy cats.

A restricted-carbohydrate diet should be started at the time of initiation of insulin therapy, and it is critical that the diet be continued after remission to minimize the demand on beta cells to secrete insulin. When changing cats already receiving insulin therapy from a moderate- or high-carbohydrate diet to a low-carbohydrate diet, it is recommended that the insulin dose be initially reduced by 30–50%, because hypoglycaemia can develop secondary to the reduction in glucose load associated with the low-carbohydrate diet.

Ultra-low-carbohydrate diets (<5% ME) are also sometimes recommended. These diets are essentially nearly all meat or fish, may not be complete or balanced and are high in phosphate, which is of concern given the frequency of kidney disease in diabetic cats. Although restricted-carbohydrate diets are recommended if remission is a goal of therapy, there are currently no studies available that compare diets of varying carbohydrate content (2%, 6% or 15% ME) to determine which is most appropriate for use in feline diabetics. Where possible, complete and balanced diets should be fed, and if CKD is present, phosphate content may be a consideration. If remission is not a realistic goal of therapy, for example, if the cat has been diabetic for several years, dietary management of other health issues takes precedence.

Feeding frequency

In healthy cats, similar blood glucose concentration curves are obtained for those that are either fed the same diet once or twice daily or fed ad libitum, because of their long postprandial period (Coradini et al., 2015). It is generally recommended that cats managed with insulin be fed at the same time as the insulin injection but, if indicated by body condition or owner preference, they can be fed more often.

Weight loss

Obesity in cats has a profound effect on insulin sensitivity, decreasing it by approximately 50% (Appleton et al., 2001). This means that more insulin is required to maintain glucose concentrations within the reference interval compared with when body condition is lean. Although many cats achieve remission in the first 4–6 weeks of insulin therapy, before substantial weight loss has occurred, obesity continues to put a high demand on beta cells to secrete insulin and likely increases the probability of relapse

in the same way as it predisposes to the development of diabetes mellitus. Thus, it is critically important to continue to address excess body condition, even if remission has been obtained. Obese cats should be energy-restricted to lose at least 1% but less than 2% of bodyweight per week (e.g. approximately 0.5 kg/month for an 8 kg cat). Because high-carbohydrate diets result in further demand on beta cells to secrete insulin, it is recommended that obese cats are fed a low-carbohydrate balanced and complete diet designed for management of feline obesity and diabetes mellitus, even though these diets are more energy-dense and have higher fat content than traditional weight-loss diets. Feeding canned food seems to increase satiety in many cats, which can facilitate owner compliance with feeding restricted amounts of food (Hoenig and Rand, 2006).

In long-term diabetic and obese cats, if a low-carbohydrate diet has not been associated with successful weight loss, a lower-energy-density diet could be used as remission is less likely. These are typically high-fibre, moderate- to high-carbohydrate diets (>25% ME), which are not recommended when remission is a realistic goal. In such cases, the reduction in insulin resistance associated with weight loss is unlikely to affect insulin dose substantially, but weight loss has other substantial health benefits that make it an important goal.

Monitoring response to therapy

Good glycaemic control is dependent upon close glycaemic and clinical monitoring and appropriate adjustment of insulin dose. Initially, close communication with owners plays a large part in this process. Crucial considerations include water intake, urine output (e.g. amount of clumping in cat litter) and bodyweight; these are evaluated along with possible signs of hypoglycaemia and developing or worsening neuropathy.

Home monitoring

Home monitoring of blood glucose concentrations provides a more accurate reflection of glycaemic control by avoiding two confounding effects often associated with a visit to a veterinary clinic:

- Depending on the amount eaten and the carbohydrate content, eating may increase the blood glucose concentration. Therefore, it is important that diabetic cats eat their normal diet and amount, so the blood glucose curve accurately reflects what is occurring at home. This may not occur in a veterinary clinic
- Stress increases the blood glucose concentration; struggling to resist blood sampling and car travel can increase blood glucose by up to 10 mmol/l (Figure 24.5).

Additionally, daily home monitoring provides more data and therefore facilitates more frequent insulin adjustments. This is advantageous because early optimization of blood glucose concentration increases the probability of remission. Home monitoring also allows immediate blood glucose assessment by the owner for confirming hypoglycaemia when vague but suggestive signs are present. Home monitoring may also be less expensive and more convenient for owners than having blood glucose curves obtained at the veterinary surgery. In addition, a feline diabetes-associated QOL survey indicated that the areas reported as most negatively impacting QOL included 'owner wanting more control', and home monitoring is associated with better glycaemic control (Niessen et al., 2010; Hazuchova et al., 2018).

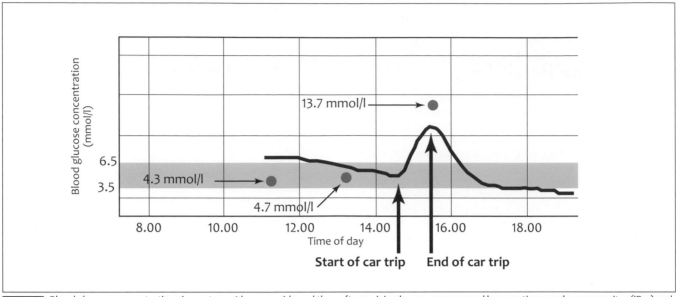

| 24.5 | Blood glucose concentrations in a cat on a 1-hour car ride and then after arriving home, as measured by a continuous glucose monitor (iPro) and with a glucometer calibrated for feline blood. Stress hyperglycaemia confounds diagnosis of diabetes in cats. In most cases, if the cat is left quietly in a cage and blood glucose is measured 3–4 hours later from an ear sample with the cat in the cage, the stress hyperglycaemia will have resolved. |

Clients still require frequent veterinary consultations in the initial stabilization phase to review the blood glucose concentrations obtained at home and the insulin dose, but these may be able to be conducted by email or telephone, with less frequent clinic visits required. Where the cat does not appear to be well controlled, a clinic visit is indicated to review insulin injection and glucose measurement methods and data, and the cat should be examined and weighed. As owners become more competent, many can confidently follow a protocol for dose adjustment without the need for frequent veterinary consultations. Home monitoring in combination with glargine treatment and a protocol for insulin dosage adjustments aimed at achieving tight glycaemic control is associated with higher remission rates compared with previous treatment with other insulins, predominantly lente and PZI (Roomp and Rand, 2009). Even among cats treated with glargine, frequent glucose monitoring and adjustment of insulin dose using a protocol to maintain blood glucose concentrations of 3.3–8.8 mmol/l was associated with significantly higher remission rates (78% *versus* 14%; relative risk ratio 5.6) compared with cats managed with less frequent monitoring and dose adjustments based primarily on the presence of clinical signs (Nack and DeClue, 2014).

For home-monitored cats treated with long-acting insulins, such as glargine, detemir or PZI, it is important to obtain measurements of blood glucose concentration before each insulin injection and, if possible, at the nadir point. A pre-insulin glucose measurement depicts the potential carry-over effect of long-acting insulins. The time of the nadir blood glucose concentration is variable between cats, and within the same cat from day to day, but can be assessed by several blood glucose measurements throughout the day or using continuous or flash glucose monitoring systems.

For intermediate-acting insulins, only a nadir blood glucose measurement is required and usually occurs 2–6 hours after insulin administration. The pre-insulin glucose measurement is useful only for indicating a dose reduction when there is impending remission, or when the blood glucose concentration is very high (>28 mmol/l), suggesting rebound hyperglycaemia.

Glucometers

Portable glucometers are frequently used for measuring blood glucose concentrations, particularly when home monitoring is being undertaken. When choosing a portable glucometer, accuracy and precision are important considerations. A number of reputable companies manufacture glucometers calibrated specifically for human blood, providing a whole-blood or plasma-equivalent value. These meters are reasonably precise. However, accuracy decreases substantially when these meters are used with feline blood. This is assumed to be a result of the different distribution of glucose between plasma and red blood cells in feline blood compared with human blood. Even among glucometers calibrated for cats, accuracy varies and some may also be affected by clinically significant erythrocytosis or anaemia (Dobromylskyj and Sparkes, 2010; Kang *et al.*, 2016; Mori *et al.*, 2017).

Whole blood glucometers calibrated for human use typically report feline blood glucose concentrations approximately 20–40% (1–2 mmol/l) lower than the actual plasma glucose concentration when concentrations are within the euglycaemic range (Wess and Reusch, 2000). This may partly explain why some cats show no or only mild signs with moderate levels of hypoglycaemia when measured with a portable human blood glucometer.

Glucometers calibrated for feline blood that provide a plasma-equivalent value are available (e.g. AlphaTRAK (Figure 24.6)) and more accurately reflect the actual glucose concentration. The blood glucose concentration reference interval in cats is approximately 4.0–6.6 mmol/l when measured using a glucometer calibrated for feline blood or a chemistry analyser. If measured with a glucometer for human use, the reference interval is 2.8–5.6 mmol/l. If a glucometer calibrated for human whole blood is used, the target blood glucose concentrations should be approximately 1.0 mmol/l lower than the feline reference interval. The newer feline glucometers are also advantageous because they require substantially smaller volumes of blood (0.3–0.6 µl *versus* 1.6 µl) and have a higher upper limit for glucose concentration. It is critical

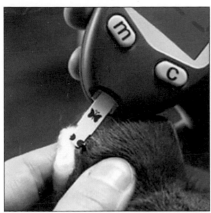

24.6 The Abbott AlphaTRAK meter is calibrated for feline blood, and requires only a 0.3 µl sample, making it ideal for measuring blood glucose concentrations in paw pad or ear samples.
(Courtesy of Zoetis)

Continuous glucose monitors

Continuous glucose monitors have historically been used for monitoring hospitalized cases and are increasingly being used for monitoring diabetic cats at home. They reduce the need for blood sampling while monitoring glucose concentrations throughout the day, allowing identification of hypo- and hyperglycaemia as well as nadir concentrations, which may be missed with traditional blood glucose monitoring (Moretti *et al.*, 2010). These sensors are commonly placed into the lateral chest wall, back of the neck (Figure 24.9) or lateral lumbar region, sometimes using tissue glue to aid in adhesion, and they measure glucose concentrations in the interstitial fluid (Hafner *et al.*, 2013; Surman and Fleeman, 2013). Meters that have been evaluated for use in cats and dogs include the MiniMed Gold, Guardian Real-Time, GlucoDay, iPro and Freestyle Libre (Surman and Fleeman, 2013; Corradini *et al.*, 2016). The majority of these require calibration three times a day using blood glucose measurements obtained from an ear, paw or jugular sample. The Freestyle Libre has the advantage that it does not require any calibrations to be performed, and additionally can last for up to 14 days (Bailey *et al.*, 2015). For these reasons, the Freestyle Libre is a good choice for home glucose monitoring. Owners can be trained to place the sensors themselves, further reducing the need to bring the cat into the veterinary clinic. Continuous glucose monitors make glucose monitoring much easier with fractious cats or unwilling clients, although financial constraints may preclude their use.

that veterinary staff and clients understand the difference between meters calibrated for human and for cat blood, especially for interpreting readings within and below the reference interval.

Typically, blood is taken from the ear or a paw pad using a needle or lancing device (Figures 24.7 and 24.8). Lancet devices may make a noise that disturbs some cats and using a needle may be better tolerated, especially for ear samples. Paw pad sampling may be well tolerated in some cats that do not like their ears being touched. Either the main pad or the pisiform (carpal) pad can be used. Warming the area by placing a moist cotton-wool ball in the microwave until warm and holding it on the paw for 20 seconds prior to sampling enhances blood flow and increases success in the early stages. Likewise, rubbing the area or using other forms of heat increases blood flow. Later, with multiple uses of an area, and particularly in the ears, vascularization appears to increase, making sampling easier.

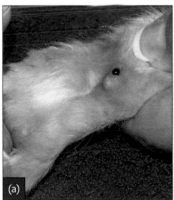
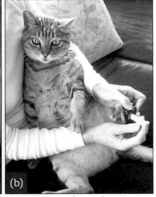

24.7 (a) Taking a blood sample from the pisiform (carpal) pad. (b) Sampling the main paw pad is well tolerated in many cats.
(a, Courtesy of S. Ford; b, Courtesy of W. Milledge)

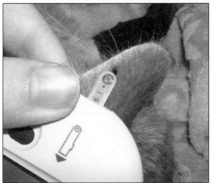

24.8 Measuring blood glucose from an ear sample. Best results are obtained if the area is rubbed or warmed first to increase blood supply.
(Courtesy of S. Ford)

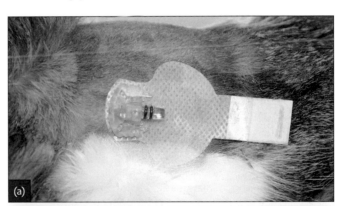
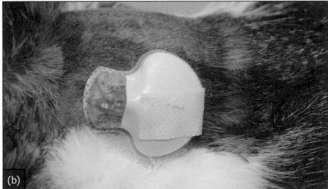

24.9 (a) Sensor for a continuous glucose monitor (iPro) mounted on the skin of a cat using tissue glue. (b) Attaching the reader to the sensor. It is not recommended to wear gloves when placing the sensor and attaching the reader, because gloves can stick to the tissue glue, leading to the sensor being accidentally dislodged. The iPro requires calibration three times daily by measuring blood glucose with a meter calibrated for feline blood. Anecdotally, it is more accurate, particularly in the low range, than the Freestyle Libre, which does not need calibration. Implantation of the sensor in the interstitium is simple and well tolerated by most cats without sedation.

Water intake and urine glucose output

Water intake and urine glucose estimations are inferior to glucose measurements obtained from blood samples or using a continuous glucose monitor, but can be useful indicators of glycaemic control in the absence of other monitoring capabilities and, as such, can be used as crude indicators for adjusting insulin doses with long-acting insulins such as glargine and detemir. Estimation of urine glucose can be achieved using special 'chips' added to cat litter, specially designed litter boxes, or urine testing strips. However, marked glucosuria can occur with both under- and overdosing, more commonly with intermediate-acting insulins than with long-acting insulins because of the short duration of action. Therefore, using urine glucose to increase the dose of intermediate-acting insulin is often problematic. Urine glucose measurements are less useful for detecting remission in cats treated with glargine or detemir because, once they are receiving the correct dose, they should have negative or trace glucosuria. Conversely, repeated negative urine glucose is more often an indicator of remission in cats treated with lente insulin. Water intake measured at home was shown to be a better indicator of mean blood glucose concentration over the past 24 hours than fructosamine concentration (Martin and Rand, 2007). Observant owners may become aware of a sudden marked increase in glucose concentration over several hours because the cat drinks substantially more.

Fructosamine and glycated haemoglobin

In general, measurement of the serum fructosamine concentration is of much less value than serial blood glucose measurements for insulin dose adjustment. However, fructosamine measurement is sometimes useful for monitoring glycaemic control, especially when reliable owner observations of clinical signs are unavailable or when clinical signs and blood glucose concentrations are conflicting (e.g. when blood glucose concentrations measured in the veterinary clinic are high, but the owner reports signs of good control at home). Because changes in fructosamine lag behind glucose concentrations by 1–3 weeks, it is considerably inferior to home monitoring in the early stages of therapy before the insulin dose has stabilized or when aiming for remission. It is more useful once the cat is stable and clinic revisits are scheduled only every 3–6 months. Similarly, HbA1c concentrations reflect blood glucose in cats over the previous 70 days and are not useful for insulin dose adjustment in the initial stages of therapy when remission is possible, but have a place in the management of long-term diabetic cats.

Outcome and prognosis

Approximately 25–30% of cats in remission will relapse and, of those, 25% can achieve a second remission and some may achieve a third (Roomp and Rand, 2009). Cats with underlying conditions associated with increasing demand on the remaining beta cells to secrete insulin are more likely to relapse. Impaired fasting blood glucose and impaired glucose tolerance have been associated with increased risk of relapse, and monitoring may help identify cats at greater risk of relapse (Gottlieb *et al.*, 2015). Therefore, important aspects of management of cats in remission include:

- Continuing to feed a low-carbohydrate diet
- Avoiding glucocorticoid administration if possible
- Normalizing body condition
- Managing underlying chronic conditions, such as dental disease.

If glucocorticoids must be administered, concurrent low-dose long-acting insulin therapy, for example, glargine 0.5–1.0 IU administered once daily, may help maintain euglycaemia. Where possible, a glucocorticoid with a high first-pass metabolism, such as budesonide, should be chosen to reduce side effects. Alternatively, immuno-suppressive drugs such as ciclosporin or chlorambucil may be used (Trepanier, 2009).

Glucose concentrations should be checked weekly for cats in remission; if this is not possible, urine glucose and water intake should be monitored closely. A second remission is more likely to be attained if beta cell loss from glucose toxicity is minimized. If insulin therapy can be instituted early before the blood glucose concentration chronically rises above the renal threshold, toxic glucose damage is reduced. If hyperglycaemia occurs (≥10 mmol/l), insulin should be reinstituted immediately to prevent further damage to beta cells.

In the absence of remission, prognosis depends on the underlying cause of the diabetes mellitus and the degree of glycaemic control that can be achieved. One study from a tertiary referral institution reported a mean survival of 17 months (Goossens *et al.*, 1998). Survival times for diabetic cats in primary-care practice have the potential to be longer for a given insulin dosing protocol. This is because, in primary-care practice, there is likely to be a smaller proportion of cats with significant underlying disease causing marked insulin resistance or impacting survival directly. Significant underlying disease decreases the probability of achieving remission, and remission is associated with longer survival in cats (Callegari *et al.*, 2013). However, the probability of remission is greatly influenced by the insulin dosing protocol, for example, whether it is aimed at just controlling clinical signs or achieving normal or near-normal blood glucose concentrations (Nack and DeClue, 2014).

In summary, whilst high remission rates (>80%) can be achieved in primary-care practice using long-acting (glargine or detemir) insulin, low-carbohydrate diets and frequent home monitoring of blood glucose concentrations together with appropriate insulin dose adjustments, these are not always possible to achieve. Where there is a legal requirement to use a veterinary-authorized insulin initially, if remission has not occurred within 4–8 weeks of initiating therapy, consideration should be given to changing the insulin to glargine or detemir to increase the probability of remission. Cats with obvious insulin resistance should be tested for other specific types of diabetes, especially hypersomatotropism (see Chapters 13 and 25).

References and further reading

American Diabetes Association (2014) Diagnosis and classification of diabetes mellitus. *Diabetes Care* **37**, S81–S90

Alejandro EU, Gregg B, Blandino-Rosano M, Cras-Méneur C and Bernal-Mizrachi E (2015) Natural history of β-cell adaptation and failure in type 2 diabetes. *Molecular Aspects of Medicine* **42**, 19–41

Appleton DJ, Rand JS and Sunvold GD (2001) Insulin sensitivity decreases with obesity, and lean cats with low insulin sensitivity are at greatest risk of glucose intolerance with weight gain. *Journal of Feline Medicine and Surgery* **3**, 211–228

Bailey T, Bode BW, Christiansen MP, Klaff LJ and Alva S (2015) The performance and usability of a factory-calibrated flash glucose monitoring system. *Diabetes Technology & Therapeutics* **17**, 787–794

Baral RM, Rand J, Catt MJ and Farrow HA (2003) Prevalence of feline diabetes mellitus in a feline private practice (abstract). *Journal of Veterinary Internal Medicine* **17**, 433–434

Barone JV, Tillman EM and Ferry RJ Jr (2011) Treatment of transient neonatal diabetes mellitus with subcutaneous insulin glargine in an extremely low birth weight neonate. *Journal of Pediatric Pharmacology and Therapeutics* **16**, 291–297

Behrend EN (2023) Velagliflozin, an SGLT2 inhibitor, as once-daily, oral solution, stand-alone therapy for feline diabetes mellitus. *ACVIM Proceedings 2023, Philadelphia*

Benedict SL, Mahony OM, McKee TS and Bergman PJ (2022) Evaluation of bexagliflozin in cats with poorly regulated diabetes mellitus. *Canadian Journal of Veterinary Research* **86**, 52–58

Bennett N (2002) Monitoring techniques for diabetes mellitus in the dog and the cat. *Clinical Techniques in Small Animal Practice* **17**, 65–69

Bennett N, Greco DS, Peterson ME et al. (2006) Comparison of a low carbohydrate–low fibre diet and a moderate carbohydrate–high fibre diet in the management of feline diabetes mellitus. *Journal of Feline Medicine and Surgery* **8**, 73–84

Berg RIM, Nelson RW, Feldman EC et al. (2007) Serum insulin-like growth factor-I concentration in cats with diabetes mellitus and acromegaly. *Journal of Veterinary Internal Medicine* **21**, 892–898

Bolli GB and Gerich JE (1984) The "dawn phenomenon" – a common occurrence in both non-insulin-dependent and insulin-dependent diabetes mellitus. *New England Journal of Medicine* **310**, 746–750

Callegari C, Mercuriali E, Hafner M et al. (2013) Survival time and prognostic factors in cats with newly diagnosed diabetes mellitus: 114 cases (2000–2009). *Journal of the American Veterinary Medical Association* **243**, 91–95

Caney SMA (2013) Pancreatitis and diabetes in cats. *Veterinary Clinics of North America: Small Animal Practice* **43**, 303–317

Carroll MF and Schade DS (2005) The dawn phenomenon revisited: implications for diabetes therapy. *Endocrine Practice* **11**, 55–64

Casella SJ, Mongilio MK, Plotnick LP, Hesterberg MP and Long CA (1993) Accuracy and precision of low-dose insulin administration. *Pediatrics* **91**, 1155–1157

Coradini M, Rand JS, Filippich LJ, Morton JM and O'Leary CA (2015) Associations between meal size, gastric emptying and post-prandial plasma glucose, insulin and lactate concentrations in meal-fed cats. *Journal of Animal Physiology and Animal Nutrition* **99**, 757–766

Corradini S, Pilosio B, Dondi F et al. (2016) Accuracy of a flash glucose monitoring system in diabetic dogs. *Journal of Veterinary Internal Medicine* **30**, 983–988

Crenshaw KL, Peterson ME, Heeb LA, Moroff SD and Nichols R (1996) Serum fructosamine concentration as an index of glycemia in cats with diabetes mellitus and stress hyperglycemia. *Journal of Veterinary Internal Medicine* **10**, 360–364

Dobromylskyj MJ and Sparkes AH (2010) Assessing portable blood glucose meters for clinical use in cats in the United Kingdom. *Veterinary Record* **107**, 438–442

Elliott DA, Nelson RW, Feldman EC and Neal LA (1997) Glycosylated hemoglobin concentration for assessment of glycemic control in diabetic cats. *Journal of Veterinary Internal Medicine* **11**, 161–165

Feldhahn JR, Rand JS and Martin G (1999) Insulin sensitivity in normal and diabetic cats. *Journal of Feline Medicine and Surgery* **1**, 107–115

Feldman EC, Nelson RW and Feldman MS (1997) Intensive 50-week evaluation of glipizide administration in 50 cats with previously untreated diabetes mellitus. *Journal of the American Veterinary Medical Association* **210**, 772–777

Fleeman LM (2007) *Clinical management of diabetes mellitus in dogs.* PhD Thesis, University of Queensland, School of Veterinary Science

Fonseca V, Bell DS, Berger S, Thomson S and Mecca TE (2004) A comparison of bedtime insulin glargine with bedtime neutral protamine Hagedorn insulin in patients with type 2 diabetes: subgroup analysis of patients taking once-daily insulin in a multicenter, randomized, parallel group study. *American Journal of the Medical Sciences* **328**, 274–280

Fulcher GR, Gilbert RE and Yue DK (2005) Glargine is superior to neutral protamine Hagedorn for improving glycated haemoglobin and fasting blood glucose levels during intensive insulin therapy. *Internal Medicine Journal* **35**, 536–542

Gal A, Trusiano B, French AF, Lopez-Villalobos N and MacNeill AL (2017) Serum fructosamine concentration in uncontrolled hyperthyroid diabetic cats is within the population reference interval. *Veterinary Sciences* **4**, 17

Galicia-Garcia U, Benito-Vicente A, Jebari S et al. (2020) Pathophysiology of type 2 diabetes mellitus. *International Journal of Molecular Sciences* **21**, 6275

Gale EAM, Kurtz AB and Tattersall RB (1980) In search of the Somogyi effect. *Lancet* **316**, 279–282

Gilor C, Culp W, Ghandi S et al. (2019) Comparison of pharmacodynamics and pharmacokinetics of insulin degludec and insulin glargine 300 U/mL in healthy cats. *Domestic Animal Endocrinology* **69**, 19–29

Gilor C, Hulsebosch SE, Pires J et al. (2021) An ultra-long-acting recombinant insulin for the treatment of diabetes mellitus in cats. *Journal of Veterinary Internal Medicine* **35**, 2123–2130

Gilor C, Ridge TK, Attermeier KJ and Graves TK (2010) Pharmacodynamics of insulin detemir and insulin glargine assessed by an isoglycemic clamp method in healthy cats. *Journal of Veterinary Internal Medicine* **24**, 870–874

Gilor C, Wasik B, Pires J et al. (2019) Comparison of pharmacodynamics between insulin glargine 100U/mL and insulin glargine 300U/mL in healthy cats (abstract). *Journal of Veterinary Internal Medicine* **33**, 2450

Goossens MM, Nelson RW, Feldman EC and Griffey SM (1998) Response to insulin treatment and survival in 104 cats with diabetes mellitus (1985–1995). *Journal of Veterinary Internal Medicine* **12**, 1–6

Gottlieb S, Rand J, Anderson ST et al. (2020) Metabolic profiling of diabetic cats in remission. *Frontiers in Veterinary Science* **7**, 218

Gottlieb S, Rand JS, Marshall R and Morton J (2015) Glycemic status and predictors of relapse for diabetic cats in remission. *Journal of Veterinary Internal Medicine* **29**, 184–192

Hadd MJ, Bienhoff SE, Little SE et al. (2023) Safety and effectiveness of the sodium-glucose cotransporter inhibitor bexagliflozin in cats newly diagnosed with diabetes mellitus. *Journal of Veterinary Internal Medicine* **37**, 915–924

Hafner M, Lutz TA, Reusch CE and Zini E (2013) Evaluation of sensor sites of continuous glucose monitoring in cats with diabetes mellitus. *Journal of Feline Medicine and Surgery* **15**, 117–123

Hazuchova K, Gostelow R, Scudder C et al. (2018) Acceptance of home blood glucose monitoring by owners of recently diagnosed diabetic cats and impact on quality of life changes in cat and owner. *Journal of Feline Medicine and Surgery* **20**, 711–720

Henson MS and O'Brien TD (2006) Feline models of type 2 diabetes mellitus. *ILAR Journal* **47**, 234–242

Herndon AM, Breshears MA and McFarlane D (2014) Oxidative modification, inflammation and amyloid in the normal and diabetic cat pancreas. *Journal of Comparative Pathology* **151**, 352–362

Hess RS and Ward CR (2000) Effect of insulin dosage on glycemic response in dogs with diabetes mellitus: 221 cases (1993–1998). *Journal of the American Veterinary Medical Association* **216**, 217–221

Hoelmkjaer KM, Spodsberg EMH and Bjornvad CR (2015) Insulin detemir treatment in diabetic cats in a practice setting. *Journal of Feline Medicine and Surgery* **17**, 144–151

Hoenig M and Rand JS (2006) Pathogenesis and management of obesity. In: *Consultations in Feline Internal Medicine, 5th edn*, ed. JR August, pp. 175–182. Saunders Elsevier, St. Louis

Imamura T, Koffler M, Helderman JH et al. (1988) Severe diabetes induced in subtotally depancreatized dogs by sustained hyperglycemia. *Diabetes* **37**, 600–609

Johnson KH, O'Brien TD, Betsholtz C and Westermark P (1992) Islet amyloid polypeptide: mechanisms of amyloidogenesis in the pancreatic islets and potential roles in diabetes mellitus. *Laboratory Investigation* **66**, 522–535

Kang MH, Kim DH, Jeong IS, Choi GC and Park HM (2016) Evaluation of four portable blood glucose meters in diabetic and non-diabetic dogs and cats. *Veterinary Quarterly* **36**, 2–9

Krämer AL, Riederer A, Fracassi F et al. (2020) Glycemic variability in newly diagnosed diabetic cats treated with the glucagon-like peptide-1 analogue exenatide extended release. *Journal of Veterinary Internal Medicine* **34**, 2287–2295

Kruth S and Cowgill L (1982) Renal glucose transport in the cat. In: *Proceedings of the American College of Veterinary Internal Medicine Forum*. American College of Veterinary Internal Medicine, Blacksburg, p. 78

Kurtzhals P (2004) Engineering predictability and protraction in a basal insulin analogue: the pharmacology of insulin detemir. *International Journal of Obesity and Related Metabolic Disorders* **28**, S23–S28

Lederer R, Rand JS, Jonsson NN, Hughes IP and Morton JM (2009) Frequency of feline diabetes mellitus and breed predisposition in domestic cats in Australia. *Veterinary Journal* **179**, 254–258

Linari G, Fleeman L, Gilor C, Giacomelli L and Fracassi F (2022) Insulin glargine 300 U/ml for the treatment of feline diabetes mellitus. *Journal of Feline Medicine and Surgery* **24**, 168–176

Link KR and Rand JS (2008) Changes in blood glucose concentration are associated with relatively rapid changes in circulating fructosamine concentrations in cats. *Journal of Feline Medicine and Surgery* **10**, 583–592

Link KRJ (2001) *Feline diabetes: diagnostics and experimental modelling.* PhD Thesis, University of Queensland, School of Veterinary Science

Link KRJ, Allio I, Rand JS and Eppler E (2013) The effect of experimentally induced chronic hyperglycaemia on serum and pancreatic insulin, pancreatic islet IGF-I and plasma and urinary ketones in the domestic cat (*Felis felis*). *General and Comparative Endocrinology* **188**, 269–281

Lutz TA and Rand JS (1996) Plasma amylin and insulin concentrations in normoglycemic and hyperglycemic cats. *Canadian Veterinary Journal* **37**, 27–34

Lutz TA, Rand JS and Ryan E (1995) Fructosamine concentrations in hyperglycemic cats. *Canadian Veterinary Journal* **36**, 155–159

Marshall RD, Rand JS, Gunew MN and Menrath VH (2013) Intramuscular glargine with or without concurrent subcutaneous administration for treatment of feline diabetic ketoacidosis. *Journal of Veterinary Emergency and Critical Care* **23**, 286–290

Marshall RD, Rand JS and Morton JM (2008a) Glargine and protamine zinc insulin have a longer duration of action and result in lower mean daily glucose concentrations than lente insulin in healthy cats. *Journal of Veterinary Pharmacology and Therapeutics* **31**, 205–212

Marshall RD, Rand JS and Morton JM (2008b) Insulin glargine has a long duration of effect following administration either once daily or twice daily in divided doses in healthy cats. *Journal of Feline Medicine and Surgery* **10**, 488–494

Marshall RD, Rand JS and Morton JM (2009) Treatment of newly diagnosed diabetic cats with glargine insulin improves glycemic control and results in higher probability of remission that protamine zinc and lente insulins. *Journal of Feline Medicine and Surgery* **11**, 683–691

Martin GJ and Rand JS (2007) Comparisons of different measurements for monitoring diabetic cats treated with porcine insulin zinc suspension. *Veterinary Record* **161**, 52–58

Matsumoto K, Nakamura H, Ueki Y, Tominaga T and Miyake S (2001) Correction of hyperglycaemia reduces insulin resistance and serum soluble E-selectin levels in patients with type 2 diabetes mellitus. *Diabetic Medicine* **18**, 224–228

McCann TM, Simpson KE, Shaw DJ, Butt JA and Gunn-Moore DA (2007) Feline diabetes mellitus in the UK: the prevalence within an insured population and a questionnaire-based putative risk factor analysis. *Journal of Feline Medicine and Surgery* **9**, 289–299

Mizisin AP, Shelton GD, Burgers ML, Powell HC and Cuddon PA (2002) Neurological complications associated with spontaneously occurring feline diabetes mellitus. *Journal of Neuropathology and Experimental Neurology* **61**, 872–884

Moretti S, Tschuor F, Osto M et al. (2010) Evaluation of a novel real-time continuous glucose-monitoring system for use in cats. *Journal of Veterinary Internal Medicine* **24**, 120–126

Mori A, Oda H, Onozawa E, Shono S and Sako T (2017) Evaluation of newly developed veterinary portable blood glucose meter with hematocrit correction in dogs and cats. *Journal of Veterinary Medical Science* **79**, 1690–1693

Mukherjee A, Morales-Scheihing D, Butler PC and Soto C (2015) Type 2 diabetes as a protein misfolding disease. *Trends in Molecular Medicine* **21**, 439–449

Nack R and DeClue AE (2014) In cats with newly diagnosed diabetes mellitus, use of a near-euglycaemic management paradigm improves remission rate over a traditional paradigm. *Veterinary Quarterly* **34**, 132–136

Nelson R (2000) Diabetes mellitus. In: *Textbook of Veterinary Internal Medicine, 5th edn*, ed. SJ Ettinger and EC Feldman, p. 1438. WB Saunders, Philadelphia

Niessen SJM, Church DB and Forcada Y (2013) Hypersomatotropism, acromegaly, and hyperadrenocorticism and feline diabetes mellitus. *Veterinary Clinics of North America: Small Animal Practice* **43**, 319–350

Niessen SJM, Petrie G, Gaudiano F et al. (2007) Feline acromegaly: an underdiagnosed endocrinopathy? *Journal of Internal Veterinary Medicine* **21**, 899–905

Niessen SJM, Powney S, Guitian J et al. (2010) Evaluation of a quality-of-life tool for cats with diabetes mellitus. *Journal of Veterinary Internal Medicine* **24**, 1098–1105

Niessen SJM, Voth R, Kroh C and Hennings L (2022) Once-daily oral therapy for feline diabetes mellitus: SGLT-2-Inhibitor velagliflozin as standalone therapy compared to insulin injection therapy in diabetic cats. *ECVIM Congress 2022, Göteborg, Sweden*

Nishii N, Maeda H, Murahata Y, Matsuu A and Hikasa Y (2012) Experimental hyperlipemia induces insulin resistance in cats. *Journal of Veterinary Medical Science* **74**, 267–269

O'Brien TD, Butler PC, Kreutter DK, Kane LA and Eberhardt NL (1995) Human islet amyloid polypeptide expression in COS-1 cells. A model of intracellular amyloidogenesis. *American Journal of Pathology* **147**, 606–616

O'Brien TD, Hayden DW, Johnson KH and Stevens JB (1985) High dose intravenous glucose tolerance test and serum insulin and glucagon levels in diabetic and non-diabetic cats: relationships to insular amyloidosis. *Veterinary Pathology* **22**, 250–261

Oda H, Mori A and Sako T (2020) The effect of Insulin Degludec on glycemic control in diabetic cats over a 12-month period. *Journal of Veterinary Medical Science* **82**, 695–698

Öhlund M, Fall T, Holst BS et al. (2015) Incidence of diabetes mellitus in insured Swedish cats in relation to age, breed and sex. *Journal of Veterinary Internal Medicine* **29**, 1342–1347

O'Neill DG, Gostelow R, Orme C et al. (2016) Epidemiology of diabetes mellitus among 193,435 cats attending primary-care veterinary practices in England. *Journal of Veterinary Internal Medicine* **30**, 964–972

Panciera DL, Thomas CB, Eicker SW and Atkins CE (1990) Epizootiologic patterns of diabetes mellitus in cats: 333 cases (1980–1986). *Journal of the American Veterinary Medical Association* **197**, 1504–1508

Poitout V and Robertson RP (2008) Glucolipotoxicity: fuel excess and β-cell dysfunction. *Endocrine Reviews* **29**, 351–366

Porte D Jr (1991) β-cells in type II diabetes mellitus. *Diabetes* **40**, 166–180

Prahl A, Guptill L, Glickman NW, Tetrick M and Glickman LT (2007) Time trends and risk factors for diabetes mellitus in cats presented to veterinary teaching hospitals. *Journal of Feline Medicine and Surgery* **9**, 351–358

Rand J (2013) Feline diabetes mellitus. In: *Clinical Endocrinology of Companion Animals*, ed. J Rand, pp. 169–190. John Wiley & Sons, Ames

Rand J and Gottlieb SA (2017) Feline diabetes mellitus. In: *Textbook of Veterinary Internal Medicine, 8th edn*, ed. S Ettinger, E Feldman and E Côté, pp. 1781–1794. Elsevier, St. Louis

Rand JS, Bobbermien LM, Hendrikz JK and Copland M (1997) Over representation of Burmese cats with diabetes mellitus. *Australian Veterinary Journal* **75**, 402–405

Rand JS and Marshall RD (2005) Diabetes mellitus in cats. *Veterinary Clinics of North America: Small Animal Practice* **35**, 211–224

Retnakaran R (2015) Novel strategies for inducing glycemic remission during the honeymoon phase of type 2 diabetes. *Canadian Journal of Diabetes* **39**, S142–S147

Reusch CE and Haberer B (2001) Evaluation of fructosamine in dogs and cats with hypo- or hyperproteinaemia, azotaemia, hyperlipidaemia and hyperbilirubinaemia. *Veterinary Record* **148**, 370–376

Reusch CE and Padrutt I (2013) New incretin hormonal therapies in humans relevant to diabetic cats. *Veterinary Clinics of North America: Small Animal Practice* **43**, 417–433

Riederer A, Zini E, Salesov E et al. (2016) Effect of the glucagon-like peptide-1 analogue exenatide extended release in cats with newly diagnosed diabetes mellitus. *Journal of Veterinary Internal Medicine* **30**, 92–100

Robertson RP, Harmon JS and Tanaka Y (2000) Glucose toxicity of the β-cell: cellular and molecular mechanisms. In: *Diabetes Mellitus: A Fundamental and Clinical Text, 2nd edn*, ed. D LeRoith, SI Taylor and JM Olefsky, pp. 125–132. Lippincott Williams & Wilkins, Philadelphia

Roomp K and Rand J (2009) Intensive blood glucose control is safe and effective in diabetic cats using home monitoring and treatment with glargine. *Journal of Feline Medicine and Surgery* **11**, 668–682

Roomp K and Rand J (2012) Evaluation of detemir in diabetic cats managed with a protocol for intensive blood glucose control. *Journal of Feline Medicine and Surgery* **14**, 566–572

Roomp K and Rand JS (2013) Management of diabetic cats with long-acting insulin. *Veterinary Clinics of North America: Small Animal Practice* **43**, 251–266

Roomp K and Rand JS (2016) Rebound hyperglycemia in diabetic cats. *Journal of Feline Medicine and Surgery* **18**, 587–596

Saini NK, Wasik B, Pires J et al. (2021) Comparison of pharmacodynamics between insulin glargine 100 U/mL and insulin glargine 300 U/mL in healthy cats. *Domestic Animal Endocrinology* **75**, 106595

Salesov E, Zini E, Riederer A, Lutz TA and Reusch CE (2018) Comparison of the pharmacodynamics of protamine zinc insulin and insulin degludec and validation of the continuous glucose monitoring system iPro2 in healthy cats. *Research in Veterinary Science* **118**, 79–85

Samuel VT and Shulman GI (2012) Mechanisms for insulin resistance: common threads and missing links. *Cell* **148**, 852–871

Scarlett JM, Donoghue S, Saidla J and Wills J (1994) Overweight cats: prevalence and risk factors. *International Journal of Obesity and Related Metabolic Disorders* **18**, S22–S28

Schaefer S, Kooistra HS, Riond B et al. (2017) Evaluation of insulin-like growth factor-1, total thyroxine, feline pancreas-specific lipase and urinary corticoid-to-creatinine ratio in cats with diabetes mellitus in Switzerland and the Netherlands. *Journal of Feline Medicine and Surgery* **19**, 888–896

Singh R, Rand JS, Coradini M and Morton JM (2015) Effect of acarbose on postprandial blood glucose concentrations in cats fed low and high carbohydrate diets. *Journal of Feline Medicine and Surgery* **17**, 848–857

Slingerland LI, Fazilova VV, Plantiga EA, Kooistra HS and Beynen AC (2009) Indoor confinement and physical inactivity rather than the proportion of dry food are risk factors in the development of feline type 2 diabetes mellitus. *Veterinary Journal* **179**, 247–253

Suh S and Kim JH (2015) Glycemic variability: how do we measure it and why is it important? *Diabetes & Metabolism Journal* **39**, 273–282

Surman S and Fleeman L (2013) Continuous glucose monitoring in small animals. *Veterinary Clinics of North America: Small Animal Practice* **43**, 381–406

Tanaka Y, Gleason CE, Tran PO, Harmon JS and Robertson RP (1999) Prevention of glucose toxicity in HIT-T15 cells and Zucker diabetic fatty rats by antioxidants. *Proceedings of the National Academy of Sciences of the United States of America* **96**, 10857–10862

Tomás E, Lin YS, Dagher Z et al. (2002) Hyperglycemia and insulin resistance: possible mechanisms. *Annals of the New York Academy of Sciences* **967**, 43–51

Trepanier L (2009) Idiopathic inflammatory bowel disease in cats. Rational treatment selection. *Journal of Feline Medicine and Surgery* **11**, 32–38

Unger RH and Grundy S (1985) Hyperglycaemia as an inducer as well as a consequence of impaired islet cell function and insulin resistance: implications for the management of diabetes. *Diabetologia* **28**, 119–121

Vuorinen-Markkola H, Koivisto VA and Yki-Jarvinen H (1992) Mechanisms of hyperglycemia-induced insulin resistance in whole body and skeletal muscle of type I diabetic patients. *Diabetes* **41**, 571–580

Weaver KE, Rozanski EA, Mahony OM, Chan DL and Freeman LM (2006) Use of glargine and lente insulins in cats with diabetes mellitus. *Journal of Veterinary Internal Medicine* **20**, 234–238

Wess G and Reusch C (2000) Assessment of five portable blood glucose meters for use in cats. *American Journal of Veterinary Research* **61**, 1587–1592

Woods JP, Panciera DL, Snyder PS, Jackson MW and Smedes SL (1994) Diabetes mellitus in a kitten. *Journal of the American Animal Hospital Association* **30**, 177–180

Zeugswetter FK, Polsterer T, Krempl H and Schwendenwein I (2019) Basal glucosuria in cats. *Journal of Animal Physiology and Animal Nutrition* **103**, 324–330

Zini E, Hafner M, Osto M et al. (2010) Predictors of clinical remission in cats with diabetes mellitus. *Journal of Veterinary Internal Medicine* **24**, 1314–1321

Zini E, Osto M, Franchini M et al. (2009) Hyperglycaemia but not hyperlipidaemia causes beta cell dysfunction and beta cell loss in the domestic cat. *Diabetologia* **52**, 336–346

Zini E, Salesov E, Dupont P et al. (2018) Glucose concentrations after insulin-induced hypoglycemia and glycemic variability in healthy and diabetic cats. *Journal of Veterinary Internal Medicine* **32**, 978–985

Chapter 25

Investigation and management of unstable diabetics

Federico Fracassi

Introduction

Diabetes mellitus is a heterogeneous group of diseases with multiple aetiologies characterized by hyperglycaemia that results from inadequate insulin secretion, inadequate insulin action or both. The classical clinical signs of diabetes mellitus in dogs and cats include polyuria and polydipsia (PU/PD), polyphagia and weight loss. When remission is not a realistic goal, the main aim of treating dogs and cats with uncomplicated diabetes mellitus is to achieve a good quality of life (QOL) for animals and their owners. A good QOL typically requires the elimination of, or a significant reduction in, the classical clinical signs, the prevention of short-term complications (e.g. hypoglycaemia, diabetic ketoacidosis (DKA)) and maintenance of stable bodyweight. Close collaboration between the veterinary surgeon (veterinarian) and the owner is essential for proper management of diabetic cases. In many animals, this collaboration contributes to excellent control of the disease and the restoration of a normal lifestyle. In some diabetics, however, adequate glycaemic control is more difficult to obtain. This can lead to a poor QOL for the animal and an increased likelihood of complications, ultimately resulting in frustration for the owner. A recent study evaluated the perceived frequency of euthanasia among cats and dogs with diabetes mellitus: in 35% of the animals, euthanasia was requested by the owners because of problems in attaining adequate control of the disease (Niessen *et al.*, 2017). This chapter describes the characteristics of the unstable diabetic, the possible reasons and investigations for this instability, and the treatment and monitoring options aimed at attaining better control of the disease.

Recognizing unstable diabetics

The primary goals of therapy in diabetic dogs and cats are the elimination of clinical signs, the prevention of short-term (e.g. hypoglycaemia, DKA) and long-term complications (e.g. cataracts in dogs, peripheral neuropathy in cats), the maintenance of a stable bodyweight and, therefore, achievement of a reasonable QOL. This can be accomplished with insulin therapy, diet, exercise, prevention or control of concurrent inflammatory, infectious, neoplastic and hormonal disorders, and the avoidance of insulin-antagonist drugs. For further details regarding the therapeutic management of uncomplicated diabetes mellitus in dogs and cats, please refer to Chapters 23 and 24.

An unstable diabetic is one that meets one or more of these criteria:

- Persistent or worsening clinical signs that are not controlled by increasing doses of insulin
- Failure to sufficiently stabilize within 2–3 months of initiation of therapy
- Recurrence of clinical signs when previously stable
- Episodes of hypoglycaemia or DKA
- Demonstrable evidence of high glucose variability despite treatment.

Causes and investigation of diabetic instability

Diabetic instability is a common reason for the referral of a diabetic animal. Investigation of diabetic instability can be a challenging and time-consuming process, requiring patience and very good client communication. It is important to review everything carried out from before the diagnosis up to the day of the consultation with the owner. Some important questions to ask the owner are listed in Figure 25.1.

Some very common causes of diabetic instability are related to management and technical problems in administering insulin, and to issues related to the insulin type, dose or frequency of administration. Other common problems include high glucose variability and insulin resistance associated with concurrent disorders.

Management and technical problems

The medical history is essential to understanding whether instability is related to mistakes or poor owner compliance. An important initial factor to determine is whether the owner is scrupulously following the instructions provided by the veterinary surgeon. It is fruitless to undertake long and expensive diagnostic procedures if the owner is not compliant. Once this has been established, aspects of instability related to diabetes management should be investigated.

Management issues

Some management factors that can influence the stability of diabetes include:

- An owner who does not exercise their dog during the week but takes it for long walks at weekends

Questions related to the pre-diabetic period and when diabetes mellitus was diagnosed
• Were there any other diseases or clinical signs before developing diabetes?
• How long before diagnosis did the clinical signs appear?
• Was there any treatment before the development of the diabetes?
• Was there a hormonal trigger (e.g. exogenous steroids, dioestrus)?
• Did diabetes arise with ketoacidosis?
• Did diabetes arise with pancreatitis?
• Are data available from any investigations carried out at the time of diagnosis (haematology, biochemistry, urinalysis, abdominal ultrasound)?
Information related to the management of diabetes
• Food: type, consistency of administration, timing with respect to insulin administration, use of food treats
• Scavenging behaviour
• Insulin: type, dose, route, frequency, storage, mixing
• Syringes: type of syringe, administration practices, injection site, who is injecting the insulin
• Dosing pen: type of pen, pen assembly and preparation, administration practices, injection site
• Exercise: frequency, intensity, consistency
• Glucose monitoring methods and monitoring frequency
• Other treatments: parenteral or topical (e.g. ophthalmic or aural products), supplements, preventive healthcare measures
Information related to the investigation and management of instability
• Clinical signs of instability and when they started
• Other clinical signs that may or may not be related to poor glycaemic control (e.g. vomiting, diarrhoea, dermatological problems, dysuria)
• Serial weight measurements
• Historical haematology, biochemistry, urinalysis and diagnostic imaging results
• Historical blood glucose curves and serial fructosamine concentrations
• Historical changes in insulin dose, frequency and preparation, along with the rationale for changes and whether they led to improvement or deterioration
• Other treatments administered (e.g. antibiotics, topical treatments, non-steroidal anti-inflammatory drugs), reasons for administration and clinical effects
• Other investigations undertaken and their results
• The historical points at which the owner reports their pet was last stable or more stable

25.1 Key considerations when taking a history from the owner of an unstable diabetic pet.

- A dog or cat that is given different snacks throughout the day (by household members or regular visitors)
- A dog or cat that has access to cohabitant pet food; for example, access to a kidney diet that is high in carbohydrates
- A dog that lives in a garden and has access to windfall fruits.

Insulin handling and insulin syringes

Errors in handling and injecting insulin are common reasons for poor glycaemic control and include failure to mix the preparation correctly, the use of an improper diluent, the use of insulin that has been frozen or heated or is outdated, incorrect injection technique with either a syringe or insulin dosing pen, and inappropriate insulin dose or syringe size (40 IU/ml *versus* 100 IU/ml). For example, if the 40 IU/ml porcine lente syringes (1 gradation = 0.025 ml) are inadvertently changed to 100 IU/ml syringes (1 gradation = 0.01 ml), there will be an underdose, with only 40% of the correct dose administered. This may result in the animal mistakenly being diagnosed as insulin resistant.

Veterinary porcine lente is an intermediate-acting, 40 IU/ml insulin that consists of 30–35% amorphous (short acting) and 65–70% crystalline ultralente (long acting). In the past, the recommendation was to gently roll the vial before use. One important change recommended by the manufacturer is that this insulin, before use, should be 'shaken thoroughly' until a homogeneous, uniformly milky suspension is obtained. This promotes better mixing of the two insulin components, allowing for more consistent pharmacokinetics. Without thorough mixing, the insulin concentration in each dose may vary widely. Some owners may not mix insulin properly before use.

Insulin should be administered immediately after being withdrawn into the syringe. Some owners may, for convenience, fill multiple syringes with insulin every 3–4 days to have them ready at the time of administration. This compromises effectiveness because the insulin settles in the syringes and adheres to the plastic.

All the above-mentioned problems can have a relevant impact on the management of the diabetic pet. They are only identified by careful evaluation of the history and by asking the owner to bring their own insulin and syringes or pen device, and to administer a dose to the animal in the clinic. If concerns arise, a veterinary surgeon or veterinary nurse should oversee the entire procedure, assisting until the owner masters correct insulin administration.

Insulin pens

Numerous dosing pens that can be used for injecting insulin have recently become available, including ones specifically designed for the veterinary porcine lente preparation. These devices were traditionally designed for humans to use without formal medical training. The aim of these devices is to dose and inject insulin easily with less pain and greater accuracy and precision. A clear advantage of using insulin dosing pens is that mistakes made with syringes, linked to different insulin concentrations (40 IU/ml *versus* 100 IU/ml), are avoided. If an owner decides to use an insulin pen, it is imperative that they are carefully informed and trained. Failure to carefully follow the steps for administration can easily lead to errors. Some recommendations are quite specific because, if the pen is incorrectly handled, the cartridges are prone to accumulating air. The pen must be stored without the needle attached because air can enter if the needle is left attached to the pen; this is also the rationale behind 'priming' before every use. One or two units must be loaded and dispelled by keeping the pen in an upright position while performing an 'air shot'. Figure 25.2 lists the main problems and possible solutions when using an insulin pen device. See Chapter 23 for more information on the administration of insulin.

Problem	Possible causes/considerations	Solution
The insulin dosing pen does not prime properly	The needle was left attached when the syringe was not in use, causing the penetration of air into the cartridge	Repeat the priming process in order to eliminate the air from the cartridge
	Needle not screwed correctly on to the end of the pen	Replace the needle
	Insulin cartridge is damaged	Replace the cartridge if the pen is rechargeable; otherwise, replace the pen
	Foreign material (e.g. fragments of a damaged cartridge) is blocking the pen mechanism	Disassemble the pen, remove the foreign material and reassemble the pen
Bent needle after use	This is not a problem, as needles are designed to bend rather than break. The insulin dose is usually administered through a bent needle	No action required
Presence of a drop of insulin on the tip of the needle after injection	This is normal. The drop can spread into the coat or be visible on the tip of the needle	Touch the injection area with fingers. If the surface is not wet, the insulin has been administered correctly
The dose selector dial does not return to '0' after the injection	The insulin dose has not been completely administered	The remaining dose can be given with another injection using the same needle without priming again. If the owner is not sure of the quantity administered, it is best to avoid giving a second injection
Difficulty in pressing the release trigger during injection	The insulin may not be delivered subcutaneously	Re-evaluate the injection technique of the owner. Check that the needles are designed for the type of pen being used. If the needles being used are too short, the insulin is administered intradermally and not subcutaneously
The insulin administration seems to be ineffective	The insulin pen is not working properly	Check the pen to make sure it is primed correctly before use
	The insulin is not appropriately resuspended	Re-evaluate the injection technique
	The insulin is not injected correctly	Re-evaluate the injection technique
	The insulin has been stored incorrectly (i.e. frozen or stored at temperatures >30°C, or exposed to light for prolonged periods)	Review the storage conditions and make sure that the insulin pen cap is replaced after every injection. Replace the cartridge
Unexpected hypoglycaemia	The insulin is not resuspended properly before the injection	Re-evaluate the injection technique

25.2 Summary of the main problems and possible solutions when using an insulin pen device.
(Modified from Thompson et al., 2015)

Inherent problems with insulin

Insulin underdose

The majority of dogs and cats are well controlled with insulin doses of approximately 1 IU/kg bodyweight administered twice daily. If the insulin dose is considerably less than 1 IU/kg, and the pet is receiving insulin twice a day, underdosing could be the reason for poor glycaemic control. In such cases, the insulin dose should be gradually increased, by approximately 10% per week in dogs and in steps of 0.5–1 IU/cat/injection per week in cats. If a dose much greater than 1 IU/kg twice a day is reached without adequate glycaemic control, an additional work-up should be pursued (Figure 25.3).

Short duration of insulin action

Short duration of insulin action is a common cause for difficulties in diabetic regulation. It is almost always observed when insulin is given once daily but may be encountered even when it is given twice daily. Neutral protamine Hagedorn (NPH) insulin preparations are notorious for their short duration of action and are rarely used today. In some diabetic dogs, and many diabetic cats, porcine lente insulin may last less than 8 hours. Whilst waning of insulin activity is expected in most animals, significant hyperglycaemia (>16 mmol/l) may occur in some animals for several hours each day, and owners usually report the persistence

of clinical signs, noted particularly as the injection interval elapses. This problem is detected by performing a blood glucose curve (BGC) (Figure 25.4) or by using a continuous glucose monitoring system (CGMS) (see 'Continuous glucose monitoring systems and the flash glucose monitoring system', below). Treatment involves switching to long-acting insulin (i.e. protamine zinc insulin (PZI), glargine or detemir) administered twice a day. Further information on the use of these insulin preparations in dogs and cats can be found in Chapters 23 and 24, respectively.

Prolonged duration of insulin action

Problems with prolonged duration of insulin action may occasionally occur. If the effect of insulin administered twice daily lasts for longer than 12 hours, the action of the insulin administrations will overlap, possibly leading to overt hypoglycaemia. Prolonged duration of insulin action is observed when the glucose nadir occurs 10 or more hours after the injection. Switching to insulin with a shorter duration of action usually resolves the problem. In some cases, a small dose reduction can counterbalance the effect. Another option is to move from twice- to once-daily insulin administration. Using an intermediate-acting insulin, such as porcine lente insulin, once-daily dosing may fail to work for close to 24 hours; in this case, switching to long-acting insulin, such as PZI, detemir or glargine (100 IU/ml or 300 IU/ml) administered once a day may be appropriate.

Step 1
• Check whether the initial work-up and treatment were correct • If not, repeat the initial work-up (haematology, biochemistry, urinalysis, ultrasonography of the abdomen) and adapt the treatment regimen
Step 2
• Check whether the insulin used is outdated or has been diluted, frozen or heated • Check whether the owner is using the right syringes (40 IU/ml *versus* 100 IU/ml) • Assess the owner's procedure of mixing, drawing up the correct dose and injecting the insulin • If the owner is using an insulin dosing pen, check that they are using it correctly • Review the dietary regimen
Step 3
• Generate blood glucose curves or use a continuous glucose monitoring system. This approach usually allows the clinician to identify whether there are problems with the duration of insulin action, hypoglycaemia, excessive glycaemic variability or insulin resistance. Insulin resistance should be considered if the glucose concentration remains high despite high insulin doses (e.g. >1 IU/kg twice a day). • If the animal is receiving low insulin doses and the glucose concentration is persistently high, increase the insulin dose every 5–7 days and continue monitoring until good glycaemic control is obtained or a dose of approximately 1 IU/kg twice a day is administered
Step 4
• If no problem has been identified to this point, carry out a work-up aimed at identifying diseases causing insulin resistance. In principle, any other concurrent disease (e.g. inflammatory, neoplastic) can cause insulin resistance. The most common causes are pancreatitis, hypercortisolism, hypersomatotropism (cats), hypothyroidism (dogs), infections (e.g. urinary tract, oral cavity), chronic kidney disease and obesity • If a cause of instability is not identified, consider the possibility of poor insulin absorption or, although quite rare, the presence of anti-insulin antibodies, particularly in dogs. At this point, it may be useful to change the insulin type • In a cat with marked glycaemic variability, if all other potential causes of instability are excluded, the addition of the glucagon-like peptide 1 analogue exenatide may be considered

25.3 Step-by-step work-up for the unstable diabetic pet.
(Modified from Reusch, 2015)

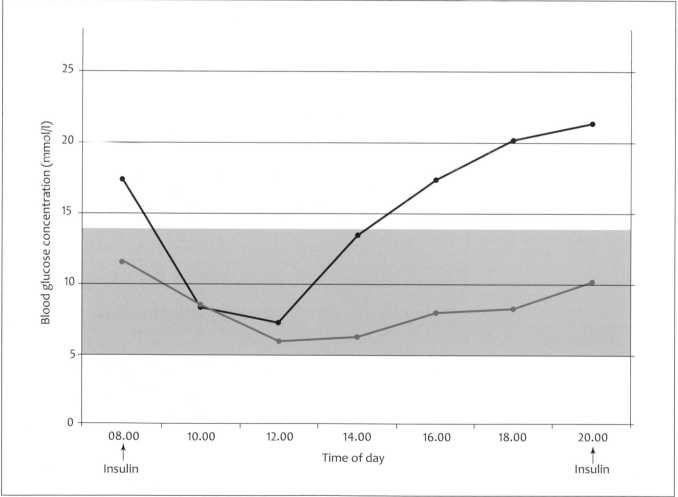

25.4 Blood glucose curves in a 10-year-old diabetic neutered female Domestic Shorthaired cat weighing 5.4 kg. The red curve indicates the blood glucose values when the cat was receiving veterinary porcine lente insulin (2.5 IU/cat twice a day). It is evident that the blood glucose values decrease to within the desired range (5–14 mmol/l) for only a few hours and then increase. The reason is a short duration of insulin action. In this cat, switching to insulin glargine (3 IU/cat twice a day) led to a marked improvement in the duration of the effect (green curve).

Anti-insulin antibodies

Canine and porcine insulins are identical, while bovine and human insulins differ. Consequently, the development of anti-insulin antibodies is rare in dogs treated with porcine insulin, and this may also be true for recombinant human insulin. By contrast, serum anti-insulin antibodies have been identified in 40–65% of dogs treated with bovine/porcine- or bovine-source insulin. The presence of anti-insulin antibodies in some cases may influence the pharmacokinetics and pharmacodynamics of exogenous insulin. Potential consequences include:

- Erratic and poor control of glycaemia
- Inability to control glycaemia for extended periods of time
- Need for frequent adjustments of the insulin dose
- Occasional development of insulin resistance.

Bovine insulin, which was widely used in the past to treat canine diabetes mellitus, is infrequently used today. For this reason, the role of anti-insulin antibodies in inducing poor glycaemic control is less relevant than in the past. Although rare, anti-insulin antibodies may develop in dogs treated with recombinant human insulin and should be suspected as the cause of poor glycaemic control if no other reason can be identified. Switching to a new insulin species (e.g. porcine-source insulin for dogs) should be considered if anti-insulin antibodies are identified in poorly controlled diabetic animals. The role of anti-insulin antibodies has not been well studied in cats, but feline insulin differs from porcine, bovine and human insulin.

Glucose variability

In healthy dogs and cats, there is very little variation of blood glucose concentration from day to day (Figure 25.5). In contrast, in diabetic animals, glucose variability is more evident even if the animal is considered to be well controlled (Figure 25.6).

In diabetic animals, blood glucose concentrations may vary substantially from day to day and also within the same day. When glucose is monitored for several consecutive days, a marked variability of the glucose trend can be observed (Figure 25.7). This happens in both dogs and cats, even if the food, the insulin dose and the environment in which the monitoring takes place (at home or in the clinic) are kept constant (Alt *et al.*, 2007; Del Baldo *et al.*, 2020). These variations are particularly marked in animals with

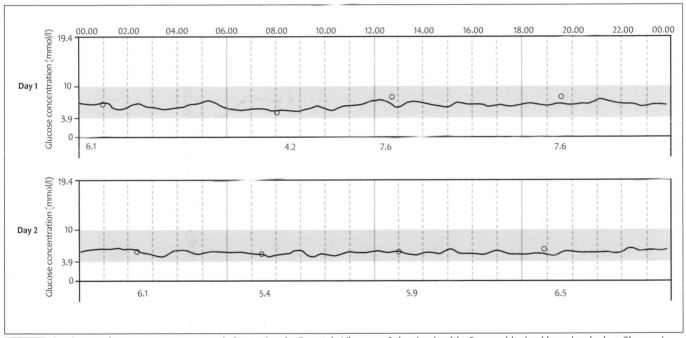

25.5 Continuous glucose measurement carried out using the Freestyle Libre over 2 days in a healthy 5-year-old mixed-breed male dog. Glycaemic variability is almost absent.

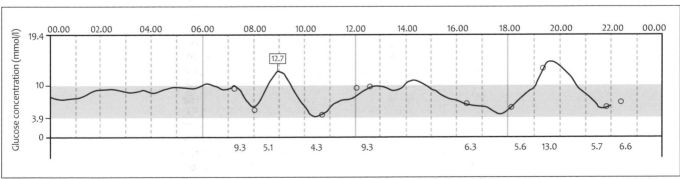

25.6 Continuous glucose measurement carried out using the Freestyle Libre in a 12-year-old neutered male Yorkshire Terrier with diabetes mellitus. The dog is given its meal and porcine lente insulin (3.5 IU) in the morning (8 am) and in the evening (6 pm). The curve shows glucose fluctuations (glycaemic variability) that are larger than those in healthy dogs (see Figure 25.5), but that can be considered appropriate for a diabetic animal.

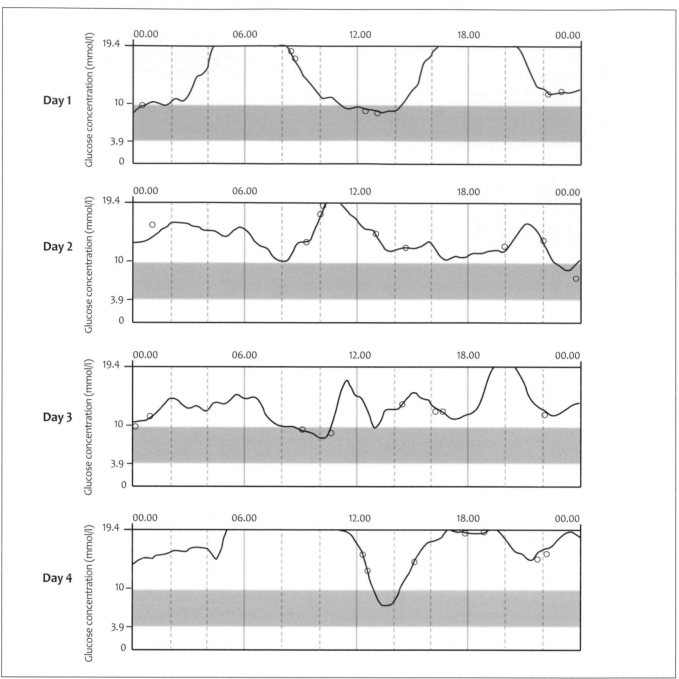

25.7 Continuous glucose measurements carried out using the Freestyle Libre over 4 days in an 8-year-old neutered male diabetic dog. Each day, the dog is given the same type and amount of food at the same time; the insulin type (porcine lente), time and amount is also kept consistent. High glycaemic variability is evident.

poor glycaemic control (Alt *et al.*, 2007) (Figure 25.8). As CGMSs are increasingly being used, the concept of glycaemic variability is being recognized and becoming increasingly important. The causes of glycaemic variability vary, and it is not always possible to identify or resolve them (Figure 25.9).

In human medicine, the concept of glycaemic variability is gaining more and more importance. Glycaemic variability refers to glycaemic excursions, including episodes of hypoglycaemia and hyperglycaemia, during a single day or on different days (Suh and Kim, 2015). High glycaemic variability in humans is considered a risk factor for hypoglycaemia, microvascular complications, neuropathy, retinopathy, stroke and all-cause mortality (Umpierrez and Kovatchev, 2018). It is unknown whether such complications are present or relevant in dogs and cats; however, a

reduction in glucose variability should be one of the aims of management of a diabetic pet.

Currently, there is a lack of consensus on the gold-standard method for measuring glucose variability, and several indicators have been proposed. Mean and standard deviation, which describes the dispersion of values around mean blood glucose concentration, a frequently used index in humans, has recently been introduced into feline diabetology (Zini *et al.*, 2018; Krämer *et al.*, 2020).

High glycaemic variability is frequently observed in poorly controlled diabetic dogs and cats. The investigations that need to be carried out to attempt to reduce the glycaemic variability are the same as those recommended for investigating the causes of diabetic instability, namely evaluating the compliance of the owner, considering possible management or technical errors, and searching for potential

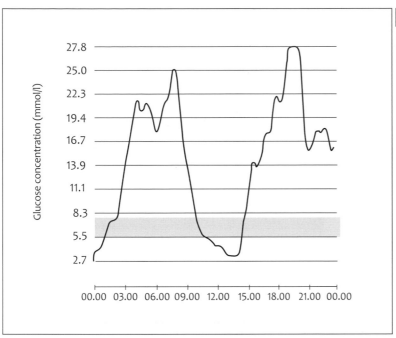

25.8 Continuous glucose measurements carried out using the Freestyle Libre in an 11-year-old neutered mixed-breed bitch weighing 6.1 kg with diabetes mellitus. The dog is given its meal and porcine lente insulin (4 IU) in the morning (7:30 am) and in the evening (7:30 pm). Post-hypoglycaemic hyperglycaemia is evident.

Controllable factors
• Level of activity
• Level of stress
• Technical problems with insulin
• Poor owner compliance with insulin regime
• Poor owner compliance with dietary recommendation
• Administration of interfering drugs (e.g. glucocorticoids)
• Other diseases (e.g. infection, pancreatitis, kidney disease, neoplasia)

Intrinsic factors
• Variable amount of remaining pancreatic beta cells
• Variable insulin absorption
• Variable insulin degradation
• Variable insulin sensitivity
• Defective counter-regulation
• Impaired gastric emptying

25.9 Causes of glycaemic variability. Controllable factors can be improved by veterinary or owner intervention; intrinsic factors usually cannot be identified and, therefore, cannot be improved. (Modified from Reusch and Salesov, 2019)

concurrent diseases (see Figure 25.3). It is sometimes not possible to identify a clear cause that explains the glycaemic variability. In such cases, a change in insulin should be considered: for example, a cat being treated with porcine lente insulin can be switched to PZI, insulin glargine (100 IU/ml or 300 IU/ml) or another insulin analogue, such as detemir insulin. In humans, the use of insulin analogues can reduce glycaemic variability in comparison with the use of other insulin preparations (e.g. NPH) (Heise *et al.*, 2004). Additionally, in some cats, the addition of exenatide, an extended-release glucagon-like peptide 1 (GLP-1) analogue, may be useful in reducing glycaemic variability and improving glycaemic control (Riederer *et al.* 2016; Krämer *et al.* 2020). If high glycaemic variability cannot be reduced in any way, insulin dose reduction should also be considered to avoid the risk of hypoglycaemia.

Rebound hypoglycaemia (Somogyi response)

The Somogyi response is defined as rebound hyperglycaemia caused by hypersecretion of counter-regulatory hormones (e.g. cortisol, glucagon and adrenaline (epinephrine))

during a hypoglycaemic episode. However, there are no studies in veterinary medicine that have measured the counter-regulatory hormones during this post-hypoglycaemic hyperglycaemia. In human diabetics, inadequate insulin action (often associated with short duration of insulin action) is considered to be responsible for the majority of these episodes of hyperglycaemia following hypoglycaemia, as opposed to true rebound hyperglycaemia associated with counter-regulatory hormones. In one study of six healthy and 133 diabetic cats, insulin-induced hypoglycaemia did not cause post-hypoglycaemic hyperglycaemia in healthy cats but did so in approximately 25% of the diabetic cats with hypoglycaemia (Zini *et al.*, 2018). Those diabetic cats with post-hypoglycaemic hyperglycaemia generally had evidence of poorer glycaemic control, with higher glycaemic variability, higher insulin doses and a reduced probability of remission compared with diabetic cats that did not have rebound hyperglycaemia. In another retrospective study evaluating 55 diabetic cats, the pattern of post-hypoglycaemic hyperglycaemia (<2.8 mmol/l followed by >16.7 mmol/l within 4–10 hours) was observed in only 0.42% of 10,767 blood glucose curves, even though biochemical hypoglycaemia frequently occurred (93% of cats) (Roomp and Rand, 2016). Although this pattern was consistent with rebound hyperglycaemia, peak glucose concentrations were not significantly different following a hypoglycaemic or normoglycaemic nadir, suggesting that the hyperglycaemia was not due to preceding hypoglycaemia and the release of counter-regulatory hormones, and was more likely due to inadequate insulin duration, as in the majority of humans.

Additional studies are required to understand the likely underlying causes of these patterns of changing glucose concentrations, but it is probable that the Somogyi phenomenon is not a specific entity, but a more severe form of glycaemic variability complex (Zini *et al.*, 2018).

Concurrent conditions causing insulin resistance

Insulin resistance is a condition in which a normal amount of insulin produces a subnormal biological response (Nelson, 2015). The majority of diabetic dogs and cats can be regulated with insulin doses of up to 1 IU/kg twice a day. In animals with higher insulin requirements, concomitant disorders should be suspected, provided that technical problems and a short duration of insulin action have been ruled out. There is no insulin dose that clearly defines insulin resistance. Insulin resistance should be suspected when glycaemic control is poor despite high insulin doses (>1.0 IU/kg twice a day), when high doses are required to maintain blood glucose concentrations below 16 mmol/l, or when glycaemic control is erratic (high glycaemic variability) and the insulin dose must be continuously adjusted. Insulin resistance may result from problems occurring prior to the interaction of insulin with its receptor (e.g. circulating anti-insulin antibodies), at the receptor site (e.g. altered insulin receptor binding affinity or concentration), or distal to the interaction of insulin and its receptor (e.g. a block in insulin signal transduction). In dogs and cats, receptor and post-receptor abnormalities are usually due to obesity, circulating acute-phase proteins or inflammatory cytokines (e.g. tumour necrosis factor-alpha, interleukin-1, interleukin-6), all of which interfere with insulin signal transduction, or a disorder causing excessive secretion of an insulin-antagonistic hormone, such as cortisol, growth hormone or progesterone, or a deficiency of thyroid hormone (DeClue *et al.*, 2012).

The severity of insulin resistance usually depends on the underlying cause. In some circumstances (e.g. obesity), insulin resistance may be mild and not well perceived because it is easily overcome by increasing the dose of insulin. Insulin resistance can sometimes be severe, causing severe hyperglycaemia despite the administration of an extreme dose of insulin, as observed in some cats with hypersomatotropism. In general, any inflammatory, infectious, neoplastic or endocrine disorder, and drugs such as glucocorticoids and progestins, can cause insulin resistance. Figure 25.10 lists causes of insulin resistance; some are easily recognizable at the time the diabetes mellitus is diagnosed, namely obesity in cats and the administration of diabetogenic drugs (e.g. glucocorticoids). Many other causes of insulin resistance are not readily apparent and require a thorough diagnostic investigation.

A detailed history and a complete physical examination are the most important steps in identifying concomitant disorders. In the majority of cases, a complete diagnostic work-up, including haematological and biochemical analyses, urinalysis with bacterial culture and susceptibility testing, abdominal ultrasonography and thoracic radiography, should be performed in order to screen for concurrent illnesses. When indicated, other diagnostic evaluations should be performed, such as the low-dose dexamethasone suppression test, measurement of serum insulin-like growth factor-1 (IGF-1), progesterone (in intact females) or pancreas-specific lipase concentrations, determination of serum trypsin-like immunoreactivity (TLI), thyroid function tests, and computed tomography (CT) or magnetic resonance imaging (MRI) (particularly when a pituitary mass is suspected). In some cases, controlling or removing the underlying cause of insulin resistance results in its reversibility. Classic examples are represented by the ovariohysterectomy of a bitch in dioestrus, a cat with hypersomatotropism treated by hypophysectomy or a hypothyroid dog treated with levothyroxine. In contrast, insulin resistance often persists with disorders that are difficult to treat, such as chronic recurring pancreatitis or many cases of hypercortisolism treated with trilostane (McLauchlan *et al.*, 2010).

Insulin therapy
• Inactive insulin
• Diluted insulin
• Improper administration technique
• Inadequate dose (too low or too high)
• Inadequate frequency of insulin administration
• Impaired insulin absorption
• Anti-insulin antibodies

Disorders typically causing severe insulin resistance
• **Hypercortisolism (dogs)**
• **Hypersomatotropism (cats)**
• **Dioestrus in intact bitches**
• **Hypothyroidism (dogs)**
• Exogenous glucocorticoids
• Progestins

Disorders typically causing mild or fluctuating insulin resistance
• **Obesity (mainly cats)**
• **Infection (especially oral or urinary tract infections)**
• Chronic inflammation
• **Chronic pancreatitis**
• Inflammatory bowel disease
• Diseases of the oral cavity
• **Chronic kidney disease**
• Hepatobiliary disease
• Cardiac disease
• Hyperthyroidism
• Exocrine pancreatic insufficiency
• **Hyperlipidaemia**
• **Neoplasia**
• Glucagonoma
• Phaeochromocytoma

25.10 Recognized causes of insulin ineffectiveness or insulin resistance in diabetic dogs and cats. Causes in bold are more common.
(Modified from Nelson, 2015)

Pancreatitis

The exocrine and endocrine components of the pancreas are interlinked, and it is not surprising that damage to the exocrine tissue can also damage the endocrine component. Pancreatitis can destroy beta cells or contribute to their loss of function and can therefore be the cause of, or a contributor to, diabetes mellitus. Pancreatitis can be acute or chronic, potentially resulting in pancreatic fibrosis. A single isolated inflammatory event of acute pancreatitis is not likely to cause diabetes mellitus (although this is possible), but the endocrine component is more likely to become affected if inflammation persists, such as in chronic pancreatitis (Davison, 2015). Very few dogs and cats with diabetes mellitus have clinical signs of pancreatitis. The concomitance of diabetes mellitus and pancreatitis has clinical implications for case management, as such cases may follow a more difficult clinical course, with glycaemic control being 'brittle' as a result of variation in the degree of pancreatic inflammation (Davison, 2015). Some animals show intermittent lethargy and inappetence, and owners report that their pet 'is not doing well'.

Diagnosis of pancreatitis: The diagnosis of pancreatitis, especially in the chronic form, can be challenging, relying on the presence of clinical signs (vomiting, lethargy, abdominal pain), ultrasonographic abnormalities and an increase in serum pancreas-specific lipase concentration.

Management of pancreatitis: Management of acute pancreatitis in diabetics uses the same therapeutic principles as the treatment of non-diabetics: fluid therapy, analgesia, antiemetics and, in dogs, a low-fat diet (see the *BSAVA Manual of Canine and Feline Gastroenterology*). Long-term treatment of chronic pancreatitis is more difficult and usually supportive, as a cure is often not possible. If gluco-corticoid therapy is deemed appropriate, it should be used with caution because glucocorticoids interfere with insulin sensitivity and a worsening of diabetic control can ensue. Higher doses of insulin are likely to be required while glucocorticoids are being administered.

Insulin antagonistic treatment

Glucocorticoids have the potential to induce severe insulin resistance in previously normoglycaemic diabetics or to worsen glycaemic control in diabetic animals that are already suboptimally controlled. Glucocorticoids impair glucose homeostasis by means of several complex physiological mechanisms but, essentially, induce insulin resistance in the muscle and adipose tissue, and increase hepatic production of glucose (Lowe *et al.*, 2009). Diabetic instability can occur after oral, parenteral or even topical administration of any of the currently available corticosteroids (Reusch, 2015). Progestins are known to exert glucocorticoid activity and they have effects similar to glucocorticoids regarding insulin sensitivity. However, the principal insulin antagonistic activity in dogs relates to stimulation of growth hormone production by mammary tissue.

Management of insulin antagonistic treatment: Whenever possible, systemic or topical corticosteroid or progestin therapy should be avoided in diabetic dogs and cats. If therapy is absolutely necessary, and no alternative drugs can be used, the insulin dose needs to be adjusted according to the severity of the insulin resistance induced. For some diseases in which the use of topical corticosteroids can be effective, this route is preferred over systemic products. Topical products or corticosteroids with a high first-pass metabolism usually have lower circulating systemic concentrations and therefore cause less insulin resistance. For example, in a dog with inflammatory bowel disease, the use of budesonide is preferable over the use of oral prednisolone. In those diabetic animals that require corticosteroids, home blood glucose monitoring or the use of a CGMS is recommended. In such animals, glycaemic control usually remains difficult. Caution is advised when insulin antagonistic treatment is withdrawn, as hypoglycaemia is a significant risk if the insulin dosage is not appropriately adjusted.

Dioestrus and other progesterone-induced insulin resistance in diabetic bitches

Dioestrus and pregnancy are associated with increased progesterone concentrations and subsequent induction of growth hormone secretion by mammary tissue in dogs (Fall *et al.*, 2010). Consequently, these conditions can lead to the development of diabetes mellitus or contribute to diabetic instability in a previously diagnosed entire diabetic bitch. The Norwegian Elkhound breed appears to be predisposed to diabetes secondary to progesterone stimulation and was proposed as a model for this condition (Fall *et al.*, 2010). However, this phenomenon seems to be frequent in several other breeds and has also been observed in dogs with ovarian remnant syndrome (Pöppl *et al.*, 2013).

Fall *et al.* (2010) described a high prevalence (17%) of pyometra in bitches with diabetes mellitus during dioestrus. In a bitch predisposed to diabetes, an episode of pyometra, especially when progesterone concentrations are increased, may worsen insulin resistance due to inflammation and consequently accelerate the development of diabetes.

Management of dioestrus: Intact bitches that develop diabetes during dioestrus should be neutered as soon as feasible, possibly 1–3 days following stabilization with insulin. Gonadectomy is associated with decreased insulin resistance and, in some cases, remission of diabetes mellitus may occur after a few days or a few weeks.

Post-pregnancy diabetic remission appears to be high. In one study of 13 bitches that developed diabetes mellitus during pregnancy, 7 of 11 dogs that survived longer than 1 day experienced diabetic remission (Fall *et al.*, 2008).

After neutering, glycaemic control should be closely monitored, and appropriate adjustment of the insulin dose is extremely important. All intact bitches with diabetes should be neutered, even if there is no obvious temporal relationship between dioestrus and the onset of the diabetes. Although neutering does not lead to diabetic remission in the majority of bitches, it is necessary to prevent progesterone-induced hypersecretion of growth hormone during the subsequent dioestrus and resultant insulin resistance and disruption of treatment. In cases where neutering is not possible, the administration of the progesterone receptor antagonist aglepristone is a possible alternative for reducing insulin resistance (Bigliardi *et al.*, 2014).

Hypercortisolism

Hypercortisolism and diabetes mellitus are two well documented diseases in dogs that are observed with greater frequency in middle-aged to elderly dogs and share some clinical signs, such as PU/PD and poly-phagia, which can make diagnosis and eventual treatment difficult. Although both diseases can appear independently, they can also be manifested concurrently. Glucocorticoids antagonize the effects of insulin, inducing a sustained increase in blood glucose concentrations and, in the most severe cases, the development of diabetes mellitus (Figure 25.11). However, the concurrence of the two endocrine disorders can also be a coincidence and, if not causative, can still result in poor glycaemic control. Hypercortisolism is observed in approximately 10–20% of all diabetic dogs, and diabetes mellitus has been reported in 10–13% of dogs with hypercortisolism (Miceli *et al.*, 2017; Hoffman *et al.*, 2018). In cats, hypercortisolism is rarer than in dogs; however, when it is present, it is associated with diabetes mellitus in approximately 80–90% of cases. These disorders are covered in greater detail in Chapters 29 and 30.

Diagnosis of hypercortisolism: The diagnosis of diabetes mellitus is quite simple, but it is not the same for naturally occurring hypercortisolism. The diagnosis of hypercortisolism is usually straightforward in highly symptomatic cases (e.g. dogs presenting with bilaterally symmetrical alopecia and calcinosis cutis, skin fragility in cats). Unfortunately, in many cases, the diagnosis of hypercortisolism in an unstable diabetic animal is challenging. Many of the clinical, biochemical and haematological signs seen in hypercortisolism (e.g. PU/PD, hepatomegaly, increased liver enzyme activities, hypercholesterolaemia, stress leucogram) are non-specific and are also present in unstable diabetics. Furthermore, endocrine tests for hypercortisolism (e.g. urinary cortisol:creatinine, adreno-corticotropic hormone (ACTH) response test, low-dose dexamethasone suppression test) can give false-positive results in chronically stressed animals, such as those with unstable diabetes mellitus. If hypercortisolism is already suspected at the time of diagnosis of diabetes mellitus,

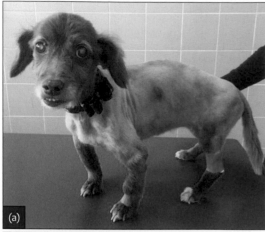

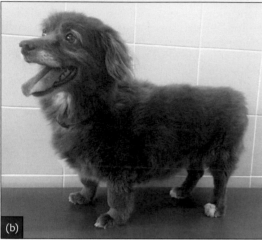

25.11 An 11-year-old neutered mixed-breed bitch. (a) After 5 months of treatment for diabetes mellitus with poor control, the dog exhibited weight loss, severe polyuria, polydipsia, polyphagia, cataracts, alopecia, and persistently high blood glucose and fructosamine concentrations despite increased insulin doses. (b) A diagnosis of concomitant hypercortisolism and treatment with trilostane twice a day resulted in resolution of the clinical signs and marked improvement in glycaemic control.

hypercortisolism in animals with only supportive endocrine test results where all other causes of diabetic instability have not been ruled out.

Treatment of hypercortisolism: Animals suffering from concomitant diabetes mellitus and hypercortisolism should be treated with the same therapeutic protocols recommended for the two diseases (see Chapters 23, 24, 29 and 30). The only caveat is that trilostane, if used for hypercortisolism in dogs, should be administered every 12 hours in order to ensure better control of cortisol concentrations over a 24-hour period. Although it is often recommended that the insulin dose is reduced (e.g. by approximately 25%) to avoid the risk of hypoglycaemia following the decline in insulin resistance, this is probably unnecessary. Insulin requirements are not consistently reduced during trilostane treatment for hypercortisolism (McLauchlan *et al.*, 2010). These cases are usually monitored by evaluating their clinical signs in association with measurement of cortisol control (Macfarlane *et al.*, 2016). If trilostane therapy is not effective, then mitotane can be considered.

Hypersomatotropism

Hypersomatotropism should be considered as a differential diagnosis in every cat with diabetes mellitus, especially those that are difficult to control. Hypersomatotropism is present in approximately 20–25%, or more, of cats with poorly controlled diabetes mellitus. In the past few decades, awareness has increased regarding the existence of hypersomatotropism in diabetic cats and, therefore, the disease is currently more commonly diagnosed. In dogs, hypersomatotropism is not often associated with diabetes mellitus. In cats, hypersomatotropism is associated with an increased production of growth hormone, typically due to a pituitary adenoma. Insulin resistance, which can be severe, is caused by growth hormone-induced postreceptor defects in insulin action at target tissues. However, insulin resistance can also be mild, especially in the initial phases of the disease, and cats with hypersomatotropism may occasionally even achieve temporary remission. Clinical manifestations of hypersomatotropism are due to the diabetogenic effect of growth hormone, and the anabolic effects of growth hormone and IGF-1 on various tissues (see Chapter 13).

Diagnosis of hypersomatotropism: Diagnosis is made based on supportive clinical signs of IGF-1 excess. However, in some cases, the only abnormality detected is a need for higher than typical insulin dosages, together with difficulties in achieving good glycaemic control. High glucose variability is commonly observed in cats with concomitant diabetes mellitus and hypersomatotropism. A diagnosis should be suspected in any unstable diabetic cat that gains weight and appears resistant to the development of DKA.

Confirmation of the diagnosis is based on documentation of an increased serum IGF-1 concentration and evidence of pituitary enlargement on CT or MRI. Insulin-like growth factor-1 should be measured using an assay validated for cats. Concentrations are typically markedly increased, but should not be measured until 2–3 weeks after initiation of insulin therapy.

Treatment of hypersomatotropism: In cats with hypersomatotropism, insulin doses exceeding 10 IU twice daily may still fail to provide anything other than poor glycaemic control. Treatment can be divided into definitive treatment

unless the clinical signs of hypercortisolism are clearly evident (e.g. consistent dermatological abnormalities), it is usually better to attempt diabetic stabilization and limit the development of ketoacidosis as a priority before starting a diagnostic work-up for hypercortisolism. Such cases often need high doses of insulin (>1–1.5 IU/kg twice daily) to control the clinical signs of diabetes mellitus.

When the animal is considered stable enough to investigate for the presence of hypercortisolism, it is recommended that biochemistry, haematology and urinalysis be repeated to look for alterations that are potentially more compatible with hypercortisolism than with diabetes mellitus. Severe thrombocytosis, low urine specific gravity (despite glucosuria) and severe proteinuria can direct the diagnostic suspicion towards concurrent hypercortisolism. Usually two endocrine tests (the low-dose dexamethasone suppression test and the ACTH response test) are recommended, on different days, together with ultrasonography of the abdomen. In the diabetic cat, the best test for diagnosing hypercortisolism is probably the low-dose dexamethasone suppression test using 0.1 mg/kg intravenous dexamethasone. The combination of consistent clinical signs, laboratory changes, specific endocrine test results and diagnostic imaging findings usually allows confirmation or exclusion of concurrent hypercortisolism in a diabetic case. Caution is advised in erroneously diagnosing (hypophysectomy, radiotherapy), targeted medical therapy (e.g. pasireotide) and conservative treatment. The highest success rate is achieved by means of surgical hypophysectomy, with the majority of such treated cats achieving diabetic remission. Stereotactic radiation therapy is associated with better glycaemic control but less frequently with diabetic remission (Wormhoudt et al., 2018). Long-acting subcutaneous pasireotide, at a dose of 6–8 mg/kg once a month for 6 months, is also associated with a reduction in the insulin dose and occasionally diabetic remission (Gostelow et al., 2017). Unfortunately, the cost of this drug is currently prohibitive. Cabergoline has had some anecdotal success and may be considered. The conservative approach focuses on the management of diabetes mellitus with insulin therapy and is reserved for cases in which definitive treatment is not available or is declined by the owner. The high insulin doses often required, combined with fluctuations in insulin resistance, predispose these cats to the development of hypoglycaemic complications. For this reason, routine home glucose monitoring is recommended.

Hypothyroidism

Hypothyroidism is a commonly diagnosed disease in dogs, characterized by dermatological abnormalities, lethargy and weight gain. Dogs with concomitant diabetes mellitus and hypothyroidism can be insulin resistant (Figure 25.12).

Insulin resistance may be related to the fact that hypothyroidism is associated with high growth hormone concentrations, and growth hormone can cause severe insulin resistance. Other possible contributors include lipid dysregulation and obesity.

Diagnosis of hypothyroidism: The diagnosis of hypothyroidism is often a challenge, and investigation should be undertaken only in those dogs with appropriate clinical signs and laboratory findings (dermatological abnormalities, lethargy, bradycardia, weight gain, severe hypercholesterolaemia, mild non-regenerative anaemia). The results of hormone concentration measurements must be evaluated very carefully as it is common to find decreased total thyroxine (T4) concentrations with unstable diabetes mellitus because of the effects of non-thyroidal illness (see Chapter 18). The majority of hypothyroid dogs have decreased T4 concentrations and increased thyrotropin (thyroid-stimulating hormone (TSH)) concentrations. In approximately 30% of hypothyroid dogs, no increase in TSH is observed. In such cases, additional diagnostic tests to confirm or exclude the diagnosis (e.g. measurement of free T4 with equilibrium dialysis, the recombinant human thyroid-stimulating hormone (rhTSH) stimulation test or thyroid scintigraphy) are recommended.

Treatment of hypothyroidism: Insulin resistance can decline rapidly, requiring a careful reduction in insulin dose when levothyroxine is started.

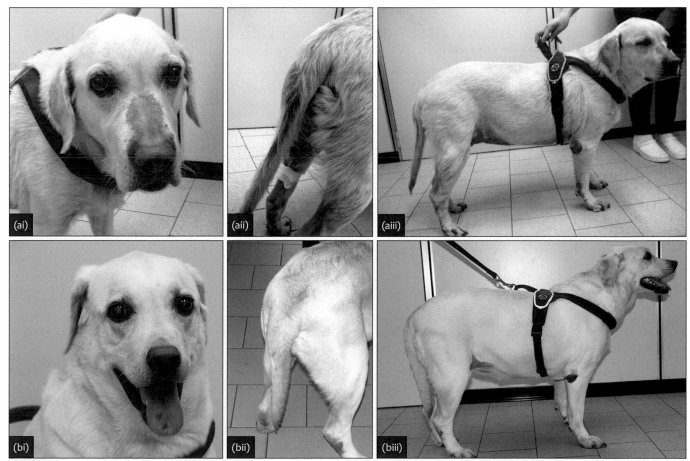

25.12 A 10-year-old neutered Labrador Retriever bitch that had been undergoing treatment for diabetes mellitus for 1 year with poor control of the disease. (ai–iii) When referred, the dog exhibited weight loss, severe polyuria, polydipsia, lethargy, cataracts, alopecia, and persistently high blood glucose and fructosamine concentrations despite receiving 22 IU of porcine lente insulin twice a day. (bi–iii) A diagnosis of concomitant hypothyroidism and treatment with levothyroxine resulted in the resolution of the majority of clinical signs after 2 months. At that time, the dog had achieved a marked improvement in glycaemic control and required a lower insulin dose (19 IU of porcine lente insulin twice a day).

Inflammation and infection

Inflammation or infections in various parts of the body can cause insulin resistance or diabetic instability. In humans, bacterial infections can contribute to decreased glucose tolerance, insulin resistance and hyperinsulinaemia. In general, diabetic cases are more prone to developing infections, which exacerbates the issue. In dogs and cats, the site of infection or inflammation is sometimes obvious (e.g. severe dental disease, nasal discharge, dermatological infections) but it can be more subtle (e.g. chronic pancreatitis, urinary tract infection, respiratory infection, prostatitis).

Diagnosis of inflammation and infection: An important step in investigating the cause of diabetic instability is ruling out sources of infection or inflammation. Screening for these should include haematology, biochemistry and urinalysis, including sediment examination and urine culture and susceptibility testing. In fact, urinary tract infections are common in dogs and cats with unstable diabetes mellitus and should always be investigated. In some cases, the use of diagnostic imaging can be helpful in identifying the site of infection. Fungal infections can also be of clinical importance and should be considered.

Treatment of inflammation and infection: Once a diagnosis has been made, appropriate treatment for that condition should be instituted. Care should be taken to consider lowering insulin doses as insulin resistance wanes. If infection is being investigated, culture and susceptibility testing is always recommended to identify the organism and guide the most appropriate antimicrobial treatment. If glucocorticoids are indicated, their effect on insulin resistance should be considered (see 'Insulin antagonistic treatment', above). Fungal infections are often difficult to eradicate in diabetic cases

The brittle diabetic

In humans, a small group of diabetic patients is characterized by severe instability of glycaemic control with frequent and unpredictable hypoglycaemic and/or ketoacidotic episodes that cannot be readily explained. These patients are often referred to as brittle diabetics. The QOL of affected patients is dramatically compromised, in particular because of the frequency of acute events, hospitalizations and the early onset of chronic complications (Bertuzzi *et al.*, 2007). Similarly, some diabetic dogs and cats have severe diabetic instability and glucose variability, and are very difficult to stabilize, despite adequate management and the absence of other detectable diseases. Examples include animals that:

- Previously had good glycaemic control and suddenly develop clinical signs of diabetes mellitus
- Develop DKA for no obvious reason
- Exhibit hypoglycaemia alternating with periods of good glycaemic control and/or hyperglycaemia.

This condition usually requires frequent hospitalizations and is extremely frustrating for both the pet owner and the veterinary surgeon. In humans, the main causes of brittle diabetes include malabsorption, certain drugs (alcohol, antipsychotics), defective insulin absorption or degradation, defects in hyperglycaemic hormones (especially glucocorticoids and glucagon) and, above all, delayed gastric emptying as a result of autonomic neuropathy (Vantyghem *et al.*,

2006). Psychological factors, such as stress and depression, are also reported to be important in humans. It is likely that some of these factors cause brittle diabetes in dogs and cats. Given that, in the majority of cases, the cause of diabetic instability is due to management problems or the presence of concomitant diseases, a thorough work-up (see Figure 25.3) should be carried out before a diagnosis of brittle diabetes mellitus is made.

In brittle diabetics, frequent monitoring (home monitoring or the use of CGMSs) and appropriate client communication are essential, as these animals frequently require insulin dose adjustments appropriate to their prevailing glucose concentration (Rand, 2019). Switching insulins and the addition of supplementary treatment may be helpful in some dogs and cats (see 'Glucose variability', above).

Glucose monitoring

The unstable diabetic is usually characterized by the presence of persistent hyperglycaemia and/or a tendency to develop hypoglycaemia and/or high glycaemic variability and DKA. For these reasons, it is clear that these cases require frequent glucose monitoring. Close monitoring can help identify the cause of diabetic instability (e.g. when the duration of action of the insulin is too short), can avoid dangerous clinical hypoglycaemia and can allow for more appropriate adjustments of the insulin dose. For these reasons, glucose monitoring in an unstable diabetic is even more important than in a well controlled diabetic.

Portable blood glucose meters and blood glucose curves

Serial BGCs provide guidelines for making rational adjustments in insulin therapy. Blood glucose concentrations are typically determined by a hand-held portable blood glucose meter (PBGM). To avoid multiple venepunctures, it is possible to collect capillary blood from the ear, the oral mucosa or other sites of the body (e.g. a paw pad). A wide range of PBGMs is available. The accuracy of commercially available PBGM devices designed for human use varies considerably when used in diabetic dogs or cats as compared with the results obtained using standard reference methods. Some PBGM devices designed for humans are sufficiently accurate and precise to monitor blood glucose concentrations in diabetic animals; however, the majority of them give lower results than the laboratory reference method. This bias may result in an incorrect diagnosis of hypoglycaemia or the misconception that the animal's glycaemic control is better than it actually is. There are now some PBGMs specifically designed for veterinary use. They give more accurate and precise blood glucose measurements for dogs and cats than the majority of the PBGMs designed for humans. Additional advantages of veterinary glucose meters are the very small sample volume needed (0.3 µl) and the extended measurement range (1.1–41 mmol/l). Conversely, they tend to overestimate blood glucose values and can potentially miss hypoglycaemia. If there is any doubt regarding the accuracy of a blood glucose concentration result, the measurement should be repeated with the same meter and, ideally, with the laboratory reference method.

When a BGC is carried out in the clinic, it is usually recommended that the animal be dropped off at the hospital early in the morning, so that blood sampling can be carried out every 1–2 hours throughout the day for glucose determination until the next insulin injection. When carrying out a BGC, the insulin and feeding schedules used by the owner should be maintained. Poor appetite can strongly affect the results of a BGC. Food and insulin can be administered at the clinic after the first blood glucose measurement. If the animal refuses to eat at the clinic, the owner should administer food and insulin at home and bring the animal to the clinic as soon as possible to start the BGC.

Glucose measurement with a PBGM using capillary blood is feasible at home and should be recommended. Home monitoring can be carried out provided that the owner is adequately instructed regarding the use of the PBGM, and that ready access to veterinary support is available if required. Once the owner is familiar with the procedure, they should produce a BGC by measuring the blood glucose concentration in the morning before giving the dog insulin and food, and then every 2 hours until the following injection. One problem can be that of overzealous owners who monitor blood glucose concentrations too frequently, and begin to interpret the results and adjust the insulin dose without consulting their veterinary practice – a situation that frequently leads to insulin overdosage.

Evaluation of the BGC determines whether the insulin administered is effective and identifies the glucose nadir (time of peak insulin action), duration of insulin action and degree of fluctuation in blood glucose concentrations in that particular animal. In a well controlled diabetic, glucose concentrations should stay between approximately 4.5 and 15 mmol/l for most of the day. The efficacy of the insulin is evaluated by determining the difference between the highest and lowest insulin concentrations and is interpreted in the light of the highest blood glucose concentration observed. A small difference (e.g. 2.5 mmol/l) is acceptable if the highest blood glucose concentration recorded is lower than 12 mmol/l but not acceptable if it is above 16 mmol/l. In interpreting the BGC, the most important parameters are the glucose nadir and the duration of insulin action. The glucose nadir should ideally be between 5 and 8 mmol/l. A lower nadir can be caused by:

- A high insulin dose
- Excessive overlap of the insulin action (common if long-acting insulin analogues are used)
- Fluctuation or variation in factors inducing insulin resistance
- Failure to eat
- Strenuous exercise.

A glucose nadir above 8 mmol/l can be caused by:

- Insufficient insulin dose
- Insulin resistance
- Stress
- Technical problems attributable to the owners.

Carrying out BGCs on multiple, consecutive days is not recommended because it promotes stress-induced hyperglycaemia. In addition, information gained from a previous BGC should never be assumed to be reproducible on subsequent curves. Variables such as the amount of insulin drawn into the syringe and subsequently absorbed at the subcutaneous site of deposition, the interaction between insulin, diet, exercise, stress and

excitement, the presence of concomitant disorders, and secretion of counter-regulatory hormones (e.g. glucagon, adrenaline, cortisol, growth hormone) change over time and affect the reproducibility of serial BGCs. Lack of consistency in the results of serial BGCs can be frustrating. It is important to remember that this lack of consistency directly reflects all the variables affecting the blood glucose concentration in a diabetic animal.

The insulin dose can be adjusted based on the results of the BGC. A change in the type of insulin may sometimes be necessary. Changes to the insulin dose should be approximately 10%, although in the case of clinical signs of hypoglycaemia the dose should be decreased by at least 25%. The insulin dose should not be modified more frequently than every 5–7 days, except in the case of hypoglycaemia.

Continuous glucose monitoring systems and the flash glucose monitoring system

Continuous glucose monitoring systems are routinely used to monitor glucose concentrations in diabetic human patients and are increasingly being used in diabetic dogs and cats. These systems allow glucose concentrations to be monitored without the need for repeated blood sampling.

The CGMS measures interstitial glucose rather than blood glucose concentrations. Interstitial fluid is easily accessible, has rapid equilibration with blood and its glucose concentration has a good correlation with blood glucose concentration. Several traditional CGMSs are available, and the use of iPro, Guardian REAL-Time, MiniMed Gold and GlucoDay has been reported in dogs and cats (Surman and Fleeman, 2013). The Guardian REAL-Time is a frequently used CGMS that measures interstitial glucose using a small, flexible sensor inserted through the skin into the subcutaneous space and secured to the skin with tape. The sensor is connected to a transmitter, which is also fixed to the skin with tape and sends data wirelessly over a maximum distance of 3 m to a pager-sized monitor. Data are collected every 10 seconds and a mean glucose value is computed every 5 minutes. The data can be downloaded to a computer for analysis. Currently, such CGMS devices present some challenges. They need to be calibrated two to three times a day, which requires blood sampling, and the sensor is quite expensive and can be used for only a few days. Furthermore, the monitor displays glucose concentrations from 2.2 to 22.2 mmol/l; concentrations outside this range are recorded but need to be downloaded to be visualized.

A newer CGMS (Freestyle Libre), produced for humans, has been used in dogs and cats (Corradini et al. 2016; Del Baldo et al. 2021). This device consists of a small, round, disposable, water-resistant sensor that continuously measures glucose in the interstitial fluid by means of a small (5 mm long x 0.4 mm wide) filament inserted subcutaneously (Figure 25.13).

The Freestyle Libre generates information every minute and the readings are automatically stored in 15-minute intervals for up to 14 days. Interstitial glucose concentrations are displayed on demand when the sensor is wirelessly scanned (or 'flashed') with a reader device, and such systems are therefore referred to as flash glucose monitoring systems (FGMSs). The reader device displays the past 8 hours of glucose information, including current glucose concentration, a trend graph and a trend arrow, which indicates the direction of change of the current

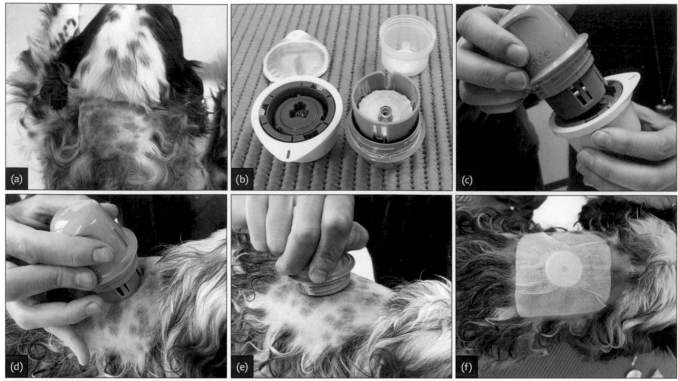

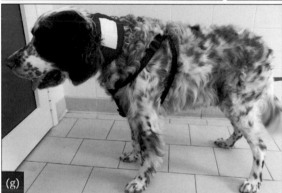

25.13 Application of the Freestyle Libre in dogs. (a) Shave a rectangular area at the level of the dorsal portion of the neck, at the point where there are fewer skin folds. The area must be large enough to allow the application of the sensor and a protective adhesive patch. Cleanse the shaved skin with chlorhexidine and alcohol, then dry with a clean gauze. (b) Assemble the sensor: open the sensor box by completely removing the cap and unscrew the cap from the sensor applicator. (c) Align the dark mark on the sensor applicator with the dark mark on the sensor box. Press firmly on the sensor applicator until a confirmation click is heard. (d) Place the sensor applicator on the clean shaved area. (e) Press firmly on the skin. Gently remove the sensor applicator from the neck. Check that the sensor is correctly positioned. (f) Apply an adhesive patch covering the sensor and the skin around it. (g) Apply a protective bandage with cotton and a cohesive layer to the area and take the first scan with the reader.

glucose concentration with respect to previous results. In dogs and cats, the FGMS is apparently painless to apply, easy to use and well tolerated. Mild erythema at the site of application can be observed at the end of the wearing period. A good correlation between interstitial and blood glucose concentrations (correlation coefficient = 0.94) has been demonstrated in dogs. The FGMS readings are less accurate for glucose concentrations below 5 mmol/l (Corradini *et al.*, 2016). The accuracy appears to be affected by skin thickness; measurements are more accurate in dogs with thick skin than in dogs with thinner skin (<5 mm). In diabetic dogs, the FGMS detects nadirs and hypoglycaemic episodes more frequently than intermittent measurement of blood glucose concentrations using a PBGM (Del Baldo *et al.*, 2020). The FGMS is also used for cats, and preliminary studies have described good clinical accuracy (Del Baldo *et al.*, 2021).

In recent years, technology has continued to evolve and CGMSs have been developed that can continuously record interstitial glucose for several months. The first implantable long-term CGMS has the tradename Eversense. This system extends the possible continuous glucose monitoring wear time up to 180 days (Eversense XL). This CGMS consists of a subcutaneously inserted sensor, a wearable transmitter and a smartphone application (Aronson *et al.*, 2019). As yet, no studies regarding this CGMS have been published in veterinary medicine. However, anecdotal use has been reported and first impressions have been positive. The Eversense XL allows remote displaying of glucose values and displays the results in intuitive graphs (Figure 25.14).

Summary

Managing an unstable diabetic can be extremely complex and requires a methodical approach and excellent communication with the owner. After ruling out management errors on the part of the owner, insulin effectiveness and duration of action should be assessed by serial glucose measurements. A work-up to detect other underlying causes may then be warranted. Chronic pancreatitis, hypercortisolism in dogs and hypersomatotropism in cats are probably the most common and relevant disorders that can cause severe insulin resistance, glucose variability and diabetic instability. Management of the underlying disease can improve diabetic stability. When detection or resolution of the underlying cause is not possible, appropriate monitoring to adapt insulin requirements in order to avoid clinical hypoglycaemia and optimize the control of the hyperglycaemia is recommended.

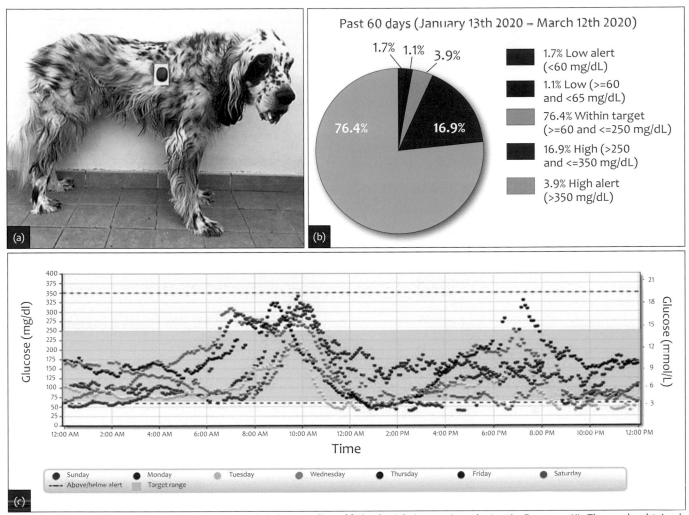

Past 60 days (January 13th 2020 – March 12th 2020)

1.7% 1.1% 3.9%

76.4%   16.9%

- 1.7% Low alert (<60 mg/dL)
- 1.1% Low (>=60 and <65 mg/dL)
- 76.4% Within target (>=60 and <=250 mg/dL)
- 16.9% High (>250 and <=350 mg/dL)
- 3.9% High alert (>350 mg/dL)

25.14 A 12-year-old neutered male English Setter with diabetes mellitus. (a) The dog is being monitored using the Eversense XL. The graphs obtained from the device software show (b) the glucose ranges recorded for 60 days and (c) the seven glucose curves recorded in a week (each day is represented by a different colour).

References and further reading

Alt N, Kley S, Haessig M and Reusch CE (2007) Day-to-day variability of blood glucose concentration curves generated at home in cats with diabetes mellitus. *Journal of the American Veterinary Medical Association* **230**, 1011–1017

Aronson R, Abitbol A and Tweden KS (2019) First assessment of the performance of an implantable continuous glucose monitoring system through 180 days in a primarily adolescent population with type 1 diabetes. *Diabetes, Obesity and Metabolism* **21**,1689–1694

Bennett N, Greco DS, Peterson ME *et al.* (2006) Comparison of a low carbohydrate–low fiber diet and a moderate carbohydrate–high fiber diet in the management of feline diabetes mellitus. *Journal of Feline Medicine and Surgery* **8**, 73–84

Bertuzzi F, Verzaro R, Provenzano V and Ricordi C (2007) Brittle type 1 diabetes mellitus. *Current Medical Chemistry* **14**, 1739–1744

Bigliardi E, Bresciani C, Callegari D *et al.* (2014) Use of aglepristone for the treatment of P_4 induced insulin resistance in dogs. *Journal of Veterinary Science* **15**, 267–271

Corradini S, Pilosio B, Dondi F *et al.* (2016) Accuracy of a flash glucose monitoring system in diabetic dogs. *Journal of Veterinary Internal Medicine* **30**, 983–988

Davison LJ (2015) Diabetes mellitus and pancreatitis – cause or effect? *Journal of Small Animal Practice* **56**, 50–59

DeClue AE, Nickell J, Chang CH and Honaker A (2012) Upregulation of proinflammatory cytokine production in response to bacterial pathogen-associated molecular patterns in dogs with diabetes mellitus undergoing insulin therapy. *Journal of Diabetes Science and Technology* **6**, 496–502

Del Baldo F, Canton C, Testa S *et al.* (2020) Comparison between a flash glucose monitoring system and a portable blood glucose meter in monitoring dogs with diabetes mellitus. *Journal of Veterinary Internal Medicine* **34**, 2296–2305

Del Baldo F, Fracassi F, Pires J *et al.* (2021) Accuracy of a flash glucose monitoring system in cats and determination of the time lag between blood glucose and interstitial glucose concentrations. *Journal of Veterinary Internal Medicine* **35**, 1279–1287

Fall T, Hedhammar Å, Wallberg A *et al.* (2010) Diabetes mellitus in elkhounds is associated with diestrus and pregnancy. *Journal of Veterinary Internal Medicine* **24**, 1322–1328

Fall T, Johansson Kreuger S, Juberget Å, Bergström A and Hedhammar Å (2008) Gestational diabetes mellitus in 13 dogs. *Journal of Veterinary Internal Medicine* **22**, 1296–1300

Frias JP, Nakhle S, Ruggles JA *et al.* (2017) Exenatide once weekly improved 24-hour glucose control and reduced glycaemic variability in metformin-treated patients with type 2 diabetes: a randomized, placebo-controlled trial. *Diabetes, Obesity and Metabolism* **19**, 40–48

Frontoni S, Di Bartolo P, Avogaro A *et al.* (2013) Glucose variability: an emerging target for the treatment of diabetes mellitus. *Diabetes Research and Clinical Practice* **102**, 86–95

Gostelow R, Scudder C, Keyte S *et al.* (2017) Pasireotide long-acting release treatment for diabetic cats with underlying hypersomatotropism. *Journal of Veterinary Internal Medicine* **31**, 355–364

Hall EJ, Williams DA and Kathrani A (2019) *BSAVA Manual of Canine and Feline Gastroenterology, 3rd edn.* BSAVA Publications, Gloucester

Heise T, Nosek L, Rønn BB *et al.* (2004) Lower within-subject variability of insulin detemir in comparison to NPH insulin and insulin glargine in people with type 1 diabetes. *Diabetes* **53**, 1614–1620

Hoffman JM, Lourenço BN, Promislow DEL and Creevy KE (2018) Canine hyperadrenocorticism associations with signalment, selected comorbidities and mortality within North American veterinary teaching hospitals. *Journal of Small Animal Practice* **59**, 681–690

Krämer AL, Riederer A, Fracassi F *et al.* (2020) Glycemic variability in newly diagnosed diabetic cats treated with the glucagon-like peptide-1 analogue exenatide extended-release. *Journal of Veterinary Internal Medicine* **34**, 2287–2295

Lachin JM, Genuth S, Nathan DM *et al.* (2008) Effect of glycemic exposure on the risk of microvascular complications in the diabetes control and complications trial – revisited. *Diabetes* **57**, 995–1001

Lin CC, Yang CP, Li CI *et al.* (2014) Visit-to-visit variability of fasting plasma glucose as a predictor of ischemic stroke: competing risk analysis in a national cohort of Taiwan Diabetes Study. *BMC Medicine* **12**, 165

Lowe AD, Graves TK, Campbell KL and Schaeffer DJ (2009) A pilot study comparing the diabetogenic effects of dexamethasone and prednisolone in cats. *Journal of the American Animal Hospital Association* **45**, 215–224

Macfarlane L, Parkin T and Ramsey I (2016) Pre-trilostane and three-hour post-trilostane cortisol to monitor trilostane therapy in dogs. *Veterinary Record* **179**, 597

Marshall RD, Rand JS and Morton JM (2009) Treatment of newly diagnosed diabetic cats with glargine insulin improves glycaemic control and results in higher probability of remission than protamine zinc and lente insulins. *Journal of Feline Medicine and Surgery* **11**, 683–691

McLauchlan G, Knottenbelt C, Augusto M *et al.* (2010) Retrospective evaluation of the effect of trilostane on insulin requirement and fructosamine concentration in eight diabetic dogs with hyperadrenocorticism. *Journal of Small Animal Practice* **51**, 642–648

Michiels L, Reusch CE, Boari A *et al.* (2008) Treatment of 46 cats with porcine lente insulin – a prospective, multicentre study. *Journal of Feline Medicine and Surgery* **10**, 439–451

Miceli DD, Pignataro OP and Castillo VA (2017) Concurrent hyperadrenocorticism and diabetes mellitus in dogs. *Research in Veterinary Science* **115**, 425–431

Nelson RW (2015) Canine diabetes mellitus. In: *Canine and Feline Endocrinology, 4th edn*, ed. EC Feldman, RW Nelson, CE Reusch, JCR Scott-Moncrieff and EP Behrend, pp. 213–257. Elsevier, St. Louis

Niessen SJM, Forcada Y, Mantis P *et al.* (2015) Studying cat (*Felis catus*) diabetes: beware of the acromegalic imposter. *PLoS ONE* **10**, e0127794

Niessen SJM, Hazuchova K, Powney SL *et al.* (2017) The big pet diabetes survey: perceived frequency and triggers for euthanasia. *Veterinary Sciences* **4**, 27

Pöppl AG, Mottin TS and González FHD (2013) Diabetes mellitus remission after resolution of inflammatory and progesterone-related conditions in bitches. *Research in Veterinary Science* **94**, 471–473

Rand J (2019) The unstable diabetic. In: *Feline Endocrinology*, ed. EC Feldman, F Fracassi and ME Peterson, pp. 556–578. Edra Publishing, Milan

Restine LM, Norsworthy GD and Kass PH (2019) Loose-control of diabetes mellitus with protamine zinc insulin in cats: 185 cases (2005–2015). *Canadian Veterinary Journal* **60**, 399–404

Reusch CE (2015) Feline diabetes mellitus. In: *Canine and Feline Endocrinology, 4th edn*, ed. EC Feldman, RW Nelson, CE Reusch, JCR Scott-Moncrieff and EP Behrend, pp 258–314. Elsevier, St. Louis

Reusch CE and Salesov E (2019) Monitoring diabetic cats. In: *Feline Endocrinology*, ed. EC Feldman, F Fracassi and ME Peterson, pp 522–541. Edra Publishing, Milan

Reusch CE, Kley S, Casella M *et al.* (2006) Measurements of growth hormone and insulin-like growth factor 1 in cats with diabetes mellitus. *Veterinary Record* **158**, 195–200

Riederer A, Zini E, Salesov E *et al.* (2016) Effect of the glucagon-like peptide-1 analogue exenatide extended release in cats with newly diagnosed diabetes mellitus. *Journal of Veterinary Internal Medicine* **30**, 92–100

Roomp K and Rand J (2016) Rebound hyperglycaemia in diabetic cats. *Journal of Feline Medicine and Surgery* **18**, 587–596

Suh S and Kim JH (2015) Glycemic variability: how do we measure it and why is it important? *Diabetes & Metabolism Journal* **39**, 273–282

Surman S and Fleeman L (2013) Continuous glucose monitoring in small animals. *Veterinary Clinics of North America: Small Animal Practice* **43**, 381–406

Thompson A, Lathan P and Fleeman L (2015) Update on insulin treatment for dogs and cats: insulin dosing pens and more. *Veterinary Medicine: Research and Reports* **6**, 129–142

Umpierrez GE and Kovatchev BP (2018) Glycemic variability: how to measure and its clinical implication for type 2 diabetes. *American Journal of the Medical Sciences* **356**, 518–527

Vantyghem MC and Press M (2006) Management strategies for brittle diabetes. *Annales d'Endocrinologie* **67**, 287–296

Wormhoudt TL, Boss MK, Lunn K *et al.* (2018) Stereotactic radiation therapy for the treatment of functional pituitary adenomas associated with feline acromegaly. *Journal of Veterinary Internal Medicine* **32**, 1383–1391

Zini E, Salesov E, Dupont P *et al.* (2018) Glucose concentrations after insulin-induced hypoglycemia and glycemic variability in healthy and diabetic cats. *Journal of Veterinary Internal Medicine* **32**, 978–985

Chapter 26

Diabetic ketoacidosis and hyperglycaemic hyperosmolar syndrome

Amanda K. Boag

Introduction

Ketoacidosis occurs when there is excessive production and accumulation of ketones (or ketoacids), notably beta-hydroxybutyrate, acetoacetate and acetone, within the circulation. Beta-hydroxybutyrate and acetoacetate are produced by the breakdown of fats that occurs under certain conditions to meet cellular energy requirements (Figure 26.1). Although low concentrations of these acids may be found in healthy animals, when excessive amounts accumulate, they overwhelm the buffering capacity of the body and a metabolic acidosis and acidaemia develop. Large concentrations of ketoacids may be produced in a few selected pathophysiological scenarios but, in small animals, significant ketoacidosis is almost invariably associated with diabetes mellitus. A much less common, but equally severe, metabolic consequence of diabetes mellitus is hyperglycaemic hyperosmolar syndrome.

Diabetic ketoacidosis

Aetiology

Ketoacidosis is a severe and potentially life-threatening complication of diabetes mellitus and can occur in both cats and dogs. It may be present at the time of initial diagnosis of diabetes mellitus, but it can also develop in a previously diagnosed diabetic dog or cat that is already undergoing treatment.

Diabetes mellitus occurs when there is an absolute or relative deficiency of insulin (see Chapters 23 and 24). Insulin is required for the movement of glucose into cells, which provides energy for metabolic processes. When glucose is unable to move into cells, alternative emergency sources of energy such as fats are mobilized, resulting in the production of ketoacids. Insulin is also required for the metabolism of ketoacids. Consequently, there may be a low rate of ketone production in untreated uncomplicated diabetes mellitus. However, this is typically insufficient to cause acidaemia. The development of ketoacidosis generally requires a concurrent relative excess of glucagon or other 'counter-regulatory' hormones (cortisol, growth hormone and adrenaline (epinephrine)). Dysregulation of inflammatory cytokines may also play a role (O'Neill et al., 2012). Therefore, diabetic ketoacidosis (DKA) most commonly occurs when there is a second triggering condition or stressor that is superimposed on the underlying diabetes

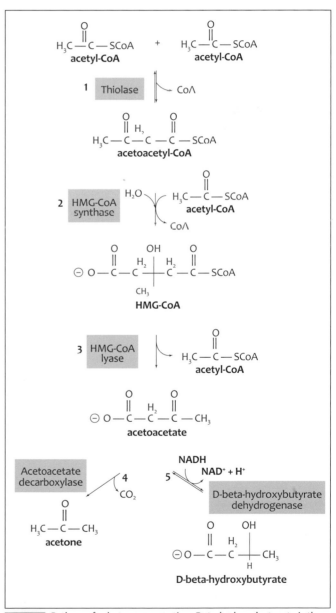

26.1 Pathway for ketone generation. Beta-hydroxybutyrate is the major ketone produced during diabetic ketoacidosis. It is converted back to acetoacetate as treatment is initiated. Concentrations of beta-hydroxybutyrate can be measured in serum. Urine dipsticks do not measure beta-hydroxybutyrate but rather measure acetone and acetoacetate. CoA = coenzyme A; HMG-CoA = beta-hydroxy-beta-methylglutaryl-CoA; NAD = nicotinamide adenine dinucleotide.

mellitus. Commonly identified triggering conditions are listed in Figure 26.2, although it should be noted that any concurrent disease or stressor could act as a trigger.

Diabetic ketoacidosis arises because there is an excess of glucagon concurrent with subnormal concentrations of endogenous insulin, and hence an increase in glucagon:insulin. High concentrations of glucagon tend to promote metabolism of free fatty acids and ketone production. Coupled with the subnormal concentrations of insulin, this leads to rapid ketogenesis. The low concentrations of insulin inhibit ketone metabolism and the rate of ketone production thus quickly overwhelms the body's excretory ability, with consequent accumulation of keto-acids and development of ketoacidosis and acidaemia.

Acidaemia has many negative physiological effects (Figure 26.3), including vomiting and anorexia. As DKA develops, affected animals tend to reduce their water intake and also undergo increased fluid and electrolyte loss through the gastrointestinal tract. This occurs alongside the obligatory polyuria seen in all diabetic animals due to the osmotic diuresis caused by glucosuria, now exacerbated by the presence of ketones in the urine. This leads to a rapid decline in intravascular volume status (development of shock), interstitial and intracellular dehydration, and mental deterioration.

Clinical features

Dogs and cats with DKA may present in a collapsed state with a relatively short (hours to several days) history of vomiting, inappetence and progressive lethargy (Figure 26.4). They may have previously been diagnosed with diabetes mellitus and already be undergoing insulin treatment, or they may not have had a prior diagnosis. In the former scenario, owners should be carefully questioned about any recent changes in the treatment regimen, including insulin storage, and the overall health of their pet. In the latter case, the owners are likely to report a more chronic history of polyuria and polydipsia (PU/PD), polyphagia and weight loss that may have been present for many months.

In consideration of the importance of triggering conditions, a thorough history should always be taken to identify any possible concurrent disorders or, at least, prioritize the differential diagnoses.

The initial physical examination should focus on the major body systems (cardiovascular, respiratory and neurological). Examination of the cardiovascular system usually reveals evidence of hypovolaemic shock, which may vary from mild to severe. Dependent on the severity of the shock, there may be varying degrees of tachycardia, with concomitant changes in pulse quality, mucous membrane colour and capillary refill time. Commonly, these cases also have an increased skin tent and dry mucous membranes, suggesting concurrent dehydration. They are usually tachypnoeic without being dyspnoeic, as the respiratory system acts to compensate for the metabolic acidosis. Auscultation of the lungs is typically unremarkable, although it should be carried out carefully as aspiration pneumonia is possible either as a consequence of the vomiting in a depressed animal or as the triggering condition. Animals are usually dull or obtunded but without specific neurological deficits. In many cases, the depression merely reflects the presence of shock but, occasionally, severe disturbances in electrolytes and osmolality may contribute to the mental depression. Other commonly identified findings on initial physical

Bacterial infections

• Any significant bacterial infection but especially consider:
  • Urinary tract infection[a][b]
  • Pneumonia
  • Pyometra
  • Pyoderma
  • Prostatitis

Inflammatory disease
• Pancreatitis[a][b]
Endocrinopathy
• Hypercortisolism[a]   • Hypothyroidism (dog)   • Hyperthyroidism (cat)   • Hypersomatotropism
Physiological endocrine changes
• Dioestrus phase of oestrous cycle
Miscellaneous
• Chronic kidney disease[b]   • Neoplasia[b]
Iatrogenic
• Administration of corticosteroids (including topical)

26.2 Conditions that may trigger diabetic ketoacidosis. [a] = Conditions identified as the most common concurrent diagnoses in a population of dogs presenting with diabetic ketoacidosis. [b] = Conditions identified as the most common concurrent diagnoses in a population of cats presenting with diabetic ketoacidosis. (Data from Bruskiewicz et al., 1997 and Hume et al., 2006)

Cardiovascular
• Reduction in cardiac output   • Reduction in cardiac contractility   • Reduced inotropic response to catecholamines   • Predisposition to dysrhythmia   • Arterial vasodilation and reduction in arterial blood pressure
Respiratory
• Tachypnoea and hyperpnoea as a compensatory mechanism (known as Kussmaul breathing in human patients)
Neurological
• Depression   • Coma
Miscellaneous
• Insulin resistance   • Anorexia   • Nausea   • Muscle weakness

26.3 Potential pathological effects of metabolic acidosis.

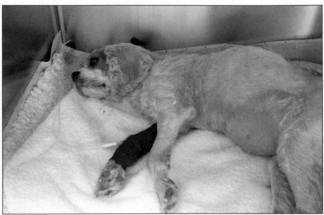

26.4 A dog with diabetic ketoacidosis. This dog was subsequently diagnosed with concurrent hypercortisolism.

examination include being overweight or underweight, cranial organomegaly and abdominal pain. Icterus is also commonly noted in cats as a consequence of concurrent disease (Bruskiewicz *et al.*, 1997).

Both DKA and its treatment are associated with a number of potentially life-threatening complications, including acute kidney injury, significant electrolyte disturbances and development of anaemia. It is important that the owner is questioned as to when the animal last urinated; an animal that has not been observed urinating for several hours, especially if previously polydipsic and polyuric, should be carefully monitored for production of urine, with placement of a urinary catheter if possible. Anuria or oliguria is a very concerning sign and should prompt urgent evaluation and potentially treatment of acute kidney injury; the detail of this is beyond the scope of this chapter (see the *BSAVA Manual of Canine and Feline Emergency and Critical Care*).

Diagnosis

Diabetic ketoacidosis should be considered in any dog or cat presenting with collapse and vomiting and with a history of PU/PD, regardless of whether there is a pre-existing diagnosis of diabetes mellitus. On initial examination, the presence of a 'pear-drop' ketone smell on the animal's breath Is highly suggestive of ketoacidosis, although not everyone is able to detect this. The index of suspicion is increased if initial in-house blood work reveals moderate to severe hyperglycaemia. Identification of metabolic acidosis on a venous blood gas and electrolyte panel further suggests DKA and necessitates assessment for ketones. Metabolic acidosis is identified when measured pH is low or just within the lower end of the reference interval and there is a negative base excess (below −4 mmol/l) or low bicarbonate concentration. The partial pressure of carbon dioxide (pCO_2) is often also low, reflecting respiratory compensation. An anion gap can also be calculated, using the formula:

$$anion\ gap = (Na^+ + K^+) - (HCO_3^- + Cl^-)$$

Diabetic ketoacidosis is typically associated with metabolic acidosis and a high anion gap. The differential diagnosis of metabolic acidosis is shown in Figure 26.5.

Diabetic ketoacidosis is confirmed when high concentrations of ketones are identified. The most relevant ketones in dogs and cats are beta-hydroxybutyrate, acetoacetate and acetone. It is important to note that the relative proportion of beta-hydroxybutyrate and acetoacetate produced is dependent upon the redox state of the liver mitochondria, which is typically reduced as a consequence of increased free fatty acid concentrations and acidosis (including both lactic acidosis secondary to shock and evolving ketoacidosis). This means that beta-hydroxybutyrate is produced in larger quantities than acetoacetate.

Beta-hydroxybutyrate concentrations are typically measured in whole blood or plasma. Traditional urine (either multi-purpose or ketone-specific) dipsticks utilize the nitroprusside reaction, which detects only acetone and acetoacetate. Historically, urinalysis was used as the principal means of confirming the diagnosis. However, serum or plasma may also be used with urine dipsticks if a sample of urine is not immediately obtainable (Brady *et al.*, 2003). This can be particularly useful in animals that do not have palpable bladders on presentation but where an urgent diagnosis is required. The serum obtained from a centrifuged packed cell volume (PCV) tube can be placed on the ketone square of a urine dipstick, with the same colour change as that expected for urine confirming the presence of ketonaemia. Point-of-care beta-hydroxybutyrate meters are also available and are widely used in human medicine; there are a small number of studies evaluating their use in small animals, but it is unclear at this time what clinical value they add to the diagnosis and treatment of DKA in cats and dogs (Di Tommaso *et al.*, 2009; Bresciani *et al.*, 2014; Weiß *et al.*, 2019). Serum can also be sent to external laboratories for more accurate assessment and characterization of ketone concentrations, although this is rarely necessary.

A possible reason accurate quantification of ketones might be considered is that it is theoretically possible to have a case of DKA that is negative for 'ketones' on serum or urine dipstick evaluation as only acetoacetate and acetone are measured. Practically, this seems to occur rarely; a more common scenario is for the ketonuria or ketonaemia to become more apparent during the first few hours or days of treatment as beta-hydroxybutyrate is metabolized to acetoacetate prior to its oxidation to acetyl coenzyme A.

Although the diagnosis of DKA is confirmed by the identification of hyperglycaemia with metabolic acidosis and ketonaemia or ketonuria, it is also strongly recommended that a number of other diagnostic tests are performed. These act either as an aid to identify the concurrent triggering condition or as a baseline to ensure stabilization and for early treatment. Diabetic ketoacidosis may be associated with a large number of potential metabolic disturbances, and success in the early phase of treatment depends as much, if not more, on consideration of these as on the primary underlying insulin abnormality. Recommended diagnostic tests are summarized in Figure 26.6 and described below.

Electrolytes

Diabetic ketoacidosis is associated with several concurrent electrolyte disturbances, some or all of which may need to be addressed during the initial treatment phase.

High anion gap (normochloraemic)
• Diabetic ketoacidosis*
• Lactic acidosis*
• Uraemic acidosis*
• Poisons (e.g. ethylene glycol, salicylates)

Normal anion gap (hyperchloraemic)
• Diarrhoea*
• Renal tubular acidosis
• Drugs (e.g. carbonic anhydrase inhibitors)
• Dilutional acidosis

26.5 Differential diagnosis of metabolic acidosis. * = Diagnoses encountered most frequently in clinical practice.

• Blood gas and electrolyte panel
• Haematology
• Biochemistry
• Urinalysis including urine culture and susceptibility
• Thoracic radiography
• Abdominal ultrasound
• Canine/feline pancreas-specific lipase

26.6 Diagnostic tests that should be considered when evaluating a dog or cat with diabetic ketoacidosis. Further endocrine testing (adrenocorticotropic hormone response test, thyroid function tests) should generally be delayed until the animal has been initially treated and is relatively stable.

Sodium: On presentation, the serum sodium concentration may be below, within or above the reference interval, reflecting the balance of free water *versus* electrolyte loss in the individual case. Hypernatraemia may be caused by a lack of water intake alongside free water loss in excess of electrolytes due to osmotic diuresis. However, hyponatraemia is most commonly due to large numbers of osmotically active particles (glucose and ketones) in the circulation. The increased serum glucose concentration has a significant osmotic effect and draws water into the vasculature, leading to dilution of serum sodium. It is expected that for every 1 mmol/l increase in glucose concentration, the serum sodium concentration is reduced by approximately 0.3–0.4 mmol/l. Hyponatraemia should thus correct with the correction of hyperglycaemia itself. Artefactual hyponatraemia may also occur when serum sodium is measured by a flame photometry methodology (used by some commercial laboratories) in the presence of hyperlipidaemia or hyperproteinaemia. In this situation, the true serum sodium concentration is likely to be within the reference interval. Measurement of serum sodium concentration is strongly recommended as, if abnormal, it may contribute to mental depression. In addition, knowledge of baseline sodium concentration is important as it is vital that the serum sodium concentration is not changed too rapidly during treatment by inappropriate fluid therapy (see 'Treatment', below).

Potassium: On presentation, the serum potassium concentration may be below, within or above the reference interval. Hyperkalaemia may occur secondary to a shift of intracellular potassium to an extracellular location due to acidosis and lack of insulin. It may also reflect reduced urine output secondary to oliguric or anuric acute kidney injury. Hypokalaemia is, however, more common and may be dramatic, especially once treatment is instituted. Regardless of the initial measured circulating values, the vast majority of affected animals exhibit whole body potassium depletion. This reflects the chronic increased renal loss of potassium that occurs because of glucose-induced osmotic diuresis exacerbated by ketonuria, combined with increased loss through the gastrointestinal tract (if there is vomiting or diarrhoea), inadequate intake (if inappetent) and hyperaldosteronism induced by volume contraction. Further, most dogs and cats will develop worsening hypokalaemia with treatment, as insulin administration and correction of acidosis cause potassium to move from the extracellular to the intracellular space. The potassium concentration should be closely monitored.

Chloride: Serum chloride concentration typically changes in the same way as sodium and does not need specific treatment.

Phosphate: Animals with DKA are at risk of hypophosphataemia. Urinary phosphate losses are increased, and gastrointestinal signs may contribute to this loss. Serum phosphate concentration may drop further with insulin treatment and correction of acidosis, as translocation from the extracellular to the intracellular space occurs.

Azotaemia

Animals with DKA are often azotaemic on presentation. Most commonly, this simply reflects a prerenal azotaemia in the face of hypovolaemia with an obligatory diuresis. Differential diagnoses, however, include both acute (oliguric or anuric) kidney injury and chronic kidney disease.

As mentioned above, it is vital to ascertain when the animal last urinated; if it has not been observed to urinate for several hours, this must be monitored very closely. Circulating urea and creatinine concentrations should also be closely monitored during early treatment to ensure resolution of azotaemia is as expected with fluid therapy. If urea and creatinine concentrations fail to decrease with appropriate fluid therapy, diagnostic tests to rule out other differentials should be considered.

Liver enzyme activities and bilirubin

Liver enzyme activities (alanine aminotransferase and alkaline phosphatase) are typically increased in diabetic cases, although such increases are more pronounced in dogs than in cats. Some of the increase may be attributable to the triggering condition (e.g. hypercortisolaemia) or secondary to the direct effects of either diabetes mellitus or the hypoperfusion that commonly accompanies DKA. Distinguishing the relative contribution of diabetes mellitus or other diseases to the increase in liver enzyme activities is difficult in DKA. However, the presence of hyperbilirubinaemia or other indices of hepatic dysfunction (hypoalbuminaemia, hyperammonaemia and markedly increased bile acid concentrations) may suggest the presence of concurrent pancreatitis or liver disease.

Haematology

The haematocrit may be below, within or above the reference interval on presentation. As it is likely to change as treatment progresses, close monitoring is warranted. Many cases have leucocytosis secondary to a mature neutrophilia on presentation. Identification of a high proportion of band cells or toxic change within the neutrophils should increase the index of suspicion for an infectious or severe inflammatory triggering condition and prompt thorough evaluation to identify any potential focus.

Urinalysis

Urinalysis should include measurement of specific gravity (SG), dipstick evaluation and sediment examination. Considering the high frequency of urinary tract infection in diabetic animals, it is strongly recommended that a urine sample is submitted for culture and susceptibility testing regardless of dipstick results; this should be considered mandatory if the sediment examination suggests infection. Urinary tract infections are a common trigger for the development of ketoacidosis.

In the presence of azotaemia, urine SG is typically used to evaluate whether the azotaemia is renal or prerenal in origin. In cases with DKA, however, this process is complicated by several factors:

* Regardless of intrinsic kidney function, diabetes mellitus leads to an osmotic diuresis that is enhanced by the presence of ketones in the urine; this could contribute to decreased urine SG
* The presence of large amounts of glucose and ketones in the urine means that the linear relationship between urine SG and urine osmolality is no longer valid and SG can no longer be taken to be a reflection of urine osmolality
* Isosthenuria is typically considered to be a urine SG of 1.008–1.012, but this is in the face of a normal serum osmolality. Significantly increased serum osmolality may occur in DKA and hence, in the absence of other factors, isosthenuria may actually be reflected by a higher SG.

The measured SG must be interpreted in the light of these considerations; it is not possible to be precise, but it is not uncommon for a case with DKA to have a prerenal azotaemia with a urine SG of 1.020 and marked (4+) glucosuria.

Tests for triggering disease

The list of potential triggering conditions for DKA is long (see Figure 26.2). Diagnostic tests should be tailored to the individual animal and based on prioritization of the differential list by signalment, history and physical examination findings. Imaging of both the thorax and abdomen should be strongly considered, as should additional diagnostic laboratory tests such as pancreas-specific lipase in appropriate cases. If infection is suspected, appropriate samples should be cultured.

Treatment

Fluid therapy and correction of electrolyte disturbances are the two most important components of initial therapy and can be started prior to a definitive diagnosis.

Disturbances in intravascular volume status, hydration and electrolytes are a key cause of morbidity in DKA and should be addressed as a priority. With appropriate use of fluid boluses, it should be possible to address hypovolaemia within 1–2 hours of admission. Insulin therapy should be started only once intravascular volume status is being addressed and is thought to be close to normal. Starting insulin therapy prior to addressing intravascular volume depletion increases the risk of rapid changes in glucose and electrolytes, and the development of metabolic complications.

Fluid therapy

Treatment for hypovolaemia: Stabilization can start prior to a confirmed diagnosis and involves the administration of one or more fluid boluses. The size and speed of administration of the bolus depend on the animal's clinical signs; suggested bolus doses for dogs are shown in Figure 26.7. In cats, it is harder to judge the severity of hypoperfusion on physical examination and high rates of fluids are less well tolerated; a more stepwise approach is recommended, with administration of incremental boluses of 5 ml/kg of isotonic crystalloid. The aim of the bolus dose is to normalize perfusion and its associated physical examination parameters. For this initial stage of fluid resuscitation, it is recommended that a balanced isotonic replacement crystalloid solution (e.g. Hartmann's solution) is used. The fluid chosen should be one with a sodium concentration close to the animal's serum sodium,

to avoid inducing rapid changes in serum sodium concentration. Unless the case is one of the more unusual cases presenting with significant hypernatraemia (Na$^+$ >165 mmol/l), 0.9% NaCl, although appropriate, may be less preferable as the high chloride content may contribute to an ongoing hyperchloraemic metabolic acidosis. As these animals invariably also suffer from interstitial and intracellular dehydration and movement of fluid from the vasculature into these compartments is also of value, there is no indication for colloids (artificial or natural).

Ongoing fluid therapy: Once any hypovolaemia is resolved, an ongoing fluid rate should be chosen. This should include consideration of:

- **Maintenance requirements** – considered to be approximately 2.5 ml/kg/h
- **Replacement of estimated hydration losses** – the animal's fluid deficit should be calculated based on the estimated percentage dehydration (fluid deficit in ml = % dehydration x bodyweight (kg) x 10). It is preferred to keep things simple and deliver this estimated fluid deficit evenly over the first 12–24 hours of treatment
- **Ongoing losses** – this should include consideration of any ongoing gastrointestinal losses (vomiting, diarrhoea) as well as the additional losses caused by the ongoing osmotic diuresis. This can be difficult to estimate; placement of a urinary catheter with accurate measurement of urine production is appropriate in some cases.

All three of the above components are estimates and hence the final fluid rate represents a judgement rather than a precise calculation. Monitoring the animal is therefore vitally important to ensure that the fluid rate is optimized as the disease and treatment progress.

Electrolytes

Sodium supplementation: Measured serum sodium concentration is variable in DKA at the time of diagnosis and will change as treatment progresses. The key challenge is to ensure that it does not change too rapidly. The maximum rate of change of sodium concentration should not exceed 12 mmol/l in 24 hours, particularly if the animal is hyponatraemic or hypernatraemic before instituting therapy. Rates of change greater than this put the animal at risk of either cerebral oedema (if the circulating sodium concentration decreases too rapidly) or cerebral dehydration (if the circulating sodium concentration increases too rapidly). Osmotic demyelination has also been suspected in a small number of cases where hyponatraemia has

Clinical parameter	Mild hypovolaemia	Moderate hypovolaemia	Severe hypovolaemia
Heart rate (bpm)	130–150	150–170	170–220
Mucous membrane colour	Normal	Pale pink	Grey, white or muddy
Capillary refill time	Rapid (<1 second)	Approximately normal (1–2 seconds)	Prolonged (>2 seconds) or absent
Pulse amplitude	Normal	Mild to moderate decrease	Severe decrease
Pulse duration	Mildly reduced	Moderately reduced	Severely reduced
Metatarsal pulse	Easily palpable	Just palpable	Absent
Suggested initial bolus dose of replacement isotonic crystalloid	5–10 ml/kg over 30 minutes to 1 hour	10–20 ml/kg over 30 minutes to 1 hour	20–30 ml/kg over 15 minutes to 1 hour

26.7 Clinical parameters of dogs with varying degrees of hypoperfusion and suggested initial bolus doses of isotonic replacement crystalloid.

undergone rapid correction. As discussed above, initial fluid resuscitation for hypovolaemia should use a crystalloid fluid with a sodium concentration similar to the animal's serum sodium concentration. Following this initial resuscitation, serum sodium concentration should be measured regularly and ongoing fluids chosen dependent on this monitoring. It is not uncommon for animals being treated for DKA to become hypernatraemic over the first few days of treatment. Along with resolution of any spurious hyponatraemia as the glucose concentration returns to normal, this occurs as ongoing fluid losses (notably large volumes of urine secondary to osmotic diuresis) contain more water than sodium. If the animal is drinking, it is likely to regain this free water loss voluntarily. However, if it is not drinking or unable to retain water taken in orally due to emesis, a hypotonic fluid (e.g. 0.45% NaCl) may be used as a component of the overall fluid therapy plan. In this case, free water deficit should ideally be calculated (see the *BSAVA Manual of Canine and Feline Emergency and Critical Care*).

Potassium supplementation: Dogs and cats with DKA may not be hypokalaemic on presentation but invariably become hypokalaemic once insulin treatment commences. Hypokalaemia may be severe enough to cause signs of muscular weakness and hypoventilation if unrecognized or untreated. Hypokalaemia should be treated by supplementation of parenteral fluids with an appropriate amount of potassium chloride (Figure 26.8) and/or potassium phosphate. Infusion rates should not exceed 0.5 mmol/kg/h except in exceptional circumstances. In an animal that requires high rates of potassium supplementation, it is recommended that a separate bag of parenteral fluids is made containing this high concentration of potassium. This should be administered through a separate intravenous line at the desired rate, thus minimizing the risk of changing the rate of potassium delivery if the ongoing fluid therapy plan changes. It should be noted that, even when maximal supplementation rates are used, hypokalaemia may persist for the first few days of treatment.

Acid–base balance

The use of sodium bicarbonate in the treatment of DKA is rarely necessary and is not routinely recommended. Generally, if appropriate fluid and insulin therapy is used, the acidosis will resolve and does not need specific treatment. The use of bicarbonate may also be associated with the development of complications such as paradoxical cerebrospinal fluid acidosis and hypernatraemia. It should not be used unless the acid–base and electrolyte status can be monitored frequently. There are, however, many negative effects of severe acidaemia (see Figure 26.3) and if the acidaemia is persistent despite appropriate treatment, bicarbonate could be considered. The dose can be calculated as:

$$NaHCO_3 \text{ (mmol/l)} = \text{base deficit} \times 0.3 \times \text{bodyweight (kg)}$$

One-third to one-half of this dose is administered by slow intravenous infusion over 15–30 minutes and the acid–base status is reassessed. The remainder can be added to the intravenous fluids and delivered over a period of hours if necessary. However, this is necessary only if there is a concurrent severe disease contributing to the acidaemia, such as acute kidney injury.

Insulin treatment

Insulin administration is an important part of the management of DKA. As discussed above (see 'Fluid therapy, electrolytes and acid–base balance'), it is not necessary to start insulin therapy immediately after diagnosis and a short period of time to start other stabilization measures is recommended. Equally, initiation of insulin therapy should not be excessively delayed. There is a longer time to resolution of DKA if insulin therapy is delayed beyond 6 hours after admission, although it has minimal impact on hospitalization time or complication rate (DiFazio and Fletcher, 2016). A short-acting insulin, such as neutral (soluble) insulin, must be used in the early stages of treatment. This has several advantages over the more familiar medium- and long-acting formulations, notably its rapid onset and short duration of action and the fact that it can be administered by numerous routes, including intravenously and intramuscularly.

Subcutaneous administration of insulin is not recommended during initial treatment of DKA as its absorption is unpredictable, especially if the animal is dehydrated. Use of neutral insulin by both the intravenous and intramuscular routes allows the clinician to titrate the delivery of insulin to the individual's needs. Both intravenous and intramuscular protocols can be used successfully, and an example of each protocol is described in Figure 26.9.

It is preferable to use the intravenous constant rate infusion (CRI) technique if suitable facilities are available, as this avoids the need for multiple intramuscular injections, which is of benefit from both a welfare and a staff

Serum potassium (mmol/l)	Potassium chloride to add to fluids (mmol/l)	Maximum recommended infusion rate for supplemented fluids (ml/kg/h)
3.5–5.0	20	25
3.0–3.5	30	18
2.5–3.0	40	12
2.0–2.5	60	8
<2.0	80	6

26.8 Guidelines for supplementation of intravenous fluids with potassium chloride for the treatment of hypokalaemia.

Intravenous constant rate infusion protocol

1. Make up insulin infusion solution in 0.9% NaCl to a concentration of 0.05 IU/ml by adding 25 IU insulin to a 500 ml bag or 2.5 IU to a 50 ml syringe
2. Infuse at 1 ml/kg/h until the blood glucose is <15 mmol/l. With normal insulin sensitivity, blood glucose typically decreases by 1–3 mmol/l/h
3. Once blood glucose is <15 mmol/l, reduce the insulin infusion rate to 0.5 ml/kg/h and add glucose supplementation of 2.5% or 5% to ongoing fluid therapy

NB: as insulin adsorbs to plastic, 50–100 ml of the insulin infusion fluid should be run through the infusion line prior to starting the infusion. The insulin infusion should be freshly made up daily

Intramuscular protocol

1. Begin treatment with an intramuscular injection of neutral insulin at 0.2 IU/kg
2. Blood glucose should be measured on an hourly basis, with repeat injections of 0.1 IU/kg as necessary until blood glucose is 8–15 mmol/l
3. If blood glucose is 8–15 mmol/l but ketoacidosis persists, intravenous fluids should be supplemented with 2.5% or 5% dextrose and intramuscular neutral insulin injections continued at 0.1 IU/kg every 1–4 hours

26.9 Examples of soluble insulin protocols to be used in the treatment of animals with diabetic ketoacidosis. Other intravenous protocols have been described (Macintire, 1993).

time management perspective. The disadvantage of the CRI technique is the need for a suitable infusion pump or syringe driver.

Regardless of which protocol is used, it is likely that the blood glucose concentration will fall towards the reference interval long before the ketoacidosis resolves. Hypoglycaemia must be avoided; therefore, it may be necessary to supplement the ongoing intravenous crystalloid fluids with 2.5% or 5% dextrose. This allows continued delivery of the insulin required for ketone metabolism whilst avoiding hypoglycaemia. Glucose supplementation should start once the blood glucose concentration falls below 15 mmol/l. It is recommended that the fluids are supplemented initially with 2.5% dextrose if the blood glucose concentration is between 10 and 15 mmol/l, and with 5% dextrose if it is below 10 mmol/l. This dextrose-supplemented fluid should then be delivered at maintenance rates alongside whatever other fluid is required to manage the overall fluid and electrolyte balance. The percentage glucose supplementation should be adjusted in light of further glucose measurements such that serum glucose is held at 10–15 mmol/l. Insulin administration may need to be temporarily discontinued if blood glucose decreases to <8 mmol/l.

More recently, newer rapid-acting insulin analogues have become available (e.g. insulin lispro, insulin aspart); these are genetically engineered modified versions of human insulin designed to have a more predictable and rapid onset of action following subcutaneous injection in humans. Their use has been explored in a small number of veterinary studies using similar doses to those described for regular insulin. Both intramuscular and intravenous CRI routes appear effective, but it is unclear at this point whether there is any real benefit to their use in small animals (Sears *et al.*, 2012; Walsh *et al.*, 2016; Malerba *et al.*, 2020a). Further, insulin glargine administered as an intermittent subcutaneous or intramuscular dose, with or without regular insulin, is emerging as a useful addition to the options available to treat DKA in cats. Relatively low numbers of cats have been involved in clinical studies to date, but the simplicity of the approach may make it a useful option to consider (Gallagher *et al.*, 2015; Zeugswetter *et al.*, 2021).

Other considerations

Hypophosphataemia: Hypophosphataemia is a common complication of DKA therapy and is often most marked 1–2 days following initiation of insulin therapy as phosphate translocates intracellularly. Severe hypophosphataemia may lead to haemolysis and can contribute to the development of anaemia. It is recommended that both PCV and serum phosphate concentration are monitored every 6–12 hours during the first 48–72 hours of treatment. Other reported negative consequences of hypophosphataemia include rhabdomyolysis, neurological dysfunction and changes in cardiac contractility, although these are rare. Phosphate supplementation is recommended if the serum phosphate concentration is below 0.35 mmol/l. The recommended phosphate supplementation rate is 0.01–0.03 mmol/kg/h for 6 hours, although on occasion this is found to be insufficient and doses up to 0.12 mmol/kg/h for 12–48 hours may be required. Regular monitoring of phosphate (every 4–12 hours) is necessary, especially if higher dose rates are used. The phosphate supplementation rate should be adjusted depending on response. Iatrogenic hyperphosphataemia and consequent hypocalcaemia should be avoided. As phosphate is generally supplied as potassium phosphate, the additional potassium supplementation should be taken into account when calculating the dose of potassium chloride supplementation required.

Hypomagnesaemia: Hypomagnesaemia is a recognized complication of DKA in human patients and is associated with clinical signs including refractory hypokalaemia, cardiac conduction disturbances and increased neuromuscular excitability. It has not been identified as a significant problem in dogs or cats with diabetes mellitus (Fincham *et al.*, 2004); however, normalization of serum magnesium concentrations is recommended if serum magnesium is low and any compatible clinical signs are present.

Antiemetics: Animals with DKA frequently exhibit profuse vomiting. Antiemetic medication containing maropitant or metoclopramide should be considered.

Nutrition: Dogs and cats with DKA are frequently inappetent on presentation. Appetite usually returns as the ketoacidosis is controlled. If appetite is poor for a prolonged period of time, alternative methods of nutritional supplementation, such as the use of feeding tubes, should be considered.

Treatment of triggering disease: As discussed above (see 'Aetiology'), DKA is frequently associated with a concurrent triggering disease process. Specific treatment for this disease may also be required. Depending on the diagnosis, specific treatment may form part of the initial treatment plan (e.g. antibiosis for an infectious trigger) or may be delayed until the initial DKA crisis is resolved and stabilization of the diabetes mellitus has started (e.g. trilostane treatment for hypercortisolism).

Monitoring

Animals with DKA are frequently critically ill on presentation, with the potential for the development of several complications during treatment. Frequent monitoring of both physical examination and clinicopathological parameters, with early intervention if complications develop, is vital for a successful outcome. The monitoring should be tailored to the individual case and should change with time. Suggested parameters to monitor are shown in Figure 26.10.

As regular repeat blood work and multiple intravenous infusions may be required, consideration should be given to placement of a central venous catheter at an early stage. These catheters have several advantages over peripheral catheters:

- Blood sampling can be performed in an easy and welfare-friendly way
- Multiple infusions can be given via the same catheter
- They can remain in place for 7–10 days
- They are generally well tolerated and easy to maintain.

Alternatively, continuous monitoring of interstitial glucose via a sensor placed in the subcutaneous space is potentially a less invasive method of monitoring and adjusting insulin therapy (see Chapter 25). Whilst ensuring calibration of these tools is important, they appear to work effectively in DKA cases and are likely to have a place in their management (Reineke *et al.*, 2010; Malerba *et al.*, 2020b). They do not, however, negate the need for blood sampling for monitoring the other parameters discussed above.

Physical examination
• Perfusion parameters (heart rate, mucous membrane colour, capillary refill time, pulse quality) initially every 1–2 hours, reducing to every 4–8 hours
• Respiratory rate and effort with thoracic auscultation every 4–8 hours
• Neurological status initially every 1–2 hours, reducing to every 4–8 hours
• Body temperature every 4–8 hours
• Bodyweight every 8–12 hours
Clinicopathological parameters
• Blood glucose concentration initially every hour, reducing to every 2–4 hours
• Packed cell volume/total solids initially every 2 hours, reducing to every 4–8 hours
• Venous blood gas and electrolyte panel initially every 2 hours, reducing to every 4–8 hours
• Urine or serum ketone dipstick evaluation every 12 hours
Other parameters
• Urine output initially every 2–4 hours; if a urinary catheter is in place, measure urine output and adjust fluids accordingly every 4 hours

26.10 Suggested parameters to be monitored in animals with diabetic ketoacidosis.

Transition to chronic therapy

The initial goal of treatment of DKA should be to manage the ketoacidotic crisis and any subsequent complications until the animal is ready for transition to a chronic management phase of their diabetes mellitus using medium- or long-acting insulin (see Chapters 23 and 24). The most important factor in deciding when to introduce subcutaneous insulin is the animal's clinical signs; it is introduced once the animal is well hydrated and eating and drinking without vomiting. Ideally, the acidosis should also have resolved and the animal should have negative or trace ketones on urine dipsticks. Dependent on the blood glucose concentration, the neutral insulin should be discontinued. Subcutaneous longer-acting insulin can be started within a few hours of that discontinuation, with the dose chosen dependent on the severity of the hyperglycaemia at that time. Care should be taken to avoid hypoglycaemia.

Prognosis

Once a diagnosis is made, informed owner consent for ongoing treatment is vital. Ketoacidotic cases can be very rewarding to treat, with approximately 70% of treated dogs and cats being discharged from the hospital (Bruskiewicz *et al.*, 1997; Hume *et al.*, 2006). However, the owners must be made aware at an early stage that treatment of the initial episode is likely to involve a moderate to prolonged period of hospitalization (average of 5–6 days), with concurrent financial and emotional impact. Any concurrent disorder may require specific treatment and could alter the prognosis; dogs with concurrent hypercortisolism have a poorer prognosis than those with uncomplicated diabetes mellitus. Dogs with a lower (more negative) base deficit also have a poorer prognosis. Furthermore, the primary underlying disease (diabetes mellitus) is chronic and requires lifelong treatment in all dogs and many cats (see Chapters 23 and 24). The owners must be prepared and willing to undertake this commitment.

Hyperglycaemic hyperosmolar syndrome

The development of hyperglycaemic hyperosmolar syndrome is much less common than DKA, but it is a similarly severe complication of diabetes mellitus. This syndrome is characterized by severe hyperglycaemia (>33 mmol/l) and a high serum osmolality (>325 mOsm/kg); pH and bicarbonate are typically within the reference interval or only mildly abnormal. There may or may not be ketones concurrently present, and co-existence of acidosis and hyperosmolarity. In one study of 1,250 diabetic dogs, only 25 dogs had a calculated high serum osmolality (>325 mOsm/kg) and were non-ketotic (Trotman *et al.*, 2013). As with DKA, these cases typically also have a concurrent disease process; the precise detail of how the pathogenesis of DKA differs from hyperosmolar syndrome is unknown. Worsening hyperosmolarity may also occur with ketosis. It is thought that lower amounts of lipolysis in these cases (either due to the particular hormonal picture in a given animal or the fact that hyperosmolarity decreases lipolysis) with consequent lower concentrations of free fatty acids mean ketone production is low, at least initially. Renal dysfunction is also more common in humans and dogs with hyperglycaemic hyperosmolar syndrome, and the reduction in glomerular filtration rate may be a factor in the development of severe hyperglycaemia.

History and physical examination features are generally similar to those for DKA, along with the recent onset of severe neurological signs (obtundation, stupor), although it appears that coma is uncommon in dogs and cats. Diagnosis is based on fulfilling the criteria mentioned above. Osmolality can rarely be measured in veterinary practice but may be calculated using the following formula:

Serum osmolality (mOsm/kg (calc)) = 2(Na⁺) (mmol/l) + urea (mmol/l) + glucose (mmol/l)

Treatment revolves around meticulous fluid, electrolyte and insulin therapy to resolve the hyperosmolarity and gain control of the underlying diabetes mellitus. Identification and treatment of any concurrent disease process are also important. Great care must be taken during the initial treatment period to ensure that hyperosmolarity does not resolve too quickly, as exacerbation of neurological signs may then occur. During hyperosmolarity, the brain generates substances known as idiogenic osmoles, which protect it from dehydration. As hyperosmolarity resolves, these idiogenic osmoles will be slowly eliminated; however, if the hyperosmolar state resolves quickly, these idiogenic osmoles act to pull water into the brain, leading to cerebral oedema.

Prognosis is guarded (Trotman *et al.*, 2013). In one study of cats, long-term (>2 month) survival was only 12% (Koenig *et al.*, 2004).

Summary

Diabetic ketoacidosis and, less commonly, hyperglycaemic hyperosmolar syndrome represent severe and potentially life-threatening complications of diabetes mellitus. Dogs and cats presenting with such complications require intensive 24-hour care in the initial stages of their management. The development of additional metabolic complications during the early part of treatment is common, and diligent monitoring is required to maximize the chance of a successful outcome.

References and further reading

Brady MA, Dennis JS and Wagner-Mann C (2003) Evaluating the use of plasma hematocrit samples to detect ketones utilizing urine dipstick colorimetric methodology in diabetic dogs and cats. *Journal of Veterinary Emergency and Critical Care* **13**, 1–6

Bresciani F, Pietra M, Corradini S, Giunti M and Fracassi F (2014) Accuracy of capillary blood 3-β-hydroxybutyrate determination for the detection and treatment of canine diabetic ketoacidosis. *Journal of Veterinary Science* **15**, 309–316

Bruskiewicz KA, Nelson RW, Feldman EC and Griffey SM (1997) Diabetic ketosis and ketoacidosis in cats: 42 cases (1980–1995). *Journal of the American Veterinary Medical Association* **211**, 188–192

DiFazio J and Fletcher DJ (2016) Retrospective comparison of early- versus late-insulin therapy regarding effect on time to resolution of diabetic ketosis and ketoacidosis in dogs and cats: 60 cases (2003–2013). *Journal of Veterinary Emergency and Critical Care* **26**, 108–115

Di Tommaso M, Aste G, Rocconi F, Guglielmini C and Boari A (2009) Evaluation of a portable meter to measure ketonemia and comparison with ketonuria for the diagnosis of canine diabetic ketoacidosis. *Journal of Veterinary Internal Medicine* **23**, 466–471

Fincham SC, Drobatz KJ, Gillespie TN and Hess RS (2004) Evaluation of plasma-ionized magnesium concentration in 122 dogs with diabetes mellitus: a retrospective study. *Journal of Veterinary Internal Medicine* **18**, 612–617

Gallagher BR, Mahony OM, Rozanski EA, Buob S and Freeman LM (2015) A pilot study comparing a protocol using intermittent administration of glargine and regular insulin to a continuous rate infusion of regular insulin in cats with naturally occurring diabetic ketoacidosis. *Journal of Veterinary Emergency and Critical Care* **25**, 234–239

Hess RS (2009) Diabetic ketoacidosis. In: *Small Animal Critical Care Medicine*, ed. DC Silverstein and K Hopper, pp. 288–291. Elsevier Saunders, St. Louis

Hume DZ, Drobatz KJ and Hess RS (2006) Outcome of dogs with diabetic ketoacidosis: 127 dogs (1993–2003). *Journal of Veterinary Internal Medicine* **20**, 547–555

King LG and Boag A (2018) *BSAVA Manual of Canine and Feline Emergency and Critical Care, 3rd edn.* BSAVA Publications, Gloucester

Koenig A, Drobatz KJ, Beale AB and King LG (2004) Hyperglycemic, hyperosmolar syndrome in feline diabetics: 17 cases (1995–2001). *Journal of Veterinary Emergency and Critical Care* **14**, 30–40

Macintire DK (1993) Treatment of diabetic ketoacidosis in dogs by continuous low-dose intravenous infusion of insulin. *Journal of the American Veterinary Medical Association* **202**, 1266–1272

Malerba E, Alessandrini F, Grossi G, Giunti M and Fracassi F (2020a) Efficacy and safety of intramuscular insulin lispro vs. continuous intravenous regular insulin for the treatment of dogs with diabetic ketoacidosis. *Frontiers in Veterinary Science* **7**, 559008

Malerba E, Cattani C, Del Baldo F et al. (2020b) Accuracy of a flash glucose monitoring system in dogs with diabetic ketoacidosis. *Journal of Veterinary Internal Medicine* **34**, 83–91

O'Neill S, Drobatz K, Satyaraj E and Hess R (2012) Evaluation of cytokines and hormones in dogs before and after treatment of diabetic ketoacidosis and in uncomplicated diabetes mellitus. *Veterinary Immunology and Immunopathology* **148**, 276–283

Reineke EL, Fletcher DJ, King LG and Drobatz KJ (2010) Accuracy of a continuous glucose monitoring system in dogs and cats with diabetic ketoacidosis. *Journal of Veterinary Emergency and Critical Care* **20**, 303–312

Sears KW, Drobatz KJ and Hess RS (2012) Use of lispro insulin for treatment of diabetic ketoacidosis in dogs. *Journal of Veterinary Emergency and Critical Care* **22**, 211–218

Trotman TK, Drobatz KJ and Hess RS (2013) Retrospective evaluation of hyperosmolar hyperglycemia in 66 dogs (1993–2008). *Journal of Veterinary Emergency and Critical Care* **23**, 557–564

Walsh ES, Drobatz KJ and Hess RS (2016) Use of intravenous insulin aspart for treatment of naturally occurring diabetic ketoacidosis in dogs. *Journal of Veterinary Emergency and Critical Care* **26**, 101–107

Weiß M, Schramm F and Dahlem D (2019) Comparative measurement using the GlucoMen®LX PLUS and a reference method to quantify β-hydroxybutyrate in dogs and cats. *Tierärztliche Praxis Ausgabe K: Kleintiere/Heimtiere* **47**, 419–424

Zeugswetter FK, Luckschander-Zeller N, Karlovits S and Rand JS (2021) Glargine versus regular insulin protocol in feline diabetic ketoacidosis. *Journal of Veterinary Emergency and Critical Care* **31**, 459–468

Chapter 27

Insulinoma

Johan P. Schoeman

Introduction

Insulinoma is an insulin-secreting tumour of pancreatic beta cells that results in excessive insulin secretion and clinical signs of hypoglycaemia. It is an uncommon condition in dogs and rare in cats. Insulinoma was first described in the dog in 1935 (Slye and Wells, 1935) and in the cat in 1974 (Priester, 1974). Subsequently, just over 300 canine cases have been described compared with 10 well documented feline cases. Consequently, this chapter will focus on canine insulinoma and conclude with a short section on the known comparative aspects of feline insulinoma.

Pathophysiology

Insulin-secreting pancreatic beta cells comprise approximately 70% of cells in the islets of Langerhans, which in turn comprise only approximately 1–2% of pancreatic volume. Most canine insulinomas are malignant. About 80% of insulinomas are solitary, located in one pancreatic lobe rather than in the body of the pancreas. Occasionally no discrete nodule is seen during gross pancreatic examination, in which case histology is required to identify the tumour.

The rate of detected metastatic lesions in dogs from different studies ranges from 45% to 64%. It is higher in studies based on post-mortem examination *versus* studies using samples obtained surgically. Clinical staging of pancreatic tumours is defined in Figure 27.1. Most dogs with insulinoma have stage II or III disease, and the most common sites of metastases are regional lymph nodes and the liver. Metastatic disease has an unlimited distribution (Moore *et al.*, 2002). Although the aetiology of insulinoma is not known, local growth hormone (GH) production that is not associated with increased plasma concentrations has been documented in primary and metastatic canine insulinoma, possibly promoting islet cell proliferation via paracrine or autocrine mechanisms (Robben *et al.*, 2002).

Neoplastic proliferation of pancreatic beta cells causes autonomous and excessive secretion of insulin with resultant episodes of hypoglycaemia. The most important compensatory mechanisms for hypoglycaemia are inhibition of insulin secretion and stimulation of counter-regulatory hormone secretion.

Glucose enters pancreatic beta cells and causes closure of ATP-sensitive K^+ channels. Closure of these channels

Stage of disease	Primary tumour	Regional lymph node involvement	Distant metastases
Stage I	T1	N0	M0
Stage II	T1	N1	M0
Stage III	T1	N0/N1	M1

27.1 World Health Organization clinical staging of insulinoma. T1 = Primary tumour present; N0 = No evidence of lymph node involvement; N1 = Lymph node involvement detected; M0 = No evidence of distant metastases; M1 = Distant metastases detected.

causes a build-up of K^+ ions inside the cell and opening of voltage-sensitive Ca^{2+} channels. The resultant increased cytoplasmic Ca^{2+} leads to insulin exocytosis into the extracellular environment and, ultimately, the blood in equimolar amounts to C-peptide (a component of the proinsulin molecule that is cleaved prior to co-secretion with insulin).

In healthy animals, insulin secretion is completely inhibited when the blood glucose concentration is less than 4.4 mmol/l. However, insulin secretion from neoplastic beta cells is independent of blood glucose concentration and persists despite low blood glucose concentrations. As a consequence, one of the biochemical hallmarks of insulinoma is high or reference interval circulating insulin concentrations despite low blood glucose concentrations. The four counter-regulatory hormones secreted in response to hypoglycaemia are glucagon, catecholamines, GH and glucocorticoids. Of these, glucagon and catecholamines are the predominant drivers of the short-term responses to low blood glucose concentrations (see Chapter 22).

Clinical features

Signalment

The mean age of dogs with insulinoma is 9 years, with a range of 3–15 years. Although any breed of dog may develop insulinoma, it has been reported most commonly in medium- to large-breed dogs. Breeds reported to be at increased risk include Boxers, German Shepherd Dogs, Golden Retrievers, Labrador Retrievers, Irish Setters, Standard Poodles, Collies, Springer Spaniels, Fox Terriers, West Highland White Terriers and Jack Russell Terriers (Coss *et al.*, 2021; Ryan *et al.*, 2021). There is no apparent sex predilection for the disease.

Clinical signs

Glucose is the single most important source of energy for the brain. Brain function is dependent on a continuous glucose supply because both carbohydrate storage and the brain's ability to utilize other fuels are limited (see Chapter 22). Clinical signs are thus usually due to the effect of episodes of hypoglycaemia on the central nervous system (neuroglycopenia) or to hypoglycaemia-induced release of catecholamines. Clinical signs attributable to neuroglycopenia include mental dullness, disorientation, weakness, proprioceptive ataxia, visual disturbances, collapse and focal or generalized seizures. Sometimes the signs might resemble those of a paroxysmal dyskinesia (Ryan et al., 2021). Clinical signs related to excess catecholamine release and stimulation of the sympathetic nervous system include hunger, nervousness and tremors.

Severity of clinical signs is partly correlated with the blood glucose nadir. Severe hypoglycaemia may ultimately result in coma and death. However, clinical signs may also be related to the duration and the rate at which hypoglycaemia develops because gradual decreases in blood glucose concentration are less likely to stimulate catecholamine secretion. Insulin secretion and clinical signs are typically episodic and the secretion of counter-regulatory hormones tends to increase the blood glucose concentration, transiently resolving the neuroglycopenic signs. Feeding can also alleviate clinical signs if the blood glucose concentration is restored to normal. However, feeding may also exacerbate clinical signs by stimulating further insulin secretion. Moreover, fasting, exercise and excitement worsen the clinical signs by decreasing the blood glucose concentration or increasing sympathetic stimulation.

The clinical signs of canine insulinoma are summarized in Figure 27.2. Although most dogs have more than one of these clinical signs, some dogs have none. Some cases may gain weight because of the anabolic effects of insulin. Postictal changes may be apparent if a seizure occurred

Clinical sign	Number of dogs (%)
Generalized weakness	128 (41)
Seizure	124 (39)
Collapse	103 (33)
Ataxia	61 (19)
Disorientation/bizarre behaviour	51 (16)
Pelvic limb weakness	43 (14)
Shaking/trembling/muscle twitching	40 (13)
Exercise intolerance	37 (12)
Focal facial seizures/muscle fasciculations	30 (10)
Polyphagia	20 (6)
Polyuria and polydipsia	20 (6)
Stupor/lethargy	12 (4)
Diarrhoea	8 (3)
Obesity or weight gain	6 (2)
Blindness	6 (2)
Anorexia	6 (2)
Head tilt	2 (1)
Nervousness	2 (1)

27.2 Clinical signs of canine insulinoma reported in 314 dogs from several studies.
(Kruth et al., 1982; Leifer et al., 1986; Dunn et al., 1993; Trifonidou et al., 1998; Tobin et al., 1999; Moore et al., 2002; Ryan et al., 2021)

quite recently. A peripheral polyneuropathy characterized by posterior paresis or tetraparesis and decreased or absent appendicular reflexes has been described in dogs with insulinoma (Ryan et al., 2021). The aetiology of this insulinoma-associated peripheral neuropathy has not been firmly established, but it may be a paraneoplastic immune-mediated disorder (Van Ham et al., 1997).

Diagnosis

Differential diagnoses

The causes of hypoglycaemia may be broadly separated into those caused by decreased glucose production, those associated with excessive glucose utilization or a combination thereof, although in some cases the exact mechanism is unknown. The differential diagnoses for hypoglycaemia and the diagnostic approach are detailed in Chapter 22.

Clinicopathological abnormalities

Clinical suspicion of insulinoma begins with the documentation of appropriate clinical signs, hypoglycaemia (blood glucose concentration less than approximately 3.5 mmol/l) and concurrent normo- or hyperinsulinaemia (serum insulin concentrations within or above the reference interval) (Figure 27.3). It is essential that the insulin assay is validated for use in the dog. A pancreatic mass may be identified with imaging studies and this strengthens the suspicion for insulinoma. The diagnosis of insulinoma is ultimately confirmed with histological examination and immunohistochemical staining of a pancreatic mass.

Aside from the hypoglycaemia observed in most dogs, the haematology, serum biochemistry and urinalysis are usually unremarkable. Mild hypokalaemia and increased alkaline phosphatase and/or alanine aminotransferase (ALT) activities have been documented (Harris et al., 2020). Although hypoglycaemia is observed in randomly obtained blood samples from the vast majority of dogs with insulinoma, especially if repeated, some are euglycaemic at the time of presentation (Leifer et al., 1986; Mellanby and Herrtage, 2002). When a dog suspected of insulinoma is euglycaemic, it should be fasted and closely

Insulin concentration	Interpretation and further action	Possible alternative diagnosis
Insulin above reference interval (>140 pmol/l)	Insulinoma	Nesidioblastosis
Insulin high end of reference interval (70–140 pmol/l)	Insulinoma	Nesidioblastosis
Insulin lower end of reference interval (35–70 pmol/l)	Equivocal; repeat insulin concentration measurement on another day; consider measuring fructosamine	Nesidioblastosis
Insulin undetectable (<35 pmol/l)	Unlikely to be insulinoma	Pancreatic or extra-pancreatic tumours secreting insulin-like growth factors

27.3 Interpretation of insulin values in hypoglycaemic dogs (glucose concentration <3.5 mmol/l), based on a reference interval of 35–140 pmol/l.

monitored for hypoglycaemia while blood glucose concentrations are measured every 30–60 minutes. Portable blood glucose meters are usually adequate for this purpose. In most dogs with insulinoma, hypoglycaemia (blood glucose concentration <3.5 mmol/l) develops within 12 hours of the previous meal.

When hypoglycaemia is documented, serum for the measurement of insulin concentration should be submitted from the same sample. However, a limited number of dogs with insulinoma do not exhibit hypoglycaemia, even with repeated measurements or after a prolonged fast of 48–72 hours (Leifer et al., 1986). Low fructosamine concentration has been used to strengthen the clinical suspicion of insulinoma in such dogs (Mellanby and Herrtage, 2002). Glycated haemoglobin (HbA1c) concentration is low in some, but not all, dogs with insulinoma (Davison et al., 2002). Repetition of serum insulin measurements at a reputable laboratory may also aid diagnosis.

Other tests have been described for the diagnosis of insulinoma in euglycaemic dogs with equivocal serum insulin concentrations. Of these, insulin:glucose and glucose:insulin are not recommended because of their low sensitivity, and the amended insulin:glucose is not recommended because of its low specificity. Additional tolerance and stimulation tests have been described, but are also not advocated because of their questionable usefulness, unnecessary complexity and/or potentially fatal side effects due to hypoglycaemia.

Diagnostic imaging
Radiography and ultrasonography

Most dogs with insulinoma appear unremarkable on abdominal and thoracic radiography; most insulinomas are quite small (<4 cm) and isoechoic on ultrasonographic examination when compared with surrounding pancreatic parenchyma. Metastases most commonly occur in the liver and regional pancreatic lymph nodes. Abdominal ultrasonography may be helpful in supporting the clinical suspicion of a pancreatic mass and metastases, with a reported sensitivity of approximately 50–75% (Lamb et al., 1995) (Figure 27.4). Nonetheless, a negative ultrasonographic examination does not rule either out. Conversely, pancreatic nodules are not specific for insulinoma and may represent changes due to chronic pancreatitis, adenomas, adenocarcinomas, endocrine-active tumours of other

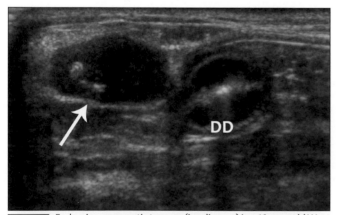

27.4 Endocrine pancreatic tumour (insulinoma) in a 16-year-old West Highland White Terrier presented with a history of trembling, seizures and hypoglycaemia. Transverse image of the right cranial abdomen demonstrating a hypoechoic nodule, approximately 8 mm in diameter, with a few hyperechoic shadowing foci associated with the right lobe of the pancreas (arrowed). DD = descending duodenum.
(Reproduced from the BSAVA Manual of Canine and Feline Ultrasonography)

cell types (gastrinoma, somatostatinoma), abscesses and cysts. Contrast-enhanced ultrasonography has been successfully employed in discriminating insulinoma from pancreatic carcinoma (Vanderperren et al., 2014; Nakamura et al., 2015).

Advanced diagnostic imaging

High-quality, dual-phase, thin-section multidetector computed tomography (CT) of the pancreas is effective in identifying a pancreatic mass in most affected humans (Tucker et al., 2006). The use of CT has been reported in a sizeable number of dogs with insulinoma. Contrast-enhanced CT proved more sensitive than ultrasonography at detecting insulinomas (Buishand et al., 2018) and the majority of cases demonstrated hyperattenuation of the pancreatic and metastatic masses during the arterial phase of the study (Coss et al., 2021). Overall arterial phase sensitivity was 94% for detecting insulinomas; nevertheless, non-contrast CT examinations still have some merit, because a high proportion of lesions deformed the shape of the pancreas, rendering them visible on pre-contrast views (Coss et al., 2021).

Treatment
Acute hypoglycaemia

During an acute hypoglycaemic crisis, 50% glucose, diluted to a 25% solution in 0.9% sodium chloride, should be given as a slow intravenous bolus of 1 ml/kg. The bolus should be followed with a constant rate infusion (CRI) of 2.5–5% glucose. The lowest amount of glucose deemed necessary to control clinical signs must be administered because glucose stimulates insulin secretion. This may cause rebound hypoglycaemia and a subsequent vicious cycle, which may be difficult to break. Glucose administration should be discontinued when clinical signs resolve, even if mild hypoglycaemia persists.

In most dogs, neuroglycopenia will resolve with administration of glucose, even without complete resolution of the hypoglycaemia. However, some animals fail to respond clinically to glucose administration alone. In such situations, intravenous dexamethasone (0.1 mg/kg twice a day) may be considered. Glucagon administration may also be helpful, because glucagon increases blood glucose concentration by promoting glycogenolysis and gluconeogenesis. While doses vary, a CRI of glucagon (approximately 10 (range 5–25) ng/kg/min with or without concurrent 2.5–5% glucose) may be successful in increasing glucose concentrations and in resolving clinical signs relatively rapidly (<1 hour in most cases). However, like glucose, glucagon also increases insulin secretion, and rebound hypoglycaemia is always possible but appears to be uncommon when these more conservative doses are used (Harris et al., 2020).

Some cases may be refractory to glucose, glucocorticoids and glucagon, and this may be due to persistently high insulin secretion and/or glycogen depletion because of chronic hyperinsulinism. Additionally, prolonged and profound hypoglycaemia may result in a series of changes that ultimately culminate in irreversible brain damage. Continued neurological signs despite normalization of blood glucose concentration are suggestive. If this is considered possible, ancillary treatment for seizures and cerebral oedema may be implemented but the prognosis is ultimately poor (see the BSAVA Manual of Canine and Feline Neurology).

Long-term treatment
Surgery

The long-term treatment of choice for insulinoma is surgical resection of both the tumour and any obvious metastases. Most tumours are readily discernible or palpable by the surgeon (Figure 27.5). Two dogs have reportedly undergone successful resection of tumour thrombi that had extended into their pancreaticoduodenal veins (Hambrook and Kudnig, 2012). In addition, one dog had a prolonged disease-free interval after primary tumour resection despite the presence of metastatic lesions (Rychel et al., 2013). Surgical exploration and biopsy of a pancreatic mass can confirm a diagnosis and may help in estimating survival time. When postoperative hyperglycaemia develops, it is usually transient and resolves once the normal beta cells, which have been suppressed by autonomous insulin secretion from neoplastic cells, regain function. Approximately 10–20% of dogs with insulinoma develop diabetes mellitus after tumour removal and require exogenous insulin for an unpredictable length of time (Del Busto et al., 2020). Other postoperative complications include pancreatitis, diabetic ketoacidosis, delayed wound healing, cardiac arrhythmias or arrest, haemorrhage, sepsis and leucopenia.

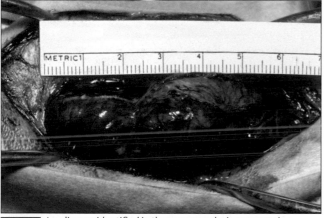

27.5 Insulinoma identified in the pancreas during surgery in a 10-year-old neutered male German Shorthaired Pointer with hypoglycaemia.
(Reproduced from the BSAVA Manual of Canine and Feline Oncology)

Medical therapy

This review of medical therapy is limited to agents that have been reported in dogs with naturally occurring insulinoma. Medical treatment is indicated prior to surgery, postoperatively if needed and in dogs in which surgery is not performed. Medical therapy can be divided into cytotoxic treatment directed at destroying insulin-secreting beta cells and treatment aimed at relieving hypoglycaemia.

Cytotoxic therapy: **Toceranib phosphate** (Palladia), a veterinary targeted multi-receptor tyrosine kinase inhibitor that has shown benefit in a range of solid-type tumours in dogs, has recently been evaluated for the treatment of canine insulinoma (Sheppard-Olivares et al., 2021). Thirty dogs were treated orally using an average dose of 2.7 mg/kg (range 2–3.3 mg/kg). Most dogs were given this dose on a Monday, Wednesday, Friday regimen and 67% of dogs with measurable disease experienced either complete remission, partial response or stable disease for a minimum of 10 weeks. The overall median survival time was 656 days. Larger dogs were at increased risk for disease

progression and the most common adverse events were mild gastrointestinal toxicities. It was concluded that toceranib afforded these dogs clinical benefit whilst causing minimal adverse events.

Streptozotocin, a nitrosourea antibiotic, selectively destroys beta cells in pancreatic or metastatic locations. The drug is nephrotoxic in dogs, but diuresis with saline will decrease drug contact time with renal tubular epithelial cells and reduces the risk of nephrotoxicity. In one study, 17 dogs, most of which underwent surgery with incomplete resection of gross lesions, were treated with intravenous 0.9% sodium chloride (18 ml/kg/h) for 3 hours prior to, 2 hours during and 2 hours following streptozotocin infusion. Streptozotocin (500 mg/m²) was given every 3 weeks for five treatments. Intramuscular butorphanol (0.4 mg/kg) was administered as an antiemetic immediately following streptozotocin therapy, but vomiting was still observed in approximately one-third of treatments. Other side effects included diabetes mellitus, transient hypoglycaemia and seizures, transient hyperglycaemia, transient increases in ALT activity, azotaemia, mild thrombocytopenia and mild neutropenia. The median duration of euglycaemia in streptozotocin-treated dogs was between 163 and 196 days. This is not significantly different from the duration of euglycaemia in dogs that have been treated with other medications (Moore et al., 2002; Northrup et al., 2013).

The adverse event profile of streptozotocin appears less tolerable than that of toceranib and further studies are necessary before streptozotocin therapy can be recommended with confidence.

Relieving hypoglycaemia: The main modes of relieving hypoglycaemia include dietary modification and treatment with prednisolone, diazoxide or synthetic somatostatin. Small, frequent meals (every 4–6 hours) of a diet high in proteins, fats and complex carbohydrates are recommended. Such a dietary profile is used for many prescription diets for diabetes mellitus. Simple sugars (present in soft moist dog foods) should be avoided.

Prednisolone, the least expensive and most commonly used drug, increases the blood glucose concentration by increasing gluconeogenesis and glucose 6-phosphatase activity, while decreasing blood glucose uptake into tissue and stimulating glucagon secretion. Prednisolone is given at an initial oral dose of approximately 0.2 mg/kg/day, increasing to 0.5 mg/kg/day as needed. Doses can be gradually increased as needed, usually until the drug is no longer perceived to be decreasing seizure episodes or in cases where intolerable signs of iatrogenic hypercortisolism (polyuria and polydipsia) develop. Prednisolone at higher doses of 1–2 mg/kg/day may also resolve the polyneuropathy in some cases (Van Ham et al., 1997).

Diazoxide is a benzothiadiazine derivative that inhibits closure of pancreatic beta cell ATP-dependent K⁺ channels, preventing beta cell depolarization and inhibiting opening of voltage-dependent Ca²⁺ channels. The resultant decreased Ca²⁺ influx causes decreased exocytosis of insulin-containing secretory vesicles. Diazoxide also increases the blood glucose concentration by increasing glycogenolysis and gluconeogenesis and inhibiting tissue uptake of glucose (Alemzadeh and Holshouser, 1999). Approximately 70% of dogs initially respond to 10–40 mg/kg/day of oral diazoxide divided into two or three daily doses. As with prednisolone, therapy should begin with the lowest dose of diazoxide and this should be gradually increased if required. Side effects in dogs are uncommon and include ptyalism, vomiting and anorexia. In some countries, diazoxide is of limited availability or high expense.

Octreotide is a long-acting synthetic somatostatin analogue that inhibits insulin secretion through its binding affinity to any of five somatostatin receptor subtypes present in insulin-secreting tumours. Dogs show a variable response to octreotide, likely because octreotide variably inhibits glucagon and GH secretion (Robben *et al.*, 1997). If the suppression of glucagon and GH secretion is of greater magnitude and duration than the suppression of insulin secretion, octreotide may worsen hypoglycaemia. While some canine insulinomas may lack somatostatin receptors, 12 dogs with insulinoma treated with a single subcutaneous octreotide dose of 50 µg/dog (median weight 23 kg) had decreases in plasma insulin concentration, yet the concentrations of glucagon, GH and adrenocorticotropic hormone were not changed (Robben *et al.*, 2006). These findings warrant studies using long-acting octreotide in dogs with insulinoma. No adverse side effects were reported with the use of octreotide. Side effects in humans include mild pain at the injection site (which is lessened if the preparation is warmed before administration), nausea, vomiting, abdominal pain, constipation or steatorrhea.

Prognosis

The median survival time of dogs that underwent partial pancreatectomy reported in several older studies was 12–14 months, with a range of 0 days to 5 years. However, a smaller, more recent study reported a median survival time of 26 months (Polton *et al.*, 2007), whilst the two latest studies (which had a combined total of 165 dogs) both demonstrated almost identical median survival times of approximately 20 months after surgery (Cleland *et al.*, 2021; Ryan *et al.*, 2021). It is postulated that earlier recognition and perhaps more radical surgery and better postoperative care account for this improved survival. Moreover, dogs with clinical stage I disease have a significantly longer disease-free interval, whilst those with persistent postoperative hypoglycaemia have a poorer prognosis (Del Busto *et al.*, 2020; Cleland *et al.*, 2021).

It was also demonstrated that tumour size and mitotic rate, as depicted by the Ki67 index (a proliferation marker), act as significant prognostic markers in canine insulinoma (Buishand *et al.*, 2010).

Feline insulinoma

To date, only approximately 16 cases of feline pancreatic islet cell tumours have been reported in cats, of which 10 cases have had detailed signalment, clinical, biochemical and/or histopathological descriptions (Schoeman, 2019). Of the 10 well described insulinoma cases, three were Siamese cats, four were Domestic Shorthaired cats, two were Domestic Longhaired cats and one was a Maine Coon. The cats were between 9 and 17 years old; eight were male and two were female.

Clinical signs associated with feline insulinoma are wide-ranging and depend on the severity of the hypoglycaemia and other concomitant disorders, but include seizures, weight loss, anorexia, episodic weakness/falling, limb and facial twitching, mental dullness, lethargy, hypothermia and bradycardia.

A diagnosis of feline insulinoma is made upon documenting hypoglycaemia in concert with inappropriate reference interval or increased serum insulin concentrations (measured using an assay validated for use in cats), followed by abdominal ultrasonography or exploratory laparotomy to identify the mass in the pancreas. In the reported cases, the left pancreatic lobe was involved in six cases, the right lobe in three cases and the angle of the pancreas in one case. Tumour size varied from 0.4 to 3 cm. The pancreatic masses in the three most recent cases have all been identified on abdominal ultrasonography, likely due to improvements in ultrasound technology and operator expertise (Schaub and Wigger, 2013; Cervone *et al.*, 2019; Gifford *et al.*, 2020).

As with dogs, prompt surgical excision is the mainstay of treatment. Cats should be monitored for transient postoperative diabetes mellitus, which may occur due to suppressed insulin secretion from the remaining atrophied pancreatic beta cells. If surgery is declined and medical management is chosen, small frequent meals and systemic glucocorticoid therapy of prednisolone at 0.5 mg/kg q12h are recommended. The prognosis depends on the stage at diagnosis, the degree of malignancy of the tumour and the success of surgical excision. Enhanced glucose sensitivity and insulin secretion, through the over-expression of glucokinase 1 by neoplastic beta cells, might also explain the varying prognosis in this disease (Jackson *et al.*, 2009). Earlier cases had survival times as short as one day to approximately 18 months, yet two more recent cases were both alive 32 months after surgery (Greene and Bright, 2008; Schaub and Wigger, 2013).

References and further reading

Alemzadeh R and Holshouser S (1999) Effect of diazoxide on brain capillary insulin receptor binding and food intake in hyperphagic obese Zucker rats. *Endocrinology* **140**, 3197–3202

Barr F and Gaschen L (2011) *BSAVA Manual of Canine and Feline Ultrasonography*. BSAVA Publications, Gloucester

Buishand FO, Kik M and Kirpensteijn J (2010) Evaluation of clinico-pathological criteria and the Ki67 index as prognostic indicators in canine insulinoma. *Veterinary Journal* **185**, 62–67

Buishand FO, Grosso FRV, Kirpensteijn J and van Nimwegen SA (2018) Utility of contrast-enhanced computed tomography in the evaluation of canine insulinoma location. *Veterinary Quarterly* **38**, 53–62

Cervone M, Harel M, Ségard-Weisse E and Krafft E (2019) Use of contrast-enhanced ultrasonography for the detection of a feline insulinoma. *Journal of Feline Medicine and Surgery Open Reports* **5**, 2055116919876140

Cleland NT, Morton J and Delisser PJ (2021) Outcome after surgical management of canine insulinoma in 49 cases. *Veterinary and Comparative Oncology* **19**, 428–441

Coss P, Gilman O, Warren-Smith C and Major AC (2021) The appearance of canine insulinoma on dual phase computed tomographic angiography. *Journal of Small Animal Practice* **62**, 540–546

Davison LJ, Podd SL, Ristic JME *et al.* (2002) Evaluation of two point-of-care analysers for measurement of fructosamine or haemoglobin A1c in dogs. *Journal of Small Animal Practice* **43**, 526–532

Del Busto I, German AJ, Treggiari E *et al.* (2020) Incidence of postoperative complications and outcome of 48 dogs undergoing surgical management of insulinoma. *Journal of Veterinary Internal Medicine* **34**, 1135–1143

Dobson JM and Lascelles BDX (2011) *BSAVA Manual of Canine and Feline Oncology, 3rd edn.* BSAVA Publications, Gloucester

Dunn J, Bostock D, Herrtage M, Jackson K and Walker M (1993) Insulin-secreting tumours of the canine pancreas: Clinical and pathological features of 11 cases. *Journal of Small Animal Practice* **34**, 325–331

Gifford CH, Morris AP, Kenney KJ and Estep JS (2020) Diagnosis of insulinoma in a Maine Coon cat. *Journal of Feline Medicine and Surgery Open Reports* **6**, 2055116919894782

Greene SN and Bright RM (2008) Insulinoma in a cat. *Journal of Small Animal Practice* **49**, 38–40

Hambrook LE and Kudnig ST (2012) Tumor thrombus formation in two dogs with insulinomas. *Journal of the American Veterinary Medical Association* **241**, 1065–1069

Harris ME, Weatherton L and Bloch CP (2020) Glucagon therapy in canines with insulinoma: a restrospective descriptive study of 11 dogs. *Canadian Veterinary Journal* **61**, 737–742

Jackson TC, Debey B, Lindbloom-Hawley S, Jones BT and Schermerhorn T (2009) Cellular and molecular characterization of a feline insulinoma. *Journal of Veterinary Internal Medicine* **23**, 383–387

Kruth SA, Feldman EC and Kennedy PC (1982) Insulin-secreting islet cell tumors: establishing a diagnosis and the clinical course for 25 dogs. *Journal of the American Veterinary Association* **181**, 54–58

Lamb CR, Simpson KW, Boswood A and Matthewman LA (1995) Ultrasonography of pancreatic neoplasia in the dog: a retrospective review of 16 cases. *Veterinary Record* **137**, 65–68

Leifer CE, Peterson ME and Matus RE (1986) Insulin-secreting tumor: diagnosis and medical and surgical management in 55 dogs. *Journal of the American Veterinary Medical Association* **188**, 60–64

Mellanby RJ and Herrtage ME (2002) Insulinoma in a normoglycaemic dog with low serum fructosamine. *Journal of Small Animal Practice* **43**, 506–508

Moore AS, Nelson RW, Henry CJ et al. (2002) Streptozocin for treatment of pancreatic islet cell tumors in dogs: 17 cases (1989–1999). *Journal of the American Veterinary Medical Association* **221**, 811–818

Nakamura K, Lim SY, Ochiai K et al. (2015) Contrast-enhanced ultrasonographic findings in three dogs with pancreatic insulinoma. *Veterinary Radiology and Ultrasound* **56**, 55–62

Northrup NC, Rassnick KM, Gieger TL et al. (2013) Prospective evaluation of biweekly streptozotocin in 19 dogs with insulinoma. *Journal of Veterinary Internal Medicine* **27**, 483–490

Polton GA, White RN, Brearley MJ and Eastwood JM (2007) Improved survival in a retrospective cohort of 28 dogs with insulinoma. *Journal of Small Animal Practice* **48**, 151–156

Platt SR and Olby NJ (2013) *BSAVA Manual of Canine and Feline Neurology, 4th edn*. BSAVA Publications, Gloucester

Priester WA (1974) Pancreatic islet cell tumors in domestic animals. Data from 11 colleges of veterinary medicine in the United States and Canada. *Journal of the National Cancer Institute* **53**, 227–229

Robben JH, van den Brom WE, Mol JA, van Haeften TW and Rijnberk A (2006) Effect of octreotide on plasma concentrations of glucose, insulin, glucagon, growth hormone, and cortisol in healthy dogs and dogs with insulinoma. *Research in Veterinary Science* **80**, 25–32

Robben JH, Van Garderen E, Mol JA, Wolfswinkel J and Rijnberk A (2002) Locally produced growth hormone in canine insulinomas. *Molecular and Cellular Endocrinology* **197**, 187–195

Hobben JH, Visser-Wisselaar HA, Rutteman GR et al. (1997) In vitro and in vivo detection of functional somatostatin receptors in canine insulinomas. *Journal of Nuclear Medicine* **38**, 1036–1042

Ryan D, Pérez-Accino J, Gonçalves R et al. (2021) Clinical findings, neurological manifestations and survival of dogs with insulinoma: 116 cases (2009–2020). *Journal of Small Animal Practice* **62**, 531–539

Rychel J, Worley DR, Hardy CS and Webb BT (2013) Prolonged survival in an aged Labrador retriever with a metastatic insulinoma. *Journal of the American Animal Hospital Association* **49**, 224–229

Schaub S and Wigger A (2013) Ultrasound-aided diagnosis of an insulinoma in a cat. *Tierärztliche Praxis Ausgabe K, Kleintiere/Heimtiere* **41**, 338–342

Schoeman JP (2019) Hypoglycemia. In: *Feline Endocrinology*, ed. EC Feldman, ME Peterson and F Fracassi. Edra Publishing, Milan

Sheppard-Olivares S, Bello N, Johannes CM et al. (2021) Toceranib phosphate in the management of canine insulinoma: a retrospective multicentre study of 30 cases (2009–2019). *Veterinary Record Open* **9**, e27

Slye M and Wells H (1935) Tumor of islet tissue with hyperinsulinism in a dog. *Archives of Pathology* **19**, 537

Tobin RL, Nelson RW, Lucroy MD, Wooldridge JD and Feldman EC (1999) Outcome of surgical *versus* medical treatment of dogs with beta cell neoplasia: 39 cases (1990–1997). *Journal of the American Veterinary Medical Association* **215**, 226–230

Trifonidou MA, Kirpensteijn J and Robben JH (1998) A retrospective evaluation of 51 dogs with insulinoma. *Veterinary Quarterly* **20**, S114–S115

Tucker ON, Crotty PL and Conlon KC (2006) The management of insulinoma. *British Journal of Surgery* **93**, 264–275

Van Ham L, Braund KG, Roels S and Putcuyps I (1997) Treatment of a dog with an insulinoma-related peripheral polyneuropathy with corticosteroids. *Veterinary Record* **141**, 98–100

Vanderperren K, Haers H, Van der Vekens E et al. (2014) Description of the use of contrast-enhanced ultrasonography in four dogs with pancreatic tumours. *Journal of Small Animal Practice* **55**, 164–169

Chapter 28

Canine hypoadrenocorticism

Alisdair Boag

Introduction

Hypoadrenocorticism is an uncommon syndrome in dogs. The clinical signs are caused by a deficiency of the adrenocortical hormones. Most affected dogs have primary hypoadrenocorticism with loss of both glucocorticoid and mineralocorticoid production as a result of immune-mediated destruction of the adrenal cortex. Hypoadrenocorticism can be a challenging disease to recognize and diagnose and is termed 'The Great Pretender' due to its waxing and waning non-specific, variable clinical signs that can become acutely life-threatening. Dogs have a higher prevalence of spontaneous primary hypoadrenocorticism compared with other species.

Physiology

The adrenal gland consists of an outer capsule surrounding a cortex, which synthesizes and secretes steroid hormones, and an inner medulla, which synthesizes and secretes adrenaline (epinephrine) and noradrenaline (norepinephrine). The adrenal cortex comprises approximately 75% of the adrenal gland and is made up of three distinct histological regions: the outer zona glomerulosa (ZG), the middle zona fasciculata (ZF) and the inner zona reticularis (ZR).

Steroid hormones include corticosteroids (glucocorticoids and mineralocorticoids) and gonadocorticoids (sex steroids). Glucocorticoids are produced in the ZF and ZR, with cortisol being the primary biologically active form in dogs. Mineralocorticoids are produced in the ZG, with aldosterone being the primary biologically active form in dogs. Gonadocorticoids are produced in the ZR and comprise oestrogens, androgens and progestogens. These are also produced in the gonads and placenta. In hypoadrenocorticism, there is disruption of the adrenal production of the sex steroids, which is associated with decreased fertility in humans. This is rarely of clinical concern in dogs and, therefore, the sex steroids are not considered further in this chapter.

All steroid hormones are derived from cholesterol, the majority of which is sourced from the diet, although synthesis from acetate is possible within the adrenal gland. The rate-limiting step for steroid hormone synthesis is movement of cholesterol into the mitochondria for the initiation of the cascade of sequential enzymatic hydrolysis, oxidation and methylation that produces the different hormones (Figure 28.1). The enzymes in this cascade are differentially expressed in the zones of the adrenal gland. In dogs, the expression of CYP17 in the ZF but not the ZG confers zone-specific differentiation between cortisol and aldosterone production.

Control of corticosteroid production

The primary steroid hormones are each produced under different homeostatic feedback loops (Figure 28.2). The hypothalamic–pituitary–adrenal (HPA) axis controls and regulates cortisol synthesis and release. Corticotropin-releasing hormone (CRH) is produced in the hypothalamus and stimulates the secretion of adrenocorticotropic hormone (ACTH) from the pituitary. In turn, ACTH stimulates synthesis and secretion of cortisol by the adrenal glands. Circulating free cortisol inhibits both CRH and ACTH release from the hypothalamus and pituitary, respectively, via negative feedback. Adrenocorticotropic hormone can inhibit CRH release from the hypothalamus as a separate feedback loop. The HPA axis is also stimulated by stress, physical activity, trauma, surgery, illness and low glucose concentrations.

Secretion of CRH and ACTH is normally episodic and pulsatile, which results in fluctuating cortisol concentrations throughout the day. Diurnal variation is superimposed on this type of release. Anecdotally, the CRH and ACTH concentrations and, thus, cortisol concentrations are highest in the early hours of the morning. However, a true circadian rhythm of cortisol concentrations has been difficult to confirm in the dog.

The renin–angiotensin–aldosterone system (RAAS) and plasma potassium concentrations are the major regulators of aldosterone synthesis and secretion, with ACTH and sodium having lesser roles. Renin is secreted from modified smooth muscle cells in the afferent arteriole in the kidney, which form the juxtaglomerular complex along with cells of the macula densa in the distal tubule. Renin secretion is upregulated by increased sympathetic nerve activity, circulating catecholamines, deceased sodium chloride concentrations at the macula densa and decreases in blood pressure. Renin catalyses the conversion of angiotensinogen from the liver to angiotensin I. Angiotensin I is then converted to angiotensin II by angiotensin converting enzyme (ACE) in vascular beds, primarily in the lungs. Angiotensin II is the primary stimulator of aldosterone secretion but also has direct effects as a vasoconstrictor. Hyperkalaemia directly stimulates aldosterone production within the adrenal gland.

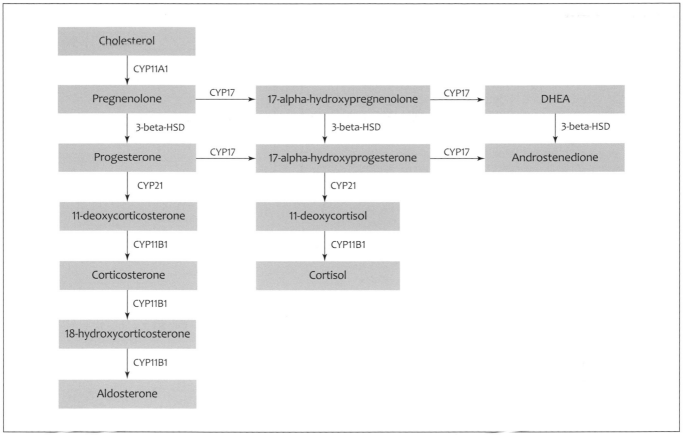

28.1 Outline of the unique steroid synthesis pathway in dogs. 3-beta-HSD = 3-beta-hydroxysteroid dehydrogenase; DHEA = dehydrocpiandrosterone.

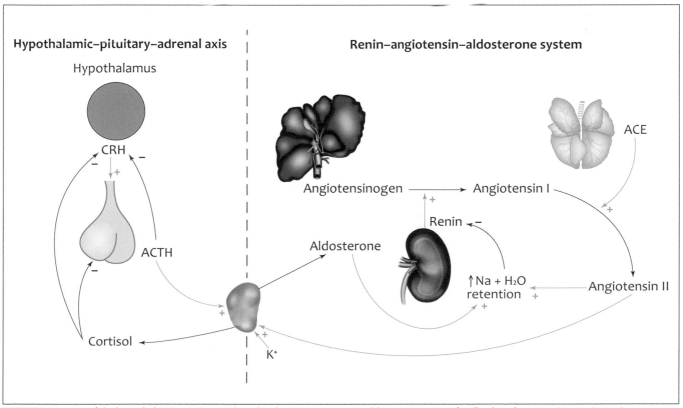

28.2 Diagram of the hypothalamic–pituitary–adrenal and renin–angiotensin–aldosterone system feedback pathways. ACE = angiotensin converting enzyme; ACTH = adrenocorticotropic hormone; CRH = corticotropin-releasing hormone; + = stimulation; − = inhibition.

Transport and metabolism

In the circulation, cortisol is largely bound to two proteins, albumin and cortisol-binding globulin, with a corresponding non-bound free cortisol fraction. Free cortisol is the active form, which can diffuse across cell membranes into the cytoplasm, where it binds to the glucocorticoid receptor (GR). This bound complex is responsible for signal transduction via direct binding to DNA response sites and alteration of transcription via non-genomic ligand-dependent steroid receptor actions.

In the circulation, less aldosterone is protein bound compared with cortisol, which contributes to its shorter half-life. As with cortisol, because steroid hormones are lipids and hydrophobic, aldosterone freely diffuses into cells where it binds to the mineralocorticoid receptor (MR) and downstream signalling follows, as with the bound cortisol–GR complex. Cortisol binds strongly to both the GR and MR, whereas aldosterone primarily binds to the MR. To prevent unnecessary activation of the MR by cortisol, cortisol is inactivated by 11-beta-hydroxysteroid dehydrogenase (11-beta-HSD) type 2. Glucocorticoid receptors are present in every cell in the body, reflecting the vital and wide-ranging functions of cortisol in body homeostasis. In contrast, MRs are present only in selected cells, primarily of the kidney, colon, salivary and sweat glands, and areas of the brain. Corticosteroids are metabolized in the liver to inactive metabolites and primarily excreted in the urine in dogs; a small amount of unaltered cortisol is excreted.

Actions

Glucocorticoids affect a wide range of normal cellular processes; major areas include:

- **Carbohydrate metabolism** – cortisol stimulates gluconeogenesis and decreases glucose uptake and usage by cells, especially skeletal muscle, via decreased glucose transporter 4 (GLUT4) expression
- **Protein metabolism** – in the liver, cortisol increases protein production. In other tissues, protein is broken down, increasing the pool of amino acids in the blood for gluconeogenesis and protein production in the liver
- **Lipid metabolism** – similar to protein, cortisol increases breakdown and release of fatty acids from adipose tissue, making these more available. Cortisol also enhances oxidation of fatty acids in the cells
- **Immune functions** – cortisol acts to depress immune function via a wide range of mechanisms, including stabilization of lysosomal membranes, decreased white cell migration, decreased phagocytosis and decreased T-cell division and turnover
- **Other functions** – maintenance of normal blood pressure, endothelial integrity and vascular permeability, and promotion of normal red blood cell production.

In contrast to the wide-ranging actions of glucocorticoids, mineralocorticoid actions are narrower in scope but even more vital to life. Aldosterone has two major actions:

- Regulation of extracellular fluid volume
- Potassium homeostasis.

The primary sites of action for aldosterone are in the distal convoluted tubules and collecting ducts of the kidney. Aldosterone stimulates Na^+/K^+ ATPase pumps in the cells of the basolateral membrane. Each pump moves three sodium ions (Na^+) out of the cell and two potassium (K^+) ions into the cell, creating an osmotic gradient which resorbs water into the systemic circulation (Figure 28.3).

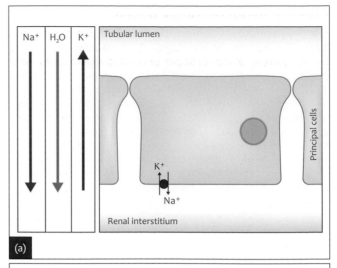

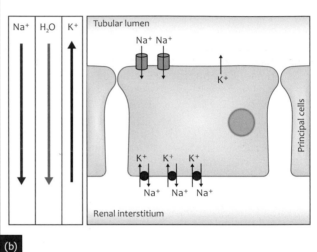

28.3 Aldosterone action in the basolateral membrane of the kidney. (a) Without aldosterone, lower concentrations of sodium and potassium ions and water move through the principal cells between the tubular lumen and the renal interstitium. (b) With aldosterone, increased Na^+/K^+ ATPase pumps create a diffusion gradient, which moves sodium and, subsequently, water from the tubular lumen through the principal cells to the renal interstitium and the body. Potassium moves in the opposite direction. Epithelial sodium channels allow more sodium to enter the principal cells, further increasing resorption.

This creates a negative potential within the lumen and facilitates potassium secretion into the tubule lumen. Aldosterone directly stimulates hydrogen ion (H^+) secretion in different cells through its effects on H^+ ATPase pumps in the luminal membrane. Hydrogen ion secretion is also indirectly increased by the effect of aldosterone on sodium resorption.

Aetiology

Hypoadrenocorticism may develop due to disease affecting any part of the HPA axis. It can be primary, resulting from disease of the adrenal glands, or secondary, due to ACTH deficiency resulting from central disease. In humans, hypoadrenocorticism can occur because of congenital disorders of steroid production or responsiveness to ACTH, but these have not yet been described in dogs. Finally, some cases with critical illness, without overt hypoadrenocorticism, may have critical-illness-related corticosteroid insufficiency (CIRCI).

Primary hypoadrenocorticism

Primary hypoadrenocorticism is the most common form of hypoadrenocorticism in dogs. It is usually manifested by concurrent glucocorticoid and mineralocorticoid deficiency; this is referred to as Addison's disease. The adrenal glands have a secretory reserve capacity, such that only after a large proportion of the steroid-producing cells are damaged does corticosteroid production become insufficient. It is widely reported that approximately 90% of the adrenal gland needs to be compromised before clinical signs arise. Various pathologies have been described.

In dogs, as in humans, the most common cause is autoimmune disease of the adrenal cortex. Affected dogs have small adrenal glands and a decreased cortical to medullary ratio. Histopathologically, the cortical destruction is associated with lymphoplasmacytic infiltration (Scott-Moncrieff, 2015). Demonstration of autoantibodies directed against the adrenal gland provides further evidence of an immunological basis. Specific antibodies against P450scc have been found in approximately 25% of dogs with hypoadrenocorticism (Boag *et al.*, 2015). There is also indirect evidence of autoimmunity, with genetic susceptibility links to immune response genes, including antigen-presenting genes (major histocompatibility complex class II) and genes involved in T-cell activation (*CTLA4* and *PTPN22*) (Boag and Catchpole, 2014).

Other causes of primary hypoadrenocorticism are rare. These include neoplastic infiltration of the adrenal glands, including lymphoma and mammary carcinoma, histoplasmosis, and bilateral infarction, abscessation and haemorrhage.

Drugs used to treat hypercortisolism, including trilostane and mitotane, can cause primary hypoadrenocorticism. Approximately 15% of dogs treated with trilostane have an episode of hypoadrenocorticism in the first 2 years (King and Morton, 2017). Trilostane can cause hypoadrenocorticism as a result of inhibition of both cortisol and aldosterone synthesis – this is usually reversible. However, trilostane has also been associated with hypoadrenocorticism resulting from acute adrenal gland necrosis. This necrosis might be mediated by ACTH, which has been associated with bilateral adrenal haemorrhage in humans; ACTH, but not trilostane, is also associated with adrenal haemorrhage in rats (Scott-Moncrieff, 2015). This mechanism is also speculated to be the reason for the spontaneous development of hypoadrenocorticism after a diagnosis of pituitary-dependent hypercortisolism in a dog (Scott-Moncrieff, 2015). Ketoconazole has also been reported to cause hypoadrenocorticism in a dog (Sullivant and Lathan, 2020).

Unusual forms of primary hypoadrenocorticism

A small proportion of dogs present with evidence of cortisol deficiency alone, and these have often been called atypical cases. Selective destruction of the ZF and ZR with relative sparing of the ZG has been reported. Isolated glucocorticoid deficiency is possible with infiltrative diseases such as lymphoma and as a consequence of drugs such as trilostane or mitotane. Isolated glucocorticoid deficiency is commonly presumed when electrolyte abnormalities are absent. However, concurrent mineralocorticoid deficiency cannot be ruled out without further testing of aldosterone production. Electrolyte concentrations may be within the reference interval in some dogs with aldosterone deficiency following prior treatment (e.g. intravenous fluids) or may be maintained because of alternative compensatory mechanisms.

Isolated hypoaldosteronism has also been described, albeit rarely, with and without increased renin activity. Isolated glucocorticoid or mineralocorticoid deficiency has the potential to progress to a deficiency of both hormones, although how likely this is or when it will occur is largely unknown and such dogs should be closely monitored.

Secondary hypoadrenocorticism

Secondary hypoadrenocorticism results from decreased ACTH production. This is most commonly iatrogenic as a result of administration of glucocorticoids and subsequent suppression of the HPA axis and atrophy of the adrenal cortices. Depending on the duration, dose and preparation of glucocorticoid therapy used, suppression of the HPA axis can be prolonged and adrenocortical atrophy can take time to reverse. Even topical glucocorticoids can affect ACTH response test results for up to 2 weeks. Other causes, such as head trauma and hypophysectomy, are recognized, but in most cases a definite cause is not found.

Loss of ACTH does not affect aldosterone production and, therefore, secondary hypoadrenocorticism consists of isolated hypocortisolism. Secondary hypoadrenocorticism is indistinguishable from atypical disease unless the endogenous ACTH concentration is measured.

Critical-illness-related corticosteroid insufficiency

A full review of CIRCI is beyond the scope of this chapter. Briefly, in humans, CIRCI refers to critically ill patients with shock who are unresponsive to fluids and vasopressors but respond positively to low-dose glucocorticoid supplementation. This positive response to glucocorticoids has been described in dogs, both clinically and experimentally. There are three potential pathophysiological pathways for CIRCI (Annane *et al.*, 2017):

- Dysregulation of the HPA axis with dissociation of ACTH from cortisol production
- Altered intracellular cortisol metabolism
- Tissue resistance to glucocorticoids.

In critically ill dogs, HPA axis dysregulation and altered cortisol metabolism have been described (Boag *et al.*, 2020). However, the potential effect of glucocorticoid supplementation and the ideal dose, timing, duration and active drug for critically ill dogs are unknown. While hydrocortisone is used in humans, its use in dogs remains controversial. Excessive glucocorticoid treatment of critically ill cases leads to worse outcomes (Annane *et al.*, 2017).

Signalment

The estimated prevalence of canine hypoadrenocorticism is between 0.1% and 1.1%, approximately 100 times higher than in humans.

Age of onset is typically between 2 and 6 years old. However, hypoadrenocorticism can develop at almost any age, with a range of 3 months to 14 years. Dogs without electrolyte abnormalities are typically reported to present at an older age. Bitches are more likely than male dogs to have hypoadrenocorticism, although this is not consistent in some breeds (Boag and Catchpole, 2014). A wide range of breeds are affected with hypoadrenocorticism, and crossbreeds are among some of the most commonly diagnosed. Some breed-specific studies report much higher prevalence estimates, including for Standard Poodles (up to 10% in one study), Portuguese Water Dogs (PWDs) (minimum of 1.5%) and Bearded Collies (3.4%) (Boag and Catchpole, 2014). Case series highlight specific breeds, including Leonbergers, Nova Scotia Duck Tolling Retrievers (NSDTRs), Soft Coated Wheaten Terriers and Pomeranians. High heritability estimates have been reported in several breeds, including 0.76 for Bearded Collies, 0.75 for Standard Poodles, 0.49 for PWDs and 0.98 for NSDTRs. The inheritance for all but a juvenile form of hypoadrenocorticism in NSDTRs is likely complex. Significantly over- and under-represented breeds are listed in Figures 28.4 and 28.5.

- Airedale Terrier
- Basset Hound
- Bearded Collie
- Border Terrier
- Cairn Terrier
- Cocker Spaniel
- English Pointer
- German Shorthaired Pointer
- Great Dane
- Griffon Bruxellois
- Portuguese Water Dog
- Pyrenean Mountain Dog
- Rottweiler
- Soft Coated Wheaten Terrier
- Springer Spaniel
- St Bernard
- Standard Poodle
- West Highland White Terrier

28.4 Breeds significantly over-represented for hypoadrenocorticism (Boag and Catchpole, 2014; Hanson *et al.*, 2016; Decôme and Blais, 2017).

- Boxer
- Bull Terrier
- Dachshund
- Dalmatian
- German Shepherd Dog
- Golden Retriever
- Labrador Retriever
- Lhasa Apso
- Pomeranian
- Shetland Sheepdog
- Shih Tzu
- Yorkshire Terrier

28.5 Breeds significantly under-represented for hypoadrenocorticism (Boag and Catchpole, 2014; Hanson *et al.*, 2016).

Clinical features

Dogs with hypoadrenocorticism can present with clinical signs ranging from an acute-onset life-threatening emergency to an insidious disease with subtle signs that may not be fully appreciated by owners. The clinical signs of hypoadrenocorticism are often described as vague, with signs primarily reflecting glucocorticoid deficiency. A high index of suspicion is required to consider hypoadrenocorticism as a differential diagnosis.

Acute presentation

Dogs presenting acutely can be critically ill, such that without emergency intervention they may die in a short time period. These dogs can be hypovolaemic, dehydrated, hypothermic, and weak or collapsed. In some cases, bradycardia may be present despite severe hypovolaemia, but this is not consistently observed. There may or may not be a history of chronic intermittent gastrointestinal signs or general malaise and a recognized stressor. Because of the acute signs and associated clinicopathological changes (see 'Diagnosis', below), they can particularly mimic dogs with acute kidney injury, acute gastrointestinal disease or hepatic failure, or may even resemble dogs with sepsis. Other emergency presentations can include substantial gastrointestinal haemorrhage and seizures secondary to hypoglycaemia that can occur in both primary and secondary hypoadrenocorticism.

As with presenting complaints, physical examination changes in hypoadrenocorticism can be variable, with no pathognomonic findings. In some dogs the physical examination may be entirely unremarkable. Hypotension has been demonstrated as a more consistent finding in dogs with hypoadrenocorticism (median 90 mmHg, range 40–150 mmHg) compared with those without (median 140 mmHg, range 50–210 mmHg) that present with similar signs (Scott-Moncrieff, 2015).

Chronic presentation

The most common chronic clinical signs are presented in Figure 28.6. Vomiting, shaking, shivering and abdominal pain are also reported. Gastrointestinal signs can also include mucoid faeces, melaena, haematemesis, haematochezia and tenesmus. Indeed, in dogs presenting for investigation of chronic gastrointestinal signs, hypoadrenocorticism was indistinguishable from other causes (Hauck *et al.*, 2020). Signs may wax and wane in intensity over time in approximately 50% of affected dogs (Scott-Moncrieff, 2015). Thus, there may be a delay between the onset of clinical signs and the time of diagnosis. Dogs may respond favourably but transiently to symptomatic therapy (e.g. intravenous fluids).

Dogs with apparent isolated glucocorticoid deficiency and reference interval electrolyte concentrations usually have a longer course of clinical signs prior to diagnosis, with anorexia, lethargy, diarrhoea and polydipsia more frequently reported. These dogs are older on average.

Hypoadrenocorticism has also been reported to present in a number of unusual ways, including megaoesophagus with regurgitation as the primary clinical sign (although published case reports are older and dogs may have been sedated for radiographs), muscle cramping and spasm with limb pain, polycythaemia and epistaxis. It has even been reported to mimic protein-losing enteropathy, including hypoalbuminaemia with ascites and peripheral oedema (Lyngby and Sellon, 2016).

Clinical sign	Reported prevalence
Lethargy	66–94%
Anorexia	54–92%
Weakness	21–66%
Diarrhoea	13–50%
Weight loss	17–48%
Hypothermia	43%
Polyuria and polydipsia	17–28%

28.6 Common clinical signs of hypoadrenocorticism.

Diagnosis

Routine clinicopathological features

Given the extensive effects of corticosteroids and variable clinical presentations, there is a wide scope of possible clinicopathological changes. Some abnormalities are more likely in dogs with hypoadrenocorticism but none is pathognomonic. Algorithms and models using routine clinicopathological data to predict or diagnose hypoadrenocorticism have been reported. Currently, these provide some help in increasing clinical suspicion but are not a replacement for definitive diagnostic tests. Common changes are outlined in Figure 28.7.

Haematology
- Non-regenerative or poorly regenerative anaemia
- Eosinophilia
- Lymphocytosis
- Lack of stress leucogram

Serum biochemistry
- Azotaemia
- Hypercalcaemia
- Hyperkalaemia
- Hyponatraemia
- Hypocholesterolaemia
- Hypochloridaemia

Urinalysis
- Inappropriately dilute urine (urine specific gravity <1.030)

28.7 Common clinicopathological abnormalities in hypoadrenocorticism.

Infectious
- Ectoparasites:
  - **Fleas**
  - **Mites**
- Endoparasites:
  - **Heartworm (where endemic)**
  - Lungworm
  - *Toxoplasma* spp.
  - *Neospora* spp.
- Fungal:
  - *Aspergillus* spp.

Hypersensitivity reactions
- **Allergic skin disease**
- **Flea allergy dermatitis**
- **Food allergy**

Eosinophilic infiltrative diseases
- **Eosinophilic bronchopneumopathy**
- Eosinophilic pulmonary granulomatosis
- Eosinophilic myositis
- Eosinophilic bronchitis
- Eosinophilic meningoencephalitis
- Eosinophilic enteritis
- Hypereosinophilic syndrome (especially in Rottweilers)

Paraneoplastic
- Mast cell tumours
- Lymphoma
- Other solid tumours

Other
- Hypoadrenocorticism

28.8 Differential diagnoses for eosinophilia. Those listed in bold are considered to be common.

Haematology

Anaemia is possible and is most often a mild to moderate normocytic normochromic non-regenerative anaemia of chronic disease. If there is significant gastrointestinal bleeding, the anaemia can be more severe with features of regeneration, albeit poor. Some dogs have evidence of haemoconcentration as a result of plasma volume depletion.

Classic changes associated with hypoadrenocorticism include a lack of stress leucogram that may or may not be accompanied by eosinophilia or lymphocytosis. Neutrophilia, monocytosis, lymphopenia and eosinopenia are all expected responses in severe illness; maintenance of white blood cell values within the reference interval may be inappropriate and should raise suspicion for hypoadrenocorticism. Lymphocyte and eosinophil counts are not always above the reference interval in hypoadrenocorticism. Whilst lymphocytosis can occur, it is less common than eosinophilia. Other causes of eosinophilia in an ill dog must be considered and are outlined in Figure 28.8.

Serum biochemistry

The most consistent electrolyte changes in hypoadrenocorticism are a combination of hyponatraemia and hyperkalaemia and, consequently, low sodium:potassium. Concurrent hypochloridaemia is also reported, mirroring the hyponatraemia. These changes are characteristic of hypoaldosteronism and reflect the failure of the kidneys to retain sodium in exchange for potassium (and hydrogen). Electrolyte abnormalities are reported in approximately 75% of dogs with hypoadrenocorticism and, although these changes are reflective of decreased aldosterone production, some dogs without electrolyte abnormalities

have hypoaldosteronism (Baumstark *et al.*, 2014). Other possible causes of hyperkalaemia are highlighted in Figure 28.9.

Decreased sodium:potassium can occur in other diseases. However, increased severity of sodium:potassium decline correlates with an increased likelihood of hypoadrenocorticism compared with other possible causes.

Dogs with hypoadrenocorticism can also develop hypercalcaemia (total, ionized or both) and this is reported in up to 40% of dogs. Whilst this is typically mild, more severe hypercalcaemia is possible, and hypoadrenocorticism should be considered as a differential diagnosis for any dog with hypercalcaemia. Hypercalcaemia may be partly driven by metabolic acidosis, decreased excretion or altered intestinal calcium absorption. It does not appear to be related to parathyroid hormone, parathyroid hormone-related protein or serum 1,25-dihydroxycholecalciferol (calcitriol, active vitamin D) concentrations. Although rare, a hypocalcaemia that is usually clinically insignificant and possibly related to hypoalbuminaemia has been described in dogs.

Azotaemia is common and usually secondary to hypovolaemia and subsequent decreased renal perfusion. In healthy dogs, hypovolaemia leads to increases in urine specific gravity (SG) to conserve fluid volume, with appropriately concentrated urine defined as having an SG greater than 1.030. In dogs with hypoadrenocorticism, urine-concentrating ability can be impaired as decreased sodium in the renal medulla impairs maximal concentrating ability in the collecting ducts. Hyponatraemia can affect arginine vasopressin (AVP) release and hypercalcaemia can also interfere with urine-concentrating ability. The combination of azotaemia with inappropriately dilute urine is particularly challenging as it mimics intrinsic kidney disease. In dogs with hypoadrenocorticism, the azotaemia may resolve more quickly with fluids than in those with kidney disease.

Artefactual
• Haemolysis • Thrombocytosis • EDTA contamination
Decreased excretion

• **Acute kidney injury**
• **Chronic kidney disease**
• Sepsis
• Effusions (pleural, peritoneal, pericardial)
• **Hypoadrenocorticism**
• **Ruptured bladder**
• **Urethral obstruction**
• Drugs:
  • ACEis
  • ARBs
  • Potassium-sparing diuretics
  • NSAIDs
  • TMPS
  • Ciclosporin
  • Heparin

Increased extracellular potassium
• Acidosis (especially hyperchloride acidosis) • Reperfusion injury • Blood transfusion • Tumour lysis syndrome • Diabetic ketoacidosis • Rhabdomyolysis • Iatrogenic (potassium-containing fluids)

28.9 Differential diagnoses for hyperkalaemia. Those listed in bold are considered to be common. ACEis = angiotensin converting enzyme inhibitors; ARBs = angiotensin receptor blockers; EDTA = ethylenediaminetetraacetic acid; NSAIDs = non-steroidal anti-inflammatory drugs; TMPS = trimethoprim and sulfamethoxazole.

Hypoglycaemia occurs in approximately 10–15% of cases of hypoadrenocorticism and can be severe enough to cause seizures. Hypoalbuminaemia is also common (Scott-Moncrieff, 2015). Hypoalbuminaemia can be severe, associated with peripheral oedema and ascites, and may be more common in dogs without classical electrolyte abnormalities. Hypocholesterolaemia is also reported in affected dogs and more commonly in those without electrolyte abnormalities.

Diagnostic imaging

Thoracic radiography may reflect changes in volume status, with decreased cardiac silhouette and diameter of the caudal vena cava. In dogs with regurgitation, a conscious lateral radiograph should be obtained to assess for megaoesophagus. The vast majority of dogs with hypoadrenocorticism have no abnormalities on thoracic radiography.

Dogs with hypoadrenocorticism typically have smaller adrenal glands than those without hypoadrenocorticism. A left adrenal gland thickness of less than 3.2 mm is more likely to be associated with hypoadrenocorticism. However, healthy dogs and those with other diseases mimicking hypoadrenocorticism can have small adrenal glands. Dogs with hypoadrenocorticism can also have normal-sized adrenal glands. Therefore, whilst adrenal gland size can be supportive of hypoadrenocorticism, it is not diagnostic.

Electrocardiography

Electrocardiography should be performed in dogs with hyperkalaemia to assess for secondary cardiac effects. Increasing concentrations of potassium produce a classic progression of changes (Figure 28.10) (Scott-Moncrieff, 2015). These changes are not consistently present and can occur at lower potassium concentrations. Other electrolyte and acid–base changes may play a role in modulating the cardiac effects of hyperkalaemia.

Specific hormone testing
Basal cortisol

Basal cortisol has emerged as a helpful screening tool to exclude hypoadrenocorticism when it is suspected in dogs. A value below approximately 55 nmol/l, assessed using a chemiluminescent immunoassay, has excellent diagnostic sensitivity (87.7–100%) but less good diagnostic specificity (58.8–70.3%). It has a negative predictive value approaching 100% at high prevalence (Gold et al., 2016). Thus, if basal cortisol is higher than 55 nmol/l, hypoadrenocorticism is excluded with few exceptions. However, a value below

Potassium	ECG	ECG description
Within referene interval		• No abnormalities
Mild hyperkalaemia (6.0–7.0 mmol/l)		• Peaking of T wave • Shortened QT interval
Moderate hyperkalaemia (7.0–9.0 mmol/l)		• Prolongation of the PR interval • Widening of the QRS complex • Decreased amplitude, widening and progressive loss of P wave (>8.0 mmol/l)

Severe hyperkalaemia (>9 mmol/l)		• Progressive widening of the QRS complex leading to:
		  • Sine wave pattern
		  • Ventricular fibrillation or standstill

28.10 Classic electrocardiogram (ECG) changes seen with increasing potassium concentrations.

55 nmol/l is of little practical use as it does not exclude non-adrenal illness. If using assays with a sufficiently low limit of detection, even lower cut-offs can be used that are more diagnostic of hypoadrenocorticism, but these assays are not widely available. If there is a strong clinical suspicion of hypoadrenocorticism, an ACTH response test remains the diagnostic test of choice (Gold *et al.*, 2016).

Adrenocorticotropic hormone response test

The definitive diagnosis of hypoadrenocorticism is made by demonstrating a failure to stimulate cortisol production after ACTH administration.

The ACTH response test is a test of the functional reserve capacity of the adrenal gland. Circulating cortisol concentrations are measured before and after the administration of a supraphysiological dose of synthetic ACTH. Healthy dogs respond with a large increase in cortisol concentration. In dogs with hypoadrenocorticism, there is little or no increase.

There are two formulations of synthetic ACTH: a short-acting formulation, which is more common, and a depot formulation, which is less widely used. With the short-acting formulation (Synacthen or CosACTHen) a blood sample is taken, then 5 μg/kg (up to a maximum of 250 μg/dog) is injected intravenously. One hour later, a second blood sample is obtained. Cortisol concentrations are measured in both blood samples.

The intravenous route is preferred for ACTH. Intramuscular and perivascular administration do not change test interpretation (Johnson *et al.*, 2017), but have not been specifically assessed in dogs with suspected hypoadrenocorticism in which dehydration may be present. The depot product (Synacthen Depot) is for intramuscular injection only and the second blood sample should be taken 1–2 hours after administration if using this formulation (Sieber-Ruckstuhl *et al.*, 2015).

In healthy dogs, post-ACTH cortisol concentrations are usually greater than approximately 250 nmol/l. A diagnosis of hypoadrenocorticism is made if a post-ACTH cortisol concentration remains low, with most affected dogs having values at or near the limit of detection of the assay (approximately 25 nmol/l for many assays). Some dogs have a demonstrable but reduced cortisol response to ACTH. This may represent a number of possibilities (Wakayama *et al.*, 2017):

- Normal for the individual
- Cortisol measurement error
- Residual effects of previous glucocorticoid use
- Possible early hypoadrenocorticism
- Failure to administer ACTH
- Use of other drugs affecting the HPA axis, including:
  - Trilostane
  - Mitotane
  - Ketoconazole
  - Etomidate.

It is important to perform an ACTH response test prior to glucocorticoid administration due to potential cross-reactivity in the cortisol assay. The only exception to this is dexamethasone, which does not cross-react. However, all the synthetic glucocorticoids, including dexamethasone, have a negative feedback effect on ACTH secretion (this is the basis of the low-dose dexamethasone suppression test), which will affect the test over time. However, a single injection of dexamethasone does not reduce post-ACTH stimulated cortisol concentrations enough to affect interpretation in healthy dogs.

A flatline cortisol response from an ACTH response test supports a diagnosis of hypoadrenocorticism, but does not distinguish naturally occurring Addison's disease, secondary disease, isolated hypocortisolism or iatrogenic disease due to prior glucocorticoid administration or trilostane/mitotane treatment. The results must be interpreted in the clinical context of the case under investigation. Other tests may be required to distinguish all possibilities (Figure 28.11).

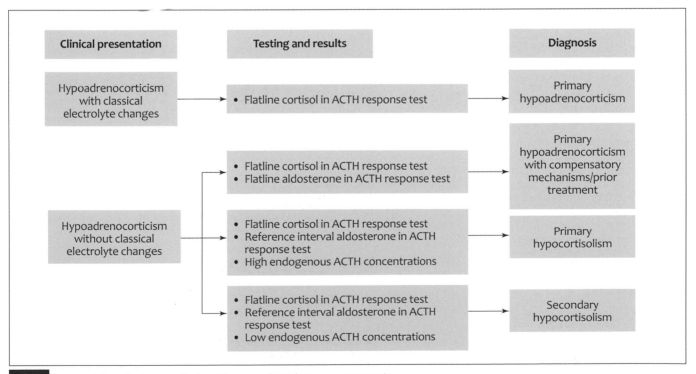

Clinical presentation	Testing and results	Diagnosis
Hypoadrenocorticism with classical electrolyte changes	• Flatline cortisol in ACTH response test	Primary hypoadrenocorticism
Hypoadrenocorticism without classical electrolyte changes	• Flatline cortisol in ACTH response test • Flatline aldosterone in ACTH response test	Primary hypoadrenocorticism with compensatory mechanisms/prior treatment
	• Flatline cortisol in ACTH response test • Reference interval aldosterone in ACTH response test • High endogenous ACTH concentrations	Primary hypocortisolism
	• Flatline cortisol in ACTH response test • Reference interval aldosterone in ACTH response test • Low endogenous ACTH concentrations	Secondary hypocortisolism

28.11 Interpretation of adrenocorticotropic hormone (ACTH) response test results.

Aldosterone can be measured with cortisol during the ACTH response test. Although ACTH plays a minor role in day-to-day aldosterone regulation, the supraphysiological dose administered for an ACTH response test is sufficient to stimulate aldosterone release. The majority of dogs with primary hypoadrenocorticism, even without electrolyte abnormalities, have low aldosterone concentrations before and after ACTH administration (Baumstark et al., 2014). Adequate aldosterone stimulation may reflect primary hypoadrenocorticism with isolated hypocortisolism or secondary hypoadrenocorticism. It is a useful test when prior glucocorticoids have been administered and there are concerns of iatrogenic cortisol suppression (Gunn et al., 2016).

Adrenocorticotropic hormone and renin concentrations

Endogenous ACTH concentration is not routinely measured, partly due to its special sample handling requirements (see Chapter 3). However, ACTH measurements can distinguish between dogs with primary versus secondary hypoadrenocorticism. This may help determine if long-term monitoring of electrolytes or repeated aldosterone measurement is required or if central disease is present. In primary hypoadrenocorticism, ACTH concentrations are high because of loss of the normal cortisol feedback. In secondary hypoadrenocorticism, ACTH concentrations are low to undetectable.

An alternative method for assessing the HPA axis is to assess both aspects of the feedback loops at the same time in a manner analogous to the thyroxine (T4) and thyrotropin (thyroid-stimulating hormone (TSH)) testing required for the investigation of hypothyroidism in dogs (see Chaper 18). Cortisol:ACTH (CAR) has shown some promise as an alternative method of assessing for hypoadrenocorticism. In dogs with primary hypoadrenocorticism, values are low and clearly distinct from values in healthy dogs. The CAR also distinguishes primary hypoadrenocorticism from non-adrenal illness, although results are not consistent across different studies (Lathan et al., 2014; Boretti et al., 2015). Similarly, aldosterone:renin (ARR) distinguishes between healthy dogs and those with primary hypoadrenocorticism (Javadi et al., 2006). Unfortunately, this has not been assessed in dogs with non-adrenal illness. Measurement of the ARR is useful in distinguishing the very rare cases of hyporeninaemic from hyperreninaemic hypoaldosteronism.

Urinary electrolytes

In healthy animals, the kidneys retain sodium in the face of hyponatraemia because of the actions of aldosterone. With aldosterone deficiency, there is sodium wastage even when hyponatraemia is present. In a small number of dogs with hyponatraemia, the urinary sodium concentration was greater than 30 mmol/l in all those with hypoadrenocorticism, and lower than 30 mmol/l in dogs with non-adrenal illness (Lennon et al., 2018). This test may be of use when testing for cortisol and aldosterone is not available.

Treatment

The initial management of dogs with hypoadrenocorticism will vary depending on the clinical presentation, its severity and the presence and magnitude of any electrolyte abnormalities. Because cortisol measurements may not be available instantly, there are times when suspected disease requires treatment before a diagnosis has been attained.

Emergency management

Initial triage and treatment of a dog with hypoadrenocorticism is the same as for any emergency (Figure 28.12). Intravenous access should be obtained and an emergency database collected. At this stage it is important to be alert to the possibility of hypoadrenocorticism in order to undertake the ACTH response test necessary for diagnosis. Treatment relies primarily on intravenous fluid administration, especially initially and in those dogs presenting in shock, and appropriate parenteral corticosteroid supplementation.

1. Triage, initial assessments with capsular history
2. Intravenous catheter placement, obtain minimum database
3. Fluid therapy
   - Initial treatment for hypovolaemia: crystalloid fluid boluses for immediate volume expansion (10 ml/kg) and reassess
   - In dogs with severe hyponatraemia (<120 mmol/l), extra care should be taken with changes in sodium
   - In dogs with hyperkalaemia, see Figure 28.13
4. If hypoglycaemic: glucose at a dose rate of 0.5–1 ml/kg of 50% glucose, diluted to a 25% solution with normal saline and delivered over 5 minutes, and then add 2.5% or 5% glucose to maintenance fluids
5. Perform ACTH response test
6. Start intravenous corticosteroid replacement therapy
   - Hydrocortisone 0.5–0.625 mg/kg/h
   OR
   - Dexamethasone 0.1–0.5 mg/kg q12h
7. Monitor (every 1–2 hours initially):
   - Heart rate, pulse quality, respiratory rate, temperature
   - Systolic blood pressure
   - Serum electrolytes
   - Glucose
   - Acid–base status
8. Continue intravenous fluids and medication until the patient is able to eat, drink and take oral medications

28.12 Emergency management of hypoadrenocorticism. ACTH = adrenocorticotropic hormone.

Intravenous fluids

The initial choice of intravenous fluid varies depending on the specific presentation. Dogs in a hypoadrenocorticoid crisis are often hypovolaemic with hyperkalaemia and hyponatraemia but may also be hypoglycaemic, hypercalcaemic or profoundly anaemic. Fluid rates, as with all emergency or critically ill cases, are tailored to the individual and may change over time depending on response.

Hypovolaemia is recognized by poor peripheral pulses, altered mentation, pale mucous membranes, prolonged capillary refill time and possibly low blood pressure as compensatory mechanisms fail to adapt. Tachycardia is an expected response to hypovolaemia but may not be present in a dog with hyperkalaemia. Correction of hypovolaemia is achieved through rapid intravenous infusion of crystalloid fluids. A typical approach is to give a bolus of 10–20 ml/kg rapidly (over 10–15 minutes) and reassess clinical parameters, repeating this process up to three times. Fluid boluses not only address hypovolaemia but also help to address electrolyte and acid–base disturbances. If there is no sustained improvement after 40–60 ml/kg of fluid is administered, other concurrent treatment such as vasopressors may need to be considered.

Following the correction of hypovolaemia, affected dogs will require continued intravenous fluid therapy based on assessment of dehydration and ongoing requirements and losses. Frequent monitoring is required until abnormalities are corrected.

The ideal choice of fluids is not known as there are no studies directly comparing different fluid types in dogs with an Addisonian crisis. Glucose boluses followed by constant rate infusion of 2.5–5% glucose are required in dogs with hypoglycaemia (see Chapter 27). Blood products may be required if the animal is severely anaemic. Some clinicians prefer to use 0.9% NaCl as it makes intuitive sense to replace sodium with no additional potassium, arguing that any acidifying effect and subsequent increase in potassium concentrations is negligible. Others prefer compound sodium lactate because of its lesser effect on acidification and slightly lower sodium concentration (130 versus 154 mmol/l), arguing that its inherent potassium content (5 mmol/l) has negligible effect. Ultimately, the timely implementation of intravenous fluid therapy is more important than choice of fluid, at least initially. Indeed, the type of fluid may change during the management of the case based on the response of both potassium and sodium concentrations.

Rapid correction of sodium (>0.5 mmol/l/h or >12 mmol/l/24h) can lead to damage to the nerve sheaths in the brain stem (central pontine myelinolysis) that manifests as neurological signs including lethargy, weakness, ataxia, hypermetria and dysphagia. This may be more likely in dogs with especially severe hyponatraemia (<120 mmol/l), particularly if of long duration (although this is rarely known at the time of diagnosis). Neurological signs have been documented in dogs treated for hypoadrenocorticism, albeit rarely (Gunn et al., 2016). These neurological signs may not be apparent for days to weeks and dogs can recover, although in rare cases these side effects are fatal. The increase in sodium concentration is dependent on the sodium content of the fluids and their rate of administration, and whether mineralocorticoid supplementation is used. However, after correction of hypovolaemia, AVP secretion decreases and allows for increased water loss, which can increase the rate of correction of hyponatraemia regardless of the fluid or hormone replacement initially used. Thus, frequent monitoring (at least every 1–2 hours initially) of sodium concentration is required and in dogs with low sodium concentrations, half-strength saline (0.45% NaCl) or 2.5–5% glucose may be required to prevent overly rapid correction of hyponatraemia.

Intravenous fluid therapy alone is often sufficient to reduce hyperkalaemia, particularly if non-life-threatening and mild to moderate (up to approximately 7.0 mmol/l). Additional treatment for hyperkalaemia may need consideration if mineralocorticoid supplementation is not being used, there is a failure to respond to intravenous fluids alone or bradyarrhythmias are present (Figure 28.13). In dogs with cardiac abnormalities, 10% calcium gluconate is cardioprotective and counteracts the impairment of myocardial membrane excitability induced by hyperkalaemia but does not reduce potassium concentrations. It is effective immediately and typically lasts for 15–20 minutes but may last for up to an hour, and therefore other treatments may be needed. Administration of glucose works by stimulating endogenous insulin release, which in turn increases cellular uptake of potassium but takes 15–20 minutes to have an effect. Insulin and supplemental glucose can also be used for added effect. However, if insulin is used, then glucose supplementation must be continued and glucose concentrations carefully monitored. Dogs with hypoadrenocorticism are exquisitely sensitive to insulin because they lack the counter-regulatory effects of cortisol. Beta-2 adrenergic agonists, such as terbutaline, can also be used to drive potassium intracellularly. However, they should be avoided in dogs with arrhythmias or heart disease.

Mild to moderate hyperkalaemia (<7 mmol/l) without ECG changes
• 10 ml/kg boluses of crystalloid intravenous fluids if hypovolaemic until stabilized and then continued for dehydration and ongoing loses AND • 1–2 g dextrose bolus followed by 2.5% dextrose in ongoing fluid therapy if needed

Hyperkalaemia with ECG changes
• 0.5–1.5 ml/kg 10% calcium gluconate by slow intravenous infusion with ECG monitoring; cardioprotective effects last for 15–20 minutes

Moderate to severe hyperkalaemia (>7 mmol/l)
• Intravenous fluid, dextrose and calcium gluconate as appropriate, as described above AND • Neutral insulin 0.2–0.5 IU intravenously in combination with 1–2 g intravenous dextrose followed by continued 2.5% dextrose in fluids; close monitoring of blood glucose concentrations is required OR • 0.01 mg/kg terbutaline by slow intravenous infusion; can take 20–40 minutes to take effect and is contraindicated in dogs with heart disease or arrhythmia

28.13 Treatment outline for hyperkalaemia. ECG = electrocardiogram.

Hormone replacement

As discussed above, if there is a strong clinical suspicion of hypoadrenocorticism and definitive testing has been performed, specific hormone replacement therapy may need to be started pending test results. Until affected cases are systemically well, hormone replacement therapy should be delivered parenterally. In the emergency situation there are two approaches: one is to give a glucocorticoid alone, the other is to give hydrocortisone, which has equipotent mineralocorticoid and glucocorticoid effects.

Dexamethasone is often started at 0.1–0.5 mg/kg as an initial intravenous dose followed by repeat doses of 0.05–0.1 mg/kg every 12 hours. This equates to approximately 0.35–0.7 mg/kg prednisolone, which is befitting of the stressful nature of the illness. Dexamethasone has no mineralocorticoid action and thus, if intravenous fluids alone are not sufficiently effective in normalizing electrolyte abnormalities, other therapies may be required.

Hydrocortisone is recommended as an intravenous infusion of 0.5–0.625 mg/kg/h (Gunn et al., 2016), although it can instead be administered in boluses of 4–10 mg/kg every 6 hours. The infusion dose is likely to achieve plasma cortisol concentrations approaching 700–1,000 nmol/l within 2–3 hours, providing adequate glucocorticoid and mineralocorticoid activity for dogs with hypoadrenocorticism and hyperkalaemia. After instituting hydrocortisone therapy, judicious rates of intravenous fluids are required but clinicians should aim for no more than 2–4 times maintenance rates, particularly if 0.9% saline is used. Hydrocortisone infusion is associated with rapid correction of hyperkalaemia without the need for any additional treatment.

Each treatment protocol has its own potential benefits. Dexamethasone is usually routinely available in any primary care practice. Whilst limited by having no mineralocorticoid activity, unlike hydrocortisone, it can be administered while an ACTH response test is ongoing. If mineralocorticoid treatment is required, oral fludrocortisone can be used as a temporary measure, if tolerated (see 'Mineralocorticoids', below). Once the diagnosis has been confirmed, subcutaneous desoxycorticosterone pivalate (DOCP), a pure mineralocorticoid, can be used. Hydrocortisone is not as routinely available in primary care practice, although it has a prolonged shelf life of several years. Its main advantage is its potent mineralocorticoid action, but it cannot be used during the ACTH response test. It has a relatively short half-life compared with dexamethasone, which may confer an advantage if a diagnosis of hypoadrenocorticism is not subsequently confirmed and glucocorticoids are not indicated for the actual diagnosis. In one retrospective study of dogs with hypoadrenocorticism treated with intravenous prednisolone/dexamethasone *versus* hydrocortisone, there was no clear benefit of either treatment (Mitropoulou *et al.*, 2022). However, case numbers were limited and lower doses of hydrocortisone than usually recommended were used in some dogs.

Whatever treatment is used, rechecking, reappraising and changing plans for intravenous fluids, supplementation and supportive care are essential for success. Basic parameters, including heart rate, pulse quality, respiratory rate, temperature and blood pressure, should be monitored every 1–2 hours initially, spacing out to every 4–6 and then 8–12 hours as the dog responds and becomes more stable. Electrolytes should also be rechecked every 1–2 hours initially, spacing out to every 6–12 hours dependent on the severity of abnormality and rate of change.

Chronic management

Transition to long-term management and hormone replacement can start once the dog is stable. Given the permanent, irreversible nature of the underlying pathology, treatment is lifelong and should not be stopped. It can take time to find the best management solution for a particular dog and this may change over time (e.g. due to the development of concurrent conditions).

There are two commonly used approaches for chronic management of dogs with hypoadrenocorticism:

- Desoxycorticosterone pivalate for mineralocorticoid replacement and prednisolone or cortisone for glucocorticoid replacement
- Fludrocortisone for mineralocorticoid replacement; sufficient inherent glucocorticoid activity may be present to avoid additional prednisolone/cortisone treatment.

In dogs with isolated hypocortisolism, whether from primary or secondary disease, only glucocorticoid replacement is required and, in those rare cases with isolated hypoaldosteronism, only mineralocorticoid replacement is required.

Glucocorticoids

Prednisolone is the most frequently used glucocorticoid supplement in dogs with hypoadrenocorticism. Prednisolone is a widely used synthetic oral glucocorticoid, with different doses having distinct pharmacological outcomes:

- Physiological replacement (0.1–0.2 mg/kg/day)
- Anti-inflammatory (0.5–1 mg/kg/day)
- Immunosuppression (2 mg/kg/day).

For dogs with hypoadrenocorticism, physiological replacement is the goal. A starting dose of approximately 0.1–0.2 mg/kg/day is used, but higher doses of 0.3–0.5 mg/kg/day can be used if the dog is recovering from a severe crisis (Sieber-Ruckstuhl *et al.*, 2019). Higher doses are then usually adjusted downwards. Finding the optimal prednisolone dose that is adequate for replacement whilst avoiding adverse effects has been described as 'the art of hypoadrenocorticism management'.

Dose reductions are required if there are any signs of iatrogenic hypercortisolism – typically polyuria and polydipsia (PU/PD), polyphagia or panting. More subtle effects on hair growth and bodyweight/composition changes can be present and even subtle signs warrant dose reduction.

Dose increments are required if there are signs attributable to a lack of glucocorticoids, typically gastrointestinal signs, lethargy, inappetence or weakness. Increases and decreases are usually between 25% and 50% of the prior dose. In most dogs, maintenance doses are 0.01–0.4 mg/kg/day (Farr *et al.*, 2020). Some dogs treated with DOCP require glucocorticoid therapy only every other day.

At periods of known stress (e.g. non-adrenal disease, elective surgery, fireworks, kennelling), it is important to remember that dogs with hypoadrenocorticism cannot increase endogenous cortisol secretion in response to the stress. Therefore, dose increases to 0.3–0.5 mg/kg/day are often recommended for a few days before tapering back down.

Cortisone can be used instead of prednisolone. It is rapidly hydroxylated to cortisol and therefore provides some mineralocorticoid activity, although this is limited at the replacement glucocorticoid doses used. Dosages usually start at 0.5–1.0 mg/kg either once or twice daily. Once stable, a dosage of 0.5 mg/kg either once or twice daily provides adequate glucocorticoid supplementation. Finding tablets of appropriate size for small dogs can be challenging.

Mineralocorticoids

Dogs with mineralocorticoid deficiency, diagnosed based on the presence of supportive electrolyte changes or known aldosterone deficiency, should receive replacement hormone therapy.

Desoxycorticosterone pivalate is an extremely potent and receptor-specific synthetic mineralocorticoid available as a suspension for injection. It has a peak action at approximately 10 (range 7–14) days and a prolonged duration of action of approximately 4 weeks. Dose adjustments are based on sodium and potassium concentrations measured at 10 days and immediately prior to the next injection (Figure 28.14). Desoxycorticosterone pivalate has been available in the USA as an authorized intramuscular injection (Percortan V) for some time. Recently, a new subcutaneous formulation (Zycortal) has been authorized in the UK, the European Union and the USA. A non-inferiority randomized study demonstrated no major difference between these two formulations (Farr *et al.*, 2020). Desoxycorticosterone pivalate has no glucocorticoid effects and, therefore, concurrent prednisolone or other glucocorticoid medication must always be used. The currently authorized initial dose for DOCP is 2.2 mg/kg. However, long-term studies have demonstrated success with lower doses for almost all dogs, with average doses of 1.69 mg/kg and 1.3 mg/kg for intramuscular DOCP, and 1.1 mg/kg for subcutaneous DOCP (Sieber-Ruckstuhl *et al.*, 2019). Studies starting at lower doses have shown that increases are infrequently required (Sieber-Ruckstuhl *et al.*, 2019).

As well as dose adjustments, the dosing interval of DOCP therapy can be altered. Reported dosing intervals range between 14 days and 90 days, with the latter often recommended for financial reasons (Jaffey *et al.*, 2017). However, prolonged dosing intervals are based on

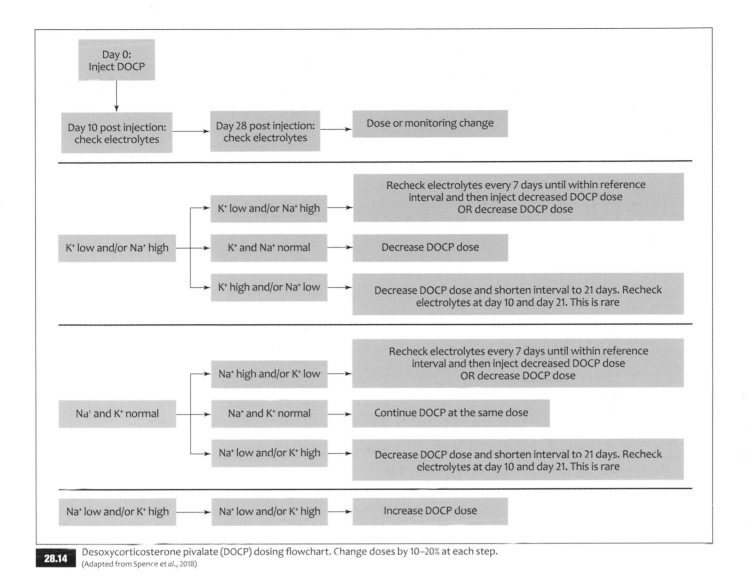

28.14 Desoxycorticosterone pivalate (DOCP) dosing flowchart. Change doses by 10–20% at each step. (Adapted from Spence *et al.*, 2018)

electrolyte measurements rather than circulating DOCP concentrations. The manufacturers' recommended dosing interval is 25 days. The preferred dosing interval is approximately 28–31 days for repeatably reliable injection frequency (every 4 weeks or once a month) and to minimise the risks of a crisis (Scott-Moncrieff, 2015). Owners can be taught to inject their own dogs once a stable dosage is found.

Side effects are not typically seen with DOCP but PU/PD at the time of peak action have been reported. This usually resolves with a dose reduction but must be distinguished from excessive prednisolone dosing.

Fludrocortisone, the main alternative mineralocorticoid, was used almost exclusively in the UK and European Union until DOCP was specifically authorized for dogs. It is a synthetic mineralocorticoid given orally, initially once a day (Roberts *et al.*, 2016). A key difference from DOCP is that fludrocortisone possesses some glucocorticoid activity and only half of dogs treated with it require concurrent prednisolone (Roberts *et al.*, 2016). Some cases will have clinical signs of iatrogenic hypercortisolism on fludrocortisone alone (Scott-Moncrieff, 2015). In the acutely presenting dog, fludrocortisone should be given only once the dog is stable and no longer vomiting.

The starting fludrocortisone dose is 0.01–0.03 mg/kg once a day, using the lower dosage initially. Dose requirements may increase over time and, as with DOCP, are based on electrolyte measurements. Electrolytes are measured every week and the dose adjusted by 0.05–0.1 mg/day until they are maintained within the reference interval. The dose is increased if there is hyponatraemia and/or hyperkalaemia and decreased if there is hypernatraemia and/or hypokalaemia. Dogs that maintain electrolyte abnormalities on once-daily dosing may eventually benefit from twice-daily dosing. Once a stable dose is found, electrolytes can be checked every 3–6 months. There is some evidence that DOCP is superior to fludrocortisone as a replacement for aldosterone in dogs. This, combined with it being an authorized product, makes DOCP the first choice for treating dogs with hypoadrenocorticism.

Prognosis

The prognosis for primary hypoadrenocorticism is usually excellent, with reported median survival times of between 2.5 and 5.4 years post diagnosis (Ramsey *et al.*, 2016). In one large epidemiological study (Hanson *et al.*, 2016), dogs with hypoadrenocorticism had an increased risk of death overall compared with dogs without hypoadrenocorticism, but long-term cohort studies are currently lacking. Most dogs with hypoadrenocorticism return to a good quality of life for many years, provided medications are reliably administered. As the majority of dogs with hypoadrenocorticism have an immune-mediated disease, it is not yet known whether they have an increased risk of developing other immune-mediated disorders (see Chapter 36).

References and further reading

Annane D, Pastores SM, Arlt W *et al.* (2017) Critical illness-related corticosteroid insufficiency (CIRCI): a narrative review from a Multispecialty Task Force of the Society of Critical Care Medicine (SCCM) and the European Society of Intensive Care Medicine (ESICM). *Intensive Care Medicine* 43, 1781–1792

Baumstark ME, Sieber-Ruckstuhl NS, Müller C *et al.* (2014) Evaluation of aldosterone concentrations in dogs with hypoadrenocorticism. *Journal of Veterinary Internal Medicine* 28, 154–159

Boag AM, Brown A, Koenigshof A *et al.* (2020) Glucocorticoid metabolism in critically ill dogs (*Canis lupus familiaris*). *Domestic Animal Endocrinology* 72, 106437

Boag AM and Catchpole B (2014) A review of the genetics of hypoadrenocorticism. *Topics in Companion Animal Medicine* 29, 96–101

Boag AM, Christie MR, McLaughlin KA *et al.* (2015) Autoantibodies against cytochrome P450 side-chain cleavage enzyme in dogs (*Canis lupus familiaris*) affected with hypoadrenocorticism (Addison's disease). *PLoS ONE* 10, e0143458

Boretti FS, Meyer F, Burkhardt WA *et al.* (2015) Evaluation of the cortisol-to-ACTH ratio in dogs with hypoadrenocorticism, dogs with diseases mimicking hypoadrenocorticism and in healthy dogs. *Journal of Veterinary Internal Medicine* 29, 1335–1341

Decôme M and Blais MC (2017) Prevalence and clinical features of hypoadrenocorticism in Great Pyrenees dogs in a referral population: 11 cases. *Canadian Veterinary Journal* 58, 1093–1099

Farr H, Mason BL and Longhofer SL (2020) Randomised clinical non-inferiority trial comparing two formulations of desoxycortone pivalate for the treatment of canine primary hypoadrenocorticism. *Veterinary Record* 187, e12

Gold AJ, Langlois DK and Refsal KR (2016) Evaluation of basal serum or plasma cortisol concentrations for the diagnosis of hypoadrenocorticism in dogs. *Journal of Veterinary Internal Medicine* 30, 1798–1805

Gunn E, Shiel RE and Mooney CT (2016) Hydrocortisone in the management of acute hypoadrenocorticism in dogs: a retrospective series of 30 cases. *Journal of Small Animal Practice* 57, 227–233

Hanson J, Tengvall, K, Bonnett B and Hedhammar Å (2016) Naturally occurring adrenocortical insufficiency – an epidemiological study based on a Swedish-insured dog population of 525,028 dogs. *Journal of Veterinary Internal Medicine* 30, 76–84

Hauck C, Schmitz SS, Burgener IA *et al.* (2020) Prevalence and characterization of hypoadrenocorticism in dogs with signs of chronic gastrointestinal disease: a multicenter study. *Journal of Veterinary Internal Medicine* 34, 1399–1405

Jaffey JA, Nurre P, Cannon AB *et al.* (2017) Desoxycorticosterone pivalate duration of action and individualized dosing intervals in dogs with primary hypoadrenocorticism. *Journal of Veterinary Internal Medicine* 31, 1649–1657

Javadi S, Galac S, Boer P *et al.* (2006) Aldosterone-to-renin and cortisol-to-adrenocorticotropic hormone ratios in healthy dogs and dogs with primary hypoadrenocorticism. *Journal of Veterinary Internal Medicine* 20, 556–561

Johnson CM, Kass PH, Cohen TA and Feldman EC (2017) Effect of intravenous or perivascular injection of synthetic adrenocorticotropic hormone on stimulation test results in dogs. *Journal of Veterinary Internal Medicine* 31, 730–733

King JB and Morton JM (2017) Incidence and risk factors for hypoadrenocorticism in dogs treated with trilostane. *Veterinary Journal* 230, 24–29

Lathan P, Scott-Moncrieff JC and Wills RW (2014) Use of the cortisol-to-ACTH ratio for diagnosis of primary hypoadrenocorticism in dogs. *Journal of Veterinary Internal Medicine* 28, 1546–1550

Lennon EM, Hummel JB and Vaden SL (2018) Urine sodium concentrations are predictive of hypoadrenocorticism in hyponatraemic dogs: a retrospective pilot study. *Journal of Small Animal Practice* 59, 228–231

Lyngby JG and Sellon RK (2016) Hypoadrenocorticism mimicking protein-losing enteropathy in 4 dogs. *Canadian Veterinary Journal* 57, 757–760

Mitropoulou A, Haüser K, Lehmann H and Hazuchova K (2022) Comparison of hydrocortisone continuous rate infusion and prednisolone or dexamethasone administration for treatment of acute hypoadrenal (Addisonian) crisis in dogs. *Frontiers in Veterinary Science* 8, 818515

Ramsey I, Roberts E and Spence S (2016) Management of Addison's disease in dogs. *Veterinary Record* 178, 478

Roberts E, Boden LA and Ramsey IK (2016) Factors that affect stabilisation times of canine spontaneous hypoadrenocorticism. *Veterinary Record* 179, 98

Scott-Moncrieff JCR (2015) Hypoadrenocorticism. In: *Canine and Feline Endocrinology, 4th edn*, ed. EC Feldman, RW Nelson, CE Reusch and JCR Scott-Moncrieff, pp. 485–520. Elsevier, St. Louis

Sieber-Ruckstuhl NS, Burkhardt WA, Hofer-Inteeworn N *et al.* (2015) Cortisol response in healthy and diseased dogs after stimulation with a depot formulation of synthetic ACTH. *Journal of Veterinary Internal Medicine* 29, 1541–1546

Sieber-Ruckstuhl NS, Reusch CE, Hofer-Inteeworn N *et al.* (2019) Evaluation of a low-dose desoxycorticosterone pivalate treatment protocol for long-term management of dogs with primary hypoadrenocorticism. *Journal of Veterinary Internal Medicine* 33, 1266–1271

Spence S, Gunn E and Ramsey I (2018) Diagnosis and treatment of canine hypoadrenocorticism. *In Practice* 40, 281–290

Sullivant AM and Lathan P (2020) Ketoconazole-induced transient hypoadrenocorticism in a dog. *Canadian Veterinary Journal* 61, 407–410

Wakayama JA, Furrow E, Merkel LK and Armstrong PJ (2017) A retrospective study of dogs with atypical hypoadrenocorticism: a diagnostic cut-off or continuum? *Journal of Small Animal Practice* 58, 365–371

Chapter 29

Canine hypercortisolism

Ian K. Ramsey and Michael E. Herrtage

Introduction

Hypercortisolism describes a clinical disorder caused by an absolute or relative excess of cortisol or other steroids that mimic the actions of cortisol. The term hyperadrenocorticism is regarded as a synonym for hypercortisolism but the more specific term hypercortisolism is now preferred. The term Cushing's syndrome is also used synonymously but should be retained to describe the constellation of signs associated with chronic exposure to cortisol excess.

Physiology of the adrenal gland

Adrenal gland anatomy and physiology are covered in Chapter 28.

Functions of cortisol

Cortisol has more diverse effects on the body than any other hormone (see Chapter 28). It is best regarded as a hormone that has evolved to play a pivotal role in the body's response to long-term stresses such as starvation, chronic inflammation and infection. During periods of stress, both adrenocorticotropic hormone (ACTH) and cortisol are maintained at high concentrations, because the effects of stress tend to override the normal negative feedback control. Challenges to the immune system also activate the hypothalamic–pituitary–adrenal (HPA) axis.

In many respects, cortisol counteracts the effects of insulin. In response to stress, cortisol stimulates gluconeogenesis and protein and fat catabolism. As a result, when cortisol is present in excessive quantities, protein and fat stores are reduced in all tissues of the body except the liver. The catabolic actions of glucocorticoids on protein result in muscle wastage and weakness. The catabolic effects on fat stores are countered by insulin, which inhibits lipolysis and stimulates lipogenesis. As a result, adipose tissue tends to be redistributed to the abdomen and back of the neck in dogs with excess concentrations of glucocorticoids and an adequate nutritional supply.

In response to chronic immunological and inflammatory stresses, cortisol has multiple profound effects that serve to prevent the body's pro-inflammatory reactions from becoming excessive or harmful. As a result, when cortisol is present in excess, it is anti-inflammatory, antipyretic and immunosuppressive.

Causes of hypercortisolism

Hypercortisolism can be spontaneous or iatrogenic. In humans, spontaneous hypercortisolism is classified as ACTH dependent (previously referred to as pituitary dependent) or ACTH independent (adrenal dependent), each with multiple potential causes. In dogs, both ACTH-dependent and -independent hypercortisolism have been identified, although, compared with humans, fewer potential causes have been identified in each of these categories.

ACTH-dependent hypercortisolism

Adrenocorticotropic hormone-dependent hypercortisolism accounts for approximately 80–85% of dogs with naturally occurring hypercortisolism. Excessive ACTH secretion results in bilateral adrenocortical hyperplasia and excess cortisol secretion (Figure 29.1a). There is a failure of the negative feedback control of cortisol on ACTH. However, ACTH secretion may remain episodic, resulting in fluctuating cortisol concentrations, which may at times fall within the reference interval.

More than 90% of dogs with ACTH-dependent hypercortisolism have an identifiable pituitary tumour. Adenomas are the most common type of canine pituitary tumour reported. Invasive adenomas, characterized by local invasion of brain parenchyma, are less common and adenocarcinomas, with evidence of metastatic disease, are rare (Pollard et al., 2010). Pituitary tumours are often classified by size as microtumours (<10 mm in diameter) and macrotumours (>10 mm in diameter). Classification by comparing tumour height to brain area may be more appropriate to account for differences in dog size (microtumours <0.40 x 10^{-2} mm^{-1} and macrotumours ≥0.40 x 10^{-2} mm^{-1}). Macrotumours may compress the remaining pituitary gland and extend dorsally into the hypothalamus (Figure 29.2).

Hypersecretion of pituitary ACTH in the absence of recognizable neoplasia has also been suggested as a potential cause of ACTH-dependent hypercortisolism. Suggested aetiologies have included chronic stimulation by hypothalamic corticotropin-releasing hormone or a primary failure of the normal cortisol negative feedback response. These theories lack supportive evidence and are not widely accepted.

From a clinical point of view, the precise pituitary pathology is not of great importance unless neurological signs are present at the time of diagnosis or become apparent during the initial treatment.

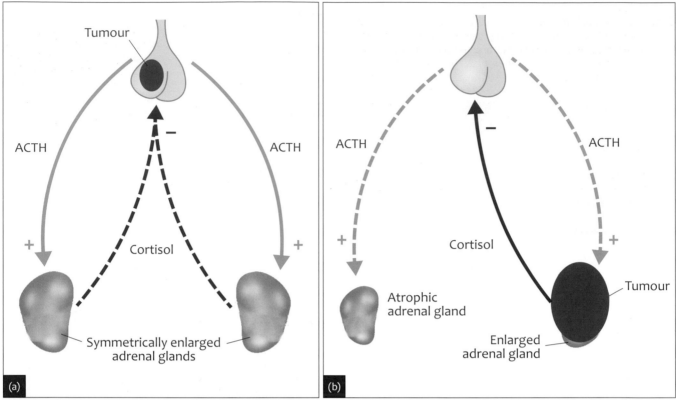

29.1 (a) The pituitary–adrenal axis in adrenocorticotropic hormone (ACTH)-dependent hypercortisolism. There is a failure of the normal negative feedback effect of cortisol on ACTH (dashed red line). (b) The pituitary–adrenal axis in ACTH-independent hypercortisolism. The excess cortisol produced by the abnormal adrenal gland suppresses ACTH secretion (dashed green lines). The contralateral adrenal gland shrinks in size due to reduced stimulation by ACTH. + = stimulation; − = inhibition.

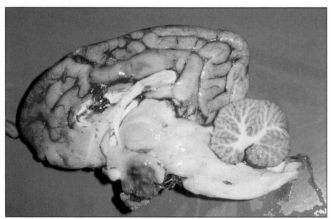

29.2 Pituitary macroadenoma found on post-mortem examination of a 13-year-old Golden Retriever that had been successfully treated with mitotane for hypercortisolism for 5 years. There were no neurological signs associated with this tumour.

In humans, ectopic ACTH secretion can occur with a variety of neoplastic disorders but most commonly small cell lung carcinoma. Ectopic ACTH production is a rare cause of hypercortisolism in the dog; only three suspected cases have been reported, of which only one was intensively investigated (Galac *et al.*, 2005).

ACTH-independent hypercortisolism

The remaining 15–20% of spontaneous cases of hypercortisolism are usually caused by unilateral adrenal tumours, with an approximately equal frequency of adenomas and carcinomas (see Figure 29.1b). Autonomous and excessive production of cortisol results in negative feedback on the pituitary gland and hypothalamus, suppressed ACTH

production and subsequent atrophy of the remaining cortisol-secreting cells within the non-neoplastic contralateral adrenal gland (Figure 29.3).

Bilateral adrenocortical tumours have also been reported but appear to be rare and need to be distinguished from unilateral adrenocortical tumours with concurrent phaeochromocytomas or incidentalomas. Adrenocortical tumours may be benign or malignant, although distinction can be difficult histologically, unless there is evidence of invasion or metastasis. Several new markers of malignancy and prognosis include an adapted version of the Ki67 proliferation index and differential expression of certain genes (such as pituitary tumour-transforming gene-1, topoisomerase II alpha and steroidogenic factor-1), although these

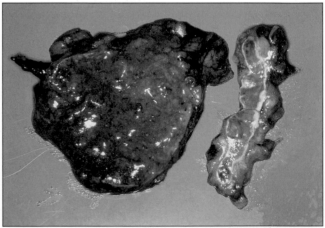

29.3 The cut surface of both adrenal glands from a case of adrenocortical carcinoma of the right adrenal gland, seen to the left of the image (see Figure 29.4). Note the severe cortical atrophy (pale rim) in the contralateral adrenal gland.

are not yet commercially available (Sanders *et al.*, 2019a,b). Clinically, benign tumours are usually small and well circumscribed, and are commonly partly calcified. In contrast, adrenocortical carcinomas are usually larger, locally invasive, haemorrhagic and necrotic. They are also often calcified. Right adrenal gland carcinomas frequently invade the phrenicoabdominal vein and caudal vena cava (Figure 29.4). Carcinomas can also metastasize to the liver, lung and kidney.

In humans, aberrant expression of receptors within the adrenal gland may enhance responsiveness to other factors and result in hypercortisolism. There is one report of food-associated hypercortisolaemia in a dog arising from ectopic adrenocortical expression of gastric-inhibitory polypeptide receptors (Galac *et al.*, 2008).

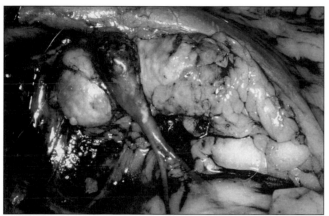

29.4 Intraoperative photograph of the same case as Figure 29.3. The carcinoma is invading the phrenicoabdominal vein. The caudal vena cava can be seen at the top of the image.

Combined ACTH-dependent and -independent hypercortisolism

A few reports exist in which dogs with ACTH-dependent hypercortisolism had concurrent adrenal tumours (Beatrice *et al.*, 2018).

Prevalence

Hypercortisolism is one of the most commonly diagnosed endocrinopathies in the dog. One epidemiological study estimated the prevalence as 0.28% in primary-care practices in the UK (O'Neill *et al.*, 2016). Another study, which used stricter inclusion criteria, reported a prevalence of 0.20% in four primary-care practices in Italy (Carotenuto *et al.*, 2019).

Signalment

Age

The large majority of dogs with hypercortisolism are older than 6 years of age. Adrenocorticotropic hormone-dependent hypercortisolism has a reported age range of 2–16 years and a median age of 7–9 years. Dogs with ACTH-independent hypercortisolism tend to be slightly older, ranging from 6 to 16 years, with mean age reported as approximately 11 years.

Breed

Any breed can develop hypercortisolism; however, small breeds such as the Toy Poodle, Dachshund, Yorkshire, Jack Russell and Staffordshire Bull Terrier, and Bichon Frise appear at greater risk of developing ACTH-dependent hypercortisolism. Adrenocortical tumours occur more frequently in larger breeds, with approximately 50% of affected dogs weighing more than 20 kg.

Sex

Both males and females can develop hypercortisolism. However, there is controversy regarding a significant sex predisposition. On balance, females are slightly more likely to develop hypercortisolism than males.

Clinical features

Affected dogs usually develop a combination of clinical signs associated with increased cortisol concentrations (Figure 29.5). Some dogs, however, may show only a few characteristic signs, rather than the classic array of clinical signs.

Hypercortisolism has an insidious onset and is slowly progressive over many months or even years. Many owners consider the early signs (e.g. thinning hair coat, lethargy) as part of the normal ageing process of their dog or misinterpret the signs (e.g. increased appetite) as indicating good health. In a few cases, clinical signs may be intermittent, with periods of remission and relapse; in others there may be an apparent rapid onset and progression of clinical signs.

Polyuria and polydipsia

Polyuria and polydipsia are noted in nearly all cases of hypercortisolism. Polydipsia is noticeable in most dogs when water consumption exceeds approximately 100 ml/kg/day. However, some astute owners may note polydipsia even if water consumption does not exceed this amount. Excessive thirst, nocturia, incontinence and/or urination in the house are usually reported by owners. The polydipsia occurs secondary to the polyuria. The precise cause of the polyuria remains obscure, but it may be due to increased glomerular filtration rate, inhibition of the release of arginine vasopressin (AVP), inhibition of the action of AVP on the renal tubules or possibly accelerated metabolism of AVP.

- Polyuria and polydipsia
- Polyphagia
- Abdominal distension
- Liver enlargement
- Muscle wasting/weakness
- Lethargy, poor exercise tolerance
- Skin changes
- Alopecia
- Excessive panting
- Hypertension
- Persistent anoestrus or testicular atrophy
- Calcinosis cutis
- Myotonia
- Neurological signs
- Hypertensive retinopathy

29.5 Clinical signs of hypercortisolism in dogs in approximate order of frequency.

Polyphagia and weight gain

Increased appetite is common and, although many owners dismiss it as a sign of good health, a voracious appetite or scavenging/stealing of food may give rise to concern, especially if the dog previously had a poor appetite. Polyphagia is assumed to be a direct effect of glucocorticoids acting on the central nervous system.

Hypercortisolism is also associated with an increase in weight in many cases, despite a concurrent loss of muscle mass. The weight gain is partly due to polyphagia, but even dogs fed normal maintenance rations may gain weight if they develop hypercortisolism. This may be because cortisol decreases the maintenance energy requirement and overall metabolic rate or because of its effect on exercise tolerance. Cortisol also has effects on fat distribution, such that increased fat deposits tend to occur in the neck area, over the dorsum and within the abdomen.

Abdominal distension

A pot-bellied appearance (Figure 29.6) is common in hypercortisolism but may be so insidious that owners fail to recognize its significance. Abdominal distension is associated with the redistribution of fat to the abdomen, liver enlargement, a chronically distended bladder and weakness of the abdominal muscles. The weakness of the abdominal muscles makes palpation of the pendulous abdomen easier and more rewarding.

Muscle wasting/weakness

The gradual onset of lethargy and poor exercise tolerance is initially considered by many owners as compatible with ageing. Owners may become concerned only when muscle weakness leads to an inability to climb stairs or jump into a car. Lethargy, excessive panting and poor exercise tolerance are probably an expression of muscle wasting and weakness. Apart from the development of a pendulous abdomen, decreased muscle mass may be noted around the limbs, over the spine or over the temporal region. Muscle weakness is the result of muscle wasting caused by protein catabolism and a direct effect of cortisol on cell membrane excitability.

Occasionally, dogs with hypercortisolism develop myotonia, characterized by persistent active muscle contractions that continue after voluntary or involuntary stimuli. All limbs may be affected, but the signs are usually more severe in the hindlimbs. Animals with myotonia walk with a stiff, stilted gait or 'bunny hop'. The

affected limbs are rigid and rapidly return to extension after being passively flexed. In some cases, passive flexion may be difficult or impossible because of the persistently increased muscle tone. Spinal reflexes are difficult to elicit because of the rigidity but pain sensation is normal. The muscles are usually slightly hypertrophied, rather than being atrophied, and a myotonic dimple can be elicited by percussion of the affected muscle. Bizarre high-frequency discharges are noted on electromyography. These bizarre myotonic discharges may also be found in some dogs with hypercortisolism that do not show obvious clinical manifestations of myotonia.

Dermatological features

The skin, particularly over the ventral abdomen, becomes thin and inelastic because of atrophy of the dermal connective tissues. Elasticity can be assessed clinically by tenting the skin between the thumb and forefinger (Figure 29.7). In healthy dogs, the skin will rapidly return to a smooth contour, whereas in hypercortisolism it remains tented. Striae (stretch marks) can form as a result of this inelasticity. The abdominal veins are prominent and easily visible through the thin skin (Figure 29.8).

There is often excessive surface scale, and comedones caused by follicular plugging are seen, especially around the nipples (Figure 29.9). Hyperpigmentation of the skin is a rare sign of canine hypercortisolism.

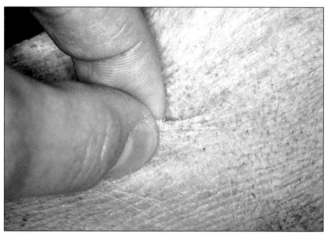

29.7 The skin on the ventral abdomen can be tented to assess elasticity.

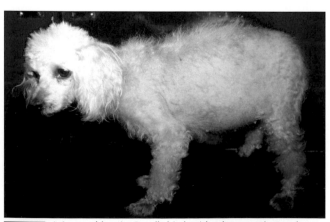

29.6 A 6-year-old entire Poodle bitch with adrenocorticotropic hormone-dependent hypercortisolism. Note the abdominal distension, muscle wasting, alopecia and thin skin.

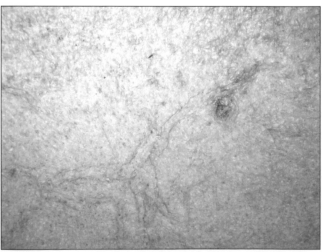

29.8 In hypercortisolism, the abdominal veins are visible through the thin skin.

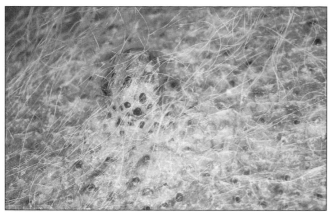

29.9 Comedones around a nipple. The skin is thin and abdominal veins are visible.

Protein catabolism, causing atrophic skin collagen, also leads to excessive bruising following venepuncture or other minor trauma (Figure 29.10). Wound healing is extraordinarily slow, presumably because of inhibition of fibroblast proliferation and collagen synthesis. Healing wounds often undergo dehiscence and even old scars may start to break down (Figure 29.11).

Calcinosis cutis is a frequent finding in biopsy material from the skin. Clinical evidence of calcinosis cutis is less common but is pathognomonic for hypercortisolism. The gross appearance can vary but predilection sites are the neck, axillae, ventral abdomen and inguinal areas (Figure 29.12). Calcinosis cutis usually appears as a firm, slightly raised, white or cream plaque surrounded by a rim of erythema. Large plaques tend to crack, become secondarily infected and develop a crust containing white powdery material.

Thinning of the hair coat leading to bilaterally symmetrical alopecia is frequently seen with hypercortisolism and occurs because of the inhibitory effect of cortisol on the anagen (growth) phase of the hair cycle. The remaining hair is dull and dry because it is in the telogen (resting) phase of the hair cycle. The alopecia is non-pruritic and affects mainly the flanks, ventral abdomen, chest, perineum and neck. The head, feet and in some cases the tail are usually the last areas to be affected (see Figure 29.6). The coat colour is often lighter than normal. Occasionally, affected dogs do not lose their hair coat but retain it, becoming hypertrichotic. When hair has been clipped in dogs with hypercortisolism, it will frequently fail to regrow, or the regrowth will be poor or sparse.

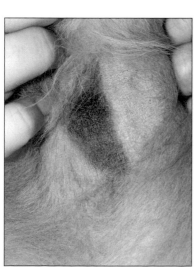

29.10 Extensive bruising on the neck of a Pomeranian with hypercortisolism. This resulted from a single needle insertion with minimal restraint and pressure being applied for a minute or so afterwards.

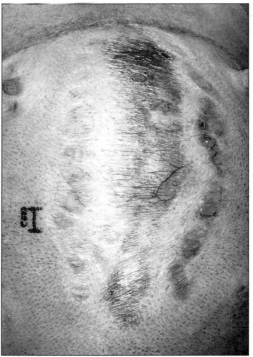

29.11 Partial breakdown of an abdominal incision in a Boxer with hypercortisolism.

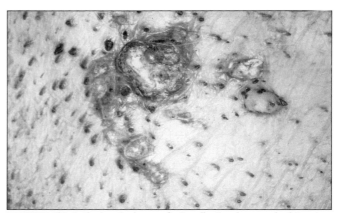

29.12 Skin in the inguinal area of a Poodle. Focal areas of calcinosis cutis can be seen eroding through the epidermis. Comedones are also present.

Occasionally, these skin and hair coat changes may be the owner's main reason for presentation (Zur and White, 2011) .

Respiratory signs

The most frequent respiratory abnormality noted is excessive panting, usually related to muscle weakness and wastage. Fat redistribution and the increasing size of the abdomen may also play a role.

Anoestrus or testicular atrophy

Entire bitches with hypercortisolism usually cease to have regular oestrous cycles. The length of anoestrus, which is often years, indicates the duration of the disease process. In the intact male, both testes become soft and spongy. Anoestrus or testicular atrophy occurs due to the negative feedback effect of high concentrations of cortisol on the pituitary gland, which also suppresses the secretion of gonadotropic hormones.

Signs associated with ACTH-dependent and -independent hypercortisolism

The clinical signs are similar in dogs with ACTH-dependent and -independent hypercortisolism, with a few exceptions. A few cases will develop neurological signs associated with a functional pituitary tumour, although a correlation between pituitary tumour size and the presence or development of neurological signs is not clear cut. Large pituitary tumours can be present without causing neurological signs, and neurological signs may be present in dogs with smaller tumours. In one study of advanced imaging (computed tomography (CT) or magnetic resonance imaging (MRI)) in dogs with ACTH-dependent hypercortisolism, a similar percentage of dogs with and without neurological signs had a detectable pituitary tumour (66% versus 71%, respectively) (Wood et al., 2007). Indeed, 56% of dogs that had neurological signs did not have a detectable pituitary tumour or had a pituitary micro-tumour. The size of the tumour thus appears less important than the rate of growth in determining the development of neurological signs. The fact that neurological signs may not be present even with large tumours suggests that many are, at least initially, slow growing. Nevertheless, neurological signs were present in 65% of dogs with macrotumours compared with 27% of those with microtumours (Wood et al., 2007).

The most common neurological signs are vague, such as lethargy, mental dullness, depression, disorientation, loss of learned behaviour and anorexia, rather than more specific signs, such as aimless wandering or pacing, head pressing, circling, ataxia, blindness, anisocoria and seizures. More often, however, neurological signs develop during initial treatment of ACTH-dependent hypercortisolism with trilostane or mitotane. This is thought to involve removal of the negative feedback inhibition of cortisol on the pituitary gland and hypothalamus, which then allows some pituitary tumours to enlarge rapidly, resulting in oedema and increased intracranial pressure. Additionally, intracranial haemorrhage from the pituitary tumour may lead to pituitary apoplexy, which is characterized by an acute severe depression and possible diabetes insipidus that is often, although not universally, fatal (Long et al., 2003; Bertolini et al., 2007). Trigger factors for pituitary apoplexy are not known in dogs, but in humans there is an association with recent endocrine testing (including ACTH response tests). The reason for this is not known.

Neurological signs are not a feature in dogs with functional adrenal tumours. Nevertheless, signs related to the rupture of an adrenal mass (e.g. acute weakness, pale mucous membranes, abdominal pain) can occur, albeit rarely. Signs related to neoplastic invasion of the phrenico-abdominal vein and/or caudal vena cava usually indicate an adrenal tumour. However, thromboembolic disease may cause similar signs.

Complications associated with hypercortisolism

Hypertension

Systemic hypertension occurs in more than 80% of dogs with untreated hypercortisolism and is severe in over 40% (>180 mmHg) (García San José et al., 2020). The mechanisms underlying hypertension are varied and potentially include cortisol-induced activation of the mineralocorticoid receptors and enhanced vascular sensitivity to vasoconstrictors (see Chapter 5). In most cases, the hypertension is not associated with clinical signs, but hypertension-induced blindness due to intraocular haemorrhage and retinal detachment has been reported, albeit rarely. In general, hypertension does not resolve following treatment of hypercortisolism. The explanation for this is not currently known.

Diabetes mellitus

Approximately 10% of cases with hypercortisolism develop overt diabetes mellitus. This is caused by antagonism to the action of insulin by the gluconeogenic effects of excess glucocorticoids. Clinical signs of the two disorders are similar, although ketones are only demonstrable in dogs that have concurrent diabetes mellitus. Some affected dogs develop diabetic ketoacidosis or hyperosmolar hyperglycaemic syndrome, in which case they will present as sick animals (see Chapter 26).

Biliary disease

There appears to be an association between hypercortisolism and development of gall bladder mucocoeles. Hypercortisolism is reported in up to approximately 25% of dogs with mucocoeles, and approximately 20% of hypercortisolaemic dogs have mucocoeles (Mesich et al., 2009; Kim et al., 2017). Whilst the underlying cause is unclear, breed, genetics, female sex predisposition, hypercholesterolaemia, cholestatic liver disease and cortisol-induced disturbances in bile acid metabolism may all play a role.

Pancreatic disease

Any association between hypercortisolism and pancreatitis is unclear. Hypercortisolism has been previously diagnosed in a small proportion of dogs with fatal acute pancreatitis. Increased canine pancreas-specific lipase concentrations and DGGR lipase activities have been identified in approximately 35% and 50% of dogs with hypercortisolism, respectively (Mawby et al., 2014; Bennaim et al., 2018). However, clinical signs associated with acute pancreatitis are not often observed in dogs with hypercortisolism.

Lower urinary tract disease

Urinary tract infection (UTI) occurs in approximately 50% of cases of hypercortisolism. There is an increased risk of UTI because urine is retained in an over-distended bladder due to incomplete voiding resulting from muscle weakness and because of the immunosuppressive effect of excess cortisol. Few clinical signs of UTI are apparent. Urinary tract infections can also ascend to the kidneys to cause pyelonephritis.

Increased calcium excretion is a feature of hypercortisolism and, consequently, dogs with hypercortisolism are more likely to have calcium oxalate urolithiasis. There may be no associated clinical signs.

Thromboembolic disease

Hypercortisolism is associated with hypercoagulability, and thromboembolic disease is a potential but rare complication. Pulmonary thromboembolism is well recognized and associated with the acute onset of clinical signs of tachypnoea progressing to overt dyspnoea. Thromboembolic disease may also involve the aorta, vena cava, and portal and splenic vessels.

Central diabetes insipidus

Dogs with pituitary macrotumours may develop concurrent central diabetes insipidus due to compression of the posterior lobe of the pituitary gland and the hypothalamus. In such cases, there will be a less than optimal reduction in thirst in response to standard therapy for hypercortisolism. See Chapter 10 for further information on central diabetes insipidus.

Routine clinicopathological features

The main haematology, biochemistry and urinalysis findings in dogs with hypercortisolism are listed in Figure 29.13.

Haematology

The most common haematological finding is a stress leucogram with an absolute lymphopenia ($<1.5 \times 10^9$/l) and eosinopenia ($<0.2 \times 10^9$/l). Lymphopenia is most likely the result of steroid lymphocytolysis and eosinopenia results from bone marrow sequestration of eosinophils. A mild to moderate neutrophilia and monocytosis may be found and is thought to result from decreased capillary margination and diapedesis associated with excess cortisol concentrations.

The red cell count is usually normal, although mild polycythaemia may occasionally be noted. Platelet counts may also be increased. These findings are thought to result from stimulatory effects of glucocorticoids on the bone marrow.

Haematology
• Lymphopenia ($<1.5 \times 10^9$/l)
• Eosinopenia ($<0.2 \times 10^9$/l)
• Neutrophilia
• Monocytosis
• Erythrocytosis
• Thrombocytosis
Biochemistry
• Increased alkaline phosphatase activity (often markedly increased)
• Increased alanine aminotransferase activity
• High reference interval or mildly increased fasting blood glucose concentration
• Decreased urea concentration
• Increased cholesterol concentration (>8 mmol/l)
• Increased triglyceride concentration (lipaemic plasma/serum)
• Increased bile acid concentrations
Urinalysis
• Urine specific gravity <1.015 and often <1.008
• Urinary tract infection
• Proteinuria
• Glucosuria (<10% of cases)
Other findings
• Low total thyroxine concentration
• Subnormal thyroxine response to thyrotropin (thyroid-stimulating hormone) administration
• Increased parathyroid hormone concentration
• Reduced growth hormone concentration
• Increased insulin and C-peptide concentrations

29.13 Typical clinicopathological and other hormonal features of canine hypercortisolism.

Biochemistry

Alkaline phosphatase

Alkaline phosphatase (ALP) activity is increased in more than 90% of dogs with hypercortisolism. The increase is commonly 5–40 times the upper limit of the reference interval and ALP activity is perhaps the most sensitive biochemical screening test for hypercortisolism. However, it is also the least specific. The increased activity occurs because glucocorticoids, whether endogenous or exogenous, induce a specific hepatic isoenzyme of ALP – an effect unique to the dog, although vacuolar hepatopathy may contribute. A reference interval serum ALP activity does not exclude a diagnosis of hypercortisolism. Equally, increases in ALP activity may be due to other conditions.

Measurement of the glucocorticoid-induced isoenzyme of ALP is as sensitive for hypercortisolism as measuring total ALP but is no more specific. This is because the glucocorticoid-induced isoenzyme can be increased in other disorders, including primary hepatopathies and diabetes mellitus, and in dogs treated with anticonvulsants and glucocorticoids (Teske *et al.*, 1989).

Alanine aminotransferase

Alanine aminotransferase (ALT) activity is commonly increased in hypercortisolism, but the increase is usually only mild. Any increase is believed to be secondary to hypercortisolism-induced vacuolar hepatopathy.

Glucose

Blood glucose concentration is usually at the high end of, or just above, the reference interval. More marked hyperglycaemia is present in dogs with concurrent diabetes mellitus (see Chapter 23).

Urea and creatinine

Blood urea concentration is usually within or below the reference interval due to the continual urinary loss associated with glucocorticoid-induced diuresis. The serum creatinine concentration also tends to be at the low end of the reference interval. Urea and creatinine concentrations at the high end of the reference interval are therefore of some concern, as affected animals may become overtly azotaemic when treatment for the hypercortisolism is instituted.

Cholesterol and triglycerides

Cholesterol and triglyceride concentrations are increased because of glucocorticoid stimulation of lipolysis. The cholesterol concentration is usually >8 mmol/l. This is not a specific finding, as hypercholesterolaemia also occurs in certain breeds and in hypothyroidism, diabetes mellitus, cholestatic liver disease and protein-losing nephropathy. Hypertriglyceridaemia can also occur, although less frequently. The resultant plasma lipaemia can interfere with the accurate assessment of a number of other laboratory parameters.

Electrolytes

Sodium, potassium, calcium and phosphate concentrations are usually within their respective reference intervals. However, phosphate concentrations may be increased when compared with age-matched controls (Ramsey *et al.*, 2005).

Bile acids

Resting and postprandial serum bile acid concentrations may show a mild to moderate increase in some cases of hypercortisolism because of the vacuolar hepatopathy. When abnormal results are obtained, it may prove difficult to differentiate hypercortisolism from primary liver disorders. This distinction can almost always be made using the dog's appetite, thirst, weight change and other clinical signs. In cases where the distinction cannot be made on clinical presentation, then a fine needle aspirate or biopsy may be needed but the risks of poor wound healing, hypertension and haemorrhage need to be assessed carefully.

Urinalysis

Specific gravity

The specific gravity (SG) of urine is usually below 1.015 and the urine is often hyposthenuric (<1.008), provided water has not been withheld. A urine SG above 1.030 is rare in dogs with hypercortisolism. However, some dogs with hypercortisolism can produce concentrated urine if water is withdrawn or if they refuse to drink because of strange surroundings. Thus, urine SG should be assessed in samples taken when the dog has had free access to water and before hospitalization. In a small number of cases of ACTH-dependent hypercortisolism with a macro-tumour, compression of the posterior lobe of the pituitary gland and suprasellar extension into the hypothalamus may cause disruption to AVP production and release and, subsequently, signs of central diabetes insipidus (see Chapter 10).

Proteinuria

Up to 45% of dogs with untreated hypercortisolism have a urine protein:creatinine above 1.0 in the absence of UTI (Hurley and Vaden, 1998). Proteinuria is usually mild and may be associated with systemic hypertension.

Glucosuria

Glucosuria is present in cases with overt diabetes mellitus, which constitute less than 10% of dogs with hypercortisolism.

Culture

Urine culture and susceptibility testing may be recommended given the high prevalence of UTIs with hypercortisolism. There is often little evidence of blood or inflammatory cells in the urine sediment because of the immunosuppressive action of excess cortisol.

Coagulation parameters

Hypercoagulability in hypercortisolism may be related to increased procoagulant activity and/or decreased fibrinolysis. One or more abnormalities of an extended hypercoagulability panel are common in hypercortisolism but without a consistent pattern.

Effects on other endocrine test results

Thyroid hormones

Glucocorticoids are known to have a profound effect on tests of thyroid function, which can include reduced circulating concentrations of total and free thyroxine (T4) and triiodothyronine (T3), and reduced thyroid responsiveness to exogenous thyrotropin (thyroid-stimulating hormone (TSH)) and thyrotropin-releasing hormone (TRH) stimulation. Excess glucocorticoids can also potentially decrease TSH concentrations. Accurate evaluation of thyroid function is therefore difficult in hypercortisolaemic dogs and, if any parameters suggest hypothyroidism, repeat testing may be required 2–3 months after sufficient control of the hypercortisolaemia is achieved (see Chapter 18).

Parathyroid hormone

Hypercortisolism is associated with hyperphosphataemia and increased urinary calcium excretion in dogs. Parathyroid hormone (PTH) concentrations are increased in more than 80% of cases of hypercortisolism, which may be related in part to increased calcium excretion (Ramsey et al., 2005). Increased PTH concentrations occur early in the course of the disease in both ACTH-dependent and -independent hypercortisolism. Trilostane results in a reduction in PTH concentrations; however, many values do not return to the reference interval (Tebb et al., 2005). The consequences of adrenal secondary hyperparathyroidism are unclear. It does not appear to be associated with a decrease in bone formation or an increase in bone resorption as measured by markers of bone turnover (Mooney et al., 2020).

Growth hormone and insulin-like growth factor-1

Chronic glucocorticoid excess reduces spontaneous and stimulated growth hormone (GH) secretion by enhancing the release of somatostatin from the hypothalamus (Lee et al., 2003). Reduced GH secretion from the pituitary gland could result in reduced serum insulin-like growth factor-1 concentrations, although this has not been clearly demonstrated.

Insulin and C-peptide

It has been shown that both insulin and C-peptide (released in equimolar concentrations to insulin) concentrations are increased in dogs with hypercortisolism and that their response to glucagon is exaggerated when compared with healthy dogs (Montgomery et al., 1996). This observation is explained by cortisol inducing peripheral insulin resistance, which may ultimately result in overt diabetes mellitus.

Diagnostic imaging

Advances in diagnostic imaging have improved the ability of clinicians to identify the cause of spontaneous hypercortisolism and the extent of the underlying pathology so that treatment can be directed more specifically to the individual case. However, finding a pituitary or adrenal mass does not necessarily mean that a functional tumour is present. Therefore, diagnostic imaging should always be interpreted in association with the clinical signs and endocrine test results. Diagnostic imaging can also provide supportive evidence for hypercortisolism. Additionally, it may provide evidence for significant concurrent disease or complications from hypercortisolism that might require treatment or affect prognosis.

Radiography

Radiographic changes associated with hypercortisolism are listed in Figure 29.14.

Abdominal radiographs
• Liver enlargement • Good radiographic contrast • Pot-bellied appearance • Calcinosis cutis/soft tissue mineralization • Distended bladder • Cystic or urethral calculi • Adrenal enlargement/mineralization • ± Osteopenia
Thoracic radiographs
• Tracheal and bronchial wall mineralization • Pulmonary metastases from adrenocortical carcinoma • ± Osteopenia • Pulmonary thromboembolism (rare)

29.14 Radiographic signs compatible with hypercortisolism.

General radiographic features

Calcinosis cutis may be apparent and tends to have a nodular mineralization pattern, whereas calcification in the fascial planes, for example, just dorsal to the thoracolumbar spine, tends to be linear. Mineralization may also be seen in the lung, renal pelvis, liver, gastric mucosa and abdominal aorta. Tracheal and bronchial wall mineralization is frequently seen radiographically. Calcification of these structures, however, can also be seen in ageing animals and is not considered to be clinically significant. Occasionally, the impression of osteopenia is gained from a distinct reduction in radiographic opacity of the vertebral bodies relative to the vertebral end plates (Figures 29.15 and 29.16).

Abdominal radiography

Hepatomegaly is the most consistent radiographic finding, easily identifiable because of the large deposits of intra-abdominal fat. Abdominal distension and a pendulous abdomen are usually obvious on the recumbent lateral view (Figure 29.15).

Normal adrenal glands are not visible on abdominal radiographs. Adrenomegaly is a rare finding but, if present, it suggests gross enlargement which is typical of, although not diagnostic for, an adrenocortical functional mass. Unilateral mineralization in the region of an adrenal gland also suggests the possibility of an adrenal tumour, although the presence of mineralization cannot be used to distinguish benign from malignant tumours as both may become mineralized (Figure 29.16).

A distended urinary bladder may be seen radiographically, even when the animal has been allowed to urinate prior to the radiographic examination. Cystic or urethral uroliths may also be present (Figure 29.16).

Thoracic radiography

Thoracic radiographs may provide evidence of lung metastasis from an adrenocortical carcinoma or pulmonary thromboembolism (although in many cases of pulmonary thromboembolism, the radiographs may appear normal). Comorbidities, such as congestive heart failure, that may have an impact on treatment may also be detected.

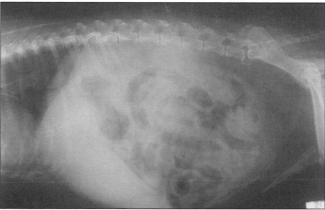

29.15 Abdominal radiograph of a Cairn Terrier with adrenocorticotropic hormone-dependent hypercortisolism. The radiographic signs include hepatomegaly, abdominal distension, calcinosis cutis, dystrophic calcification in the soft tissues along the spine, an enlarged bladder and osteopenia.

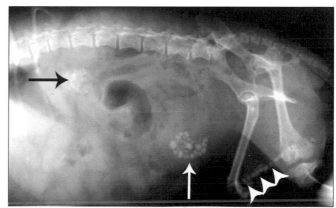

29.16 Abdominal radiograph of a Yorkshire Terrier with an adrenal tumour. A calcified mass can be seen in the dorsocranial area of the abdomen (black arrow). In addition, cystic (white arrow) and urethral (arrowheads) calculi are present. Despite this extensive urolithiasis, the dog was able to urinate normally, possibly due to the anti-inflammatory effects of the excessive glucocorticoids.

Abdominal ultrasonography

Ultrasound examination of the abdomen may reveal a diffusely hyperechoic enlarged liver or the presence of urolithiasis. Evidence of associated diseases, such as gall bladder mucocoele or pyelonephritis, may also be identified. However, abdominal ultrasonography is most important for evaluation of the adrenal glands. The best images of the adrenal glands are obtained by scanning from the right and left lateral intercostal, subcostal and abdominal approaches.

Location of the adrenal glands

The right adrenal gland is more difficult to image than the left because of its deeper and more cranial location under the ribs. The right adrenal gland is located craniomedial to the right kidney, lying between the cranial pole of the kidney, dorsal or dorsolateral to the caudal vena cava and just cranial to the cranial mesenteric artery. The left adrenal gland is more variable in location. It may be found anywhere from craniomedial to the left kidney to a more midline position ventrolateral to the aorta and adjacent to the first or second lumbar vertebra. The left adrenal gland is located between the origin of the cranial mesenteric artery and the left renal artery.

Appearance of the adrenal glands

The normal adrenal glands are usually well defined and appear hypoechoic relative to the surrounding fat. The right adrenal gland is usually folded or V-shaped with an elongated caudal pole. The left adrenal gland is bilobed or peanut-shaped. The medulla of the normal adrenal gland is slightly hyperechoic relative to the cortex. A wide range of adrenal gland sizes has been reported in healthy dogs of different breeds and, recently, a correlation has been shown between adrenal size and bodyweight (Soulsby *et al.*, 2015; Bento *et al.*, 2016; Melián *et al.*, 2021). The measurement of adrenal gland length is usually considered less accurate because of difficulty in aligning the ultrasound beam along the long axis of the gland. The dorsoventral thickness measured on the sagittal plane of the adrenal gland is generally considered to be the most reliable measurement. By grouping healthy dogs into four separate bands by bodyweight, it has been shown that the upper limit for the thickness of the left adrenal gland in clinically healthy dogs is 5.1 mm for dogs weighing 2.5–5.0 kg, 5.5 mm for dogs weighing >5–10 kg, 6.4 mm for dogs weighing >10–20 kg, and 7.3 mm for dogs weighing >20–40 kg. For the right adrenal gland, the upper limit is 5.3 mm for dogs weighing 2–5 kg, 6.8 mm for dogs weighing >5–10 kg, 7.5 mm for dogs weighing >10–20 kg, and 8.7 mm for dogs weighing >20–40 kg (Melián *et al.*, 2021). It is challenging to consistently distinguish between healthy, hyperplastic and neoplastic glands.

ACTH-dependent hypercortisolism: Although the adrenal glands of dogs with ACTH-dependent hypercortisolism have been characterized as symmetrically enlarged and of normal conformation, the diagnosis of adrenal hyperplasia is still a somewhat subjective evaluation. Hyperplastic adrenal glands are usually easier to image than normal adrenal glands and usually maintain the normal, homogeneous hypoechoic pattern (Figure 29.17a). The thickness of the adrenal gland should exceed the upper limit for healthy dogs of the same bodyweight. However, whilst the detection of adrenomegaly is considered of high diagnostic sensitivity for hypercortisolism, the finding of an adrenal gland of normal thickness does not rule it out. Additionally, it is not diagnostically specific, and adrenal gland enlargement may occur with other illnesses. Overall, ultrasonographic identification of both adrenal glands of similar size with normal architecture in a dog with clinical signs of hypercortisolism and positive endocrine test results confirms ACTH-dependent hypercortisolism. Mild adrenal asymmetry can occur in some cases of ACTH-dependent hypercortisolism but may also be seen in some dogs with chronic non-adrenal disease.

ACTH-independent hypercortisolism: The ultrasonographic appearance of adrenal nodules and masses is not specific for the underlying pathology. Differentials for solid nodules or masses within the adrenal gland include adrenocortical adenoma/carcinoma, phaeochromocytoma, myelolipoma, metastasis, nodular hyperplasia and granuloma. Adrenal masses exceeding 2 cm in diameter generally predict neoplasia rather than hyperplasia, and increasing size is associated with an increased probability of malignancy (Figure 29.17b). Mineralization is frequently associated with both benign and malignant adrenocortical tumours in the dog, and acoustic shadowing may aid in localizing the adrenal tumour.

Evaluation of asymmetry between the adrenal glands is helpful in diagnosing adrenal neoplasia. Several calculations can be made (e.g. dorsoventral ratios and differences exceeding 5 mm). However, a maximal dorsoventral thickness of the smaller gland of less than 5 mm provides a highly sensitive and specific distinction between ACTH-dependent and -independent hypercortisolism, indicating the latter (Benchekroun *et al.*, 2010). There is a propensity for malignant adrenal tumours to invade nearby vessels and surrounding tissues; therefore, a thorough ultrasonographic examination of adjacent vessels and tissues should be performed (Figure 29.17c). Additionally, if adrenal neoplasia is suspected, the liver, spleen and kidneys should also be examined for evidence of metastasis.

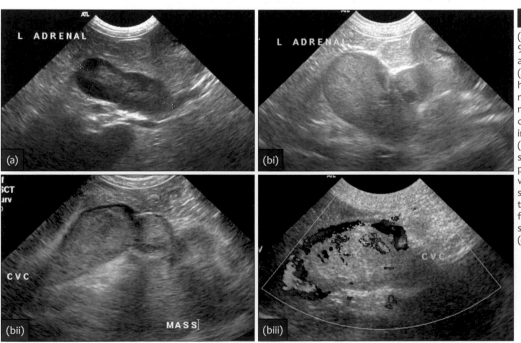

29.17 Ultrasonography of the canine adrenal gland. (a) The left adrenal gland of a 9-year-old Jack Russell Terrier with adrenocorticotropic hormone (ACTH)-dependent hypercortisolism. The gland measures 40 mm in length and 16 mm in width. (b) A 7-year-old male crossbreed with ACTH-independent hypercortisolism. (bi) The left adrenal tumour can be seen and (bii) extends into the phrenicoabdominal vein and caudal vena cava (CVC). (biii) Despite the size of the neoplastic thrombus in the caudal vena cava, some blood flow around the thrombus can be seen using colour flow mapping. (continues) ▶

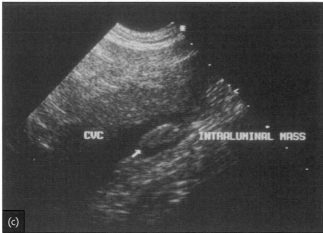

29.17 (continued) Ultrasonography of the canine adrenal gland. (c) The cranial abdomen of a 10-year-old Labrador Retriever bitch with an adrenocortical carcinoma that has invaded the caudal vena cava (CVC).

Advanced diagnostic imaging

Cross-sectional imaging using CT and MRI has proved useful in the diagnosis and assessment of adrenal tumours, adrenal hyperplasia and pituitary tumours, but both techniques are more expensive than abdominal ultrasonography and not always available. Whilst there is a perception that advanced imaging is always more accurate, adrenal gland measurements from cross-sectional or reformatted CT scans overlapped in dogs with ACTH-dependent and -independent hypercortisolism (Rodríguez Piñeiro *et al.*, 2011). Nevertheless, abdominal CT can provide important additional information, particularly in dogs with adrenal neoplasia, as the presence of vascular or tissue invasion and distant metastasis can be more readily identified than with any other imaging modality (Figure 29.18).

Pituitary imaging is essential for treatment planning before either hypophysectomy or pituitary irradiation but has some limitations regarding diagnosis and differentiation of cause. Magnetic resonance imaging is superior to CT in detecting ACTH-secreting tumours of the pituitary gland in humans, where it is considered to be the modality of choice for this evaluation. A comparison of CT and low-field MRI in a small series of dogs with ACTH-dependent hypercortisolism showed that, whilst both techniques provided comparable information on the presence of pituitary tumours, MRI produced better image quality (Auriemma *et al.*, 2009). Additionally, MRI is more sensitive and can detect pituitary tumours as small as 3 mm in height. Despite this, only approximately 50% of dogs with ACTH-dependent hypercortisolism have a detectable pituitary mass on MRI (Figure 29.19).

Similarly, the size of the pituitary gland as assessed by CT was considered normal in 56% of dogs with ACTH-dependent hypercortisolism (Rodríguez Piñeiro *et al.*, 2011). Dynamic CT and MRI procedures, involving thinly collimated image acquisition of the pituitary gland every few seconds for 2–5 minutes following intravenous contrast administration, can detect displacement of the posterior lobe by small pituitary tumours (Graham *et al.*, 2000; van der Vlugt-Meijer *et al.*, 2003).

Computed tomography or MRI is particularly indicated to assess the size of the pituitary gland (see above) if neurological signs are present, as prognosis and treatment will vary depending on results.

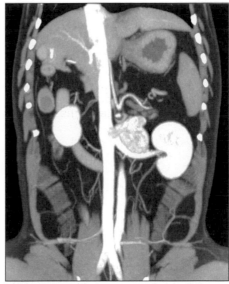

29.18 Computed tomographic dorsal plane reconstruction using maximum intensity projection that shows a left adrenal mass displacing the renal vein caudally. A small thrombus can be seen extending into the lumen of the caudal vena cava.

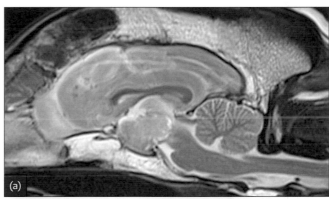

29.19 (a) Sagittal and (b) transverse T2-weighted magnetic resonance images of a pituitary macroadenoma in a 10-year-old entire crossbreed bitch with adrenocorticotropic hormone-dependent hypercortisolism and central diabetes insipidus.

Diagnostic endocrine tests

A presumptive diagnosis of hypercortisolism can be made from clinical signs, routine clinicopathological features and diagnostic imaging findings, but the diagnosis must be confirmed by performing endocrine tests (Figure 29.20). A single resting or basal plasma or serum cortisol determination is of limited diagnostic value because of the overlap in cortisol concentrations obtained from animals in healthy and diseased states (including adrenal and non-adrenal illnesses). The most commonly used diagnostic

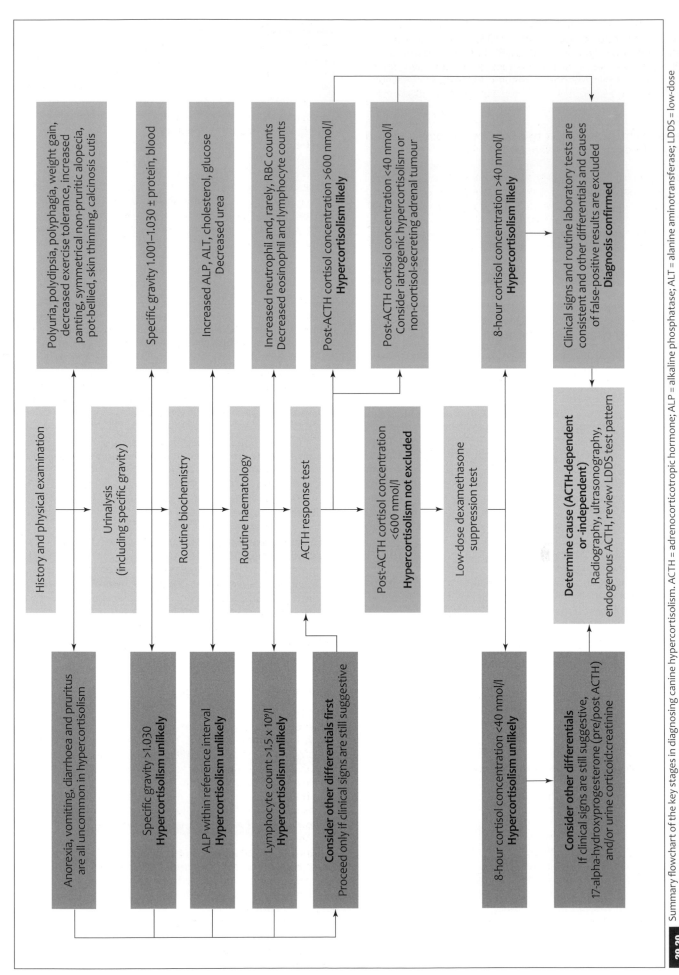

29.20 Summary flowchart of the key stages in diagnosing canine hypercortisolism. ACTH = adrenocorticotropic hormone; ALP = alkaline phosphatase; ALT = alanine aminotransferase; LDDS = low-dose dexamethasone suppression; RBC = red blood cell.

tests are the ACTH response test and the low-dose dexamethasone suppression (LDDS) test; however, the urine corticoid:creatinine (UCCR) has also been used. All of these tests are imperfect and can give false-positive and false-negative results. False-positive results are typically obtained in dogs suffering from non-adrenal disease. If there is a marked difference in the diagnostic sensitivity or specificity of tests, a combination of two tests might be selected to maximize performance. If a dog with clinical signs compatible with hypercortisolism produces a negative result with one test, an alternative test should be considered. A definitive diagnosis of hypercortisolism should never be made purely based on results of any of these diagnostic tests, especially in dogs without classic signs of hypercortisolism or in dogs with known non-adrenal disease.

The protocols for the different tests are given in Figure 29.21, and their approximate sensitivities and specificities in Figure 29.22. The relative merits of each test and interpretation are discussed below.

Where absolute cortisol values are quoted, they are intended as a general guide. Cortisol assays vary in performance and it is important to consult individual laboratories and assay manufacturers regarding their precise cut-offs (see Chapter 3).

ACTH response test
1. Collect a blood sample for basal cortisol concentration[a]
2. Inject 5 µg/kg of synthetic ACTH (tetracosactide, cosyntropin) i.v.[b]
3. Collect a second sample for cortisol concentration 60 minutes later. Care must be taken to time the post-ACTH sample correctly

Low-dose dexamethasone suppression test
1. Collect a blood sample for cortisol determination
2. Inject 0.01–0.015 mg/kg of dexamethasone i.v.
3. Collect a second sample for cortisol concentration 3–4 hours later and a third sample 8 hours after dexamethasone administration

Urine corticoid:creatinine
1. Collect a urine sample in the morning for corticoid and creatinine measurements. It is preferable for the dog to be at home for this test so that it is minimally stressed
2. Determine the urine corticoid:creatinine by dividing the urine corticoid concentration (µmol/l) by the urine creatinine concentration (µmol/l)

29.21 Protocols for screening tests for hypercortisolism. [a] The recent administration of glucocorticoids such as hydrocortisone, prednisolone or prednisone may result in increased cortisol concentrations due to cross-reactivity in many cortisol assays. For this reason, glucocorticoids should be withheld for at least 24 hours before testing. There is no cross-reactivity with dexamethasone but, as with other glucocorticoids, dexamethasone will suppress cortisol concentrations in dogs with an intact hypothalamic–pituitary–adrenal axis. [b] Synthetic adrenocorticotropic hormone (ACTH) can be given i.m. if needed but may sting. Fixed doses of 125 µg for dogs <5 kg and 250 µg for dogs 5–50 kg have also been used successfully.

Test	Sensitivity	Specificity
ACTH response test (overall)	80%	95%
ACTH response test (ACTH-dependent)	85%	95%
ACTH response test (ACTH-independent)	50%	95%
Low-dose dexamethasone suppression test (overall)	95%	67%

29.22 Approximate sensitivity and specificity of commonly used tests. Values for urine corticoid:creatinine are not provided as this depends on the assay used and some have not been fully evaluated. ACTH = adrenocorticotropic hormone.

ACTH response test

The ACTH response test is specific but lacks sensitivity for diagnosing spontaneous hypercortisolism (Figure 29.22). Positive test results are found in approximately half of dogs with ACTH-independent hypercortisolism and the majority of dogs with ACTH-dependent hypercortisolism. Occasional false-positive results do occur, although false-negative results are more common.

The test is simple, robust and quick to perform, and documents excessive production of cortisol by the adrenal cortex. The information gained is useful in providing baseline information for monitoring subsequent trilostane or mitotane therapy, although different criteria are used to interpret cortisol results during treatment. The cost of ACTH varies considerably in different countries and, when expensive, can limit the widespread use of this test. Doses as low as 5 µg/kg have been tested and, at least in healthy dogs, appear adequate (Martin et al., 2007).

The ACTH response test does not, however, reliably differentiate ACTH-dependent and -independent hypercortisolism. A diagnosis of hypercortisolism should not be excluded based on a negative ACTH response if clinical signs are compatible with the disease. Occasionally, an animal under chronic stress may develop some degree of adrenal hyperplasia, which produces an abnormal ACTH response. This may be seen, for example, with diabetes mellitus or pyometra, and in these cases a normal cortisol response to ACTH stimulation will be obtained after treatment of the underlying disease.

In healthy dogs, pre-ACTH cortisol concentrations are usually 20–250 nmol/l and post-ACTH cortisol concentrations are usually 200–450 nmol/l. Regardless of the pre-ACTH cortisol value, a diagnosis of hypercortisolism is supported by demonstrating a post-ACTH cortisol concentration greater than 600 nmol/l in dogs with compatible clinical signs and without evidence of concurrent non-adrenal disease (Figure 29.23). For cases with a high suspicion of hypercortisolism and a negative test result, a suggested approach is to lower the diagnostic cut-off (in so doing sacrificing specificity for an increase in sensitivity and increasing the number of false-positive results), potentially to as low as 450 nmol/l (Frank et al., 2015).

The ACTH response test is the best test for distinguishing spontaneous from iatrogenic hypercortisolism. A limited cortisol response is expected in iatrogenic disease.

Low-dose dexamethasone suppression test

The LDDS test is sensitive but lacks specificity for diagnosing spontaneous hypercortisolism. Positive test results are found in the majority of ACTH-independent cases and in 85–90% of dogs with ACTH-dependent hypercortisolism. Occasional false-negative results do occur, although false-positive results are more common.

The LDDS test is affected by more variables than the ACTH response test, takes 8 hours to complete and does not provide pre-treatment information that may be used in monitoring the effects of mitotane or trilostane therapy. It cannot be used for the detection of iatrogenic hypercortisolism. Samples for cortisol estimation should be collected just before, as well as 3–4 and 8 hours after, the intravenous administration of short-acting dexamethasone preparations.

Recent studies reviewing two series of 123 and 177 LDDS tests (in both cases, approximately half the tests came from dogs that were subsequently confirmed to have hypercortisolism, the other half coming from dogs with a

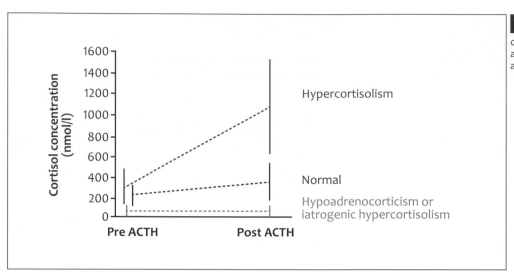

29.23 Interpretation of measurements of plasma cortisol concentrations before and after administration of synthetic adrenocorticotropic hormone (ACTH).

range of non-adrenal illnesses) have provided useful data on the interpretation of these tests (Bennaim *et al.*, 2018; Zeugswetter *et al.*, 2021). Several different patterns have been defined (Figure 29.24), including:

- Complete suppression, with 3–4 and 8-hour cortisol concentrations <27 nmol/l
- Lack of suppression, with 3–4 and 8-hour cortisol concentrations >27 nmol/l and both >50% of basal value
- Partial suppression, with 3–4 and 8-hour cortisol concentrations >27 nmol/l and either or both <50% of basal value
- Escape, with 3–4-hour cortisol concentration <27 nmol/l and 8-hour cortisol concentration >27 nmol/l
- Inverse, with 3–4-hour cortisol concentration >27 nmol/l and 8-hour cortisol concentration <27 nmol/l.

If there is a complete suppression pattern, hypercortisolism is highly unlikely (4–17% of dogs that have this pattern are subsequently diagnosed with hypercortisolism). If the dexamethasone completely fails to suppress cortisol,

then hypercortisolism is highly likely (0–6% of dogs with non-adrenal illness have this pattern of response). However, between these two extremes the picture is less clear cut. The partial suppression pattern is strongly suggestive of hypercortisolism but 6–27% of dogs with such a pattern will turn out to have non-adrenal disease. The escape pattern is less reliable, with 14–64% of dogs with this pattern subsequently found to have non-adrenal illness. The inverse pattern is essentially non-diagnostic for hypercortisolism – such results should be ignored and alternative methods of diagnosis used.

Key to the successful use of the LDDS test is the strict exclusion of dogs with signs (e.g. fever, jaundice, vomiting, diarrhoea and coughing) that are not compatible with hypercortisolism, dogs with intercurrent diseases (e.g. untreated or unstable diabetes mellitus, acute pancreatitis) and obese dogs with no other clinical signs that have not yet been properly dieted. The better the pre-test screening, the better the test performs.

Results of the LDDS test can help distinguish between ACTH-dependent and -independent forms of hypercortisolism. It is generally considered that suppression of

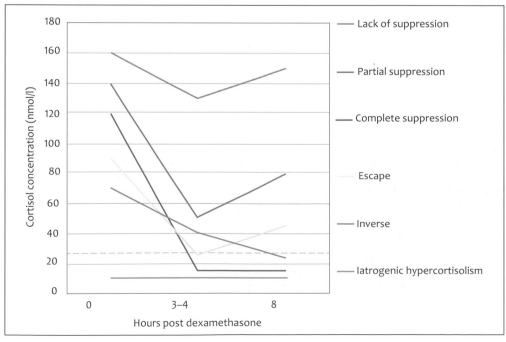

29.24 Interpretation of measurements of plasma cortisol concentrations before and after the administration of a low dose of dexamethasone. The dashed line represents the lower limit of cortisol (27 nmol/l).
(Data from Bennaim *et al.*, 2018 and Zeugswetter *et al.*, 2021).

plasma cortisol concentration during an LDDS test (partial, escape or inverse pattern) supports a diagnosis of ACTH-dependent hypercortisolism (concurrent adrenal tumours may still occur in this group). If there is no cortisol suppression during the test then the cause of the hypercortisolism cannot be determined.

Urine corticoid:creatinine

Evaluation of UCCR, rather than the more laborious 24-hour urinary corticoid excretion, can be used to evaluate for hypercortisolism.

Cortisol and its metabolites are excreted in urine. Measuring urinary corticoids in a morning sample ensures the concentration will reflect release over a period of several hours, thereby adjusting for fluctuations in plasma corticoid concentrations. Relating the urine corticoid concentration to urine creatinine concentration provides a correction for any differences in urine concentration. The UCCR is determined by dividing the urine corticoid concentration (in μmol/l) by the urine creatinine concentration (in μmol/l).

Urine is collected in the morning for corticoid and creatinine estimations. It is preferable for the dog to be at home for this test to minimize stress as far as possible, otherwise abnormal cortisol concentrations will be present in the urine.

There are considerable differences between laboratories in the measurement of UCCR that are likely to be due to differences in the antibodies used, extraction techniques and recommendations for sample handling (Galeandro et al., 2014). The reference interval for healthy dogs varies accordingly, with values as low as 10×10^{-6} and as high as 30×10^{-6} being used.

The UCCR is increased in most dogs with hypercortisolism. However, it is also increased in many dogs with non-adrenal illness. For example, dogs with congestive heart failure have UCCR values that are similar to those seen in dogs with hypercortisolism (Quilez et al., 2020). Therefore, while this simple test appears to be highly sensitive for detecting hypercortisolism in dogs, it is not specific and false-positive results are common. The test does provide a good screening test for hypercortisolism, in that values within the reference interval make a diagnosis of hypercortisolism unlikely. The UCCR does not reliably differentiate ACTH-dependent from ACTH-independent hypercortisolism unless the ratio exceeds 100×10^{-6} (based on one laboratory), in which case it is likely that the dog is suffering from ACTH-dependent hypercortisolism (Galac et al., 1997). The test is of little value in monitoring the response to mitotane or trilostane therapy.

Ancillary diagnostic tests

Some dogs with classic clinical signs of hypercortisolism and typical haematological and biochemical features have negative ACTH response and LDDS test results. These cases have been termed as having 'atypical' or 'subdiagnostic' hypercortisolism. In such cases with ACTH-dependent hypercortisolism, it has been suggested that measurement of 17-alpha-hydroxyprogesterone during an ACTH response test may be helpful. In healthy dogs, pre-ACTH 17-alpha-hydroxyprogesterone concentrations range from less than 1.0 to 1.9 nmol/l and increase to between 1.0 and 5.5 nmol/l after ACTH administration. Circulating 17-alpha-hydroxyprogesterone concentrations exhibit an exaggerated response to ACTH stimulation in both typical and atypical hypercortisolism, with 17-alpha-hydroxyprogesterone concentrations increasing to between 6.5 and 38 nmol/l after stimulation (Ristic et al., 2002). However, abnormal 17-alpha-hydroxyprogesterone responses can be found in cases of non-adrenal illnesses (Chapman et al., 2003; Sieber-Ruckstuhl et al., 2008a). Thus, whilst evaluation of 17-alpha-hydroxyprogresterone may improve diagnostic sensitivity of the ACTH response test, this is to the detriment of specificity.

It is recognized that some less common cases of ACTH-independent hypercortisolism have a derangement of the steroid production pathway such that cortisol concentrations before and after ACTH administration are unexpectedly low. In some such cases, cortisol concentrations are <27 nmol/l before administration of dexamethasone, making any further decrease unmeasurable with many commonly used assays. Measurement of 17-alpha-hydroxyprogesterone before and after ACTH administration in these cases may be useful, as it typically remains high (Norman et al., 1999; Syme et al., 2001; Ristic et al., 2002).

Tests to differentiate the cause of hypercortisolism

The ability to differentiate between ACTH-dependent and -independent hypercortisolism can have important implications for provision of the most effective method of management. A diagnosis of ACTH-dependent hypercortisolism may be apparent from the results of the LDDS test (see above). The high-dose dexamethasone suppression test was historically recommended, but its accuracy is questionable and it is no longer used. Canine ACTH assays and abdominal ultrasound facilities are now readily available, and both methods are more reliable.

Plasma endogenous ACTH concentration

Stringent and meticulous sample handling is crucial, as ACTH activity in the plasma will reduce rapidly, resulting in falsely low values and incorrect interpretation (see Chapter 3). The endogenous ACTH assay used must be validated for dogs.

Measurement of basal endogenous ACTH concentration is of no value in the diagnosis of hypercortisolism because of the episodic secretion of ACTH in healthy dogs and the overlap of values in dogs with hypercortisolism.

With one validated assay, endogenous ACTH concentrations in healthy dogs ranged from 2.91 to 11 pmol/l (Rodríguez Piñeiro et al., 2009). Dogs with ACTH-independent hypercortisolism have very low endogenous ACTH concentrations (<1.1 pmol/l), whereas those with ACTH-dependent hypercortisolism tend to have high reference interval to increased concentrations of endogenous ACTH (>6 pmol/l), which discriminates the cause with high diagnostic sensitivity and specificity. It has also been recognized that there is a positive correlation between the plasma endogenous ACTH concentration and the size of the pituitary mass in ACTH-dependent hypercortisolism (Théon and Feldman, 1998).

Diagnostic imaging

Abdominal radiography, abdominal ultrasonography, and abdominal and brain CT/MRI can be used to differentiate between ACTH-dependent and -independent hypercortisolism (see 'Diagnostic imaging', above).

Treatment of ACTH-dependent hypercortisolism

Many dogs with hypercortisolism remain bright and have a good appetite, and it has been suggested that survival time is similar whether or not a dog with hypercortisolism is treated. Although it might seem intuitive, it has now been documented that medical treatment with trilostane prolongs the survival time of dogs with ACTH-dependent hypercortisolism compared with untreated dogs, and that untreated dogs have an odds ratio of death five times higher than dogs treated with trilostane (Nagata *et al.*, 2017). Reasons for improved survival might be related to reducing the complications associated with the disease (e.g. thromboembolism, hypertension, infections). Interestingly in this study, the most frequent cause of death was dyspnoea; although post-mortem examinations were not performed in any of these dogs, pulmonary thromboembolism could have been the cause and is a known complication and cause of death in humans with hypercortisolism.

Trilostane

Trilostane is a synthetic steroid with no inherent hormonal activity. The clinical use of trilostane in canine hypercortisolism, and in particular ACTH-dependent disease, has been evaluated in several published clinical studies from centres across the world (including Neiger *et al.*, 2002; Ruckstuhl *et al.*, 2002; Braddock *et al.*, 2003). It is currently the only authorized preparation for the treatment of hypercortisolism in the dog.

Mode of action

Trilostane primarily acts as a competitive, and therefore reversible, inhibitor of the 3-beta-hydroxysteroid dehydrogenase enzyme system, which blocks adrenal synthesis of glucocorticoids, mineralocorticoids and sex hormones. However, 17-alpha-hydroxyprogesterone concentrations do not change, or may increase, in dogs treated with trilostane. In addition, trilostane appears to have a more marked suppressive effect on cortisol than on cortisone. This has been suggested as evidence of an effect on 11-beta-hydroxylase and possibly on the interconversion of cortisol and cortisone by 11-beta-hydroxysteroid dehydrogenase (Sieber-Ruckstuhl *et al.*, 2006, 2008b).

Safety

Handling trilostane does not require any special safety precautions; however, as a drug with antiprogesterone effects, it should be avoided or handled with extra care (e.g. wearing gloves) by people who are pregnant or intending to become pregnant.

Starting dose

The starting dose recommended by the manufacturer is approximately 2 mg/kg orally q24h. A range of capsule sizes (5, 10, 30, 60 and 120 mg) is available in the UK, but in other countries reformulation may be necessary for low doses. Absorption of trilostane is more effective if the capsules are administered with food. The authorized dose frequency is once daily. Although this frequency is usually effective, it is known that the suppressive effect of trilostane on cortisol lasts less than 24 hours and switching from once- to twice-daily dosing is beneficial in some cases (Bell *et al.*, 2006). Many endocrinologists now recommend starting doses of 1 mg/kg twice daily.

Monitoring

Dogs receiving trilostane should be assessed 10 days, 4 weeks and 12 weeks after starting treatment and thereafter every 3–6 months and after each dose adjustment. Previously, ACTH response test results, biochemical monitoring and clinical signs were used as the primary methods of assessing control. However, other methods of monitoring can be used successfully. Regardless of the method(s) chosen, it is important to interpret all monitoring tests in the light of clinical findings.

Clinical signs: The role of an accurate and complete assessment of clinical signs in the management of hypercortisolism cannot be overemphasized. However, examining a dog and developing an understanding of owners' current concerns, whilst also being aware of the significance of less overt clinical signs and ensuring that every owner is asked the same questions, every time, can be challenging in the midst of most busy primary-care practices. The use of owner questionnaires that are completed (usually in the waiting room) before the consultation for this condition (and indeed for all chronic medical conditions) can be helpful in terms of efficiency, good record-keeping and accuracy.

Although such questionnaires can be used to produce scoring systems, a global assessment of the animal's progress since a previous visit can also be valuable. Cases should be divided as follows:

- Clinically well and showing minimal or residual signs of hypercortisolism
- Still showing signs of hypercortisolism
- Clinically unwell with signs (such as vomiting, abdominal pain) that are not generally associated with hypercortisolism.

Any effective treatment for hypercortisolism should resolve all the clinical signs of hypercortisolism, with perhaps the exceptions of those that are expected to improve but resolve only rarely (e.g. myotonia, hypertension) and in milder cases.

ACTH response tests: Trilostane causes significant reductions in both the mean basal and post-ACTH cortisol concentrations in dogs with hypercortisolism in the first month of treatment.

As the effects of trilostane are relatively short lived, the results obtained by an ACTH response test vary considerably with the time of testing relative to dosing (Bell *et al.*, 2006). It is recommended that ACTH response tests are performed 4–6 hours after dosing to enable accurate interpretation of results. However, ACTH response tests can also be performed 2–4 hours after dosing, as this is more likely to reflect the nadir of cortisol production following trilostane administration. It is important that the same timing is used for serial tests in the same dog.

Various cortisol target concentrations for the ACTH response test have been used to monitor trilostane therapy. The lower the target range, the greater the possibility of the animal developing signs of hypoadrenocorticism. A commonly recommended target range for the post-ACTH cortisol concentration is 40–120 nmol/l for ACTH response tests started 2–4 hours after dosing. However, all results must be interpreted in light of clinical signs. If dogs are responding well to treatment and have a post-ACTH cortisol concentration of 120–200 nmol/l, then repeat monitoring at a later date may be more acceptable to the owners than increasing the trilostane dose. Minimal cortisol responses to ACTH may indicate overdose, particularly in dogs that are clinically unwell. However, many dogs with such results do not develop signs of hypoadrenocorticism (Midence et al., 2015). The short duration of action of trilostane can have a protective effect against the development of hypoadrenocorticism. In contrast, some dogs that have a post-ACTH cortisol concentration in the target range will maintain signs of hypercortisolism (Braddock et al., 2003; Bell et al., 2006). In this situation, switching from once- to twice-daily administration (if not already using twice-daily administration) of trilostane can potentially help.

Pre-trilostane cortisol measurements: Pre-trilostane cortisol measurements were developed as a clinical tool when ACTH became temporarily unavailable in the UK, and have proven to be of value in monitoring response to therapy. For dogs that are clinically well, with or without signs of hypercortisolism, cortisol is measured in a single sample obtained just before (or within at least 2 hours of) the normal time of trilostane administration; results correlate well with assessments of clinical control by owners (Macfarlane et al., 2016). Dogs that are markedly stressed at the time of blood sampling may have artefactual increases in cortisol. In such dogs, repeated sampling 1 hour later may be beneficial, although the exact interpretation of such results is unclear.

- **Pre-trilostane cortisol concentration less than 40 nmol/l:**
  - If the dog is well controlled, then serious consideration should be given to decreasing the dose of trilostane and, regardless of any change in dose, a re-examination should be scheduled after 1 month
  - If the dog is unwell, see below.
- **Pre-trilostane cortisol concentration greater than 140 nmol/l:**
  - If the dog is still showing signs of hypercortisolism, then the dose of trilostane likely needs to be increased. If a dog is being treated once daily, then the first consideration may be to increase the frequency of administration to twice daily, providing acceptable capsule sizes are available. If increasing dose frequency, the total daily dose should increase by no more than 50%
  - If the dog is showing minimal or residual signs of hypercortisolism, then this should be confirmed with the owner and the next monitoring visit scheduled earlier than normal (e.g. 1 month) as it is likely that a dose increase will shortly be required.
- **Pre-trilostane cortisol concentration between 40 and 140 nmol/l:**
  - If the dog appears to be clinically well controlled, then the trilostane dose should be maintained
  - If the dog is clinically well but still has signs of hypercortisolism, the trilostane dose may need to be increased.

In dogs that are presented as clinically unwell with signs that cannot be explained by hypercortisolism, trilostane should be stopped. In this circumstance, an ACTH response test and potentially other diagnostic tests should be performed to determine whether the clinical signs are due to hypoadrenocorticism or some other disease (e.g. pancreatitis). If the post-ACTH cortisol concentration is lower than 40 nmol/l, then hypocortisolism is likely to be the cause of the signs; electrolyte concentrations should be checked for evidence of aldosterone deficiency and glucocorticoid supplementation should be started for at least 3 days. Trilostane should be stopped for at least 7 days and reintroduced (at a lower dose) only when the dog is well.

If post-ACTH cortisol concentrations are greater than 60 nmol/l, then hypocortisolism is less likely and alternative causes of the clinical signs should be investigated. Until the cause has been determined or the dog is well enough to return home and has a good appetite, trilostane administration should be suspended. Post-ACTH cortisol concentrations between 40 and 60 nmol/l should be regarded as equivocal and the clinical effect of trilostane withdrawal without glucocorticoid supplementation should be assessed.

Other methods of monitoring: Pre- and post-ACTH circulating 17-alpha-hydroxyprogesterone concentrations can be used to monitor mitotane treatment of ACTH-independent hypercortisolism associated with derangement of the cortisol synthesis pathway (see 'Mitotane', below). However, measurement of 17-alpha-hydroxyprogesterone is not helpful in monitoring cases treated with trilostane as the concentrations remain the same or increase further as treatment is instituted.

Measurement of the UCCR, pre-trilostane cortisol to endogenous ACTH ratio, urine SG, liver enzyme activities (ALT, ALP, gamma glutamyl transferase (GGT)) and haptoglobin concentration have all been examined as potential monitoring tools. None is consistently better than the above monitoring techniques, but all could have at least some value in the assessment of individual dogs. Of these, increased haptoglobin concentration appears to be the best predictor of poor versus good control, with ALT and GGT also providing some differentiation (Golinelli et al., 2021). At the time of writing, none of these can be recommended as first-choice methods of monitoring and none provide information on dogs that are overdosed.

Dose adjustments

Dose adjustments should be moderate and should be in the range of 25–75% higher or lower than the current dose. Very small adjustments are expensive in time and owner resources and there is no evidence that they increase safety. Most animals will stabilize within the range of a total daily dose of 2–7 mg/kg/day. However, a small number of animals may require doses significantly in excess of 10 mg/kg/day.

Efficacy and survival

Trilostane has been found to be up to 90% effective in resolving the various signs of hypercortisolism over 3–6 months.

The reported median survival times of dogs treated with trilostane ranged from 662 to 900 days in two studies that compared the outcome with that of mitotane treatment (which ranged from 708 to 720 days) (Barker et al., 2005; Clemente et al., 2007). One study compared twice-daily trilostane with a non-selective adrenocorticolytic protocol: in those countries that do not currently regard either routine twice-daily dosing with trilostane or non-selective adrenocorticolysis with mitotane as first-choice protocols, this study has more relevance to animals that have failed a conventional first-choice protocol (Clemente et al., 2007).

In primary-care practice in the UK, the median survival time from first diagnosis was 510 days (95% confidence interval: 412–618 days) in one study in which 94% of the cases were treated with trilostane (Schofield *et al.*, 2020). In another study from Japan, untreated dogs had a median survival time of 506 days (95% confidence interval: 292–564 days) and dogs treated with trilostane had significantly longer survival times (median survival time not reached during study period, 95% confidence interval: 443 days–not applicable) (Nagata *et al.*, 2017).

Side effects

Approximately 15% of dogs treated with trilostane develop adverse effects that are directly attributable to the drug. This figure compares favourably to those reported for mitotane (see 'Mitotane', below). If failure to respond is regarded as an adverse effect, then this is probably the most common adverse effect of trilostane administration. In these cases, an increase in the dose (and/or frequency) or a change to an alternative medication (e.g. mitotane) is indicated. Other side effects are summarized in Figure 29.25.

Other common side effects include an increase in the size of the adrenal glands and a change in their echotexture (Mantis *et al.*, 2003).

Adrenal necrosis: Acute adrenal necrosis is the most serious side effect of trilostane identified to date (Chapman *et al.*, 2004; Ramsey *et al.*, 2008; Aldridge *et al.*, 2016). Although deaths are rare, histopathological evidence of adrenal necrosis is more common (Reusch *et al.*, 2007). Necrosis of the adrenal cortex cannot be directly explained by the competitive inhibition of steroidogenesis but could be due to the hypersecretion of ACTH, which, together with increasing the size of the adrenal glands, may also, paradoxically, result in necrosis and haemorrhage of the adrenal glands. Treatment of the ensuing hypoadrenocorticism is required, and although this may be permanent, recurrence of hypercortisolism is a possibility.

Hypoadrenocorticism: Overdosing with trilostane can result in signs of hypocortisolaemia. Most affected dogs recover rapidly following temporary cessation of trilostane and glucocorticoid supplementation but will continue to require the drug, albeit at a lower dose, to control the clinical signs of hypercortisolism. Some dogs have evidence of both cortisol and aldosterone deficiency with typical electrolyte changes (hyponatraemia, hyperkalaemia). In such cases, trilostane therapy should be stopped and appropriate therapy for hypoadrenocorticism instituted (see Chapter 28). Trilostane therapy may be required again if clinical signs of hypercortisolism recur.

Transient hyperkalaemia: Some clinical studies of trilostane have recorded a mild increase in serum potassium concentrations. Dogs that develop hyperkalaemia but whose cortisol concentrations are adequate do not appear to have low aldosterone concentrations. The mechanism of action of this hyperkalaemia has not yet been identified. An ACTH response test, rather than an empirical dose reduction, should be performed for any trilostane-treated dog with a mild increase in potassium concentration. Trilostane can be safely withheld whilst waiting for the results of the test.

Other side effects: Trilostane is associated with vomiting and diarrhoea in some dogs, independently of any effects on cortisol concentration. The best treatment is to administer the tablets with food or to change to an alternative medication.

Successful treatment with trilostane might also lead to the emergence of previously suppressed immune-mediated, inflammatory or neoplastic diseases. There is also a theoretical risk that trilostane-induced adrenal hyperplasia could undergo neoplastic transformation. However, no evidence for this has been published to date.

Mitotane

Mitotane (o,p'-DDD) is an adrenocorticolytic drug. It selectively destroys the zona fasciculata and zona reticularis, whilst tending to preserve the zona glomerulosa. Mitotane requires a Special Treatment Authorization from the Veterinary Medicines Directorate for its use in the UK. In this country, it should be used only in the treatment of ACTH-dependent hypercortisolism when trilostane has been shown to be ineffective, when adverse effects have meant that trilostane cannot be used or when pre-existing disorders preclude the use of trilostane.

Pre-treatment assessment

Mitotane therapy should be considered only once the diagnosis of hypercortisolism has been confirmed. Because of its powerful effects, it should never be used empirically.

Problem	Management
Profound weakness, depression and anorexia	Discontinue trilostane and reassess dog. Check sodium and potassium concentrations and institute once-daily oral prednisolone (0.2 mg/kg). Reassess ACTH response test
Acute onset of neurological signs	Reassess dog. Continue trilostane unless dog is anorexic, vomiting or depressed. Give once-daily oral prednisolone (1–2 mg/kg) or dexamethasone (0.1 mg/kg) and decrease dose slowly once neurological signs have resolved. If no response, consider radiotherapy
Failure to resume normal water intake	Recheck urinalysis and creatinine concentration. Reassess ACTH response test. Increase trilostane by 50% if post-ACTH cortisol concentration is >200 nmol/l. If post-ACTH cortisol concentration is <120 nmol/l, consider increasing the frequency of medication. Consider central diabetes insipidus in association with a macroadenoma
Failure of hair to regrow	Reassess ACTH response test. Increase trilostane by 50% if post-ACTH cortisol concentration is >200 nmol/l. If post-ACTH cortisol concentration is <120 nmol/l, consider increasing the frequency of medication. Consider concurrent hypothyroidism (determine baseline total T4 and cTSH concentrations)
Failure to respond despite ACTH response test results that suggest adequate dose of trilostane	Consider switching to twice-daily administration. Consider switching to mitotane after 2 weeks of treatment

29.25 Possible problems that may be encountered during trilostane therapy and their management. ACTH = adrenocorticotropic hormone; cTSH = canine thyroid-stimulating hormone; T4 = thyroxine.

Before treatment is instigated, the dog's daily water consumption should be measured over at least two consecutive 24-hour periods. If the water intake and appetite are not increased, then pre-treatment cortisol concentrations, both before and after ACTH stimulation, should be recorded in order for the effects of treatment to be monitored.

Initial treatment

It is preferable to have dogs hospitalized for the initial course of treatment, although many clinicians commence therapy at home, with the owners doing the necessary monitoring.

Mitotane is given orally at a dose of 50 mg/kg/day. It should be administered with food as it is a fat-soluble drug and its absorption is poor when administered orally to fasted animals. Daily mitotane therapy should be continued until any of the following are noted:

- The water intake of a polydipsic dog decreases to 60 ml/kg/day or lower
- The dog takes longer to consume its meals than before treatment or stops eating completely
- The dog develops vomiting or diarrhoea
- The dog becomes listless and depressed
- Nine days of therapy have been completed.

The initial mitotane course is then stopped and maintenance therapy is initiated (see below) if cortisol production has been adequately suppressed. The importance of close monitoring of the dog during this period cannot be overemphasized.

The majority of dogs with ACTH-dependent hypercortisolism require between 7 and 14 days of treatment, with an average of 10 days, before water consumption reduces to 60 ml/kg/day or lower. If the dog is not polydipsic or polyphagic, treatment should continue until the serum cortisol concentrations, both before and after ACTH administration, are below 120 nmol/l. Some dogs respond in 2–3 days; others require upwards of 60 consecutive days of treatment but these extremes are rare. It is important to emphasize that each dog must be treated as an individual if the therapy is to be successful, and that an ACTH response test should be performed to check that the induction course of therapy has adequately suppressed adrenal function before maintenance therapy is introduced. If serum cortisol concentrations are less than 27 nmol/l and do not respond to ACTH stimulation, a delay in the introduction of maintenance therapy should be considered until the cortisol concentrations are between 27 and 120 nmol/l after ACTH administration.

Maintenance therapy

Having produced sufficient adrenocortical damage with daily mitotane treatment, it is important to continue therapy, albeit at a lower dose, otherwise the adrenal cortex will regenerate a hyperplastic zona fasciculata and zona reticularis and the clinical signs will recur.

Mitotane is given at a dose of 50 mg/kg/week with food. Dogs whose conditions are well controlled may sleep for a few hours after the weekly dose, and for that reason it is often recommended that the treatment is given in the evening. More profound depression or weakness requires re-evaluation using the ACTH response test and possibly a reduction or splitting of the maintenance dose. Poorly controlled polydipsia may require an increased dose of mitotane.

Re-examination

Treated dogs should be re-examined 4–8 weeks after initiation of maintenance therapy, unless problems are encountered. Marked improvement should be noted at this time. The most obvious and rapid response is a reduction in water intake, urine output and appetite, which is usually obvious at the end of the initial course of therapy. Muscle strength and exercise tolerance improve over the first 3–4 weeks. Skin and hair coat changes take longer and their progress is variable. Alopecia may get markedly worse before improving. Although improvement should be noted at 8 weeks, the skin and hair coat may not return to normal for 3–6 months (Figure 29.26).

Re-evaluation every 3–6 months is recommended for the remainder of the animal's life. The dosage of mitotane should be adjusted according to the results of ACTH response testing. The goal of therapy is to achieve an ACTH test result with serum cortisol concentrations between 27 and 120 nmol/l. Relapses (serum cortisol >200 nmol/l) do occur in up to 55% of cases (Kintzer and

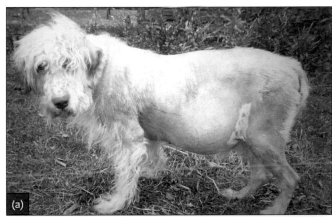

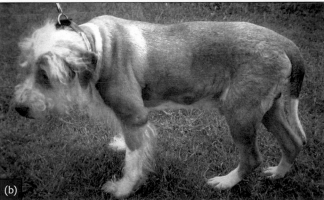

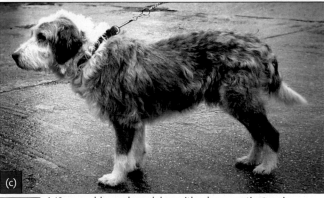

29.26 A 10-year-old crossbreed dog with adrenocorticotropic hormone-dependent hypercortisolism. (a) Before treatment; (b) after commencing treatment with mitotane; (c) 6 months later.

Peterson, 1991). These should be treated with a short course of daily mitotane therapy or an increase in the maintenance dose. Overdose (serum cortisol <20 nmol/l) is less frequent (5–10% of cases) and requires a reduction in the frequency or dose of maintenance therapy (Kintzer and Peterson, 1991; Dunn et al., 1995).

Side effects

Mitotane therapy is comparatively safe and the most frequent adverse effects (anorexia, vomiting and diarrhoea) are rarely serious, provided they are noticed early on so that mitotane therapy can be withheld. Some of the problems that can be encountered during treatment are summarized in Figure 29.27, together with their suggested management.

The use of prednisolone and other glucocorticoids is not necessary; although they are often recommended during induction to prevent signs of hypocortisolaemia, there is limited evidence of a true reduction in the incidence of adverse effects and they may mask the indicators of the endpoint of daily induction. In addition, at least for prednisolone, the interpretation of subsequent ACTH response test results is difficult due to the cross-reactivity of prednisolone in most cortisol assays (Dunn et al., 1995). However, if the dog is being treated at home, the owner should be given a small supply of prednisolone tablets to be used in an emergency.

Successful treatment with mitotane might also lead to the emergence of previously suppressed immune-mediated, inflammatory or neoplastic diseases.

Neurological signs: Rarely, dogs will develop persistent neurological signs during the induction course of treatment with mitotane because of enlargement of a pituitary tumour. Most of these cases will respond favourably to treatment with glucocorticoids. If the glucocorticoid therapy is slowly withdrawn over several weeks, the brain can often adapt to the enlargement of the pituitary tumour. If there is no response to glucocorticoid therapy, radiotherapy should be considered.

Hypoadrenocorticism: Mitotane can be associated with signs of hypocortisolism and, when noted, post-ACTH cortisol vales are usually extremely low (<27 nmol/l). A reduction in the frequency or dose, or both, is recommended (Kintzer and Peterson, 1991; Dunn et al., 1995). Addison's disease, with both glucocorticoid and mineralo-corticoid insufficiency, occurs in 5–17% of treated dogs during maintenance therapy (see Chapter 28). Although hypoadrenocorticism can develop at any time during treatment, most cases of primary hypoadrenocorticism occur during the first year of treatment. There is no way to predict which dogs will develop complete adrenocortical insufficiency but, if hypoadrenocorticism does develop, maintenance mitotane therapy should be stopped and the dog should be treated with mineralocorticoid and glucocorticoid supplementation, as for primary hypoadrenocorticism (see Chapter 28). Mitotane may have to be re-introduced if clinical signs of hypercortisolism recur.

Survival data

The mean survival time of treated dogs was 30 months in one study, with a range of a few days to over 7 years (Dunn et al., 1995). The highest mortality was seen in the first 16 weeks of treatment and dogs that survived this period had a longer mean survival time. Other studies have shown similar survival times (Kintzer and Peterson, 1991).

Other treatments
Selegiline

Selegiline (L-deprenyl) is a monoamine oxidase inhibitor (MAOI) and, as such, it should inhibit ACTH secretion. Selegiline is not authorized for use in ACTH-dependent hypercortisolism in the UK but is authorized for behavioural disorders in dogs.

Selegiline is not recommended for dogs with concurrent diabetes mellitus, pancreatitis, heart failure, kidney disease or other severe illness. It should not be used in cases of ACTH-independent hypercortisolism.

Preliminary trials with selegiline in cases of ACTH-dependent hypercortisolism have shown that the efficacy is poor, with approximately 80% of dogs failing to show improvement of clinical signs. However, selegiline is not associated with any severe adverse effects. Monitoring therapy with endocrine testing is difficult, since there are only minor reductions in serum cortisol concentrations during ACTH response tests (Reusch et al., 1999). The recommended dose of selegiline for canine hypercortisolism is 1 mg/kg orally q24h. If there is an inadequate response after 2 months, the dosage is increased to 2 mg/kg q24h.

Problem	Management
Vomiting or anorexia within the first 3 days of treatment (gastric irritation)	Discontinue mitotane and reassess dog. Divide dose and give 2–4 times a day
Profound weakness, depression and anorexia, usually after the fourth or fifth day of treatment with mitotane	Discontinue mitotane and reassess dog. Reassess ACTH response test. Check sodium and potassium concentrations and institute prednisolone (0.2 mg/kg orally q24h). Start maintenance therapy with mitotane
Acute onset of neurological signs	Reassess dog. Continue mitotane unless dog is anorexic, vomiting or depressed. Give prednisolone 1–2 mg/kg orally q24h or dexamethasone 0.1 mg/kg orally q24h and decrease dose slowly once neurological signs have resolved. If no response, consider radiotherapy
Failure to resume normal water intake	Recheck urinalysis and creatinine concentration. Reassess ACTH response test. Increase mitotane by 50% if post-ACTH cortisol is >200 nmol/l. Consider central diabetes insipidus in association with a macroadenoma
Failure of hair to regrow	Reassess ACTH response test. Increase mitotane by 50% if post-ACTH cortisol concentration is >200 nmol/l. Consider concurrent hypothyroidism. Determine baseline total T4 and cTSH
Excessive depression, weakness or ataxia related to weekly maintenance therapy using mitotane	Reassess dog. Check sodium and potassium concentrations. Repeat ACTH response test. If post-ACTH cortisol concentration is <27 nmol/l, reduce maintenance dose or give every other week. If post-ACTH cortisol is indicative of reasonable control, divide dose and administer twice weekly

29.27 Possible problems that may be encountered during mitotane therapy and their management. ACTH = adrenocorticotropic hormone; cTSH = canine thyroid-stimulating hormone; T4 = thyroxine.

Ketoconazole

Ketoconazole has a similar mode of action to trilostane. Ketoconazole has been used effectively in the management of canine hypercortisolism but has more side effects than trilostane (Lien and Huang, 2008). Adverse effects include anorexia, vomiting, diarrhoea, hepatopathy and jaundice.

Ketoconazole treatment is expensive and not always effective – about 25% of dogs fail to respond adequately. Ketoconazole should not be used unless trilostane and mitotane have failed or are not available.

Other drugs

Various other drugs have been suggested for the treatment of hypercortisolism, including pasireotide, phosphatidyl-serine, retinoic acid, cyproheptadine, cabergoline, metyrapone and aminoglutethimide. Some of these drugs have been found to be ineffective, some are associated with unacceptable side effects and some have not yet been properly investigated. They are not currently recommended treatment options for canine hypercortisolism.

Pituitary irradiation

Pituitary irradiation is indicated for dogs with neurological signs associated with pituitary tumours. Computed tomography or MRI of the brain is required to plan the treatment protocol. Radiotherapy using megavoltage irradiation from a linear accelerator is required to penetrate to the depth of the pituitary gland without seriously injuring overlying soft tissues. Most treatment protocols involve the administration of 40–50 Gy in 3–4 Gy fractions (Théon and Feldman, 1998). However, increasing the number of fractions and reducing the dose per fraction, whilst keeping the total dose at the low end of the range, can lead to increased survival times (Marcinowska et al., 2015). There is often a dramatic response, although in some cases improvement takes several weeks (Sawada et al., 2018). The resolution of neurological signs parallels the reduction in size of the tumour, which can continue to decrease for a year or more after completion of the radiotherapy. Reduction in ACTH secretion by the tumour is less predictable, occurring in about 20% of cases, and may not be evident for 6–12 months after therapy. Therefore, concurrent medical management of hypercortisolism with trilostane or mitotane is indicated, at least initially.

Hypophysectomy

Hypophysectomy has been successfully performed in the dog for the treatment of ACTH-dependent hypercortisolism using the transsphenoidal approach (van Rijn et al., 2016). The operation is technically difficult and should only be carried out by a surgeon with considerable skill and experience of the technique, otherwise it is associated with high morbidity and mortality. In experienced hands, transsphenoidal hypophysectomy has proved an effective treatment for ACTH-dependent hypercortisolism in dogs, with an acceptable long-term outcome. In one large study of 306 cases, 91% of dogs were alive 4 weeks after surgery, with a median survival time of 781 days and median disease-free interval of 951 days. However, over time, 27% developed recurrence of hypercortisolism after a median period of 555 days. Dogs with recurrence had significantly higher pituitary height:brain area. Survival time and disease-free intervals were negatively correlated with pituitary gland size, making pituitary height:brain area an important preoperative prognostic factor (van Rijn et al., 2016).

Haemorrhage and incomplete visualization and removal of larger lesions are common complications. Diabetes insipidus, which may be transient, develops in about 50% of cases and requires treatment and all dogs will require lifelong thyroid hormone and glucocorticoid replacement therapy.

Bilateral adrenalectomy

Bilateral adrenalectomy has been employed successfully but involves the risk of putting an ill animal with a compromised immune system and poor wound healing through a difficult surgical procedure (Oblak et al., 2016). With other, more effective, treatments available there is little benefit to this technique except where both adrenal glands have tumours and at least one is suspected to be a phaeochromocytoma. Dogs treated by this approach will require lifelong treatment for hypoadrenocorticism (see Chapter 28).

Treatment of ACTH-independent hypercortisolism

There are three main treatment options for ACTH-independent hypercortisolism.

Surgical adrenalectomy

Dogs with ACTH-independent hypercortisolism carry the best prognosis if the tumour can be completely removed surgically. However, animals with untreated ACTH-independent hypercortisolism represent difficult surgical candidates because of increased anaesthetic risk (due to poor respiratory and hepatic function), hypercoagulability (leading to an increased risk of pulmonary thromboembolism) and poor vascular tone (leading to poor haemostasis). Primary wound healing is delayed but wound breakdown is rare. The anatomical location and surrounding blood vessels make surgical exposure and removal difficult. Furthermore, many adrenal tumours are quite friable and haemorrhagic. Unilateral adrenalectomy, therefore, requires considerable experience and expertise. Acute postoperative hypoadrenocorticism due to preexisting contralateral adrenal atrophy is common and glucocorticoid supplementation should be started at the time of induction. Postoperative intensive care facilities are, therefore, essential.

Inexperienced surgeons or those without adequate facilities, including assistance in anaesthesia, should not attempt adrenalectomy. Even in referral institutes, perioperative mortality rates are often in the range of 20–30% (van Sluijs et al., 1995; Schwartz et al., 2008).

If surgery is an option, then preoperative staging of the adrenal tumour should include thoracic radiography and abdominal ultrasonography or, preferably, CT to assess for the presence of vascular invasion and metastatic spread. Administration of trilostane or mitotane is recommended by some authors in order to attempt to control the hypercortisolism before surgery. Preoperative stabilization probably improves survival, but this has not been clearly demonstrated. Mitotane may be less useful than trilostane or ketoconazole in this respect because it may make the tumour more friable, but objective data are not available.

Adrenalectomy is best performed by a ventral midline laparotomy (Scavelli et al., 1986; Anderson et al., 2001). The paracostal approach that has been advocated by some authors provides inadequate exposure. The contralateral adrenal gland should be checked for the presence of bilateral tumours, and other abdominal organs should be checked for metastases. The renal vessels and caudal vena cava should be carefully examined for the presence of tumours. If there is local invasion, debulking surgery is still worthwhile, providing this can be accomplished safely; if not, a small biopsy sample should be taken. The abdomen should be closed with suture materials that are slowly absorbed.

During and for up to 24 hours following surgery, glucocorticoid supplementation is generally provided by treatment with hydrocortisone (4–10 mg/kg q6h or 0.5 mg/kg/h constant rate infusion). Dogs that receive such treatment have a better chance of survival. Theoretically, mineralocorticoid supplementation should not be required unless hypotension or supportive electrolyte abnormalities develop. For this reason, intravenous dexamethasone (0.1–0.5 mg/kg q12h) has been used as an alternative perioperative treatment but there are no specific data on its effect on survival. Glucocorticoid therapy should be slowly discontinued over a period of weeks to months, depending on the assessment of the dog's appetite and results of ACTH response tests.

If surgery is successful and the dog survives the perioperative period, then the prognosis is good, but recurrence can be seen (some studies suggest 40% will recur eventually). In one study, the median survival time was just less than 2 years, although some dogs survived for longer than 4 years (van Sluijs et al., 1995).

Mitotane

Mitotane is effective and relatively safe in dogs with ACTH-independent hypercortisolism. Dogs with adrenal tumours, however, tend to be more resistant to mitotane than dogs with ACTH-dependent hypercortisolism (Feldman et al., 1992). Generally, dogs with ACTH-independent hypercortisolism require higher daily induction doses (50–75 mg/kg orally q24h) and a longer period of induction (>14 days) than dogs with ACTH-dependent hypercortisolism (Kintzer and Peterson, 1994). Frequent monitoring of treatment by ACTH response testing is important to ensure adequate control of the hypercortisolism.

Maintenance doses are also generally higher (75–100 mg/kg/week) and, again, frequent monitoring of the cortisol response to ACTH stimulation is required to maintain optimal control of the disease. Adverse effects of treatment are similar to those described for ACTH-dependent hypercortisolism. Those dogs requiring higher dose rates tend to be more prone to adverse effects. The adrenal tumour and metastatic mass will often reduce in size, due the cytotoxic effects of mitotane, but in other cases the tumour will continue to grow despite the use of mitotane. In one study of adrenocortical tumours treated using mitotane therapy, the median survival time was 11 months, with a range of a few weeks to more than 5 years (Kintzer and Peterson, 1994).

Trilostane

Trilostane has also been used to control clinical signs in ACTH-independent hypercortisolism with some success (Helm et al., 2011; Arenas et al., 2014). Comparisons of dogs treated with mitotane and with trilostane suggest survival times are not significantly different. There is currently limited evidence that higher trilostane doses are required compared with those for ACTH-dependent hypercortisolism. As an enzyme inhibitor, however, trilostane provides control of only the clinical signs without treating the underlying neoplastic disease process.

Future options

With our developing understanding of pituitary and adrenal pathology in hypercortisolism, new options for therapeutic interventions, such as abiraterone acetate, melanocortin 2 receptor antagonists and steroidogenic factor-1 inverse agonists, are being actively considered (Sanders et al., 2018). These may be used in addition to or instead of current treatments. However, at the time of publication none of these is available for routine clinical use.

References and further reading

Aldridge C, Behrend EN, Kemppainen RJ et al. (2016) Comparison of 2 doses for ACTH stimulation testing in dogs suspected of or treated for hyperadrenocorticism. Journal of Veterinary Internal Medicine 30, 1637–1641

Anderson CR, Birchard SJ, Powers BE et al. (2001) Surgical treatment of adrenocortical tumors: 21 cases (1990–1996). Journal of the American Animal Hospital Association 37, 93–97

Arenas C, Melian C and Perez-Alenza MD (2014) Long-term survival of dogs with adrenal-dependent hyperadrenocorticism: a comparison between mitotane and twice daily trilostane treatment. Journal of Veterinary Internal Medicine 28, 473–480

Auriemma E, Barthez PY, van der Vlugt-Meijer RH, Voorhout G and Meij BP (2009) Computed tomography and low-field magnetic resonance imaging of the pituitary gland in dogs with pituitary-dependent hyperadrenocorticism: 11 cases (2001–2003). Journal of the American Veterinary Medical Association 235, 409–414

Barker EN, Campbell S, Tebb AJ et al. (2005) A comparison of the survival times of dogs treated with mitotane or trilostane for pituitary-dependent hyperadrenocorticism. Journal of Veterinary Internal Medicine 19, 810–815

Beatrice L, Boretti FS, Sieber-Ruckstuhl NS et al. (2018) Concurrent endocrine neoplasias in dogs and cats: a retrospective study (2004–2014). Veterinary Record 182, 323

Bell R, Neiger R, McGrotty Y and Ramsey IK (2006) Study of the effects of once daily doses of trilostane on cortisol concentrations and responsiveness to adrenocorticotrophic hormone in hyperadrenocorticoid dogs. Veterinary Record 159, 277–281

Benchekroun G, de Fornel-Thibaud P, Rodríguez Piñeiro MI et al. (2010) Ultrasonography criteria for differentiating ACTH dependency from ACTH independency in 47 dogs with hyperadrenocorticism and equivocal adrenal asymmetry. Journal of Veterinary Internal Medicine 24, 1077–1085

Bennaim M, Shiel RE, Forde C and Mooney CT (2018) Evaluation of individual low-dose dexamethasone suppression test patterns in naturally occurring hyperadrenocorticism in dogs. Journal of Veterinary Internal Medicine 32, 967–977

Bento PL, Center SA, Randolph JF, Yeager AE and Bicalho RC (2016) Associations between sex, body weight, age, and ultrasonographically determined adrenal gland thickness in dogs with non adrenal gland illness. Journal of the American Veterinary Medical Association 248, 652–660

Bertolini G, Rossetti E and Caldin M (2007) Pituitary apoplexy-like disease in 4 dogs. Journal of Veterinary Internal Medicine 21, 1251–1257

Braddock JA, Church DB, Robertson ID and Watson ADJ (2003) Trilostane treatment in dogs with pituitary-dependent hyperadrenocorticism. Australian Veterinary Journal 81, 600–607

Carotenuto G, Malerba E, Dolfini C et al. (2019) Cushing's syndrome–an epidemiological study based on a canine population of 21,281 dogs. Open Veterinary Journal 9, 27–32

Chapman PS, Kelly DF, Archer J, Brockman DJ and Neiger R (2004) Adrenal necrosis in a dog receiving trilostane for the treatment of hyperadrenocorticism. Journal of Small Animal Practice 45, 307–310

Chapman PS, Mooney CT, Ede J et al. (2003) Evaluation of the basal and post-adrenocorticotrophic hormone serum concentrations of 17-hydroxyprogesterone for the diagnosis of hyperadrenocorticism in dogs. Veterinary Record 153, 771–775

Clemente M, De Andrés PJ, Arenas C et al. (2007) Comparison of non-selective adrenocorticolysis with mitotane or trilostane for the treatment of dogs with pituitary-dependent hyperadrenocorticism. Veterinary Record 161, 805–809

Dunn KJ, Herrtage ME and Dunn JK (1995) Use of ACTH stimulation tests to monitor the treatment of canine hyperadrenocorticism. Veterinary Record 137, 161–165

Feldman EC, Nelson RW, Feldman MS and Farver TB (1992) Comparison of mitotane treatment for adrenal tumor versus pituitary-dependent hyperadrenocorticism in dogs. Journal of the American Veterinary Medical Association 200, 1642–1647

Frank LA, Henry GA, Whittemore JC et al. (2015) Serum cortisol concentrations in dogs with pituitary-dependent hyperadrenocorticism and atypical hyperadrenocorticism. Journal of Veterinary Internal Medicine 29, 193–199

Galac S, Kars VJ, Voorhout G, Mol JA and Kooistra HS (2008) ACTH-independent hyperadrenocorticism due to food-dependent hypercortisolemia in a dog: a case report. The Veterinary Journal 177, 141–143

Galac S, Kooistra HS, Teske E and Rijnberk A (1997) Urinary corticoid/creatinine ratios in the differentiation between pituitary-dependent hyperadrenocorticism and hyperadrenocorticism due to adrenocortical tumour in the dog. *Veterinary Quarterly* **19**, 17–20

Galac S, Kooistra HS, Voorhout G *et al.* (2005) Hyperadrenocorticism in a dog due to ectopic secretion of adrenocorticotropic hormone. *Domestic Animal Endocrinology* **28**, 338–348

Galeandro L, Sieber-Ruckstuhl NS, Riond B *et al.* (2014) Urinary corticoid concentrations measured by 5 different immunoassays and gas chromatography-mass spectrometry in healthy dogs and dogs with hypercortisolism at home and in the hospital. *Journal of Veterinary Internal Medicine* **28**, 1433–1441

García San José P, Arenas Bermejo C, Clares Moral I, Cuesta Alvaro P and Pérez Alenza MD (2020) Prevalence and risk factors associated with systemic hypertension in dogs with spontaneous hyperadrenocorticism. *Journal of Veterinary Internal Medicine* **34**, 1768–1778

Golinelli S, de Marco V, Leal RO *et al.* (2021) Comparison of methods to monitor dogs with hypercortisolism treated with trilostane. *Journal of Veterinary Internal Medicine* **35**, 2616–2627

Graham JP, Roberts GD and Newell SM (2000) Dynamic magnetic resonance imaging of the normal canine pituitary gland. *Veterinary Radiology & Ultrasound* **41**, 35–40

Helm JR, McLauchlan G, Boden LA *et al.* (2011) A comparison of factors that influence survival in dogs with adrenal-dependent hyperadrenocorticism treated with mitotane or trilostane. *Journal of Veterinary Internal Medicine* **25**, 251–260

Hurley KJ and Vaden SL (1998) Evaluation of urine protein content in dogs with pituitary-dependent hyperadrenocorticism. *Journal of the American Veterinary Medical Association* **212**, 369–373

Kim KH, Han SM, Jeon KO *et al.* (2017) Clinical relationship between cholestatic disease and pituitary-dependent hyperadrenocorticism in dogs: a retrospective case series. *Journal of Veterinary Internal Medicine* **31**, 335–342

Kintzer PP and Peterson ME (1991) Mitotane (o,p'-DDD) treatment of 200 dogs with pituitary-dependent hyperadrenocorticism. *Journal of Veterinary Internal Medicine* **5**, 182–190

Kintzer PP and Peterson ME (1994) Mitotane treatment of 32 dogs with cortisol-secreting adrenocortical neoplasms. *Journal of the American Veterinary Medical Association* **205**, 54–61

Lee WM, Meij BP, Bhatti SFM *et al.* (2003) Pulsatile secretion pattern of growth hormone in dogs with pituitary-dependent hyperadrenocorticism. *Domestic Animal Endocrinology* **24**, 59–68

Lien YH and Huang HP (2008) Use of ketoconazole to treat dogs with pituitary-dependent hyperadrenocorticism: 48 cases (1994–2007). *Journal of the American Veterinary Medical Association* **233**, 1896–1901

Long SN, Michieletto A, Anderson TJ, Williams A and Knottenbelt CM (2003) Suspected pituitary apoplexy in a German shorthaired pointer. *Journal of Small Animal Practice* **44**, 497–502

Macfarlane L, Parkin T and Ramsey I (2016) Pre-trilostane and three hour post-trilostane cortisol to monitor trilostane therapy in dogs. *Veterinary Record* **179**, 597

Mantis P, Lamb CR, Witt AL and Neiger R (2003) Changes in ultrasonographic appearance of adrenal glands in dogs with pituitary-dependent hyperadrenocorticism treated with trilostane. *Veterinary Radiology & Ultrasound* **44**, 682–685

Marcinowska A, Warland J, Brearley M and Dobson J (2015) Comparison of two coarse fractionated radiation protocols for the management of canine pituitary macrotumor: an observational study of 24 dogs. *Veterinary Radiology & Ultrasound* **56**, 554–562

Martin LG, Behrend EN, Mealey KL, Carpenter DM and Hickey KC (2007) Effect of low doses of cosyntropin on serum cortisol concentrations in clinically normal dogs. *American Journal of Veterinary Research* **68**, 555–560

Mawby DI, Whittemore JC and Fecteau KA (2014) Canine pancreatic-specific lipase concentrations in clinically healthy dogs and dogs with naturally occurring hyperadrenocorticism. *Journal of Veterinary Internal Medicine* **28**, 1244–1250

Melián C, Pérez-López L, Saavedra P *et al.* (2021) Ultrasound evaluation of adrenal gland size in clinically healthy dogs and in dogs with hyperadrenocorticism. *Veterinary Record* **188**, e80

Mesich MLL, Mayhew PD, Paek M, Holt DE and Brown DC (2009) Gall bladder mucoceles and their association with endocrinopathies in dogs: a retrospective case-control study. *Journal of Small Animal Practice* **50**, 630–635

Midence JN, Drobatz KJ and Hess RS (2015) Cortisol concentrations in well-regulated dogs with hyperadrenocorticism treated with trilostane. *Journal of Veterinary Internal Medicine* **29**, 1529–1533

Montgomery TM, Nelson RW, Feldman EC, Robertson K and Polonsky KS (1996) Basal and glucagon-stimulated plasma C-peptide concentrations in healthy dogs, dogs with diabetes mellitus, and dogs with hyperadrenocorticism. *Journal of Veterinary Internal Medicine* **10**, 116–122

Mooney CT, Shiel RE, Sekiya M, Dunning M and Gunn E (2020) A preliminary study of the effect of hyperadrenocorticism on calcium and phosphate concentrations, parathyroid hormone and markers of bone turnover in dogs. *Frontiers in Veterinary Science* **7**, 311

Nagata N, Kojima K and Yuki M (2017) Comparison of survival times for dogs with pituitary-dependent hyperadrenocorticism in a primary-care hospital: treated with trilostane *versus* untreated. *Journal of Veterinary Internal Medicine* **31**, 22–28

Neiger R, Ramsey I, O'Connor J, Hurley KJ and Mooney CT (2002) Trilostane treatment of 78 dogs with pituitary-dependent hyperadrenocorticism. *Veterinary Record* **150**, 799–804

Norman EJ, Thompson H and Mooney CT (1999) Dynamic adrenal function testing in eight dogs with hyperadrenocorticism associated with adrenocortical neoplasia. *Veterinary Record* **144**, 551–554

O'Neill DG, Scudder C, Faire JM *et al.* (2016) Epidemiology of hyperadrenocorticism among 210,824 dogs attending primary-care veterinary practices in the UK from 2009 to 2014. *Journal of Small Animal Practice* **57**, 365–373

Oblak ML, Bacon NJ and Covey JL (2016) Perioperative management and outcome of bilateral adrenalectomy in 9 dogs. *Veterinary Surgery* **45**, 790–797

Pollard RE, Reilly CM, Uerling MR, Wood FD and Feldman EC (2010) Cross-sectional imaging characteristics of pituitary adenomas, invasive adenomas and adenocarcinomas in dogs: 33 cases (1988–2006). *Journal of Veterinary Internal Medicine* **24**, 160–165

Quilez E, Burchell RK, Thorstensen EB *et al.* (2020) Cortisol urinary metabolites in dogs with hypercortisolism, congestive heart failure, and healthy dogs: pilot investigation. *Journal of Veterinary Diagnostic Investigation* **32**, 317–323

Ramsey IK, Richardson J, Lenard Z, Tebb AJ and Irwin PJ (2008) Persistent isolated hypocortisolism following brief treatment with trilostane. *Australian Veterinary Journal* **86**, 491–495

Ramsey IK, Tebb A, Harris E, Evans H and Herrtage ME (2005) Hyperparathyroidism in dogs with hyperadrenocorticism. *Journal of Small Animal Practice* **46**, 531–536

Reusch CE, Sieber-Ruckstuhl N, Wenger M *et al.* (2007) Histological evaluation of the adrenal glands of seven dogs with hyperadrenocorticism treated with trilostane. *Veterinary Record* **160**, 219–224

Reusch CE, Steffen T and Hoerauf A (1999) The efficacy of L-Deprenyl in dogs with pituitary-dependent hyperadrenocorticism. *Journal of Veterinary Internal Medicine* **13**, 291–301

Ristic JME, Ramsey IK, Heath EM, Evans HJ and Herrtage ME (2002) The use of 17-hydroxyprogesterone in the diagnosis of canine hyperadrenocorticism. *Journal of Veterinary Internal Medicine* **16**, 433–439

Rodríguez Piñeiro MI, Benchekroun G, de Fornel-Thibaud P *et al.* (2009) Accuracy of an adrenocorticotropic hormone (ACTH) immunoluminometric assay for differentiating ACTH-dependent from ACTH-independent hyperadrenocorticism in dogs. *Journal of Veterinary Internal Medicine* **23**, 850–855

Rodríguez Piñeiro MI, de Fornel-Thibaud P, Benchekroun G *et al.* (2011) Use of computed tomography adrenal gland measurement for differentiating ACTH dependence from ACTH independence in 64 dogs with hyperadrenocorticism. *Journal of Veterinary Internal Medicine* **25**, 1066–1074

Ruckstuhl NS, Nett CS and Reusch CE (2002) Results of clinical examinations, laboratory tests, and ultrasonography in dogs with pituitary-dependent hyperadrenocorticism treated with trilostane. *American Journal of Veterinary Research* **63**, 506–512

Sanders K, Cirkel K, Grinwis GCM *et al.* (2019a) The Utrecht Score: a novel histopathological scoring system to assess the prognosis of dogs with cortisol-secreting adrenocortical tumours. *Veterinary and Comparative Oncology* **17**, 329–337

Sanders K, van Staalduinen GJ, Uijens MCM *et al.* (2019b) Molecular markers of prognosis in canine cortisol-secreting adrenocortical tumours. *Veterinary and Comparative Oncology* **17**, 545–552

Sanders K, Kooistra HS and Galac S (2018) Treating canine Cushing's syndrome: current options and future prospects. *Veterinary Journal* **241**, 42–51

Sawada H, Mori A, Lee P *et al.* (2018) Pituitary size alteration and adverse effects of radiation therapy performed in 9 dogs with pituitary-dependent hypercortisolism. *Research in Veterinary Science* **118**, 19–26

Scavelli TD, Peterson ME and Matthiesen DT (1986) Results of surgical treatment for hyperadrenocorticism caused by adrenocortical neoplasia in the dog: 25 cases (1980–1984). *Journal of the American Veterinary Medical Association* **189**, 1360–1364

Schofield I, Brodbelt DC, Wilson ARL *et al.* (2020) Survival analysis of 219 dogs with hyperadrenocorticism attending primary care practice in England. *Veterinary Record* **186**, 348

Schwartz P, Kovak JR, Koprowski A *et al.* (2008) Evaluation of prognostic factors in the surgical treatment of adrenal gland tumors in dogs: 41 cases (1999–2005). *Journal of the American Veterinary Medical Association* **232**, 77–84

Sieber-Ruckstuhl NS, Boretti FS, Wenger M, Maser-Gluth C and Reusch CE (2006) Cortisol, aldosterone, cortisol precursor, androgen and endogenous ACTH concentrations in dogs with pituitary-dependant hyperadrenocorticism treated with trilostane. *Domestic Animal Endocrinology* **31**, 63–75

Sieber-Ruckstuhl NS, Boretti FS, Wenger M, Maser-Gluth C and Reusch CE (2008a) Evaluation of cortisol precursors for the diagnosis of pituitary-dependent hypercortisolism in dogs. *Veterinary Record* **162**, 673–678

Sieber-Ruckstuhl NS, Boretti FS, Wenger M, Maser-Gluth C and Reusch CE (2008b) Serum concentrations of cortisol and cortisone in healthy dogs and dogs with pituitary-dependent hyperadrenocorticism treated with trilostane. *Veterinary Record* **163**, 477–481

Soulsby SN, Holland M, Hudson JA and Behrend EN (2015) Ultrasonographic evaluation of adrenal gland size compared to body weight in normal dogs. *Veterinary Radiology & Ultrasound* **56**, 317–326

Syme HM, Scott-Moncrieff JC, Treadwell NG *et al.* (2001) Hyperadrenocorticism associated with excessive sex hormone production by an adrenocortical tumor in two dogs. *Journal of the American Veterinary Medical Association* **219**, 1725–1728

Tebb AJ, Arteaga A, Evans H and Ramsey IK (2005) Canine hyperadrenocorticism: effects of trilostane on parathyroid hormone, calcium and phosphate concentrations. *Journal of Small Animal Practice* **46**, 537–542

Teske E, Rothuizen J, de Bruijne JJ and Rijnberk A (1989) Corticosteroid-induced alkaline phosphatase isoenzyme in the diagnosis of canine hypercorticism. *Veterinary Record* **125**, 12–14

Théon AP and Feldman EC (1998) Megavoltage irradiation of pituitary macrotumors in dogs with neurologic signs. *Journal of the American Veterinary Medical Association* **213**, 225–231

van der Vlugt-Meijer RH, Meij BP, van den Ingh TSGAM, Rijnberk A and Voorhout G (2003) Dynamic computed tomography of the pituitary gland in dogs with pituitary-dependent hyperadrenocorticism. *Journal of Veterinary Internal Medicine* **17**, 773–780

van Rijn SJ, Galac S, Tryfonidou MA *et al.* (2016) The influence of pituitary size on outcome after transsphenoidal hypophysectomy in a large cohort of dogs with pituitary-dependent hypercortisolism. *Journal of Veterinary Internal Medicine* **30**, 989–995

van Sluijs FJ, Sjollema BE, Voorhout G, van den Ingh TSGAM and Rijnberk A (1995) Results of adrenalectomy in 36 dogs with hyperadrenocorticism caused by adrenocortical tumour. *Veterinary Quarterly* **17**, 113–116

Wood FD, Pollard RE, Uerling MR and Feldman EC (2007) Diagnostic imaging findings and endocrine test results in dogs with pituitary-dependent hyperadrenocorticism that did or did not have neurologic abnormalities: 157 cases (1989–2005). *Journal of the American Veterinary Medical Association* **231**, 1081–1085

Zeugswetter FK, Carranza Valencia A, Glavassevich K and Schwendenwein I (2021) Patterns of the low-dose dexamethasone suppression test in canine hyperadrenocorticism revisited. *Veterinary Clinical Pathology* **50**, 62–70

Zur G and White SD (2011) Hyperadrenocorticism in 10 dogs with skin lesions as the only presenting clinical signs. *Journal of the American Animal Hospital Association* **47**, 419–427

Chapter 30

Feline hypercortisolism

Ellen Behrend and Brett Wasik

Introduction

Generally speaking, the term hyperadrenocorticism refers to excess production of any hormone synthesized and secreted by the adrenal cortex. Adrenal gland physiology and hormone secretion is discussed in Chapter 28. The hormone that is encountered most frequently in excess in dogs is cortisol (see Chapter 29). Hypercortisolism occurs in cats but is rare, with fewer than 200 cases reported since 1973. Although feline hypercortisolism resulting from endogenous cortisol synthesis is the primary focus of this chapter, hyperadrenocorticism can occur due to an adrenal tumour secreting excess cortisol precursors such as progesterone. Hyperadrenocorticism involving over-production of sex hormones such as oestradiol, testosterone and androstenedione has also been reported. These presentations are briefly discussed below.

Naturally occurring feline hypercortisolism is caused by hyperfunction of either the pituitary or adrenal glands. Similar to humans and dogs, adrenocorticotropic hormone (ACTH)-dependent hypercortisolism accounts for 80–85% of feline cases. The vast majority are pituitary dependent, where a pituitary adenoma arising from the pars distalis or pars intermedia secretes excess ACTH, resulting in bilateral adrenocortical hyperplasia and overproduction of cortisol. Pituitary carcinomas are rare. Extra-pituitary tumours secreting ACTH have not been identified in cats. The remaining 15–20% of cases are ACTH independent and typically occur when an adrenal tumour autonomously secretes excess cortisol. Approximately 50% of adrenal tumours in cats are adenomas and 50% are carcinomas (Boland and Barrs, 2017). Other ACTH-independent causes of hypercortisolism have not been identified in cats.

Iatrogenic hypercortisolism can be caused by chronic administration of exogenous glucocorticoids by any route. Because cats are relatively resistant to the effects of glu-cocorticoids, iatrogenic disease is uncommon.

Clinical features

Feline hypercortisolism is a disease of older cats with a mean age at diagnosis of approximately 10 years. Domestic Shorthaired and Longhaired cats constitute the majority of reported cases, and most cases are neutered. No obvious sex predisposition exists. Clinical signs of naturally occurring hypercortisolism are listed in Figure 30.1.

Clinical signs	Prevalence (%)
Polyuria and polydipsia	81
Abdominal enlargement ('pot belly')	61
Polyphagia	60
Skin atrophy	59
Muscle wasting	47
Weight loss	47
Lethargy	41
Alopecia	37
Skin fragility (skin tears)	32
Unkempt hair coat	30
Weakness/plantigrade stance	18
Hepatomegaly	13
Weight gain	12

30.1 Clinical signs collated from reports of 167 cats with hypercortisolism.
(Reproduced from Boland and Barrs (2017), with permission from the publisher)

Cats are more tolerant of higher glucocorticoid con-centrations (either endogenous or exogenous) compared to dogs. Therefore, owners may not report clinical signs early in the development of hypercortisolism, which can delay definitive diagnosis until later in the course of disease. Recurrent bacterial or fungal infections second-ary to hypercortisolism-induced immunosuppression may be an early indicator of disease prior to the development of more obvious polyuria and polydipsia (PU/PD). Infections can involve the urinary tract, respiratory tract and oral cavity in addition to the development of subcutaneous abscesses and paronychia (Boland and Barrs, 2017).

Differences in clinical presentation in cats *versus* dogs

Although similarities exist in cats and dogs with hypercor-tisolism, some major differences in clinical presentation are worth noting.

Dermatological changes

Dermatological changes occur in both dogs and cats but a more severe form, termed feline skin fragility syndrome, occurs in approximately one third of cats with hyper-cortisolism. Hypercortisolism causes skin atrophy with a subsequent reduction in elasticity, making skin very fragile, thin and papery. Skin tears can occur easily with routine handling, minor trauma or grooming (Figure 30.2). Extreme care should be taken when handling cats with suspected hypercortisolism to avoid iatrogenic trauma to the skin.

Bilaterally symmetrical alopecia involving the thoracic, ventral abdominal, flank and limb regions can develop, and may be patchy or generalized. An 'unkempt' hair coat can occur due to growth of brittle and sparse hair, scaling and seborrhoea. To date, calcinosis cutis has not been documented in cats with hypercortisolism.

Polyuria and polydipsia

In contrast to dogs, cats do not generally have PU/PD and polyphagia from glucocorticoid effects alone. When these clinical signs occur in cats with hypercortisolism, they are typically attributable to secondary diabetes mellitus. Therefore, PU/PD (and increased appetite) may develop months to years after the initial increase in cortisol and are not often present in the early stages of the disease in cats. Diabetes mellitus occurs in almost 80% of cats with hypercortisolism (Boland and Barrs, 2017).

A few case reports exist of cats with PU/PD and hypercortisolism without concurrent diabetes mellitus, but the mechanism for PU/PD in non-diabetic cats is unclear. It could be related to concurrent disease such as chronic kidney disease (CKD) or hyperthyroidism in some instances. Whether hypercortisolism can cause central or secondary nephrogenic diabetes insipidus, as it is believed to do in dogs, has not been established in cats.

Weight loss

Although common in cats with hypercortisolism, weight loss may not be apparent to owners because of abdominal distension resulting from hepatomegaly, abdominal fat deposition and abdominal muscle wasting. Generalized muscle wasting due to increased protein catabolism occurs with concurrent diabetes mellitus and contributes to weight loss. Insulin resistance can occur with feline hypercortisolism, making management of concurrent diabetes mellitus difficult.

Diagnosis

A suspicion of hypercortisolism should be established from the history, physical examination findings, results of routine clinicopathological analyses (haematology, biochemistry and urinalysis), and radiographs and/or ultrasonography (preferred). The initial results not only help to ensure the correct diagnosis is being pursued, they also might identify concomitant medical problems.

Routine clinicopathological analyses

Certain clinicopathological changes are consistent with a diagnosis of hypercortisolism, but none is pathognomonic. Laboratory test results must always be interpreted within the context of the history and physical examination findings. A stress leucogram is not as consistent a finding in cats as it is in dogs. Lymphopenia is the most common component identified, yet it is not specific to hypercortisolism. Mild to moderate mature neutrophilia, eosinopenia and/or monocytosis may also be found (Boland and Barrs, 2017). Serum biochemical abnormalities are also non-specific (Figure 30.3). Concurrent diabetes mellitus is common. In contrast to dogs with hypercortisolism, increases in alkaline phosphatase (ALP) activity are less common. As cats lack a glucocorticoid-induced isoenzyme of ALP, increases in the activity of this enzyme occur secondary to diabetes mellitus or other concurrent diseases.

If diabetes mellitus is present, glucosuria will be observable. Unlike dogs, the majority of cats with hypercortisolism have a urine specific gravity greater than 1.020. Proteinuria commonly occurs in dogs with hypercortisolism; proteinuria has been reported in cats with hypercortisolism but the frequency is not known.

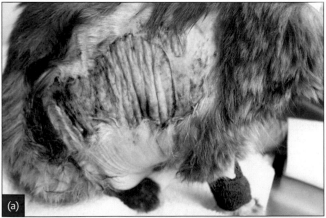
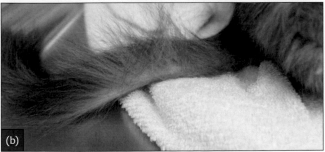

30.2 Uncontrolled hypercortisolism in a cat. (a) Note the alopecia, thin inelastic skin and large wound. (b) Tail of the same cat – note the partial alopecia.

Biochemical abnormality	Prevalence (%)
Hyperglycaemia	84
Hypercholesterolaemia	34
Mild to moderate increase in urea concentration	30
Mild to moderate increase in ALT activity	30
Hyperglobulinaemia	21
Mild to moderate increase in ALP activity	17
Increased creatinine concentration	13
Hypokalaemia	10
Increased total protein concentration	7
Hyperphosphataemia	7
Hypertriglyceridaemia	7
Hypernatraemia	4

30.3 Abnormalities in serum biochemistry collated from reports of 138 cats with hypercortisolism. ALP = alkaline phosphatase; ALT = alanine aminotransferase.
(Reproduced from Boland and Barrs (2017), with permission from the publisher)

Endocrine testing

Confirmation of a diagnosis of hypercortisolism requires the performance of specific endocrine tests. The evaluation for hypercortisolism proceeds through two basic steps of diagnosing and differentiating. Diagnostic tests (i.e. low-dose dexamethasone suppression (LDDS) test, ACTH response test and determination of urine corticoid:creatinine (UCCR)) can help to rule in or rule out the existence of hypercortisolism. If a diagnosis is confirmed, the second step is to differentiate between ACTH-dependent and -independent hypercortisolism by either endocrine tests or diagnostic imaging. Unfortunately, the sensitivity and specificity of the tests are not well documented in cats. Protocols for the tests are presented in Figure 30.4. Since no test is perfect, the decision to test and interpretation of test results must always take clinical signs into account.

Urine corticoid:creatinine

The UCCR can be used to screen for hypercortisolism. Determination of the UCCR is safe, easy and relatively inexpensive. As stress can increase the UCCR, a urine sample should be collected at home before or at least 2 days after a visit to a veterinary clinic. The presence of other diseases, such as diabetes mellitus or hyperthyroidism, can increase the UCCR.

Overall, the UCCR has a high sensitivity and low specificity for diagnosing hypercortisolism in cats. It can help rule out the presence of hypercortisolism; a reference interval UCCR makes hypercortisolism highly unlikely. However, due to its low specificity, an increased UCCR is not diagnostic for hypercortisolism. In cats with an increased UCCR, a diagnosis of hypercortisolism must be confirmed with the LDDS or ACTH response test.

Low-dose dexamethasone suppression test

The LDDS test is considered to be the best screening test for spontaneous hypercortisolism in cats. Compared with the LDDS test in dogs, the dose of dexamethasone used for cats is tenfold higher, as cats are less sensitive to the effects of glucocorticoids than dogs. Unaffected cats should have an 8-hour post-dexamethasone cortisol concentration below approximately 30 nmol/l (depending on the individual laboratory).

The sensitivity of the LDDS test for diagnosing hypercortisolism in cats appears to be high (>90%); the specificity is largely unknown. In one study of diabetic cats without evidence of hypercortisolism, none had a false-positive LDDS test result even in the face of poor glycaemic control (Kley et al., 2007). Whilst this suggests that the LDDS test may have good specificity, a single study including only a small number of cats is insufficient to make definitive conclusions.

Adrenocorticotropic hormone response test

The ACTH response test is the gold standard for diagnosis of iatrogenic disease. The preferred form of ACTH is synthetic tetracosactide (cosyntropin). It can be frozen in aliquots at –20°C in plastic syringes for 6 months without loss of activity in dogs; the same is likely to be true for cats. As the effect of thawing and refreezing is not known, freezing in aliquots and thawing only those needed for a single test is recommended, as opposed to freezing the whole vial. Depot and compounded forms of ACTH should not be used.

The sensitivity of the ACTH response test for diagnosing hypercortisolism in cats may be as low as 33–60% (Valentin et al., 2014; Boland and Barrs, 2017). Thus, it is

Test	Test protocol and comments
Screening tests	
ACTH response test	Administer 125 µg/cat of short-acting ACTH (i.e. tetracosactin or cosyntropin (intravenous route preferred)). Samples should be taken before injection and both 60 and 90 minutes after injection for serum cortisol measurement. The same forms of ACTH can be given intramuscularly but post-injection samples should be taken at 30 and 60 minutes. This test has relatively low sensitivity for naturally occurring hypercortisolism. It is the only test that can diagnose iatrogenic hypercortisolism
UCCR	Owner collects a urine specimen at home. Highly sensitive test with very low specificity. Can be used to rule out hypercortisolism
LDDS test	Collect a baseline sample for serum cortisol measurement. Administer dexamethasone (0.1 mg/kg i.v.). Collect samples at 3 or 4 hours and 8 hours post-dexamethasone. Dilution of dexamethasone with sterile saline to 0.2 mg/ml or less may be needed. Screening test of choice for spontaneous hypercortisolism in cats. Dexamethasone or dexamethasone sodium phosphate can be used as long as calculations are based on the concentration of active ingredient. May also serve to differentiate between ACTH-dependent and -independent forms
Differentiating tests	
HDDS test	Collect a baseline sample for serum cortisol measurement. Administer dexamethasone (1.0 mg/kg i.v.). Collect samples at 3 or 4 hours and 8 hours post-dexamethasone. Unlikely to provide differentiation if the LDDS test did not. Cannot prove that a cat has an adrenal tumour, only that it has pituitary-dependent hypercortisolism
Combined UCCR and oral dexamethasone suppression test	Owner collects a urine specimen at home on two consecutive mornings for determination of the UCCR. On the second day, owner administers three doses of dexamethasone (0.1 mg/kg orally) at 16:00, 20:00 and 00:00. On the third day, the owner collects a third urine sample at 08:00. Not recommended as analysis requires a specific assay that is not widely available
Plasma endogenous ACTH concentration	Blood should be collected into chilled, silicone-coated glass or plastic tubes containing EDTA and centrifuged within 15 minutes, ideally in a cooled centrifuge. The plasma must be transferred to plastic tubes and frozen immediately. Samples must stay frozen until analysis; if a courier is used for quick transport to a reference laboratory, ice may be sufficient. If samples are shipped, they should be sent overnight packed in dry ice. Although the addition of protease inhibitors (e.g. aprotinin) to plasma as a preservative has been recommended for dogs, it is not recommended in cats
Abdominal ultrasonography	Requires equipment and a skilled operator who can reliably identify both adrenal glands

30.4 Summary of diagnostic test protocols used in cats with suspected hypercortisolism. ACTH = adrenocorticotropic hormone; EDTA = ethylenediaminetetraacetic acid; HDDS = high-dose dexamethasone suppression; LDDS = low-dose dexamethasone suppression; UCCR = urine corticoid:creatinine.

not recommended as the initial screening test for hypercortisolism in cats; however, if the LDDS test provides negative results, especially if borderline, and clinical suspicion remains high, an ACTH response test should be considered. Diagnostic specificity was approximately 86% in one study (Valentin *et al.*, 2014).

Occasionally, a less-than-normal cortisol response to ACTH occurs in cats being screened for hypercortisolism. The most likely cause is that the cat has recently received exogenous glucocorticoids, including topical preparations. If glucocorticoid therapy has been ruled out, other possibilities include:

- Recent treatment with progestins
- Inactive ACTH (e.g. incorrectly stored previously reconstituted tetracosactide)
- The post-ACTH sample was collected at an inappropriate time
- The ACTH dose was miscalculated and was too low
- The presence of a functional adrenal tumour.

In the case of a functional adrenal tumour, the adrenal-dependent hypercortisolism is likely due to secretion of either a progestin or another cortisol intermediate, such as corticosterone. Progestins and some cortisol precursors can, through various mechanisms, cause clinical signs of apparent hypercortisolism and exert negative feedback on the pituitary gland, decreasing ACTH secretion. As a result, normal adrenocortical tissue atrophies and endogenous total cortisol concentrations fall below the reference interval.

Differentiation of ACTH-dependent from -independent hypercortisolism

It is important to differentiate pituitary-dependent hypercortisolism and functional adrenal tumours because their treatment and prognosis differ. Laboratory tests for differentiation include the high-dose dexamethasone suppression (HDDS) test and measurement of endogenous ACTH (eACTH) concentration. In some cases, the LDDS test may provide differentiation as well as diagnosis. Imaging can be performed to distinguish pituitary-dependent hypercortisolism and adrenal-dependent hypercortisolism. As with screening tests, no test is 100% accurate.

Low-dose dexamethasone suppression test

In dogs, the LDDS test can be used to differentiate between ACTH-dependent and -independent hypercortisolism, and the same may be true in cats (Behrend *et al.*, 2013). If the 8-hour post-dexamethasone concentration is above the laboratory cut-off, results are consistent with hypercortisolism. In dogs, if the 3-hour or 4-hour post-dexamethasone concentration is below the laboratory cut-off or if one or both post-dexamethasone concentrations are below 50% of baseline, ACTH-dependent hypercortisolism is likely. Unfortunately, there are no studies evaluating whether the same criteria apply to cats; if the criteria are appropriate, the LDDS test may diagnose and provide differentiation in approximately 50% of cats with pituitary-dependent hypercortisolism (Feldman, 2015). If both post-dexamethasone concentrations are above the laboratory cut-off and neither is below 50% of baseline, either ACTH-dependent or -independent hypercortisolosm is possible.

High-dose dexamethasone suppression test

For the HDDS test, suppression of the 3-hour or 4-hour and/or the 8-hour post-dexamethasone cortisol concentration to less than the laboratory cut-off or to below 50% of the baseline is consistent with ACTH-dependent hypercortisolism and occurs in approximately 50% of cats with pituitary-dependent hypercortisolism (Boland and Barrs, 2017). The likelihood of the HDDS test result providing much more information than the LDDS test result is limited. As for the LDDS test, if none of these criteria is fulfilled, either cause of hypercortisolism is possible.

Combined UCCR and oral dexamethasone suppression test

The UCCR can be combined with an oral dexamethasone suppression test as a way to screen and differentiate simultaneously. Diagnosis of hypercortisolism is based on the mean of the UCCR from the first two morning urine samples. If the results are consistent with hypercortisolism, and the UCCR in the third sample collected following administration of oral dexamethasone is less than 50% of the mean of the first two, the result is consistent with ACTH-dependent hypercortisolism. This test correctly differentiated 10/13 (77%) cats with pituitary-dependent hypercortisolism (Boland and Barrs, 2017). Unfortunately, the urine corticoid assay used in the study is not widely available and other assays have not been similarly evaluated.

Combined dexamethasone suppression and ACTH response test

The test combines a diagnostic test (ACTH response test) and a differentiating test (dexamethasone suppression test), with the aim of diagnosing and differentiating in one test. The diagnosis of hypercortisolism is made on the basis of the ACTH response test results; if the test is positive for hypercortisolism, the response to dexamethasone can be used to try to differentiate between ACTH-dependent and -independent hypercortisolism.

This test is not recommended for use in cats to diagnose hypercortisolism. The ACTH response test is limited as a diagnostic test, as explained above. In addition, the dexamethasone suppression portion is incomplete in that only a 4-hour post-dexamethasone sample is collected and not an 8-hour sample. Also, although sporadic reports of its use appear in the literature, the utility and accuracy of the test have never been assessed.

Endogenous ACTH measurement

Feline eACTH can be difficult to measure as eACTH is species specific. Some human assays validated for dogs do not detect feline eACTH, so care must be taken to use an assay specifically validated for cats. In addition, eACTH is labile and strict guidelines for handling samples must be followed. As in dogs, measurement of eACTH may be a good means of differentiating ACTH-dependent and -independent hypercortisolism. In a study involving 10 cats with hypercortisolism, two with adrenal-dependent hypercortisolism had eACTH concentrations below the reference interval and eight with pituitary-dependent hypercortisolism had concentrations that were within the reference interval or increased (Tardo *et al.*, 2021). Advantages of measuring eACTH include the requirement for only a single sample and the ability to definitively diagnose

ACTH-independent hypercortisolism. If the sample is handled appropriately, measurement of eACTH is the most accurate stand-alone biochemical test for differentiating ACTH-dependent from -independent hypercortisolism.

Cytology of adrenal masses

Fine-needle aspiration cytology of adrenal masses can potentially determine whether an adrenal tumour is cortical or medullary (i.e. a phaeochromocytoma) in origin (Bertazzolo *et al.*, 2014). However, due to difficulties in aspirating adrenal glands, results can be non-diagnostic. Cytology cannot determine whether a mass is benign or malignant or whether it is functional. The presence of an adrenocortical mass in and of itself does not mean a cat has hypercortisolism – endocrine testing is required to determine this.

Diagnostic imaging

Diagnostic imaging of the adrenal and pituitary glands can be used to differentiate ACTH-dependent and -independent hypercortisolism. Imaging should never be used to diagnose hypercortisolism, as glandular enlargement does not necessarily equate with increased function.

Abdominal ultrasonography or radiography: Abdominal radiography can identify non-specific changes consistent with hypercortisolism and may be helpful for differentiation. Consistent findings include abdominal distension (i.e. a 'pot belly'), hepatomegaly and increased intra-abdominal fat (Boland and Barrs, 2017). Sufficiently large adrenal masses may be visible in cats (Figure 30.5). Compared with dogs, adrenal gland mineralization occurs in healthy older cats and is of no significance in the work-up of hypercortisolism.

On ultrasound examination, healthy feline adrenal glands are hypoechoic compared to surrounding tissue and surrounded by a thin hyperechoic halo (Combes *et al.*, 2013). They are usually bean-shaped but may be ovoid or fusiform. Hyperechoic loci of various shapes occur in up to 20% of healthy cats; their significance is unknown. In healthy cats, the adrenal glands range from 3.9 to 4.8 mm in maximum dorsoventral thickness, dependent on bodyweight, with variable length (approximately 9–11 mm) (see Chapter 34). The measurement with the least inter- and intraobserver variability is adrenal thickness (Combes *et al.*, 2014).

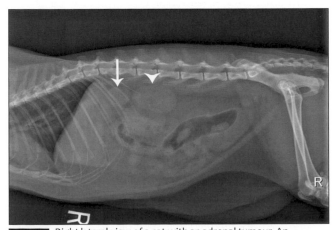

30.5 Right lateral view of a cat with an adrenal tumour. An abnormal circular structure (arrowed) can be seen cranial to the right kidney (arrowhead); it is a large adrenal tumour.

With an experienced ultrasonographer, the accuracy of ultrasonography for differentiation may be 90% or higher (Valentin *et al.*, 2014). Most cats with pituitary-dependent hypercortisolism have bilaterally symmetrical adrenal gland enlargement; however, adrenal size can be within the reference interval and, rarely, adrenomegaly can be asymmetric (Boland and Barrs, 2017). Chronically ill cats can have bilateral adrenomegaly (Combes *et al.*, 2013), especially those with hyperthyroidism, hypersomatotropism or hyperaldosteronism. Cats with functional adrenal tumours typically have a unilateral mass; although the function of the contralateral gland will be suppressed and the gland is expected to be atrophied, objective criteria for defining atrophy by ultrasonography have not yet been determined for cats. With a malignant tumour, invasion of the vena cava or evidence of metastasis to regional lymph nodes or the liver may be obvious.

Computed tomography or magnetic resonance imaging: Brain imaging is used to confirm the presence of a pituitary mass and determine its size. An enlarged pituitary gland or displacement of the contrast medium in a normal-sized pituitary gland during dynamic computed tomography (CT) occurs in approximately two thirds of cats with pituitary-dependent hypercortisolism (Galac and Rosenberg, 2019). The appearance of adrenal glands from healthy cats on CT has been described as similar in shape and dimensions to that observed on ultrasonography but with no clear corticomedullary differentiation (Mallol *et al.*, 2020). A CT examination of the abdomen can be used to identify an adrenal tumour and for surgical planning if adrenalectomy is to be performed.

Treatment

Feline hypercortisolism is difficult to treat consistently and effectively (Figure 30.6). Medical therapy has historically focused on the adrenocorticolytic agent mitotane and cortisol-synthesis enzyme inhibitors such as metyrapone and ketoconazole. Trilostane is now considered the medical treatment of choice. Potentially curative options such as adrenalectomy (unilateral or bilateral) and hypophysectomy exist, but adrenalectomy poses significant morbidity and mortality risks, and lack of availability limits the usefulness of hypophysectomy. External beam radiation therapy can be considered for pituitary-dependent hypercortisolism.

Medical therapy

Trilostane

Trilostane is a synthetic steroid analogue that competitively inhibits the adrenocortical enzyme 3-beta-hydroxysteroid dehydrogenase, reducing the production of mineralocorticoids and glucocorticoids. Trilostane appears to be well tolerated in cats and is the most efficacious medical treatment currently available for feline hypercortisolism (Figure 30.7), despite the lack of knowledge regarding its pharmacokinetics in cats (Boland and Barrs, 2017).

Most trilostane-treated cats have a reduction in, but not resolution of, their clinical signs in addition to improved ACTH response test results. Diabetic remission appears to be rare, although the required insulin dose may decrease in those cats with concurrent diabetes mellitus. The optimal way to monitor trilostane therapy is unknown and is currently controversial in dogs (see Chapter 29). Current

Treatment	Indication	Comments
Medical therapy		
Trilostane	ACTH-dependent hypercortisolism or adrenal tumour	1–2 mg/kg/day orally, although 10–30 mg/cat orally q12–24h has also been reported. Twice-daily dosing may be required in some cats. Useful for long-term medical management and preoperative preparation for adrenalectomy. Side effects include anorexia, weight loss, lethargy, pancreatitis and hypoadrenocorticism
Mitotane	ACTH-dependent hypercortisolism or adrenal tumour	25–50 mg/kg/day orally for induction; 25–50 mg/kg/week for maintenance therapy. Not recommended for medical treatment of feline hypercortisolism. Adverse effects (lethargy, vomiting, anorexia) are common. Trilostane is more effective
Radiation therapy		
Pituitary radiation	ACTH-dependent hypercortisolism	Best option to alleviate neurological signs secondary to ACTH-dependent hypercortisolism when hypophysectomy is not possible. Gamma knife/stereotactic-capable linear accelerators reduce the number of treatments (in comparison to standard multiple fractionated plans) but availability of these methods is limited. Use of trilostane is recommended prior to and following radiation to control signs of hypercortisolaemia. Can be expensive
Surgery		
Unilateral adrenalectomy	Adrenal tumour	Treatment of choice for unilateral tumour with chance of cure. Preoperative treatment with trilostane is recommended. Relatively high postoperative complication rate. Clinical signs should resolve within 1–4 months. Glucocorticoid supplementation may be required until the contralateral atrophied gland recovers
Bilateral adrenalectomy	ACTH-dependent hypercortisolism	Preoperative treatment with trilostane is recommended. Relatively high postoperative complication rate. Clinical signs should resolve within 1–4 months. Lifelong replacement therapy with glucocorticoids and mineralocorticoids is required. Pituitary tumour remains and may result in future neurological signs
Hypophysectomy	ACTH-dependent hypercortisolism	Offers potential cure for ACTH-dependent hypercortisolism. Highly specialized treatment requiring a skilled, highly experienced surgeon in addition to advanced imaging capabilities. Stabilization with trilostane is recommended preoperatively. Postoperative diabetes insipidus is common, requiring temporary desmopressin administration; long-term administration may be required. Lifelong substitution therapy with levothyroxine and glucocorticoids is necessary

30.6 Summary of treatment options for cats with hypercortisolism. ACTH = adrenocorticotropic hormone.

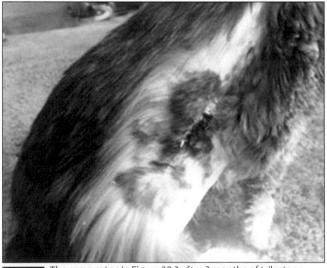

30.7 The same cat as in Figure 30.2 after 2 months of trilostane therapy. Note the healing of the skin wound and partial regrowth of hair. The required insulin dose for the concurrent diabetes mellitus also decreased when trilostane therapy was initiated.

recommendations for cats are to perform an ACTH response test beginning 2–4 hours after trilostane dosing; the ideal post-ACTH cortisol concentration is 50–150 nmol/l (Feldman, 2015). Routine monitoring is required, for example, at 10, 30 and 90 days after starting therapy and regularly thereafter, depending on the clinical response. Clinical signs of hypoadrenocorticism and cortisol excess must be taken into consideration in determining whether a dose adjustment is required. Use of compounded

trilostane is discouraged; in one study, 38% of compounded trilostane products tested were either not the prescribed strength or had variable dissolution characteristics (Cook *et al.*, 2012).

If a cat receiving trilostane presents with clinical signs consistent with hypoadrenocorticism (see Chapter 31), trilostane should be discontinued and an ACTH response test performed to determine whether the clinical signs are due to hypocortisolaemia. If hypoadrenocorticism is confirmed and serum electrolyte concentrations are unaffected, trilostane should be stopped and glucocorticoids administered. If hyperkalaemia or hyponatraemia are documented, trilostane should be discontinued and both glucocorticoid and mineralocorticoid therapy administered. Further ACTH response testing should be undertaken to assess if and when adrenal function returns, and therapy should be reinitiated accordingly at a lower dose.

Prolonged survival is possible; in the largest study of 15 cats with hypercortisolism treated with trilostane, 13 demonstrated improvement and median survival was 20 months (range 2–42 months) (Mellett Keith *et al.*, 2013).

Mitotane and other medical therapies

Mitotane is an adrenocorticolytic agent targeting and destroying the zona fasciculata and zona reticularis. Short-term success has been limited to a few cases and long-term results are discouraging.

Other steroid hormone synthesis inhibitors (e.g. metyrapone and ketoconazole) have been used in a small number of cats. They are not recommended due to adverse effects, lack of efficacy or, in the case of metyrapone, lack of commercial availability.

Surgery

Unilateral and bilateral adrenalectomy

Adrenalectomy appears to be a successful method of treating cats with hypercortisolism and represents a potential cure. Unilateral adrenalectomy is considered the treatment of choice for cats with a unilateral cortisol-secreting tumour; bilateral adrenalectomy is required in cats with pituitary-dependent hypercortisolism.

Unfortunately, cats with hypercortisolism tend to present in a debilitated and catabolic state resulting from chronic glucocorticoid secretion. Adrenalectomy can be associated with a relatively high complication rate due to poor wound healing, immunosuppression and skin fragility. Common postoperative complications include haemorrhage, sepsis, hypoglycaemia, pancreatitis, thromboembolism and hypoadrenocorticism. As many cats with hypercortisolism are older, comorbidities such as CKD and hyperthyroidism are common. The severity of concurrent disease, owner willingness to pursue surgery, size and invasiveness of adrenal tumours, and age of the cat should factor into the decision to pursue surgery. Careful case selection, preoperative planning, and intra- and postoperative management are essential in minimizing complications and achieving optimum outcomes. In cats with adrenal-dependent hypercortisolism, abdominal CT prior to surgery facilitates identification of tumour invasion and thrombosis of the phrenicoabdominal vein, caudal vena cava or renal vein. Presurgical medical stabilization with trilostane may help improve postoperative outcomes.

Adrenalectomy should be undertaken only by experienced surgeons in a hospital with a well equipped intensive care unit and 24-hour observation and care. Even so, the mortality rate is approximately 10%. After bilateral adrenalectomy, lifelong therapy for hypoadrenocorticism is required. Clinical signs of hypercortisolism resolve 1–4 months postoperatively, and insulin requirements usually decrease in cats with concurrent diabetes mellitus. Successful long-term outcome following bilateral adrenalectomy is dependent on client compliance with chronic therapy for hypoadrenocorticism.

Hypophysectomy

Microsurgical transsphenoidal hypophysectomy is an effective treatment method for cats with pituitary-dependent hypercortisolism. It remains a specialized form of treatment requiring an experienced, highly skilled surgeon and advanced imaging capabilities. Complications include oronasal fistulae, soft palate dehiscence, transient reduction in tear production and recurrence of hypercortisolism due to regrowth of pituitary remnants (Owen et al., 2018).

Careful peri- and postoperative management are required, including frequent electrolyte monitoring and desmopressin, glucocorticoid and levothyroxine replacement therapies. Although this procedure is potentially curative, the availability of the surgical expertise required is limited. Successful long-term outcomes depend on client compliance with postoperative treatment and monitoring.

Radiation therapy

Radiation therapy has been used to treat a small number of cats with hypercortisolism and may decrease tumour size and prolong survival in cats with a large or invasive pituitary tumour. The main goal is to control pituitary tumour size. If hypophysectomy is not possible, radiation therapy is the only option available to alleviate neurological signs due to a large pituitary tumour. Radiation therapy for pituitary-dependent hypercortisolism generally involves multiple fractionated treatments, requiring frequent anaesthesia and extended hospitalization periods. However, reductions in tumour size and ACTH secretion are often delayed.

Cats with concurrent diabetes mellitus may have a reduction in insulin requirements or enter diabetic remission following treatment. Neurological signs secondary to a pituitary mass typically show improvement over weeks to months.

Radiation side effects can be early or late in onset and consist of epilation, fur depigmentation, otitis externa, brain necrosis, cataract development and hearing loss. Some side effects may be manageable with anti-inflammatory glucocorticoids but others, such as late-onset brain necrosis, are irreversible.

Iatrogenic hypercortisolism

Although cats appear resistant to the side effects of chronic exogenous glucocorticoid administration, iatrogenic hypercortisolism can occur. Clinical signs and clinicopathological findings are identical to those in the naturally occurring spontaneous disease. Most reports involve cats receiving long-term or high-dose glucocorticoids such as methylprednisolone acetate, topical and subcutaneous triamcinolone, subcutaneous dexamethasone and oral prednisolone.

An ACTH response test is required to make a diagnosis of iatrogenic hypercortisolism. Basal cortisol concentration is low with a lack of stimulation following ACTH administration. Gradual discontinuation of exogenous glucocorticoid administration is the treatment. Resolution of abnormalities is expected to occur over the ensuing several months.

Sex-hormone-secreting adrenocortical tumours

Adrenal tumours can secrete hormones besides cortisol that have glucocorticoid activity, including cortisol precursors such as progesterone, corticosterone or sex hormones. Cats with excessive secretion of corticosterone or progesterone may have clinical signs similar to those caused by hypercortisolaemia. Diabetes mellitus usually develops. Such hormones can cause clinical signs of apparent hypercortisolism and can suppress the hypothalamic–pituitary–adrenal axis. Cats with such adrenal tumours have low serum cortisol concentrations on ACTH response tests, similar to results obtained in cats with hypoadrenocorticism, despite clinical signs of hypercortisolaemia. An increased index of suspicion and use of adrenal hormone panels are required for diagnosis.

Overproduction of oestrogens or androgens can result in clinical signs of oestrus or male secondary sexual behaviours (e.g. urine spraying, aggression, penile spines) in previously neutered cats, respectively. Hormones can be secreted alone or in combination with other adrenocortical hormones, leading to a mixture of clinical signs (e.g. clinical signs of both hypercortisolism and hyperaldosteronism). If concurrent hyperaldosteronism is present, clinical signs of hypokalaemic polymyopathy and hypertension may be observed (see Chapter 32).

Adrenalectomy is the treatment of choice for cortisol precursor or sex-hormone-secreting tumours, leading to resolution of clinical signs over weeks to months. If adrenalectomy is not an option, therapy with trilostane may be attempted.

Prognosis

Feline hypercortisolism is a serious disease and the prognosis for cats with untreated spontaneous disease is poor; most cats succumb to complications within weeks to months of diagnosis. Comorbidities may further limit survival times. Prolonged survival times and cure are possible following adrenalectomy or transsphenoidal hypophysectomy. Radiation therapy may provide prolonged survival times in cats that respond to treatment. Cats with concurrent diabetes mellitus may enter diabetic remission or have reduced insulin requirements if they respond to treatment for hypercortisolism.

References and further reading

Behrend EN, Kooistra HS, Nelson R, Reusch CE and Scott-Moncrieff JC (2013) Diagnosis of spontaneous canine hyperadrenocorticism: 2012 ACVIM consensus statement (small animal). *Journal of Veterinary Internal Medicine* **27**, 1292–1304

Bertazzolo W, Didier M, Gelain ME *et al.* (2014) Accuracy of cytology in distinguishing adrenocortical tumors from pheochromocytoma in companion animals. *Veterinary Clinical Pathology* **43**, 453–459

Boland LA and Barrs VR (2017) Peculiarities of feline hyperadrenocorticism: update on diagnosis and treatment. *Journal of Feline Medicine and Surgery* **19**, 933–947

Combes A, Pey P, Paepe D *et al.* (2013) Ultrasonographic appearance of adrenal glands in healthy and sick cats. *Journal of Feline Medicine and Surgery* **15**, 445–457

Combes A, Stock E, Van der Vekens E *et al.* (2014) Ultrasonographical examination of feline adrenal glands: intra- and inter-observer variability. *Journal of Feline Medicine and Surgery* **16**, 937–942

Cook AK, Nieuwoudt CD and Longhofer SL (2012) Pharmaceutical evaluation of compounded trilostane products. *Journal of the American Animal Hospital Association* **48**, 228–233

Feldman EC (2015) Hyperadrenocorticism in cats. In: *Canine and Feline Endocrinology, 4th edn*, ed. EC Feldman, RW Nelson, C Reusch, JCR Scott-Moncrieff and E Behrend, pp. 452–484. Elsevier, St. Louis

Galac S and Rosenberg D (2019) Cushing's syndrome (hypercortisolism). In: *Feline Endocrinology, 1st edn*, ed. EC Feldman, F Fracassi and ME Peterson, pp. 363–380. Edra, Milan

Kley S, Alt M, Zimmer C, Hoerauf A and Reusch CE (2007) Evaluation of the low-dose dexamethasone suppression test and ultrasonographic measurements of the adrenal glands in cats with diabetes mellitus. *Schweizer Archiv für Tierheilkunde* **149**, 493–500

Mallol C, Altuzarra R, Espada Y *et al.* (2020) CT characterisation of feline adrenal glands. *Journal of Feline Medicine and Surgery* **22**, 285–291

Mellett Keith AM, Bruyette D and Stanley S (2013) Trilostane therapy for treatment of spontaneous hyperadrenocorticism in cats: 15 cases (2004–2012). *Journal of Veterinary Internal Medicine* **27**, 1471–1477

Owen TJ, Martin LG and Chen AV (2018) Transsphenoidal surgery for pituitary tumors and other sellar masses. *Veterinary Clinics of North America: Small Animal Practice* **48**, 129–151

Tardo AM, Reusch CE, Galac S *et al.* (2021) Feline plasma adrenocorticotropic hormone: validation of a chemiluminescent assay and concentrations in cats with hypercortisolism, primary hypoadrenocorticism and other diseases. *Journal of Feline Medicine and Surgery* **23**, 67–73

Valentin SY, Cortright CC, Nelson RW *et al.* (2014) Clinical findings, diagnostic test results, and treatment outcome in cats with spontaneous hyperadrenocorticism: 30 cases. *Journal of Veterinary Internal Medicine* **28**, 481–487

Chapter 31

Feline hypoadrenocorticism

Samuel Fowlie and Ian K. Ramsey

Introduction

Only a few cases of feline hypoadrenocorticism have been reported since it was first described (Johnessee *et al.*, 1983). The true prevalence of the disease in the cat is not known, although its incidence is certainly less than in dogs, even amongst cases with low sodium:potassium (Bell *et al.*, 2005). Feline hypoadrenocorticism is similar in many aspects to the disease in other species and should be considered in cases with compatible clinical signs and clinicopathological changes. However, developing an initial index of suspicion can be more challenging as some key clinical signs, such as lethargy, are less noticeable in cats

Aetiology and pathophysiology

Hypoadrenocorticism is caused by reduced adrenocortical secretion of glucocorticoids, usually with a concurrent deficiency of mineralocorticoids (see Chapter 28). It can be either naturally occurring or iatrogenic. Both primary (due to adrenocortical disease) and secondary (due to failure or suppression of pituitary adrenocorticotropic hormone (ACTH) production) forms have been reported in cats.

Primary hypoadrenocorticism

Primary hypoadrenocorticism involves the destruction (upwards of 85–90%) of all three adrenocortical zones. In cats, autoimmune destruction (with a lymphocytic infiltrate on histopathology), neoplastic infiltration (e.g. lymphoma or metastases) and abdominal trauma (suspected due to adrenal haemorrhage) have been reported as causes of adrenocortical destruction (Peterson *et al.*, 1989; Berger and Reed, 1993; Brain, 1997; Romine *et al.*, 2016). Other reported causes include drugs that suppress adrenocortical hormone production (e.g. trilostane, ketoconazole) (Mellett Keith *et al.*, 2013). Iatrogenic primary hypoadrenocorticism was previously a well recognized complication of bilateral adrenalectomy for treatment of pituitary-dependent hyperadrenocorticism in cats, but this is currently rarely performed (Duesberg *et al.*, 1995; see Chapter 30). Neither the existence of anti-adrenal antibodies nor genetic markers have been studied in cats with primary hypoadrenocorticism.

Atypical hypoadrenocorticism

Atypical hypoadrenocorticism, defined as primary hypocortisolism with adequate aldosterone and reference interval electrolyte concentrations, has not been conclusively diagnosed in cats. A single case report describes a cat with suspected atypical disease, but aldosterone concentrations were not measured and dexamethasone had been administered prior to ACTH response testing. Additionally, the cat did not fully respond to glucocorticoid supplementation (Hock, 2011).

Secondary hypoadrenocorticism

Secondary hypoadrenocorticism results from a lack of pituitary ACTH causing atrophy of the adrenal cortex (zona fasciculata and zona reticularis) and a subsequent decrease in glucocorticoid production. Adrenocorticotropic hormone has little stimulatory effect on mineralocorticoid production and, therefore, the zona glomerulosa is preserved. Secondary hypoadrenocorticism is most commonly iatrogenic following rapid cessation of glucocorticoid or progestin treatment (Church *et al.*, 1994, Smith *et al.*, 2002). It is also a well recognized complication of hypophysectomy to treat feline hypersomatotropism and pituitary-dependent hypercortisolism (Meij *et al.*, 2010). A single case of naturally occurring hypoadrenocorticism secondary to lymphocytic panhypophysitis has been documented in a cat (Rudinsky *et al.*, 2015). Adrenocorticotropic hormone deficiency associated with neoplastic pituitary disease has not yet been confirmed in a cat, although a congenital cause was suspected in one kitten (Giudice *et al.*, 2016).

Clinical features

Cats of any age, breed or sex can develop primary hypoadrenocorticism. There is no reported sex predisposition and the median age at the time of diagnosis is 4 years (range 1.5–14) (Peterson *et al.*, 1989; Parnell *et al.*, 1999; Fowlie *et al.*, 2018). Cats with hypoadrenocorticism are reported to display similar clinical signs to those recognized in other species (Figure 31.1). They may present with a spectrum of disease ranging from mild to severe, acute or chronic, continuous or 'waxing and waning'. As with dogs, many of the clinical signs are vague or consistent with many other conditions, such as lethargy, weight loss, weakness, and inappetence or anorexia. Most affected

Clinical features	Clinicopathological abnormalities
• Lethargy • Anorexia • Weight loss • Vomiting • Weak peripheral pulses • Weakness • Collapse • Shock • Diarrhoea • Polyuria and polydipsia • Muscle cramps • Bradycardia (<120 bpm) • Regurgitation • Seizures	• Hyperkalaemia • Hyponatraemia • Hypoalbuminaemia • Azotaemia • Non-regenerative anaemia • Absence of stress leucogram • Minimally concentrated urine (specific gravity <1.030) • Neutropenia • Lymphocytosis • Eosinophilia • Hypercalcaemia • Hypoglycaemia • Hypocholesterolaemia

31.1 Clinical and clinicopathological features of feline hypoadrenocorticism in approximate order of frequency based on reported cases (Ramsey, 2019). Note that bradycardia and hypercalcaemia are less commonly reported than in dogs.

cats are dehydrated and in poor body condition at presentation (see Figure 31.4). They typically have a normal heart rate and rhythm on examination and bradycardia is rare. Hypothermia is reported and may be more common than in dogs. Approximately one third of cats have a history of gastrointestinal signs, with vomiting being more common than diarrhoea. Melaena, haematochezia and haematemesis have not been recorded to date. Approximately one quarter of cats are reported to be polyuric and polydipsic.

Many cats present following acute collapse with no other clinical signs. Stressful events (e.g. kennelling, house move) might trigger this deterioration but so far this has not been specifically reported. The clinical signs often respond well to symptomatic treatment but quickly recur soon after the cessation of treatment and, as such, cases can be easily missed initially. The acute presentation of the condition contrasts with clinical findings suggesting a more chronic course.

Hypoadrenocorticism may be difficult to differentiate from other more common diseases, such as hyperthyroidism or chronic kidney disease (CKD), based on history and physical examination alone (Figure 31.2). Physical examination findings can be variable and may be completely unremarkable. Hypoadrenocorticism is a frequent differential diagnosis but a rare diagnosis; routine diagnostic testing should be performed before carrying out any more expensive endocrine tests.

Condition	Clinical features	Clinicopathological abnormalities
Inflammatory bowel disease	• Vomiting • Diarrhoea • Weight loss • Lethargy	• Hypoalbuminaemia • Anaemia • Hypocholesterolaemia
Chronic kidney disease	• Anorexia • Dehydration • Weight loss • Polyuria and polydipsia	• Azotaemia • Anaemia • Hypercalcaemia • Urine specific gravity <1.030
Hyperthyroidism	• Weight loss • Weakness • Polyuria and polydipsia	
Diabetes mellitus	• Weight loss • Lethargy • Polyuria and polydipsia	

31.2 Summary of the similarities between hypoadrenocorticism and four common feline medical conditions. This emphasizes the importance of screening for hypoadrenocorticism by regular measurement of electrolyte concentrations.

Diagnosis
Routine clinicopathological features
Haematology

The haemogram is characterized by the absence of a stress leucogram despite the cat being ill and therefore 'stressed'. It is expected that cats with primary hypoadrenocorticism have a lymphocytosis or eosinophilia with concurrently normal to low neutrophil numbers. In practice, however, this 'classic' haemogram is identified in only a moderate proportion of affected cats and some even present with a stress leucogram. A mild normocytic normochromic non-regenerative anaemia has been found in approximately one quarter of cases. As with many other features of this disease, haematological findings can be completely unremarkable.

Biochemistry

All cats reported to date have had hyponatraemia, hyperkalaemia or both. Historically, a low sodium:potassium (<27:1) has been used to support a diagnosis of hypoadrenocorticism. However, some cases may be missed when using the ratio and the absolute concentrations should be considered separately. There are several other causes of hyperkalaemia with or without hyponatraemia in the cat (Figure 31.3) (Bell et al., 2005). Hypochloraemia and hyperphosphataemia have also been reported in affected cats. Electrolyte abnormalities may correct rapidly following initiation of fluid therapy alone, increasing the risk of missing a diagnosis of hypoadrenocorticism.

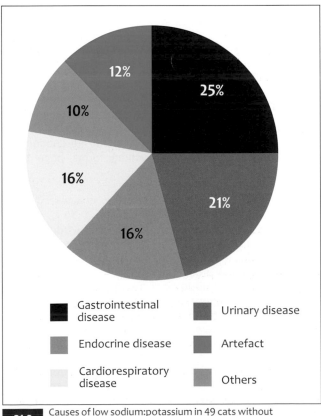

31.3 Causes of low sodium:potassium in 49 cats without hypoadrenocorticism. All 49 cats had hyperkalaemia; nine also had hyponatraemia. No cats with hypoadrenocorticism were identified while these cases were collected, emphasizing the rarity of feline hypoadrenocorticism as a cause of sodium and potassium abnormalities. (Data from Bell et al., 2005)

Prerenal azotaemia is the second most common finding and occurs because of water loss and dehydration due to aldosterone deficiency. Gastrointestinal bleeding can lead to disproportionate increases in urea concentrations relative to creatinine concentrations. More chronic cases may develop irreversible kidney damage, although this has not been fully recognized in cats.

Less commonly, cats may present in a hypoglycaemic state because of glucocorticoid deficiency. Rarely, hypo-albuminaemia and hypocholesterolaemia are noted and may be due to poor hepatic function or gastrointestinal disease. Hypercalcaemia has been reported, especially in cats with concurrent severe hyperkalaemia. The exact mechanism for this is unknown and is likely multifactorial; however, hypocortisolaemia may reduce calcium excretion.

Urinalysis

Pre-treatment urine specific gravity (SG) is often inappropriate (<1.030) in the presence of prerenal azotaemia and dehydration. The cause of this loss of renal concentrating ability is not fully understood but it may be a result of renal sodium loss and medullary washout. Care must be taken to differentiate hypoadrenocorticism from azotaemia caused by kidney disease (e.g. CKD or acute kidney injury (AKI)). Cats with CKD are rarely hyperkalaemic or hyponatraemic and often have a stress leucogram. Cats with AKI usually have reduced urine output and may produce hypersthenuric (SG >1.035) or isosthenuric urine prior to starting fluid therapy.

Diagnostic imaging

No systematic studies reporting the diagnostic imaging findings in cats with hypoadrenocorticism exist. Extrapolating from findings in dogs, identification of small adrenal glands on ultrasonographic assessment may support a diagnosis of hypoadrenocorticism, but affected cats frequently have normal adrenal gland size. Some cats with lymphoma causing hypoadrenocorticism may in fact have enlarged adrenal glands. Reference intervals for feline adrenal gland dimensions are based on healthy and chronically sick cats (Zimmer et al., 2000; Combes et al., 2013). Depending on the reference used, feline adrenal glands may be approximately 9–11 mm in length and 3.9–4.8 mm in maximum dorsoventral thickness, depending on bodyweight. Radiography may reveal hypoperfusion of the pulmonary vessels and microcardia.

Electrocardiography and echocardiography

Electrocardiographic changes consistent with hyperkalaemia (bradycardia, widened QRS complexes, larger spiked T waves and reduced P-wave amplitude) have been reported in only one cat diagnosed with hypoadrenocorticism despite electrocardiography being performed in several others (Spalla et al., 2014). Sinus bradycardia and premature atrial contractions have been reported in a handful of other cats (Peterson et al., 1989). Hyperkalaemia has also been associated with wide complex tachycardias in cats (Norman et al., 2006). Experimental data suggest that cats may be more resistant to the cardiac effects of hyperkalaemia than other species (Coulter et al., 1975). No reports exist of echocardiography being performed in cats with hypoadrenocorticism, likely due to the small number of cases reported; however, reduced fractional shortening may be expected and is commonly seen in dogs due to volume depletion.

Pituitary–adrenal function tests
Adrenocorticotropic hormone response test

The most accurate test for diagnosing feline hypoadrenocorticism is the ACTH response test. However, healthy cats tend to respond to ACTH with a smaller rise in peak serum cortisol than that seen in dogs. The minimum dose of ACTH required to elicit a maximal cortisol response is 5 µg/kg i.v. with a second sample taken between 60 and 75 minutes later. Lower doses of ACTH risk overdiagnosis because of a failure to adequately stimulate cortisol production. Where cost is not an issue, 125 µg/cat is often used but is not strictly necessary (DeClue et al., 2011). A failure of ACTH to stimulate an increase in cortisol concentration above approximately 40 nmol/l confirms hypoadrenocorticism but does not discriminate between primary or secondary causes. As for dogs, exogenous glucocorticoids and progestins may suppress cortisol release and potentially give rise to false-positive results (i.e. misdiagnosis of hypoadrenocorticism). The clinical history should therefore be examined closely for any recent drug administration.

Basal cortisol concentrations have not been investigated as a screening test for hypoadrenocorticism in cats and are not currently recommended. In an ill cat suspected of having hypoadrenocorticism, an ACTH response test should be performed.

Aldosterone

Human aldosterone assays have been validated in cats (Yu and Morris, 1998). For cats with decreased cortisol and abnormal electrolyte concentrations, aldosterone measurement is rarely indicated. Values would be expected to be low but have been measured in only one case (Fowlie et al., 2018). However, in a cat with normal electrolyte concentrations but a suspicion of hypoadrenocorticism, aldosterone measurement may be useful to determine mineralocorticoid status. A single suspected case of aldosterone deficiency without hypocortisolaemia has been reported but post-ACTH cortisol concentration was not measured (Romine et al., 2016).

Endogenous adrenocorticotropic hormone concentration

Cases with primary hypoadrenocorticism have increased endogenous ACTH concentrations because of loss of glucocorticoid-induced negative feedback (Figure 31.4) (Fowlie et al., 2018). By contrast, cats with secondary disease have undetectable ACTH concentrations.

Most commercial veterinary laboratories offer assays for canine ACTH and some of those validated for dogs appear to work well in cats (Church et al., 1994; Eiler et al., 2013). Samples should be collected prior to treatment with glucocorticoids and special sample handling is required (see Chapter 3). Several case reports have demonstrated a marked increase in endogenous ACTH concentration, as expected (Brain 1997; Battaglia and Agnoli 2012; Fowlie et al., 2018).

Cortisol:adrenocorticotropic hormone

Cortisol:ACTH has not been examined in cats and therefore recommendations as to its diagnostic utility cannot be made. One case has been reported in which the ratio was measured when an ACTH response test could not be performed, and it was appropriately low (Brain, 1997).

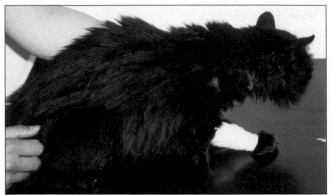

31.4 A thin (2.2kg) cat with history of waxing and waning lethargy, reduced appetite and soft faeces that was diagnosed with primary hypoadrenocorticism on the basis of hyponatraemia with normal potassium concentration, a failure of cortisol secretion to respond to ACTH stimulation and a greatly increased endogenous ACTH concentration (323 pmol/l; reference interval 8–39 pmol/l).

Differential diagnosis

Clinical features

The clinical signs of hypoadrenocorticism are vague and varied (e.g. weight loss, weakness, lethargy, reduced appetite). They may, therefore, be confused for those of many other much more common conditions such as CKD, liver disease, hyperthyroidism and inflammatory bowel disease (see Figure 31.2). There are no pathognomonic features.

Electrolyte abnormalities

The classical abnormalities of hyponatremia and hyperkalaemia, and resultant low sodium:potassium, may also be seen in cats with gastrointestinal disease, kidney disease, urinary obstruction, cardiac disease, body cavity effusions and diabetes mellitus (Bissett *et al.*, 2001; Bell *et al.*, 2005) (see Figure 31.3). Additionally, gross lipaemia and potassium EDTA contamination can cause artefactual changes in electrolyte concentrations.

Low cortisol concentration

Exogenous glucocorticoid administration results in low basal cortisol concentrations. Transiently high concentrations may occur because of cross-reaction between cortisol and administered hydrocortisone or prednisolone in many cortisol assays. Dexamethasone does not cross-react but will suppress adrenal function through reduced production of ACTH.

Iatrogenic hypercortisolism causing cortisol concentrations that are low enough to be confused with hypoadrenocorticism is less common in cats than in dogs. Cats are relatively resistant to glucocorticoid side effects and iatrogenic hypercortisolism is rarely reported. Doses of 2 mg/kg of prednisolone given daily for 2 weeks have been shown to suppress the cortisol response to ACTH for 3–4 weeks after cessation of treatment (Middleton *et al.*, 1987). Similarly, treatment with synthetic progestins (e.g. megoestrol acetate 5 mg/cat daily, or proligestone 100 mg/cat weekly, for 2 weeks) can suppress ACTH response tests (Watson *et al.*, 1989). In cases where there is doubt in the history of steroid administration, endogenous ACTH concentrations may provide helpful information to avoid the misdiagnosis of hypoadrenocorticism.

Treatment

Initial treatment

Fluid therapy

Acute treatment of hypoadrenocorticism involves the administration of intravenous fluids to restore plasma volume whilst reducing potassium and increasing sodium concentrations. Normal saline (0.9% NaCl) is an excellent initial fluid choice. If this is not available, other crystalloids are still of benefit because of their relatively low potassium concentrations. Fluid resuscitation should be performed in a goal-directed manner, taking into consideration the degree of dehydration and clinical status of the cat. This may dictate the rate and volume of fluids administered. However, 'shock rates' (5–10 ml/kg incremental boluses administered over 15–30 minutes) are frequently recommended, at least initially. Fluid boluses should be slowed or stopped if any adverse effects are observed or perfusion parameters improve (i.e. improvement in mucous membrane colour and pulse quality, normalization of heart rate and improved mentation).

Electrolyte concentrations should be closely monitored (every 2–6 hours) to ensure potassium concentrations are declining and that hyponatraemia, if present, is not corrected too rapidly. Correcting sodium concentrations too rapidly may lead to central pontine myelinolysis (sometimes called osmotic demyelination syndrome) and can result in acute severe neurological signs such as ataxia, postural deficits, dysphagia and decreased mentation. Signs may develop many days later. This syndrome has not yet been reported as a complication in cats with hypoadrenocorticism. Sodium concentrations should not increase by more than 12 mmol/l/day (0.5 mmol/l/hour) in chronic cases of hyponatraemia, such as those seen in hypoadrenocorticism. In cats with very low sodium concentrations (<120 mmol/l), 0.45% NaCl or other low-sodium fluids may be more appropriate.

Specific treatment for hyperkalaemia has not been reported in cats with hypoadrenocorticism and is only necessary if there are associated cardiac complications (i.e. severe bradycardia <60 bpm). As for hyperkalaemia associated with urinary obstruction, management with intravenous 10% calcium gluconate (0.5–1 ml/kg given slowly) may be used to reduce the excitability of the myocardial tissues.

Glucose, urea, creatinine, calcium and albumin concentrations should all be monitored at least every 6–12 hours depending on the clinical status of the cat (e.g. glucose concentration should be measured more frequently if insulin and dextrose are given). Fluid therapy is expected to reduce urea concentrations, which may be used to help assess fluid volume status. Aggressive rehydration will correct most acid–base abnormalities and, although most cats with hypoadrenocorticism will be acidotic, specific treatment is not usually required. Care should be taken not to overcorrect any sodium abnormalities. Fluid therapy can be decreased and tapered to maintenance rates after the initial crisis has passed. Fluids can be stopped once the azotaemia has resolved and the cat is eating and drinking voluntarily.

Glucocorticoid therapy

Glucocorticoids are indicated in the acute management of severe hypoadrenocorticism. Dexamethasone and prednisolone are most commonly reported; both lack any mineralocorticoid activity. There is no evidence that high doses of glucocorticoids are needed, and they may even be contraindicated because of the risk of inducing or exacerbating gastrointestinal haemorrhage. A single bolus of intravenous dexamethasone is recommended (0.2–0.4 mg/kg) and will not interfere with concurrent ACTH response testing. Alternatively, hydrocortisone may be administered, although this drug has been reported in only one cat with hypoadrenocorticism (Fowlie et al., 2018). Hydrocortisone has both mineralocorticoid and glucocorticoid activity and aids effective correction of sodium and potassium concentrations. Initial doses may be extrapolated from those used in dogs and a constant rate infusion of 0.5–0.625 mg/kg/h could be considered. Alternatively, boluses of 2 mg/kg every 6 hours have been reported in a cat (Fowlie et al., 2018). If hydrocortisone is used, it should be given only after collecting samples for endocrine testing and should be used carefully, especially to avoid rapid overcorrection in the face of severe hyponatraemia.

There is a relatively slow response to acute management in cats compared with dogs, with several reported cases taking 3–5 days to respond fully.

Mineralocorticoid therapy and long-term treatment

Long-term mineralocorticoid treatment options for cats are either oral fludrocortisone or a combination of injectable desoxycorticosterone pivalate (DOCP) and oral prednisolone. Neither fludrocortisone nor DOCP is specifically authorized for cats. Fludrocortisone is administered at a starting dose of 0.1 mg/cat/day. Once- and twice-daily fludrocortisone dosing has been described, although there are no data to suggest which is more effective in cats. During stabilization, fludrocortisone should be supplemented with prednisolone, as this has been shown to produce faster stabilization in dogs (Roberts et al., 2016). Fludrocortisone has two potential limitations. Firstly, the oral route of administration may be challenging for some owners. Secondly, fludrocortisone is administered daily and missed doses can rapidly result in clinical deterioration. The main advantage, however, is that fludrocortisone may be considerably cheaper than DOCP in some countries. Some cats treated with fludrocortisone may require additional glucocorticoid support.

There are a few reported cases of feline hypoadrenocorticism treated with DOCP. It has the potential advantage of easier administration, as it is injectable and owners can be trained to administer DOCP at home after initial stabilization. Desoxycorticosterone pivalate doses can be adjusted in a similar manner to that used in dogs (see Chapter 28), with a starting dose of 2.2 mg/kg (Spence et al., 2018). Final doses of DOCP tend to be higher in the few cats reported than are usually required in dogs. Desoxycorticosterone pivalate is very effective at increasing sodium retention and may lead to a rapid increase in plasma volume. Therefore, 30–50% lower starting doses are advised in cats with pre-existing heart disease. Spironolactone should be avoided in cats receiving either DOCP or fludrocortisone.

Cats treated with DOCP require separate glucocorticoid support. Oral prednisolone is the most common choice (0.2 mg/kg/day). However, long-acting methylprednisolone ester injections have been reported (10 mg/cat/month). Care must be taken to avoid chronic overdosing, and any clinical signs of hypercortisolism (poor hair regrowth, symmetrical alopecia or diabetes mellitus) should prompt a dose reduction of approximately 50%. During stressful events (e.g. boarding, illness or surgery), oral prednisolone dose increases of 100–400% are recommended.

Prognosis

Provided the condition is recognized and treated, the outcome is generally positive and rewarding. Of the approximately 30 cases reported to date, 10 died during hospitalization, and several of these deaths were related to underlying lymphoma. Survival times for cats that survive to discharge are long, with many lost to follow-up before death, so it is not possible to provide a median survival time. The prognosis is therefore excellent if lymphoma is excluded as a cause.

References and further reading

Battaglia L and Agnoli C (2012) Two cases of feline hypoadrenocorticism. Veterinaria 26, 43–49

Bell R, Mellor DJ, Ramsey I and Knottenbelt C (2005) Decreased sodium:potassium ratios in cats: 49 cases. Veterinary Clinical Pathology 34, 110–114

Berger SL and Reed JR (1993) Traumatically induced hypoadrenocorticism in a cat. Journal of the American Animal Hospital Association 29, 337–339

Bissett SA, Lamb M and Ward CR (2001) Hyponatremia and hyperkalemia associated with peritoneal effusion in four cats. Journal of the American Veterinary Medical Association 218, 1590–1592

Brain PH (1997) Trauma-induced hypoadrenocorticism in a cat. Australian Veterinary Practitioner 27, 178–181

Church DB, Watson AD, Emslie DR et al. (1994) Effects of proligestone and megestrol on plasma adrenocorticotrophic hormone, insulin and insulin-like growth factor-1 concentrations in cats. Research in Veterinary Science 56, 175–178

Combes A, Pey P, Paepe D et al. (2013) Ultrasonographic appearance of adrenal glands in healthy and sick cats. Journal of Feline Medicine and Surgery 15, 445–457

Coulter DB, Duncan RJ and Sander PD (1975) Effects of asphyxia and potassium on canine and feline electrocardiograms. Canadian Journal of Comparative Medicine 39, 442–449

DeClue AE, Martin LG, Behrend EN et al. (2011) Cortisol and aldosterone response to various doses of cosyntropin in healthy cats. Journal of the American Veterinary Medical Association 238, 176–182

Duesberg CA, Nelson RW, Feldman EC, Vaden SL and Scott-Moncrieff CR (1995) Adrenalectomy for treatment of hyperadrenocorticism in cats: 10 cases (1988–1992). Journal of the American Veterinary Medical Association 207, 1066–1070

Eiler KC, Bruyette DS, Behrend EN, Kemppainen RJ and Kass PH (2013) Comparison of intravenous versus intramuscular administration of corticotropin-releasing hormone in healthy cats. Journal of Veterinary Internal Medicine 27, 516–521

Fowlie SJ, McKenzie J and Ramsey I (2018) Hypoadrenocorticism in an aged cat. Veterinary Record Case Reports 6, e000565

Giudice E, Macrì F, Crinò C, Viganò F and di Pietro S (2016) Hypoadrenocorticism in a young dwarf cat – case report. Veterinarski Arhiv 86, 591–600

Hock CE (2011) Atypical hypoadrenocorticism in a Birman cat. Canadian Veterinary Journal 52, 893–896

Johnessee JS, Peterson ME and Gilbertson SR (1983) Primary hypoadrenocorticism in a cat. Journal of the American Veterinary Medical Association 183, 881–882

Meij BP, Auriemma E, Grinwis G, Buijtels JJCWM and Kooistra HS (2010) Successful treatment of acromegaly in a diabetic cat with transsphenoidal hypophysectomy. Journal of Feline Medicine and Surgery 12, 406–410

Mellett Keith AM, Bruyette D and Stanley S (2013) Trilostane therapy for treatment of spontaneous hyperadrenocorticism in cats: 15 cases (2004–2012). Journal of Veterinary Internal Medicine 27, 1471–1477

Middleton DJ, Watson AD, Howe CJ and Caterson ID (1987) Suppression of cortisol responses to exogenous adrenocorticotrophic hormone, and the occurrence of side effects attributable to glucocorticoid excess, in cats during therapy with megestrol acetate and prednisolone. Canadian Journal of Veterinary Research 51, 60–65

Norman BC, Côté E and Barrett KA (2006) Wide-complex tachycardia associated with severe hyperkalemia in three cats. Journal of Feline Medicine and Surgery 8, 372–378

Parnell NK, Powell LL, Hohenhaus AE, Patnaik AK and Peterson ME (1999) Hypoadrenocorticism as the primary manifestation of lymphoma in two cats. Journal of the American Veterinary Medical Association 214, 1208–1211, 1200

Peterson ME, Greco DS and Orth DN (1989) Primary hypoadrenocorticism in ten cats. Journal of Veterinary Internal Medicine 3, 55–58

Ramsey I (2019) Feline hypoadrenocorticism. In: Feline Endocrinology, 1st edn, ed. EC Feldman, F Fracassi and ME Peterson. Edra Publishing, Milan

Roberts E, Boden LA and Ramsey IK (2016) Factors that affect stabilisation times of canine spontaneous hypoadrenocorticism. Veterinary Record 179, 98

Romine JF, Kozicki AR and Elie MS (2016) Primary adrenal lymphoma causing hypoaldosteronism in a cat. *Journal of Feline Medicine and Surgery Open Reports* **2**, 2055116916684409

Rudinsky AJ, Clark ES, Russell DS and Gilor C (2015) Adrenal insufficiency secondary to lymphocytic panhypophysitis in a cat. *Australian Veterinary Journal* **93**, 327–331

Smith SA, Freeman LC and Bagladi-Swanson M (2002) Hypercalcemia due to iatrogenic secondary hypoadrenocorticism and diabetes mellitus in a cat. *Journal of the American Animal Hospital Association* **38**, 41–44

Spalla I, Spinelli D, Lucatini C *et al.* (2014) ECG of the Month. Hypoadrenocorticism. *Journal of the American Veterinary Medical Association* **244**, 45–47

Spence S, Gunn E and Ramsey I (2018) Diagnosis and treatment of canine hypoadrenocorticism. *In Practice* **40**, 281–290

Watson AD, Church DB, Emslie DR and Middleton DJ (1989) Comparative effects of proligestone and megestrol acetate on basal plasma glucose concentrations and cortisol responses to exogenous adrenocorticotrophic hormone in cats. *Research in Veterinary Science* **47**, 374–376

Yu S and Morris JG (1998) Plasma aldosterone concentration of cats. *The Veterinary Journal* **155**, 63–68

Zimmer C, Hörauf A and Reusch C (2000) Ultrasonographic examination of the adrenal gland and evaluation of the hypophyseal-adrenal axis in 20 cats. *Journal of Small Animal Practice* **41**, 156–160

Chapter 32

Feline hyperaldosteronism

Ghita Benchekroun

Introduction

Primary hyperaldosteronism is an uncommon but emerging endocrine disorder in cats and extremely rare in dogs, with only a few isolated case reports. It is characterized by autonomous secretion of aldosterone arising from adrenal neoplasia or hyperplasia. The condition is referred to as Conn's syndrome in humans, after Jerome Conn, the physician who first described it, in a woman experiencing episodic weakness as a result of recurrent hypokalaemia.

Since the first description of primary hyperaldosteronism in a cat in 1983, four case series have been published describing 10, 11, 13 and 17 cats (Ash *et al.*, 2005; Javadi *et al.*, 2005; Daniel *et al.*, 2016; Harro *et al.*, 2021). Together with several single-case reports, approximately 100 cases have been reported. The author has diagnosed 21 cats with primary hyperaldosteronism over the past 15 years. It is likely under-diagnosed because of non-specific clinical features coupled with the difficulties of definitive diagnosis. The most commonly reported clinical manifestations of primary hyperaldosteronism relate to hypokalaemic myopathy and/or systemic hypertension, both occurring secondary to excess circulating aldosterone concentrations, leading to target organ damage (TOD). Chronic kidney disease (CKD) and primary hyperaldosteronism can be associated, and it is suggested that CKD may be a frequently unrecognized consequence of primary hyperaldosteronism. Hypokalaemia and systemic hypertension can occur in cats with primary CKD and are often not investigated any further as CKD is considered to be the causal disease.

Aetiology and pathophysiology

Primary hyperaldosteronism is defined by autonomous and excessive secretion of aldosterone by neoplasia or hyperplasia of the zona glomerulosa of the adrenal cortex. In most cases, the underlying aetiology is an adrenocortical tumour that can be benign or malignant with or without local invasion and distant metastasis. This contrasts with primary hyperaldosteronism in humans, which usually occurs due to benign lesions. Primary hyperaldosteronism must be distinguished from secondary hyperaldosteronism, in which aldosterone secretion occurs in response to stimulation of the renin–angiotensin–aldosterone system (RAAS) as a result of another underlying condition (e.g. heart disease, hyperthyroidism, CKD).

Aldosterone secretion is regulated by the RAAS (see Chapter 28). The main effects of aldosterone are potassium excretion and water and salt retention. Both extracellular volume expansion and increased total peripheral resistance contribute to systemic hypertension. Aldosterone may also mediate inflammation and stimulate fibroblasts, leading to renal, vascular and myocardial fibrosis (Ames *et al.*, 2019). Aldosterone (and angiotensin II) is known to be both cardiotoxic and nephrotoxic, and hyperaldosteronism has been investigated as a mediator of progressive kidney disease in cats (Javadi *et al.*, 2005). It is important to note, however, that the antinatriuretic actions of aldosterone are counteracted by changes in renal perfusion pressure that prevent sodium resorption. Because the greater part of the filtered sodium is resorbed at the level of the proximal tubule by a constitutive mechanism (i.e. without hormonal modulation), only a small fraction of the sodium filtered by the glomerulus is affected by distal tubule adaptive resorption. In primary hyperaldosteronism, excess distal resorption is counteracted by simultaneous blood volume expansion that reduces proximal resorption of sodium. Thus, the final amount of excreted sodium in the collecting duct stays approximately the same. This phenomenon is called 'escape' and it explains the absence, in most cases, of major water and sodium retention, in particular hypernatraemia, peripheral oedema and effusion.

Unilateral tumours (adenomas or carcinomas) are the main cause of primary hyperaldosteronism in cats; they account for 85% of cases, with the other 15% attributed to bilateral micronodular hyperplasia or bilateral tumours. It is likely that bilateral hyperplasia is underdiagnosed in cats because ultrasonography reveals only minor changes of the adrenal glands and because CKD is often present and taken as the sole diagnosis. In some cases, aldosterone secretion may be coupled with secretion of other adrenal hormones (cortisol or progesterone), leading to a different clinical presentation (Harro *et al.*, 2021; Langlois *et al.*, 2021).

Clinical features

Details of cases reported in the largest case series and those seen by the author are presented in Figure 32.1.

Signalment

Primary hyperaldosteronism is mainly seen in older cats (median age 12.5 years), although two cases have been

Parameter		Prevalence and clinicopathological values			
		Ash et al., 2005 (n=13)	*Javadi et al., 2005 (n=11)*	*Djajadiningrat-Laanen et al., 2013 (n=9)*	*Cases seen at EnvA (n=21)*
Age (years): mean (min, max)		10 (6, 13)	14 (11, 18)	13 (8, 19)	13 (6, 18)
Sex	Male	8	3	3	13
	Female	5	8	6	9
Weakness		6	6	3	9
Cervical ventroflexion		7	–	–	6
Retinopathy, blindness		2	7	–	3
Clinical signs: other		PU/PD (3), polyphagia (2)	–	–	Decreased appetite (11), weight loss (11), PU/PD (8), vomiting (5), neurological signs as manifestation of hypertensive encephalopathy (3)
Underlying cause	Adrenal mass	13	0	7	19
	Adrenal hyperplasia	0	11	2	2
Comorbidities	Chronic kidney disease	3	8	–	10
	Hyperthyroidism	1	0	0	4
	Hypercortisolism	0	0	0	2
Potassium (mmol/l): mean (min, max)		2.5 (1.9, 3.2)	3.1 (2.3, 3.7)	3.1 (1.8, 4.3)	2.8 (1.4, 4)
Hypokalaemia		13	6	5	19
Sodium (mmol/l): mean (min, max)		155 (148, 168)	153 (149, 156)	151 (147, 155)	154 (144, 169)
Hypernatraemia		1	0	0	3
Systolic blood pressure (mmHg): mean (min, max)		193 (160, 250)	212 (185, 230)	193 (160, 280)	190 (135, 300)
Systemic hypertension		11	11	9	14
Aldosterone (pmol/l): mean (min, max)		5,820 (877, 14,653)	510 (130, 830)	1,056 (556, 2,778)	3,388 (659, 13,178)

32.1 Signalment and clinical and clinicopathological features of primary hyperaldosteronism in 54 cats collected from published case series and cases seen at the Alfort University Veterinary Hospital (EnvA). – = no data; PU/PD = polyuria and polydipsia.

described in young adults (5 and 6.5 years old). Domestic Shorthaired cats are the most commonly affected breed, but any breed can develop the disease. No sex predisposition has been identified.

Clinical signs

The main clinical signs of primary hyperaldosteronism are due to dysregulated and autonomous secretion of aldosterone, which leads to:

- Hypokalaemia (due to excess kaliuresis)
- Systemic arterial hypertension (due to excessive sodium retention).

Hypokalaemia

Hypokalaemic polymyopathy is common in cats with primary hyperaldosteronism. Its pathogenesis is poorly understood but might involve potassium-related disturbance of muscular microcirculation and perturbation of plasma membrane ion pumps. Associated manifestations include generalized weakness and cervical ventroflexion in most cases (Figure 32.2). A plantigrade stance, flaccid paresis, apparent ataxia and dyspnoea are also described. However, in some cases with severe hypokalaemia, neuromuscular manifestations are not present. It is possible that the variation in the response to hypokalaemia depends on its chronicity, or that the circulating potassium concentration does not accurately represent total body potassium status.

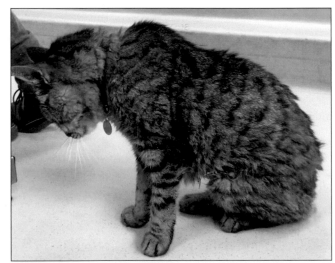

32.2 Cervical ventroflexion caused by hypokalaemic polymyopathy in a cat with primary hyperaldosteronism. Cervical ventroflexion is a specific sign of hypokalaemia in cats and its recognition during clinical examination can direct the diagnostic approach.

Systemic hypertension

Systemic hypertension is frequent in feline primary hyperaldosteronism and will lead to TOD if sustained. Evidence of TOD includes progression of kidney disease, retinopathy, encephalopathy and left ventricular hypertrophy. Clinical signs are not always present – regular monitoring of blood pressure is recommended.

Ocular signs are the most commonly described complications of systemic hypertension in cats (Maggio *et al.*, 2000). Such cases present with ocular lesions of varying degrees of severity, including (in order of increasing severity) sinuous retinal vessels, retinal oedema, retinal detachment, retinal haemorrhage and intraocular haemorrhage. Subsequent clinical signs range from a mild reduction in visual acuity to complete blindness with unresponsive mydriasis (Figure 32.3). Exudative retinal detachment is the most commonly observed ophthalmological finding in cats with systemic hypertension (Figure 32.4). Sudden-onset blindness is a frequent clinical complaint of feline primary hyperaldosteronism and should immediately prompt blood pressure measurement.

Primary hyperaldosteronism may also manifest as hypertensive encephalopathy. In one case, neurological manifestations comprised short episodes of head tilt, prostration and ataxia; in another, there was a sudden onset of vestibular syndrome (head tilt, circling and ataxia).

In addition, systemic hypertension is the cause of major cardiovascular and renal sequelae. Hypertrophic cardiomyopathy has been observed in several cases of primary hyperaldosteronism with systemic hypertension.

Non-specific clinical signs

Occasionally, cats with primary hyperaldosteronism present with only non-specific clinical signs, such as polyuria and polydipsia, gastrointestinal signs, lethargy and weight loss. In a few cases, an abdominal mass can be palpated. The diagnostic approach to such cases is difficult but, once again, the identification of hypokalaemia and/or systemic hypertension, or the presence of an adrenal mass, should raise the index of suspicion for primary hyperaldosteronism. Polyuria and polydipsia in cats with primary hyperaldosteronism can occur in association with CKD but may also arise from nephrogenic diabetes insipidus caused by hypokalaemia.

If there is concurrent secretion of cortisol or progesterone by the adrenal tumours, cats show clinical signs of hypercortisolism and thus can be diabetic or exhibit cutaneous signs characterized by non-pruritic alopecia, a thin hair coat and skin fragility (see Chapter 30).

Uncommon and misleading clinical signs are possible. Three cats presented with signs related to acute haemoabdomen as a consequence of adrenal haemorrhage. In

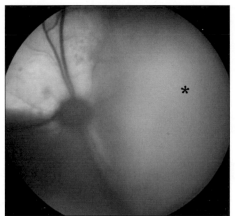

32.4 Fundus examination in a Domestic Shorthaired cat showing a large peripapillary retinal detachment (the hazy area indicated by the asterisk).
(Courtesy of Dr Chahory, Ophthalmology Unit, ChuvA)

each case, the presence of an adrenal mass guided the diagnostic approach. Another cat presented with oxygen-dependent respiratory failure; thoracic radiographs failed to detect any lesions and the signs were later attributed to respiratory muscle paresis. Positive pressure ventilation was required to support respiratory function. The cat had a moderately low plasma potassium concentration (2.7 mmol/l, reference interval: 3.8–5.4) and demonstrated profound hindlimb weakness.

Diagnosis
Routine clinicopathological features
Haematology

There are usually no significant haematological abnormalities in cats with primary hyperaldosteronism.

Biochemistry

Hypokalaemia is the main biochemical abnormality encountered in primary hyperaldosteronism (84% of published cases). The differential diagnoses for hypokalaemia are extensive (Figure 32.5), but in unmedicated cats with

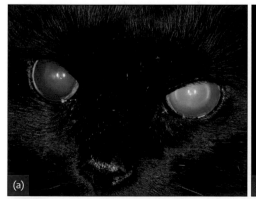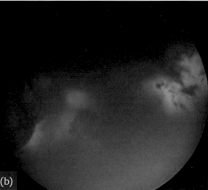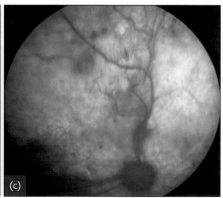

32.3 A 14-year-old Domestic Shorthaired cat presented for blindness and bilateral mydriasis. (a) The red colour of the eye through the pupil is consistent with vitreal haemorrhage. Mydriasis was unresponsive to light and blindness was associated with bilateral retinal detachment and retinal haemorrhage. (b) Fundus examination of the right eye showed a large vitreous and subretinal haemorrhage with retinal detachment. (c) Fundus examination of the left eye revealed retinal oedema, partial perivascular retinal detachment and small retinal haemorrhage. Blindness is one of the major clinical complaints of primary hyperaldosteronism. If there is retinal haemorrhage and/or retinal detachment, blood pressure should be measured. In cases of systemic hypertension, differential diagnoses include primary hyperaldosteronism, which should be investigated by potassium measurement and adrenal ultrasonography.
(Courtesy of Dr Chahory, Ophthalmology Unit, ChuvA)

Increased renal loss
- Kidney disease
- Renal tubular acidosis
- Hyperaldosteronism
- Iatrogenic (furosemide)
- Post-obstructive diuresis
- Diabetic ketoacidosis
- Urine-acidifying diet

Increased intestinal loss
- Vomiting
- Diarrhoea

Decreased intake
- Anorexia
- Unsupplemented fluid therapy

Intracellular shift
- Burmese hypokalaemia
- Metabolic alkalosis
- Iatrogenic (salbutamol, insulin)

32.5 Differential diagnoses for hypokalaemia in cats.

no gastrointestinal signs, kidney or endocrine disease is most likely. Because aldosterone causes sodium resorption and potassium excretion, it would be logical to expect cats with hyperaldosteronism to have both hypokalaemia and hypernatremia. However, sodium concentrations tend to remain within the reference interval. Hypernatraemia is only rarely found (6% of cases with primary hyperaldosteronism). Metabolic alkalosis is the most widely described acid–base change in primary hyperaldosteronism. It is usually mild, but its prevalence is unknown in cats with primary hyperaldosteronism. To date, severe alkalosis causing related clinical signs (e.g. respiratory or muscular) or electrolyte imbalances (hypocalcaemia) has not been reported in cats, but it could be underdiagnosed.

Azotaemia is observed in approximately 50% of cats with primary hyperaldosteronism. Interestingly, phosphate concentration tends to be within or slightly below the reference interval in these cases, probably secondary to enhanced phosphaturia and volume expansion. Therefore, the combination of azotaemia, hypokalaemia and low-normal phosphate concentrations should prompt investigations for primary hyperaldosteronism rather than being interpreted solely as an indication of CKD. Although 30% of cats with CKD may develop hypokalaemia due to loss of tubular resorption or secondary hyperaldosteronism, recurrent hypokalaemia in an azotaemic cat should not be trivialized, and attention should be directed to the possibility of concurrent primary hyperaldosteronism.

An increase in creatine kinase activity is also frequently seen, related to hypokalaemic myopathy. The increase is usually marked, with values above 1,000 IU/l. Increased creatine kinase activity can also occur secondary to prolonged recumbency, restraint or recent intramuscular injection.

Urinalysis

Urinalysis may be used to calculate the fractional excretion of potassium in the face of hypokalaemia of unknown origin. A value above 4–6% in a potassium-deficient cat indicates inappropriate potassium loss from the kidneys and should prompt investigation of primary hyperaldosteronism.

Blood pressure measurement

Measurement of systolic blood pressure is essential because demonstrating hypertension helps to guide diagnosis. It is important to exclude conditions other than primary hyperaldosteronism that may cause systemic hypertension, including CKD and other endocrine diseases (hypercortisolism and phaeochromocytoma) (Figure 32.6). Systolic blood pressure should be measured on several occasions to confirm the presence of systemic hypertension. The main difficulty in interpreting blood pressure in cats is the presence of situational hypertension (also called white-coat hypertension). It is important to note that increased blood pressure usually remains asymptomatic in cats until severe TOD prompts veterinary consultation. It is therefore likely that primary hyperaldosteronism in cats is underdiagnosed because it can sometimes manifest as nothing more than a chronic, mild systemic hypertension that is not routinely detected during annual visits. It is important to incorporate blood pressure measurements in regular check-ups of cats. This will accustom the cat to the procedure, help to detect systemic hypertension at an early stage and will probably help in the diagnosis of primary hyperaldosteronism. The presence of TOD justifies immediate initiation of treatment and investigation of the underlying cause of hypertension. If prehypertension (140–159 mmHg) or moderate hypertension (160–179 mmHg) is found, a second measurement can be performed 4–8 weeks later. If the hypertension is severe (≥180 mmHg), blood pressure measurement should be repeated within 1–2 weeks and investigation of conditions associated with secondary hypertension should be initiated.

Challenging differential diagnoses

Primary hyperaldosteronism can easily be confused with CKD. Indeed, CKD is a common cause of hypokalaemia and systemic hypertension. Moreover, CKD leads to secondary hyperaldosteronism. To a lesser extent, hyperthyroidism can manifest with hypokalaemia and systemic hypertension and can also lead to secondary hyperaldosteronism. For these reasons, diagnosis of primary hyperaldosteronism may be challenging, especially when no adrenal mass is identified by diagnostic imaging. As mentioned above (see 'Aetiology and pathophysiology'), bilateral adrenal hyperplasia is a possible cause of primary hyperaldosteronism in cats and may be a mediator of progressive CKD. In cats with concurrent

- Chronic kidney disease
- Idiopathic hypertension
- Endocrine disease
  - Hypercortisolism
  - Primary hyperaldosteronism
  - Phaeochromocytoma (very rare)
  - Hyperthyroidism
  - Hypersomatotropism
  - Diabetes mellitus
- Iatrogenic
  - Steroids
  - Dobutamine
  - Darbepoetin
  - Epoetin
  - Erythropoietin
  - Fludrocortisone
  - Phenylpropanolamine
  - Situational hypertension (white-coat hypertension)

32.6 Differential diagnoses for systemic hypertension in cats.

primary hyperaldosteronism and CKD, it is challenging to determine whether kidney disease is primary or secondary to systemic hypertension and the direct effects of aldosterone.

> - Primary hyperaldosteronism should be included as a differential diagnosis for systemic hypertension.
> - Other causes include CKD, idiopathic hypertension, hypercortisolism and phaeochromocytoma.
> - Integration of blood pressure measurement in annual visits is recommended, especially in elderly cats.

Diagnostic confirmation

Once a clinical suspicion of primary hyperaldosteronism is established, strong support for the diagnosis is provided by plasma aldosterone concentration and plasma renin activity.

The diagnosis of primary hyperaldosteronism is usually based on supportive clinical signs, increased plasma aldosterone concentration in the presence of hypokalaemia, and the visualization of an adrenal mass on diagnostic imaging. However, none of these signs is pathognomonic. Aldosterone:renin (ARR) is currently considered to be the gold standard for diagnosing primary hyperaldosteronism and helps distinguish it from secondary hyperaldosteronism. Unfortunately, measurement of renin activity is not widely available and there are strict pre-analytical conditions, making its evaluation difficult. Moreover, studies comparing ARR measurement in cats with primary hyperaldosteronism and cats with secondary hyperaldosteronism are lacking.

The lack of a practical and inexpensive confirmatory test can render the diagnosis of primary hyperaldosteronism challenging, especially if comorbidities are present (e.g. hyperthyroidism, CKD) and if an adrenal mass is not present (e.g. cases of bilateral adrenal hyperplasia).

Plasma aldosterone concentration

A validated radioimmunoassay is recommended for aldosterone measurement. As an example, in a study of 130 healthy cats aged from 0.3 to 14.5 years, plasma aldosterone concentrations ranged from 10 to 800 pmol/l and the reference interval was set between 110 and 540 pmol/l. These values overlap with those of cats with primary or secondary hyperaldosteronism.

When all published cases of primary hyperaldosteronism are analysed, aldosterone concentration appears to be higher in cats presenting with an adrenal mass than in cats with bilateral adrenal hyperplasia. In approximately 25% of primary hyperaldosteronism cases, plasma aldosterone concentrations are within the reference interval. In conditions such as CKD, hyperthyroidism or idiopathic hypertension, which cause stimulation of the RAAS, the aldosterone concentration may be above the reference interval (Williams *et al.*, 2013; Jepson *et al.*, 2014). Evaluation of the potassium concentration at the same sampling time can aid interpretation: an increase in aldosterone concentration, even if slight, in the presence of hypokalaemia is inappropriate. In physiological situations, negative feedback from hypokalaemia would suppress aldosterone secretion (see Chapter 28). Thus, the finding of an increased aldosterone concentration in the face of hypokalaemia increases the suspicion of primary hyperaldosteronism.

> Interpret plasma aldosterone concentrations carefully. They can be:
> - Within the reference interval in cats with primary hyperaldosteronism
> - Higher in cases of primary hyperaldosteronism caused by adrenal neoplasia compared with those caused by bilateral adrenal hyperplasia
> - Increased in cases of hyperthyroidism or CKD.

Plasma renin activity

Assessment of plasma renin activity is of major importance because, combined with the aldosterone concentration, it allows discrimination between primary and secondary hyperaldosteronism. Decreased plasma renin activity in the presence of an increased aldosterone concentration indicates that aldosterone is being secreted autonomously. Theoretically, this hormonal profile should be characteristic of primary hyperaldosteronism; however, in some cases of primary hyperaldosteronism, plasma renin activity is high, which might indicate suboptimal ability to discriminate between primary and secondary hyperaldosteronism, a concurrent condition leading to RAAS activation and overwhelming the negative feedback of aldosterone on renin secretion, or an erroneous diagnosis. On the other hand, it has been shown that plasma renin activity can also be reduced in cats with systemic hypertension with or without concurrent azotaemia, further complicating the diagnostic challenges (Jepson *et al.*, 2014).

Assessment of active renin is preferred in humans, but this has not yet been validated in cats.

> - Renin activity is usually suppressed in primary hyperaldosteronism.
> - Analysis of renin activity is not readily available and requires strict pre-analytical conditions.

Aldosterone:renin

In theory, the use of ARR solves the challenges of using individual measurements to diagnose primary hyperaldosteronism. In healthy cats, a reference interval ARR has been reported as between 0.3 and 3.8 when plasma aldosterone in pmol/l was divided by renin activity in fmol/l/s (Javadi *et al.*, 2005). In cats with primary hyperaldosteronism, it is expected to be above 3.8. The ARR is commonly used in human medicine and has proven useful in most cases to confirm a diagnosis of primary hyperaldosteronism. It is difficult to assess the clinical utility and accuracy of ARR for primary hyperaldosteronism diagnosis in cats because of the limited availability of plasma renin activity in this species.

Urine aldosterone:creatinine

It has been suggested that the urine aldosterone:creatinine could be a more informative diagnostic test than plasma aldosterone concentration alone. A reference interval of less than 46.5×10^{-9} for the ratio of urine aldosterone in pmol/l to creatinine in μmol/l has been suggested (Djajadiningrat-Laanen *et al.*, 2008). However, the ratio was not helpful in distinguishing healthy cats, normotensive cats with CKD, and cats with CKD and systemic hypertension (Syme *et al.*, 2007).

Suppression tests

In the diagnosis of any disease caused by autonomous hormone secretion, a suppression test can help determine whether an increased hormone concentration is due to autonomous secretion. In human medicine, several suppression tests for aldosterone have been described. The most commonly used tests are based on intravenous salt loading, but captopril (an angiotensin converting enzyme inhibitor) and losartan (an angiotensin II receptor blocker) tests have also been described.

A fludrocortisone suppression test and an oral salt-loading suppression test have been reported in cats. The principle is based on the determination of urine aldosterone:creatinine before and after the administration of fludrocortisone or sodium chloride tablets (Djajadiningrat-Laanen et al., 2008, 2013; Koutinas et al., 2015). Results were inconclusive for salt loading but demonstrated that fludrocortisone administration may be useful as a suppression test for primary hyperaldosteronism, irrespective of aetiology. Fludrocortisone is administered at a dosage of 0.05 mg/kg q12h for 4 days, and the last urine sample is collected after the ninth dose, administered on the fifth day (Djajadiningrat-Laanen et al., 2013). Although the results are encouraging, this test has two major limitations:

- Restrictive protocol – fludrocortisone is administered orally every 12 hours for 4 consecutive days
- Poor diagnostic sensitivity – urine aldosterone:creatinine was not suppressed in 6 of 9 (67%) cats with primary hyperaldosteronism.

More recently, the same test has been described but using plasma aldosterone measurement (Matsuda et al., 2015). Only three doses of fludrocortisone were required in healthy cats, with the last sample taken 4 hours after the third dose. Further studies are needed to document the usefulness of this test in cats with primary and secondary hyperaldosteronism.

Preliminary results of a telmisartan suppression test were initially encouraging (Fabrès et al., 2019). A single oral dose of 2 mg/kg telmisartan resulted in an aldosterone suppression of approximately 40–50% after 1.0–1.5 hours in healthy cats and no suppression in cats with primary hyperaldosteronism. However, this test did not discriminate primary hyperaldosteronism from diseases associated with secondary hyperaldosteronism, such as CKD, hyperthyroidism and idiopathic hypertension (Kurtz et al., 2023)

Diagnosis of primary hyperaldosteronism can be straightforward in a non-azotaemic cat with suggestive clinical signs. Diagnosis may be challenging in cases where there is azotaemia or, to a lesser extent, hyperthyroidism because hypokalaemia, systemic hypertension and increased plasma aldosterone concentration may be related to primary hyperaldosteronism, CKD, hyperthyroidism or a combination of these conditions. In such cases, in the absence of a reliable suppression test or renin activity measurement to assess the ARR, diagnostic imaging can help if an adrenal mass is identified.

Diagnostic imaging

Once hyperaldosteronism has been confirmed or is highly suspected, diagnostic imaging of the adrenal glands, interpreted together with laboratory results, helps to establish the aetiology (Figure 32.7). Abdominal ultrasonography is the most common imaging modality used. In healthy cats, the adrenal glands are of variable shape

Parameter	Primary hyperaldosteronism		Secondary hyperaldosteronism
	Adrenal tumour	*Bilateral adrenal hyperplasia*	
Aldosterone	Marked increase	Mild to moderate increase	Mild to moderate increase
Renin activity	Mild decrease	Mild decrease	Mild increase or no change
Adrenal ultrasonography	Adrenal mass, normal contralateral adrenal gland	Symmetrical, normal to moderately enlarged adrenal glands	Symmetrical, normal to moderately enlarged adrenal glands

32.7 Aldosterone, renin activity and adrenal ultrasonographic findings expected in primary and secondary hyperaldosteronism.

and size. They are uniformly hypoechoic and delineated by a thin hyperechoic halo. They are typically bean-shaped or, less commonly, ovoid or fusiform. They are variable in length (approximately 9–11 mm) and approximately 3.9–4.8 mm in maximum thickness (dorsoventral height), dependent on bodyweight (see Chapter 34). Other visualization techniques include computed tomography (CT) and magnetic resonance imaging. Whatever imaging modality is chosen, its main objective is to detect an adrenal tumour and its laterality, and to evaluate local invasion and distant metastasis in cases of neoplasia.

Ultrasonography is advantageous because of its relatively low cost, its non-invasive nature and the fact that it does not require general anaesthesia. However, it lacks sensitivity, particularly in cases of bilateral hyperplasia and also for identification of local vascular invasion. In practice, the visualization of an adrenal mass facilitates a diagnosis of primary hyperaldosteronism when other clinical findings are suggestive. In other cases, the discovery of an adrenal mass is incidental but it should nevertheless be followed up with an investigation for the presence of primary hyperaldosteronism, as this is the most common adrenal disorder in cats. When there is a functional adrenal tumour of the zona glomerulosa, the contralateral gland is usually of normal size (except in the case of bilateral tumours) (Figure 32.8a). In the case of bilateral hyperplasia, the adrenal glands are of normal or moderately increased size (Figure 32.8b).

Adrenal masses

- Some adrenal gland nodules responsible for primary hyperaldosteronism do not disrupt the normal architecture of the gland and may be detected only as areas with different echotexture.
- Finding an adrenal mass is not pathognomonic for primary hyperaldosteronism.
- Bilateral adrenal hyperplasia can be difficult to detect and can be due to diseases other than primary hyperaldosteronism (e.g. hyperthyroidism, hypersomatotropism).

Computed tomography, which is more sensitive than ultrasonography, is less commonly used given its higher cost and the need for deep sedation or, more likely, general anaesthesia. It is not 100% sensitive for detection of infiltration of the caudal vena cava. The main indication for CT is the preoperative assessment of a cat with

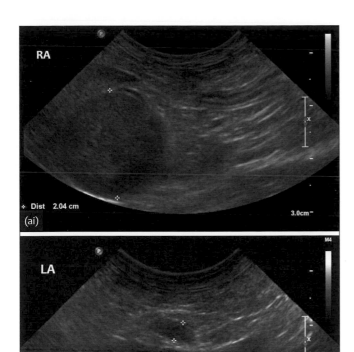

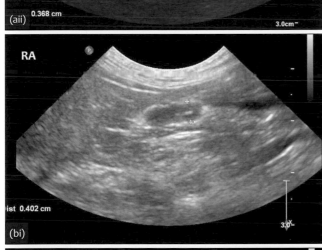

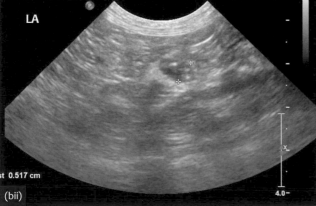

32.8 Adrenal tumours are the most commonly recognized cause of primary hyperaldosteronism in cats, but bilateral adrenal hyperplasia can also be responsible. Ultrasonography of the adrenal glands helps to determine the aetiology. (a) In this case, (ai) an adrenal mass was identified in the right adrenal gland (RA), whereas (aii) the left adrenal gland (LA) was of normal size. (b) In this case, both the (bi) right and (bii) left adrenal glands were moderately increased in size. In both cases, primary hyperaldosteronism was confirmed.
(Courtesy of the Imaging Unit, ChuvA)

primary hyperaldosteronism when surgical treatment by adrenalectomy is being considered. In this situation, a CT scan will provide the most accurate information if extended into the chest to detect distant metastases.

Histopathological analysis

Histopathological analysis requires adrenalectomy and is therefore performed only if the cat is treated surgically (Figure 32.9). It confirms the presence of an adrenocortical tumour. It also allows neoplasia to be distinguished from hyperplasia. It occasionally allows the distinction of adenoma from carcinoma, but this may be challenging, and other clinical and imaging features may help in this regard (Figure 32.10).

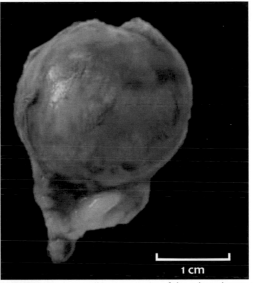

32.9 Macroscopic appearance of the adrenal mass detected by ultrasonography in Figure 32.8ai. Neither the macroscopic appearance of an adrenal tumour nor the histological examination findings are specific for primary hyperaldosteronism.

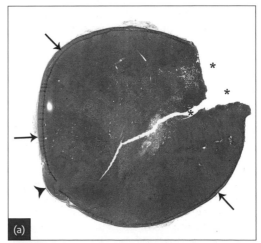

32.10 Micrographs of sections from the adrenal mass shown in Figure 32.9. Histopathology can confirm an adrenocortical tumour in cats with primary hyperaldosteronism but can rarely distinguish between the involvement of different zones of the cortex or discriminate malignant from benign tumours (carcinoma *versus* adenoma). (a) Low-power image. The adrenal gland has been partially incised (*). At the periphery, a rim of residual and compressed adrenal parenchyma (arrowed) is separated from the tumour by a thin pseudocapsule. There is a focus of capsular effraction (arrowhead). (Haematoxylin-eosin-saffron stain). (continues) ▶
(Courtesy of Dr Reyes-Gomez, Histology Unit, Biopôle)

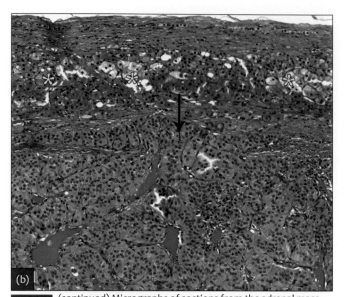

32.10 (continued) Micrographs of sections from the adrenal mass shown in Figure 32.9. Histopathology can confirm an adrenocortical tumour in cats with primary hyperaldosteronism but can rarely distinguish between the involvement of different zones of the cortex or discriminate malignant from benign tumours (carcinoma *versus* adenoma). (b) Medium-power image. At the periphery, a rim of residual and compressed adrenal parenchyma (*) is separated from the tumour by a thin pseudocapsule. Neoplastic cells are organized in convoluted trabeculae supported by a delicate fibrovascular stroma. Neoplastic cells tend to be elongated with a central nucleus, resembling cells of the zona glomerulosa. There is a focus of effraction of the tumour capsule (arrowed), suggestive of malignant behaviour. (Haematoxylin-eosin-saffron stain).
(Courtesy of Dr Reyes-Gomez, Histology Unit, Biopôle)

Treatment

Medical management

Medical treatment is required in three different situations:

- Emergencies where the signs are life-threatening
- To stabilize circulating potassium concentrations and blood pressure before adrenalectomy
- As a long-term palliative treatment if surgery is not an option.

Potassium supplementation

Initially, potassium is usually supplemented through intravenous fluid therapy (Figure 32.11), especially if intravenous supplementation is preferred. The dose should not exceed 0.5 mmol/kg/h, which dictates the maximal fluid rate depending on the amount of potassium chloride added to the fluid. It is important to bear in mind that the circulating potassium concentration does not represent the total body store of potassium, and a cat may exhibit only mild hypokalaemia despite total body stores being severely

Blood potassium concentration (mmol/l)	Potassium chloride (mmol/l of 0.9% saline)	Maximal fluid rate (ml/kg/h)
<2.0	80	6
2–2.5	60	8
2.5–3.0	40	12
3–3.5	30	18
3.5–5.0	20	25

32.11 Guidelines for supplementation of intravenous fluids with potassium chloride for the treatment of hypokalaemia.

depleted. As soon as oral intake is possible, oral potassium gluconate supplementation is recommended. The recommended dose is 2–6 mmol of potassium gluconate per cat per day, divided over two or three administrations. Doses as high as 12 mmol per cat per day have been used without side effects. Occasionally, supplementation fails to normalize circulating potassium concentrations, but it should resolve the clinical signs of hypokalaemia. If hypokalaemia is refractory to supplementation, hypomagnesaemia should be investigated and, if needed, corrected. Potassium supplementation is often required initially but can usually be withdrawn once treatment with a mineralocorticoid receptor blocker is initiated.

Mineralocorticoid antagonists

Spironolactone is an intracellular aldosterone receptor antagonist. It thus inhibits potassium secretion and promotes natriuresis. It is recommended orally at doses of 2–4 mg/kg/day. Doses above 4 mg/kg/day can cause anorexia, diarrhoea and vomiting. Administration of spironolactone in cats can cause facial ulcerative dermatitis, but this is a rare complication.

Antihypertensive drugs

Amlodipine, at an initial dose of 0.1 mg/kg once a day, is the recommended and most frequently used antihypertensive treatment in primary hyperaldosteronism, although some cases of primary hyperaldosteronism refractory to treatment have been described (Ash *et al.*, 2005). Regular monitoring of blood pressure, creatinine, urinalysis and fundus examination is essential in follow-up of these cases.

Surgical management

Unilateral adrenalectomy is the treatment of choice for primary hyperaldosteronism resulting from a non-metastasized unilateral tumour. It can be performed via a mid-line laparotomy, paracostal approach or laparoscopy. Laparoscopic adrenalectomy may be the surgical procedure of choice but is not yet widely performed. Adrenalectomy is a definitive treatment without the need for subsequent medical treatment. Nevertheless, hypertension and hypokalaemia must be carefully controlled before and during the surgery by means of oral or intravenous medications. Potential complications of surgery include haemorrhage. After surgery, the cat should be monitored for hypoaldosteronism due to contralateral adrenal suppression; mineralocorticoid supplementation and salt administration may be required, but is usually not necessary.
Contraindications to surgery are:

- Bilateral disease (bilateral hyperplasia or, more rarely, a bilateral tumour)
- Metastasis
- Tumour infiltration and local vascular adhesions
- Financial limitations
- The presence of comorbidities and significant anaesthetic risk.

Prognosis

After successful removal of an adrenal tumour, the prognosis is usually excellent. In one study describing adrenalectomy in 10 cats with primary hyperaldosteronism, median survival time was 1,297 days (Lo *et al.*, 2014). The median post-adrenalectomy survival time is considerably less when the duration of anaesthesia is more than 4 hours compared with less than 4 hours (10 and 1,329 days, respectively) (Lo *et al.*, 2014). Apart from duration of anaesthesia, no other prognostic factors have been identified. Perioperative haemorrhage is not associated with a specific type of tumour, its venous extension, or the presence or absence of systemic hypertension. In cases of malignant tumours, relapse of primary hyperaldosteronism can occur due to metastatic growth.

The prognosis for cats receiving medical treatment is less favourable than for those benefiting from surgery.

Summary

Primary hyperaldosteronism is a rare but probably under-diagnosed endocrine disease of the adult and senior cat. The clinical picture is dominated by hypokalaemic poly-myopathy and/or systemic hypertension. The diagnosis may be challenging due to the lack of specificity and sensitivity of the investigations and subsequent lack of a reliable confirmatory test, especially for cases of bilateral hyperplasia, which may not have abnormal ultrasonography findings. The treatment of choice, when feasible, remains adrenalectomy.

References and further reading

Ames MK, Atkins CE and Pitt B (2019) The renin-angiotensin-aldosterone system and its suppression. *Journal of Veterinary Internal Medicine* **33**, 363–382

Ash RA, Harvey AM and Tasker S (2005) Primary hyperaldosteronism in the cat: a series of 13 cases. *Journal of Feline Medicine and Surgery* **7**, 173–182

Daniel G, Mahony OM, Markovich JE et al. (2016) Clinical findings, diagnostics and outcome in 33 cats with adrenal neoplasia (2002–2013). *Journal of Feline Medicine and Surgery* **18**, 77–84

Djajadiningrat-Laanen SC, Galac S, Boevé MH *et al.* (2013) Evaluation of the oral fludrocortisone suppression test for diagnosing primary hyperaldosteronism in cats. *Journal of Veterinary Internal Medicine* **27**, 1493–1499

Djajadiningrat-Laanen SC, Galac S, Cammelbeeck SE *et al.* (2008) Urinary aldosterone to creatinine ratio in cats before and after suppression with salt or fludrocortisone acetate. *Journal of Veterinary Internal Medicine* **22**, 1283–1288

Fabrès V, Dumont R, Garcia M *et al.* (2019) Evaluation of telmisartan administration as a suppression test for primary hyperaldosteronism diagnosis in cats (abstract). *Journal of Veterinary Internal Medicine* **33**, 1041

Harro CC, Refsal KR, Shaw N *et al.* (2021) Retrospective study of aldosterone and progesterone secreting adrenal tumors in 10 cats. *Journal of Veterinary Internal Medicine* **35**, 2159–2166

Javadi S, Djajadiningrat-Laanen SC, Kooistra HS *et al.* (2005) Primary hyperaldosteronism, a mediator of progressive renal disease in cats. *Domestic Animal Endocrinology* **28**, 85–104

Jepson RE, Syme HM and Elliott J (2014) Plasma renin activity and aldosterone concentrations in hypertensive cats with and without azotemia and in response to treatment with amlodipine besylate. *Journal of Veterinary Internal Medicine* **28**, 144–153

Koutinas CK, Soubasis NC, Djajadiningrat-Laanen SC, Kolia E and Theodorou K (2015) Urinary aldosterone/creatinine ratio after fludrocortisone suppression consistent with PHA in a cat. *Journal of the American Animal Hospital Association* **51**, 338–341

Kurtz M, Fabrès V, Dumont R *et al.* (2023) Prospective evaluation of a telmi-sartan suppression test as a diagnostic tool for primary hyperaldosteronism in cats. *Journal of Veterinary Internal Medicine* doi.org/10.1111/jvim.16741

Langlois DK, Mazaki-Tovi M, Harro CC and Refsal KR (2021) Multiple corticosteroid abnormalities in cats with hyperaldosteronism. *Journal of Veterinary Internal Medicine* **35**, 2152–2158

Lo AJ, Holt DE, Brown DC *et al.* (2014) Treatment of aldosterone-secreting adrenocortical tumors in cats by unilateral adrenalectomy: 10 cases (2002–2012). *Journal of Veterinary Internal Medicine* **28**, 137–143

Maggio F, DeFrancesco TC, Atkins CE *et al.* (2000) Ocular lesions associated with systemic hypertension in cats: 69 cases (1985–1998). *Journal of the American Veterinary Medical Association* **217**, 695–702

Matsuda M, Behrend EN, Kemppainen R *et al.* (2015) Serum aldosterone and cortisol concentrations before and after suppression with fludrocortisone in cats: a pilot study. *Journal of Veterinary Diagnostic Investigation* **27**, 361–368

Syme HM, Fletcher MGR, Bailey SR and Elliott J (2007) Measurement of aldos-terone in feline, canine and human urine. *Journal of Small Animal Practice* **48**, 202–208

Williams TL, Elliott J and Syme HM (2013) Renin-angiotensin-aldosterone system activity in hyperthyroid cats with and without concurrent hypertension. *Journal of Veterinary Internal Medicine* **27**, 522–529

Chapter 33

Phaeochromocytoma

Sara Galac

Introduction

Phaeochromocytomas are adrenal tumours characterized by the overproduction of catecholamines such as adrenaline (epinephrine) and noradrenaline (norepinephrine) (Reusch, 2015). They have been called 'The Great Mimic', as clinical signs can be incorrectly attributed to many other more common disorders. An awareness of their existence represents a crucial initial step for diagnosis, while confirmation requires demonstration of both excessive catecholamine production and an abnormal adrenal gland. Currently, it is estimated that phaeochromocytomas account for 0.01–0.1% of all canine tumours. This prevalence might be underestimated because the biochemical diagnosis of phaeochromocytoma has only recently become possible. In cats, phaeochromocytoma is extremely rare and knowledge is limited to a few case reports. This chapter, therefore, primarily focuses on the canine disease.

Physiology

The adrenal medullary cells, called phaeochromocytes or chromaffin cells, release adrenaline and noradrenaline into the bloodstream. Catecholamines are synthesized from the amino acid tyrosine via a series of modifications with adrenaline and noradrenaline as the end products (Figure 33.1). In most sympathetic postganglionic neurons, noradrenaline is the final product, but the adrenal medulla expresses an additional enzyme, phenylethanolamine-N-methyltransferase (PNMT), allowing adrenaline production. Centripetal blood flow from the adrenal cortex exposes the medulla to sufficiently high cortisol concentrations to allow induction of *PNMT* gene expression. Within the adrenal medulla, noradrenaline is re-leased from the chromaffin vesicles to the cytoplasm and is converted to adrenaline. The amount of stored adrenaline and noradrenaline varies from species to species. In dogs, adrenaline accounts for approximately 70% of

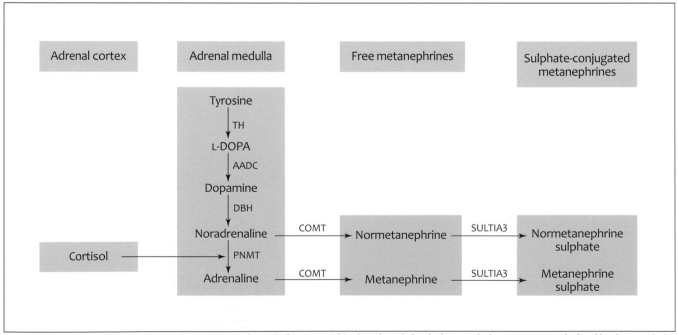

33.1 The biosynthetic pathway and metabolism of catecholamines within the adrenal gland. The catecholamines are metabolized by the catechol-O-methyltransferase (COMT) enzyme and can be measured as free normetanephrine and metanephrine in plasma. In the gastrointestinal tract, kidneys and liver, sulphate conjugation by sulphotransferase enzyme (SULTIA3) takes place. AADC = aromatic amino acid decarboxylase; DBH = dopamine beta-hydroxylase; L-DOPA = 3,4-dihydroxyphenylalanine; PNMT = phenylethanolamine-N-methyltransferase; TH = tyrosine hydroxylase. (Modified from Reusch, 2015)

catecholamines and noradrenaline for 30%. In cats, approximately 60% of catecholamines are adrenaline and 40% are noradrenaline.

The release of catecholamines is triggered by stressors such as anxiety, fear, pain, trauma, haemorrhage or other fluid loss, changes in blood pH, hypoglycaemia, or exposure to excessive heat or cold. The half-life of circulating catecholamines is short and their inactivation begins within minutes. They are metabolized in the liver and kidney but can also be inactivated by deconjugation in the gastrointestinal tract. In addition to this, there is continual metabolism of noradrenaline and adrenaline within the adrenal medulla itself. This results from leakage of noradrenaline and adrenaline from the storage granules and leads to substantial intracellular production of the metabolites metanephrine (metadrenaline) and normetanephrine (normetadrenaline) (Figure 33.2). Most of this metabolism is independent of catecholamine release and accounts for the majority of circulating normetanephrine and metanephrine concentrations (Pacak, 2011).

Catecholamines act exclusively by activating adrenergic G-protein-coupled receptors, divided into alpha and beta types and their subtypes. They are present in most cells of the body and the effect of catecholamines depends on the density of the different receptors, their subtypes and the relative concentrations of adrenaline and noradrenaline. The effects of catecholamines are responsible for reactions to stress and mediate the 'fight or flight' response by increasing heart rate and contractility, blood pressure, respiratory rate, blood glucose and fatty acid concentrations, and alertness, and by decreasing gastrointestinal motility.

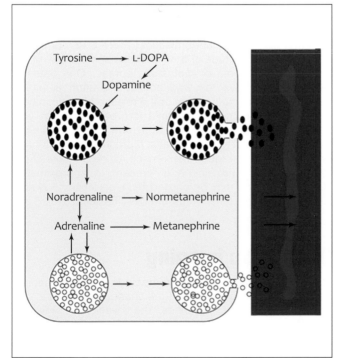

33.2 The pathway of catecholamine synthesis, metabolism and secretion in adrenal chromaffin cells. The secretion of normetanephrine and metanephrine is a continuous action independent of adrenaline and noradrenaline release.
L-DOPA = 3,4-dihydroxyphenylalanine.
(Modified from Pacak, 2011)

Aetiology

The majority of phaeochromocytomas are unilateral and vary in size from a few millimetres up to 15 cm. Local invasion to adjacent vessels, such as phrenicoabdominal veins, the caudal vena cava, renal vessels, adrenal vessels or hepatic veins, or other tissues is observed in up to 56% of dogs. Invasive growth was previously considered a sign of malignancy and was reported in 50% of affected dogs. However, based on the latest definition from the World Health Organization (WHO), phaeochromocytomas are considered malignant only when distant metastases are present. In approximately 20% of dogs with phaeochromocytoma, metastases are described in the regional lymph nodes, liver, spleen, pancreas, lungs, heart, central nervous system (CNS), kidneys or bone at initial presentation. The overall malignancy of 50% for phaeochromocytoma may be an overestimate based on local invasion (Galac and Korpershoek, 2017).

Approximately 50% of dogs with phaeochromocytoma have concurrent neoplasia. These include other endocrine tumours such as cortisol-secreting adrenocortical tumours, adrenocorticotropic hormone-secreting pituitary tumours, parathyroid tumours, thyroid tumours and insulinomas (see Chapter 35). However, other non-endocrine tumours, including lymphoma and haemangiosarcoma, have also been described (Beatrice et al., 2018).

Genetic background

The genetic alterations in dogs with phaeochromocytoma reveal mutations in genes encoding succinate dehydrogenase (SDH) subunit B and D (SDHB and SDHD) (Korpershoek et al., 2019). The SDHB-Arg38Gln and SDHD-Lys122Arg mutations could be responsible for the development of phaeochromocytoma in dogs. In humans, mutations in SDHB are associated with a high likelihood of metastasis and malignancy. The link between SDH variants and neoplasia appears to be through the stabilization of hypoxia-inducible factor (HIF), which is normally induced by hypoxia. Stabilization of HIF1-alpha results in the transcription of genes encoding vascular endothelial growth factor (VEGF) and other genes potentially involved in the development of neoplasia. Hypothetically, chronic hypoxia in brachycephalic dogs might play a role in the development of chemoreceptor neoplasia and also phaeochromocytoma, although this remains to be determined.

Clinical features

Signalment

Phaeochromocytomas occur most commonly in older dogs. However, the age at diagnosis ranges from 1.6 to 18 years. There is no apparent sex or breed predisposition, and the more frequent description of phaeochromocytoma in some breeds (Rhodesian Ridgeback, Labrador Retriever, Boxer, Golden Retriever, Shih Tzu) probably reflects their popularity more than an increased risk of the disease.

History and physical examination

Clinical signs are usually related to the direct actions of secreted catecholamines and/or the space-occupying or invasive nature of the adrenal mass. Phaeochromocytoma should be considered a potentially life-threatening disease that can result in collapse and sudden death due to massive catecholamine release or tumour rupture. There appears to be a correlation between tumour size and severity of clinical signs. Small tumours are often associated with mild signs, whereas large tumours are often found in dogs with serious and life-threatening clinical signs, invasion into the vena cava and the possibility of tumour rupture. There may be progression from mild to severe over time.

Hormone secretion from the tumour is unpredictable and episodic and, consequently, the clinical picture varies considerably. Episodes of increased catecholamine release may occur several times per day or only at intervals of weeks to months. The triggers for catecholamine secretion in dogs are usually not known.

The clinical manifestations of catecholamine excess are often non-specific, including weakness, abdominal pain, anorexia and discomfort. Those related to the cardiorespiratory system include panting, tachycardia, arrhythmias and collapse. Premature supraventricular and ventricular complexes and tachycardia are the most common arrhythmias. The conduction disturbances are due to myocardial damage, ischaemia and fibrosis, which are a result of prolonged exposure to catecholamines from the phaeochromocytoma. Rarely, phaeochromocytoma is associated with bradycardia and atrioventricular block. Myocardial lesions (necrosis, degeneration, lymphoplasmacytic myocarditis, haemorrhage, fibrosis) identified in dogs are similar to those in humans with phaeochromocytoma-associated cardiomyopathy (Edmondson et al., 2015).

Systemic hypertension, one of the hallmarks of phaeochromocytoma, is present in approximately 50% of affected dogs at the time of initial examination. Consequently, a failure to document systemic hypertension does not rule out the disease. The percentage of dogs that present with consequences of hypertension, such as nasal bleeding, retinal bleeding, retinal detachment and blindness, is low. Most likely, catecholamine release and hypertensive episodes are not sustained enough to cause such damage.

The neuromuscular system may be affected by catecholamine-induced vasospasm, haemorrhage within the CNS or brain metastases. Dogs may present with pacing, disorientation, anxiety and seizures. Paresis, lameness and pain have been reported as a result of metastases to the vertebral canal or bone.

Polyuria and polydipsia (PU/PD) are among the reported clinical signs of phaeochromocytoma. The pathophysiological mechanism is not completely understood and may be multifactorial. Catecholamines, in particular noradrenaline, suppress the release of arginine vasopressin, which may lead to PU/PD with low urine specific gravity (SG). In some dogs with phaeochromocytoma, primary polydipsia is suspected because dogs are able to produce concentrated urine and have a urine SG greater than 1.030 after water deprivation or even in a first morning urine sample (Reusch, 2015).

Clinical signs may also be caused by large tumour size, invasion of surrounding structures and metastases. The invasive nature of phaeochromocytoma commonly leads to occlusion of the caudal vena cava, which may cause ascites, hindlimb oedema and distension of the caudal epigastric veins. However, clinical signs may not be present even if there is complete occlusion of the caudal vena cava. In such cases, slow tumour growth presumably allows for the development of sufficient collateral circulation.

Spontaneous tumour rupture with retroperitoneal haemorrhage is possible in dogs with large phaeochromocytomas, and owners need to be made aware of this risk.

Dogs with tumour rupture usually present with acute-onset lethargy, tachypnoea, tachycardia, pale mucous membranes, prolonged capillary refill time and a painful abdomen. Emergency treatment is required.

The most common clinical signs in dogs with phaeochromocytoma are presented in Figure 33.3.

Clinical signs	Prevalence (%)
Weakness/lethargy	40
Cardiac arrhythmias	30
Panting/tachypnoea	25
Anorexia	25
Vomiting	24
Collapse	22
Polyuria and polydipsia	20
Weight loss	20
Abdominal pain	14
Pale mucous membranes	14
Abdominal distension	12
Seizures	8

33.3 Approximate prevalence of the most common clinical signs in dogs with phaeochromocytoma.

Clinicopathological features

There are no consistent changes in haematology, serum biochemistry or urinalysis that support the suspicion of phaeochromocytoma. However, as most affected dogs are older and may have concurrent disorders, a full clinicopathological profile should always be performed. Mild to moderate non-regenerative anaemia associated with chronic disease may be present, either because of the phaeochromocytoma or due to comorbidities. In chronically bleeding cases, thrombocytosis is present. Increased liver enzyme activities (alanine aminotransferase (ALT), alkaline phosphatase and aspartate aminotransferase) are the most common biochemical abnormalities. There is no correlation between the magnitude of their increase and the size of the phaeochromocytoma or metastatic spread. One potential explanation for liver enzyme activity elevation is hypertension-induced hepatopathy or the release of inflammatory cytokines. Hypercholesterolaemia is present in dogs with advanced disease and is most likely due to catecholamine-induced lipolysis. Hyperglycaemia, if present, is usually very mild and does not require intervention. Urine SG varies from 1.006 to 1.044. Proteinuria is present in approximately 30% of dogs and may be caused by hypertension-induced kidney damage or other comorbidities (Reusch, 2015).

Diagnostic imaging

The visualization of phaeochromocytoma with diagnostic imaging allows assessment of the shape, architecture, size and margination of the mass, the invasion of adjacent structures and the symmetry of the adrenal glands.

Ultrasonography

There is no ultrasonographic appearance that is typical for phaeochromocytoma in dogs. Most are unilateral and the contralateral adrenal gland is of normal size and shape, but approximately 10% are bilateral. It is not unusual for phaeochromocytoma to be diagnosed after an incidental adrenal mass is visualized during abdominal ultrasonography for an unrelated problem (see Chapter 34). Cortisol-secreting adrenocortical tumours remain the most challenging differential diagnosis. Both tumour types can be bilateral; even if a unilateral lesion is present, the atrophy of the contralateral adrenal gland expected with adrenal-dependent hypercortisolism is difficult to establish or may not be apparent. Contrast-enhanced ultrasonography might be helpful in differentiating phaeochromocytoma from other adrenal tumour types. A rapid wash-in and wash-out of the contrast was reported to be characteristic for phaeochromocytoma and can aid in making a definitive diagnosis (Nagumo *et al.*, 2020).

Tumour thrombi extending into local vessels may be visible. These thrombi likely invade the phrenicoabdominal vein first and then extend into the caudal vena cava. Such changes have been described in up to 50% of affected dogs. However, this relatively high percentage may be the result of delayed diagnosis of phaeochromocytoma in older studies. Invasive growth is not synonymous with malignancy as it may represent only the expansion of a large tumour into structures with minimal resistance. The correlation between tumour size, invasiveness and malignancy requires further study.

Fine-needle aspiration

Percutaneous ultrasound-guided fine-needle aspiration is one of the most used techniques for the collection of samples for cytological analysis. Adrenal cytology can discriminate between cortical and medullary cells with a diagnostic accuracy of approximately 87%, but distinguishing benign from malignant lesions is problematic. Fine-needle aspiration of functional and hormonally inactive adrenocortical and adrenomedullary tumours is considered relatively safe, with the most common complications including haemorrhage, ventricular tachycardia and respiratory distress (Pey *et al.*, 2020). However, only a small number of dogs with phaeochromocytoma have been evaluated, and therefore biochemical diagnosis is preferred (see 'Assessment of catecholamine and metabolite concentrations', below).

Computed tomography

A more precise and complete evaluation of tumour size, shape and architecture is possible using computed tomography (CT) and this is superior to detect vascular invasion (Figure 33.4). Computed tomography is also advantageous for evaluating metastases and comorbidities including hypercortisolism. When performing CT in a dog with a phaeochromocytoma, it is advised to scan the abdomen, thorax and head.

Nuclear imaging

While ultrasonography and CT have excellent sensitivity for detecting adrenal tumours, these anatomical imaging approaches lack the specificity required to unequivocally identify a mass as a phaeochromocytoma. The higher specificity of functional imaging with 131-iodine-labelled meta-iodobenzylguanidine (^{131}I-MIBG) scintigraphy offers an alternative approach. This radioisotope competes with noradrenaline for uptake and storage in neurosecretory granules of catecholamine cells and is thereby a marker of functional adrenomedullary tissue. Its use in dogs has been reported only once and the technique is not widely available (Bommarito *et al.*, 2011).

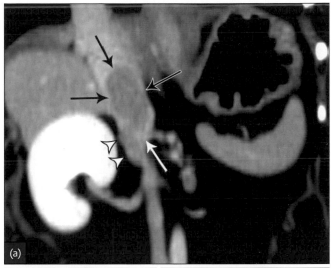

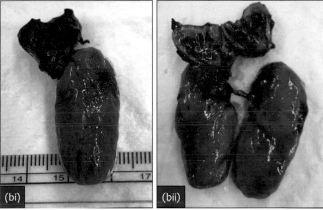

33.4 (a) Transverse computed tomographic image of a phaeochromocytoma (arrowed) after intravenous administration of contrast medium in an 8-year-old dog. Severe ingrowth in the vena cava is visible (arrowheads). (bi) The tumour was successfully removed. (bii) The cut surface of the adrenal mass, comprising the adrenal gland and tumour thrombus removed from the vena cava.

Assessment of catecholamine and metabolite concentrations

Biochemical evaluation of phaeochromocytoma includes measurement of plasma or urinary catecholamines and their metabolites, metanephrine and normetanephrine, the so-called free metanephrines (Galac and Korpershoek, 2017). The reason for measuring metanephrines is based on the intramedullary metabolism of catecholamines: the production and secretion of metanephrines in tumour cells is continuous and more accurately reflects medullary function than the release of catecholamines, which is usually episodic (see Figure 33.2).

In dogs, biochemical testing for phaeochromocytoma has recently become available. Measurement of urinary catecholamines is performed in a single voided sample that can be collected in the hospital. Concentrations are expressed as a ratio to the creatinine concentration in the same urine sample (Figure 33.5) (Salesov *et al.*, 2015). Acidification of urine to pH <2 depends on the laboratory method used and is not always required. Normetanephrine:creatinine has a higher sensitivity than metanephrine:creatinine, adrenaline:creatinine and

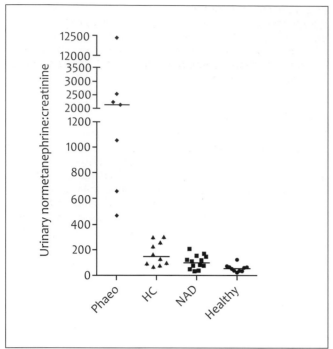

33.5 Urinary normetanephrine:creatinine in healthy dogs, dogs with hypercortisolism (HC), dogs with non-adrenal diseases (NAD) and dogs with phaeochromocytoma (Phaeo). Significantly higher urinary ratios were measured in dogs with phaeochromocytoma compared with healthy dogs and dogs with hypercortisolism.

noradrenaline:creatinine in the diagnosis of canine phaeochromocytoma and discriminates between healthy and sick dogs and dogs with phaeochromocytoma with no overlap. This is not surprising, as canine phaeochromocytomas predominantly produce noradrenaline, which is then metabolized to normetanephrine.

Measurement of plasma free normetanephrine concentration is also superior to plasma free metanephrine; plasma free normetanephrine is significantly higher in dogs with phaeochromocytoma compared with healthy dogs and dogs with other adrenal tumours (Figure 33.6; Gostelow *et al.*, 2013). Sampling conditions are critical for reliable results and it is important to follow laboratory-specific sample handling requirements (see Chapter 3). The availability of species- and laboratory-specific reference intervals is essential for accurate interpretation of results.

Currently, there is no consensus regarding the preferred use of plasma or urine, but there is a strong preference for normetanephrine determination. The sensitivity and specificity of either test in dogs is largely unknown so far. Of importance in interpretation of the results is the discrimination between phaeochromocytomas and other diseases, in particular hypercortisolism. The similarities in clinical features of phaeochromocytoma and adrenal-dependent hypercortisolism make the differentiation challenging. Screening tests for hypercortisolism can yield false-positive results in dogs with phaeochromocytoma, just as with other comorbidities. Additionally, endogenous and exogenous glucocorticoids can increase catecholamine production. In humans with phaeochromocytoma, dexamethasone used in the suppression test to diagnose hypercortisolism may induce a hypertensive crisis. This has not yet been described in dogs with phaeochromocytoma but close monitoring during testing is warranted. The best discriminatory test appears to be determination of the normetanephrine concentration in either urine or

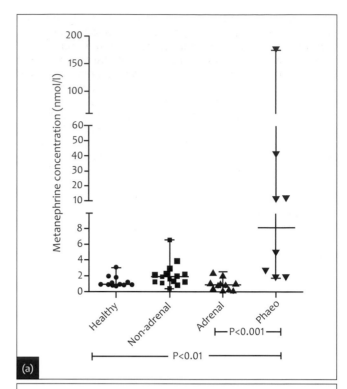

(a)

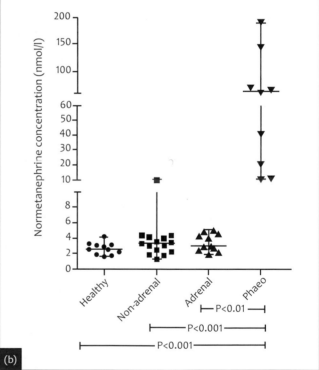

(b)

33.6 Scatter plots of free plasma (a) metanephrine and (b) normetanephrine concentrations in healthy dogs, dogs with non-adrenal disease, dogs with adrenocortical tumours (Adrenal) and dogs with phaeochromocytoma (Phaeo). The statistical significance between the phaeochromocytoma group and the other groups is shown below the X axis.
(Modified from Gostelow *et al.*, 2013)

plasma. The influence of drugs on normetanephrine and metanephrine concentrations has not been studied extensively in dogs to date. Based on the experience in human medicine, phenoxybenzamine may lead to false-positive results and should be prescribed only after samples for endocrine testing have been taken.

Alternatively, measurement of serum inhibin can be helpful in dogs. Inhibin concentrations should be undetectable in dogs with phaeochromocytoma, but not in those with hypercortisolism. This measurement is not applicable in sexually intact dogs because gonadal and adrenocortical inhibin cannot be distinguished in serum.

Recently, measuring urinary 3-methoxy-4-hydroxy-mandelic acid (vanillylmandelic acid (VMA)) concentrations has been suggested (Soler Arias et al., 2021). This is an end product of catecholamine metabolism almost exclusively produced in the liver and excreted in the urine. The urinary VMA:creatinine performed well in differentiating dogs with phaeochromocytoma from healthy dogs and those with pituitary-dependent hypercortisolism. However, there was some overlap between dogs with phaeochromocytoma and dogs with adrenal-dependent hypercortisolism. Sampling requires acidification of urine to prevent VMA degradation.

Treatment

Adrenalectomy is the preferred treatment for phaeochromocytoma because removal of the tumour will reverse the clinical signs associated with excessive catecholamine release and avoid the complications of uncontrolled tumour growth. Complications occurring during surgery are mainly catecholamine-induced effects, which may be serious and potentially life-threatening. Prerequisites for a successful outcome are appropriate preoperative medical treatment, an experienced anaesthetist, a skilled surgeon and adequate facilities for postoperative intensive care.

Preoperative medical management

Catecholamine-induced complications associated with surgical removal of phaeochromocytoma in dogs include hypertensive crisis, cardiac arrhythmias, pulmonary oedema and cardiac ischaemia. To avoid them, treatment with phenoxybenzamine should be initiated at least 2 weeks before adrenalectomy. Phenoxybenzamine is an alpha-adrenergic receptor antagonist that irreversibly binds to alpha-1 and alpha-2 adrenergic receptors and blocks the alpha-adrenergic response to circulating adrenaline and noradrenaline. Phenoxybenzamine does not block the synthesis of catecholamines. It decreases blood pressure, supports the expansion of contracted blood volume and decreases the frequency of ventricular arrhythmias. The starting dose is 0.25 mg/kg administered orally q12h and the dose should be increased incrementally every 3–5 days until a final dose of 0.75–1 mg/kg q12h is reached (Reusch, 2015). The last dose should be given in the evening the day before surgery. During treatment, blood pressure should be regularly monitored to avoid hypotension. Often, the dose titration is based on feedback from the owner. If the dog shows signs of hypotension, such as lethargy and weakness, the dose of phenoxybenzamine should be decreased. The mortality rate after adrenalectomy is significantly lower in dogs pre-treated with phenoxybenzamine than in untreated dogs.

Another option for preoperative preparation is treatment with calcium channel blockers, but these are less effective than alpha-blockers. If tachycardia or tachyarrhythmias are likely to occur during the preoperative period, a beta-blocker may be added to the treatment regimen alongside the alpha-blocker. A selective beta-1 antagonist (e.g. atenolol) is preferred over a non-selective beta-blocker (e.g. propranolol) to minimize the effect on beta-2-mediated vasodilation. Beta blockade should never be used before the dog has received phenoxybenzamine for several days. With beta blockade alone, hypertension can become more severe because alpha-1-mediated vasoconstriction is unopposed.

Adrenalectomy

Close communication between the surgeon and the anaesthetist is essential during adrenalectomy because manipulation of the tumour can cause a surge in catecholamine release. The anaesthetist should be able to anticipate these critical stages and manage them in advance. If this is not sufficient, a short-acting alpha-adrenergic antagonist (phentolamine) is administered to combat hypertension and esmolol, an ultra-short-acting beta-1 antagonist, may be added if tachycardia persists.

Laparoscopic adrenalectomy has gained popularity in veterinary medicine and observational studies have shown that it results in faster recovery, shorter hospitalization, fewer wound complications and shorter surgical time than open laparotomy. The size of the phaeochromocytoma and the extent of vascular invasion are the most important criteria in choosing between laparoscopy and open laparotomy. Masses up to 5 cm in diameter without invasion of the caudal vena cava are amenable to laparoscopy, while open adrenalectomy is indicated in cases with vascular invasion.

Significant prognostic indicators for the survival of dogs with phaeochromocytoma after adrenalectomy include lack of intraoperative arrhythmias, pre-treatment with phenoxybenzamine, younger age and short duration of surgery. There is no association between the size of the tumour or the presence of vascular invasion and survival, but it is possible that the presence of vascular invasion increases surgical time and thus indirectly influences survival. In line with this, extended invasion of the caudal vena cava beyond the hepatic hilus was associated with a higher postoperative mortality rate but did not affect long-term prognosis. A median survival time of 53 weeks has been reported in dogs following surgical removal of phaeochromocytoma, with some living for 2–3 years (Massari et al., 2011).

Complications that can occur postoperatively include cardiac arrhythmias, respiratory distress, haemorrhage and hypertension. Hypotension is also possible, due to the abrupt fall in circulating catecholamines after tumour removal in the continuing presence of alpha-adrenoreceptor blockade (by phenoxybenzamine).

Medical management

When a phaeochromocytoma is not amenable to surgical removal or surgery is prevented by concurrent disorders, metastases or other reasons, medical treatment with tyrosine kinase inhibitors (TKIs) is an option (Musser et al., 2018). This approach has been translated from use in humans with inoperable phaeochromocytomas, where TKIs appear to have a biological response of approximately 60%. In dogs, toceranib phosphate is an oral TKI approved for use in recurrent mast cell tumours, but it appears to have efficacy against multiple tumour types, including phaeochromocytoma. Toceranib phosphate blocks the two key receptors associated with angiogenesis: VEGF and platelet-derived growth factor. The recommended dosing regimen is to administer 2.75 mg/kg orally q48h or on a Monday–Wednesday–Friday schedule. Treatment may be associated with adverse reactions, such as diarrhoea, decreased appetite, lameness, muscle weakness, proteinuria and hypertension. Among laboratory abnormalities, anaemia, thrombocytopenia and neutropenia can occur, as well as increased ALT activity and creatinine concentration. Dose interruptions and dose reductions may be needed during the treatment course depending upon the severity of clinical signs. The dose should be adjusted based on regular veterinary assessments during the first 6 weeks and approximately every 6 weeks thereafter. After 2 weeks, haematology and biochemistry are required to evaluate the safety of the drug. After 6 weeks, these are combined with diagnostic imaging. The treatment is continued if the adrenal mass is stable or if partial remission is achieved. Complete remission has thus far not been reported. Treatment with toceranib phosphate may provide a survival advantage in dogs. The effect of TKIs in dogs with phaeochromocytoma is described in only one retrospective study involving five dogs (Musser *et al.*, 2018). In this study, three dogs without metastatic disease had progression-free intervals of 28, 36 and 61 weeks. Two dogs with metastatic disease had survival times of 11 and 18 weeks. Toceranib phosphate can be combined with phenoxybenzamine if indicated.

Histopathology and immunohistochemistry

Histopathologically, phaeochromocytomas are characterized by polygonal-shaped basophilic neoplastic cells with rounded nuclei, arranged in nests, surrounded by a fibrovascular stromal network. The diagnosis of phaeochromocytoma is supported by immunohistochemistry using several different markers, including chromogranin A and synaptophysin, which stain the chromaffin cells, and S-100, which is specific for the sustentacular cells (Galac and Korpershoek, 2017). These markers have high diagnostic sensitivity for phaeochromocytoma and help distinguish it from cortisol-secreting adrenocortical tumours (Beatrice *et al.*, 2018).

Histopathological criteria of tumour cells as defined by the WHO classification scheme do not predict malignant behaviour; only the presence of distant metastasis is confirmative of malignancy. Hence, the histopathological scoring system has been refined and linked to prognosis. The phaeochromocytoma of the adrenal gland scaled score (PASS) is based on the combination of 12 different histopathological parameters and is expected to be higher in cases with malignant lesions compared with those with a benign course (Zini *et al.*, 2019). In dogs with phaeochromocytoma, however, the PASS did not correlate with survival, and its significance is currently unknown. Another approach to malignancy is linked to the genetic background of phaeochromocytoma. In humans, the mutation status of *SDHB* is associated with penetrance and malignant behaviour, and the frequency of metastatic behaviour is approximately 30% in *SDHB* mutation carriers (Korpershoek *et al.*, 2019). Loss of SDHB protein expression, evaluated by immunohistochemistry, is highly correlated with SDH mutation status. Immunohistochemistry of the SDH family is a promising approach to evaluating the prognosis for dogs with phaeochromocytoma.

Prognosis

Prognosis depends on the size of the tumour, its endocrine activity, vascular invasion, and the presence of metastases. Additional prognostic factors are age, general health and the presence of concurrent disease. Dogs that undergo successful adrenalectomy can live for several years. Survival times of dogs receiving medical treatment only are not known so far. Most dogs with phaeochromocytoma die because of complications caused by catecholamine excess, tumour thrombosis, tumour invasion into surrounding tissues, tumour rupture or metastases.

References and further reading

Abed FM, Brown MA, Al-Mahmood OA and Dark MJ (2020) SDHB and SDHA immunohistochemistry in canine pheochromocytomas. *Animals* **10**, 1683

Beatrice L, Boretti FS, Sieber-Ruckstuhl NS *et al.* (2018) Concurrent endocrine neoplasias in dogs and cats: a retrospective study (2004–2014). *Veterinary Record* **182**, 323

Bommarito JA, Lattimer JC, Selting KA *et al.* (2011) Treatment of malignant pheochromocytoma in a dog using ^{131}I metaiodobenzylguanidine. *Journal of the American Animal Hospital Association* **47**, e188–e194

Edmondson EF, Bright JM, Halsey CH and Ehrhart EJ (2015) Pathologic and cardiovascular characterization of pheochromocytoma-associated cardiomyopathy in dogs. *Veterinary Pathology* **52**, 338–343

Galac S and Korpershoek E (2017) Pheochromocytomas and paragangliomas in humans and dogs. *Veterinary and Comparative Oncology* **15**, 1158–1170

Gostelow R, Bridger N and Syme HM (2013) Plasma-free metanephrine and free normetanephrine measurement for the diagnosis of pheochromocytoma in dogs. *Journal of Veterinary Internal Medicine* **27**, 83–90

Korpershoek E, Dieduksman DAER, Grinwis GCM *et al.* (2019) Molecular alterations in dog pheochromocytomas and paragangliomas. *Cancers* **11**, 607

Massari F, Nicoli S, Romanelli G, Buracco P and Zini E (2011) Adrenalectomy in dogs with adrenal gland tumors: 52 cases (2002–2008). *Journal of the American Veterinary Medical Association* **239**, 216–221

Musser ML, Taikowski KL, Johannes CM and Bergman PJ (2018) Retrospective evaluation of toceranib phosphate (Palladia®) use in the treatment of inoperable, metastatic, or recurrent canine pheochromocytomas: 5 dogs (2014–2017). *BMC Veterinary Research* **14**, 272

Nagumo T, Ishigaki K, Yoshida O *et al.* (2020) Utility of contrast-enhanced ultrasound in differential diagnosis of adrenal tumors in dogs. *Journal of Veterinary Medical Science* **82**, 1594–1601

Pacak K (2011) Pheochromocytoma: a catecholamine and oxidative stress disorder. *Endocrine Regulations* **45**, 65–90

Pey P, Diana A, Rossi F *et al.* (2020) Safety of percutaneous ultrasound-guided fine-needle aspiration of adrenal lesions in dogs: perception of the procedure by radiologists and presentation of 50 cases. *Journal of Veterinary Internal Medicine* **34**, 626–635

Reusch CE (2015) Pheochromocytoma and multiple endocrine neoplasia. In: *Canine and Feline Endocrinology, 4th edn*, ed. EC Feldman, RW Nelson, CE Reusch, JCR Scott-Moncrieff and EN Behrend, pp. 521–544. Elsevier, St. Louis

Salesov E, Boretti FS, Sieber-Ruckstuhl NS *et al.* (2015) Urinary and plasma catecholamines and metanephrines in dogs with pheochromocytoma, hypercortisolism, nonadrenal disease and in healthy dogs. *Journal of Veterinary Internal Medicine* **29**, 597–602

Soler Arias EA, Trigo RH, Miceli DD *et al.* (2021) Urinary vanillylmandelic acid:creatinine ratio in dogs with pheochromocytoma. *Domestic Animal Endocrinology* **74**, 106559

Zini E, Nolli S, Ferri F *et al.* (2019) Pheochromocytoma in dogs undergoing adrenalectomy. *Veterinary Pathology* **56**, 358–368

Chapter 34

The incidentally discovered adrenal mass

Carlos Melián and Laura Pérez-López

Introduction

An incidentally discovered adrenal mass, also known as an incidentaloma, is an adrenal mass discovered in cases involving diagnostic imaging or post-mortem examination for reasons other than adrenal disease.

Adrenal tumours may be benign or malignant, and functional or non-functional (Figure 34.1). When functional, either one or several hormones may be secreted. Based on these considerations, the finding of an adrenal mass represents a significant diagnostic and therapeutic challenge.

An adrenal incidentaloma is a common finding in humans, where its prevalence approaches 3% in middle age and increases to as much as 10% in the elderly. Most (71–84%) humans with an adrenal incidentaloma have a

benign, non-functional adrenal mass. Regular monitoring and evaluation of tumour growth is recommended (Fassnacht *et al.*, 2016).

Adrenal incidentalomas are being diagnosed with increasing frequency in small animals; however, there are no prospective studies with a large number of cases. In two retrospective studies performed in dogs that underwent ultrasound or computed tomography (CT) examinations without an initial suspicion of adrenal disease, the prevalence of incidental adrenal gland masses was 4% and 9.3%, respectively. Most (>80%) affected dogs are 9 years old or older. However, dogs examined for a reason other than neoplasia were less likely to have an incidental adrenal mass, with a prevalence of only 2–3% (Cook *et al.*, 2014; Baum *et al.*, 2016). In human medicine, the finding of an adrenal mass in a patient with known extra-adrenal malignancies does not meet the strict definition of adrenal incidentaloma, as adrenal metastases are not unexpected (Fassnacht *et al.*, 2016). Similarly, adrenal metastases should be considered in dogs and cats, as 21% of dogs and approximately 15% of cats with metastatic tumours present with adrenal metastases (Labelle and De Cock, 2005).

In small animals, the most common functional adrenal tumours cause adrenocorticotropic hormone (ACTH)-independent hypercortisolism in dogs and primary hyperaldosteronism in cats (see Chapters 29 and 32). However, other adrenal masses, including phaeochromocytoma, sex-hormone-secreting neoplasms and non-functional adrenal masses, should also be considered.

Adrenal cortex[a]
• Adenoma (non-functional or functional: glucocorticoid-secreting tumour, mineralocorticoid-secreting tumour, sex-hormone-secreting tumour)
• Adenocarcinoma (non-functional or functional: glucocorticoid-secreting tumour, mineralocorticoid-secreting tumour, sex-hormone-secreting tumour)
• Nodular hyperplasia (non-functional or functional: adrenocorticotropic hormone-dependent hypercortisolism)
Adrenal medulla
• Phaeochromocytoma
• Ganglioneuroma
• Neuroblastoma
Adrenal metastasis
• Carcinomas (most commonly mammary gland, pulmonary, prostate, bladder, gastric or pancreatic)
• Sarcomas (most commonly haemangiosarcoma, osteosarcoma or histiocytic sarcoma)
• Melanoma
• Mast cell tumour
• Lymphoma
• Mesothelioma
Other adrenal masses
• Myelolipoma
• Granulomatous disease (fungal, feline infectious peritonitis)
• Teratoma
• Cyst
• Haematoma

34.1 Differential diagnoses in a case with a suspected adrenal mass. [a] Tumours arising from the adrenal cortex may secrete more than one type of hormone (i.e. glucocorticoids, mineralocorticoids, sex hormones or combinations thereof).

Diagnostic approach

In clinical practice, it is essential to separate adrenal nodules or masses that require intervention (functional or malignant tumours) from those that can safely be left untreated and simply monitored (non-functional and benign incidentalomas). The first consideration is to ensure that an adrenal nodule or mass truly exists. Ultrasonography is the most commonly used tool for visualizing an adrenal tumour, although it may be difficult to distinguish adrenal tumours from other primary adrenal lesions (nodular hyperplasia, haematoma, granuloma, cyst) or adrenal metastases. An adrenal mass or nodule should be a reliably repeatable finding on abdominal ultrasonography.

Ultrasonographic appearance

Normal adrenal glands appear as hypoechoic and ovoid, fusiform, peanut- or bean-shaped structures on ultrasonographic examination. In healthy dogs and cats, reference intervals for maximum thickness (dorsoventral height) on ultrasonographic evaluation depend on bodyweight (Figures 34.2 and 34.3) (Melián et al., 2021; Pérez-López et al., 2021).

Bodyweight (kg)	Maximal thickness (mm)					
	Lower limit		Median		Upper limit	
	Left	Right	Left	Right	Left	Right
2–5	3.2	2.8	4.2	4.1	5.1	5.3
5–10	3.0	3.4	4.3	5.2	5.5	6.8
10–20	3.8	3.5	5.0	5.6	6.4	7.5
20–40	4.7	5.1	6.1	7.1	7.3	8.7

34.2 Reference intervals for the maximal dorsoventral thickness of the left and right adrenal glands in dogs, based on data from 86 clinically healthy dogs.
(Data from Melián et al., 2021)

Bodyweight (kg)	Maximal thickness (mm)		
	Lower limit	Median	Upper limit
≤4	2.4	3.2	3.9
4–8	2.6	3.7	4.8

34.3 Reference intervals for the maximal dorsoventral adrenal gland thickness in cats, based on data from 39 clinically healthy cats.
(Data from Pérez-López et al., 2021)

An adrenal incidentaloma is suspected when significant enlargement or altered shape of an adrenal gland is unexpectedly found (Figure 34.4). The changes may vary from small nodules to large masses. Echogenicity is variable, ranging from solidly homogeneous to a mixed heterogeneous and possibly cystic appearance. An adrenal mass can be considered as an irregular enlargement and loss of the normal shape of the adrenal gland. Adrenal masses may invade or compress adjacent structures.

Adrenal nodules are focal, well defined rounded lesions within the parenchyma of the adrenal gland but without loss of adrenal shape. Adrenal nodules can be solitary lesions or can appear as multifocal lesions. Nodules are commonly hyperplastic cortical lesions, but they can also

be a sign of an adrenocortical tumour or phaeochromocytoma (Pagani et al., 2016).

In humans, an adrenal mass is arbitrarily defined as a mass of at least 1 cm in diameter; no further work-up is recommended if the lesion is less than 1 cm unless clinical signs suggestive of endocrine disease are present (Fassnacht et al., 2016). By contrast, in dogs, the size of incidentalomas should be interpreted depending on the dog's size. There is a large variation in the size of dogs, and it is more difficult to define the size of what should be considered abnormal. An adrenal gland with a thickness of 1 cm could represent a significant increase of adrenal gland size in a 5 kg dog but it might represent a mild increase in a 30 kg dog.

Functional or non-functional

Once an adrenal incidentaloma has been confirmed, the diagnostic and therapeutic approach is based on clinical presentation (age, clinical signs, laboratory features, blood pressure measurement) and the characteristics of the adrenal mass (size, hormonal activity, invasion of other structures and presence of metastases) (Figure 34.5). A detailed history and physical examination are of immense value in determining the diagnostic plan, as some clinical signs may have been largely unnoticed or their significance may have been misinterpreted.

Functional tumours should be differentiated from non-functional tumours. As such, measurement of blood pressure is important for diagnostic investigation and treatment planning. Persistently or intermittently increased blood pressure increases the likelihood of a functional adrenal mass. Phaeochromocytoma and functional cortical tumours leading to hypercortisolism are well recognized causes of hypertension in dogs and aldosteronoma in cats (see Chapters 29, 32 and 33). To confirm the diagnosis, endocrine function tests should be performed based on the clinical signs in each case.

Evaluation of the contralateral adrenal gland thickness is also important. In cases with ACTH-independent hypercortisolism, excess cortisol can chronically suppress ACTH release, leading to atrophy of the contralateral adrenal gland. This finding supports the suspicion of a functional adrenocortical tumour. However, imaging techniques have some limitations; for example, it may be difficult, if not impossible, to differentiate a cortisol-producing adrenal tumour from other adrenal tumours, such as phaeochromocytoma, aldosteronoma, and metastatic and non-functional tumours.

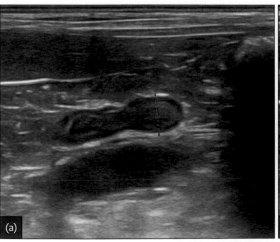
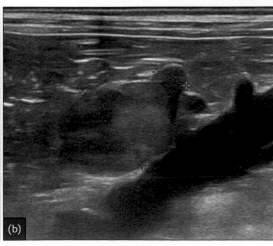

34.4 (a) Normal left adrenal gland shape and thickness (5.2 mm) in a dog weighing 5.3 kg. (b) Unexpectedly discovered enlargement (15.5 mm) in the cranial pole of the left adrenal gland in a dog weighing 8 kg.

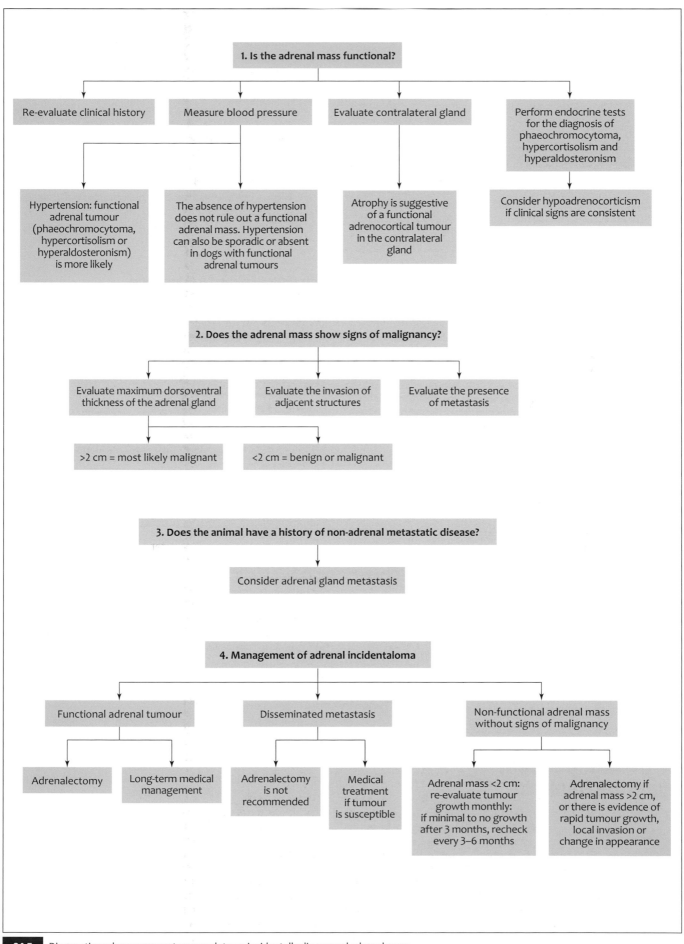

34.5 Diagnostic and management approach to an incidentally discovered adrenal mass.

Benign or malignant

Once the functionality of the adrenal tumour has been evaluated, signs of malignancy of the tumour should be investigated. Tumours of the adrenal gland larger than 2 cm are more likely to be malignant, and those larger than 4 cm are almost always malignant. In canine ACTH-independent hypercortisolism, dogs with a tumour diameter above 3 cm had a reduced survival time compared with dogs with a tumour diameter below 3 cm (Sanders *et al.*, 2019). Advanced imaging studies such as CT and magnetic resonance imaging (MRI) may be helpful in detecting adrenal masses, in lesion localization and also in better determining the extent of disease with regards to local invasion and metastases. In humans, CT and MRI have standardized criteria used to differentiate benign from malignant adrenal masses (Fassnacht *et al.*, 2016; Mayo-Smith *et al.*, 2017). Such criteria are lacking in veterinary medicine. Interestingly, a recent study in dogs suggested that CT features may be helpful to predict tumour type. Precontrast attenuation value of the adrenal tumour, long axis of the thrombus, presence of tumour rupture and size of the contralateral adrenal gland might assist in the differentiation between adrenal carcinoma and phaeochromocytoma (Pey *et al.*, 2022).

Fine-needle aspiration and biopsy

In dogs, ultrasound-guided percutaneous fine-needle aspiration (FNA) has good diagnostic accuracy in distinguishing neoplasms of cortical origin from those of medullary origin. However, benign and malignant tumours cannot be accurately distinguished by cytology alone (Bertazzolo *et al.*, 2014). Recently, one study suggested that ultrasound-guided FNA may be a low-risk procedure in dogs. In that study, 58 cytological analyses were performed in 50 dogs (23 with phaeochromocytoma): adverse effects (haemorrhage and acute respiratory distress) were noted in only four (8%) dogs, although one died (2%) (Pey *et al.*, 2020). Cytological results were inconclusive in approximately 30% of cases. Risk–benefit analysis should be considered before performing this procedure in dogs.

In humans, adrenal biopsy in the diagnostic work-up for adrenal masses is not recommended unless there is a history of extra-adrenal malignancy or the lesion has not been conclusively characterized as benign. However, its use also requires a careful risk–benefit evaluation and functional tumours, especially phaeochromocytoma, should be ruled out first as severe adverse effects such as fatal haemorrhage or hypertensive crises have been described. Additionally, dissemination of adrenocortical carcinoma after biopsy has been reported in humans (Fassnacht *et al.*, 2016).

ACTH-independent hypercortisolism

A cortisol-producing adrenal mass causing clinical signs of hypercortisolism is the most common adrenal neoplasm in dogs. If there are any supportive clinical or clinicopathological features, adrenal function tests should be performed to confirm or rule out hypercortisolism (see Chapters 29 and 30). In a dog with clinical signs of hypercortisolism and a confirmed adrenal mass, a post-ACTH cortisol concentration within the reference interval does not rule out a cortisol-producing adrenal tumour.

Most cases of ACTH-independent hypercortisolism are caused by a unilateral adrenal mass with atrophy of the contralateral gland. However, some dogs with unilateral ACTH-independent hypercortisolism do not develop obvious contralateral adrenal atrophy. In these dogs, ultrasonographic differentiation between ACTH-dependent or -independent hypercortisolism is challenging and might rely on further diagnostic tests including endogenous ACTH measurement.

Other forms of ACTH-independent hypercortisolism may occur. Bilateral adrenocortical neoplasia is not uncommon, occurring in approximately 10% of cases. Concurrent ACTH-dependent and -independent hypercortisolism has also been described in 5% of dogs with hypercortisolism (van Bokhorst *et al.*, 2019). Additionally, dogs with a cortisol-producing adrenocortical mass may present concurrently with other non-functional or functional adrenal tumours, such as phaeochromocytoma.

Hyperaldosteronism

Hyperaldosteronism is extremely rare in dogs and is an uncommon but emerging disorder in cats (see Chapter 32). Primary hyperaldosteronism is characterized by autonomous excessive production of aldosterone, generally caused by a functional tumour (carcinoma or adenoma) arising from the adrenal cortex (zona glomerulosa).

Supportive clinical manifestations in cats with hyperaldosteronism include weakness, hypokalaemia and signs related to systemic hypertension. However, not all cats have evidence of hypokalaemia or hypertension. Additionally, chronic kidney disease might progress in the presence of excessive aldosterone production.

Confirmation of primary hyperaldosteronism requires demonstration of an increased circulating aldosterone concentration in the face of low renin activity. Pitfalls include difficulties in the preservation of renin activity in samples and a lack of availability of methods to measure renin activity among laboratories. Most cats with primary hyperaldosteronism have a significant increase of basal aldosterone concentration and, in the presence of supportive clinical signs and an adrenal mass, this is sufficient to diagnose primary hyperaldosteronism. Measuring urinary aldosterone:creatinine after fludrocortisone administration might work as an alternative diagnostic approach to confirm hyperaldosteronism in cats.

On rare occasions, the effects of mineralocorticoid excess can also be mimicked by high concentrations of an aldosterone precursor, such as deoxycorticosterone. The plasma deoxycorticosterone concentration should be evaluated in dogs or cats with a suspected aldosteronoma that have reference interval or low plasma aldosterone concentrations. Cats with an adrenocortical tumour causing hyperaldosteronism can present with concurrent hyperprogesteronism (see below) and signs associated with hypercortisolism (Briscoe *et al.*, 2009; Guerios *et al.*, 2015).

Sex-hormone-secreting adrenal neoplasia

Adrenocortical tumours can potentially produce and secrete excessive concentrations of several hormones other than aldosterone and cortisol including a variety of cortisol and aldosterone precursors and sex hormones. For example, tumours may also secrete progestogens, oestrogens or androgens (see Chapter 28). In humans, adrenal carcinomas are usually inefficient in the conversion of cholesterol to cortisol. This might result from aberrant biosynthetic pathways or enzyme deficiencies and can give rise to high circulating concentrations of hormone precursors. By contrast, adrenal adenomas exhibit more efficient steroidogenesis and the production of precursors may be low or normal in relation to cortisol production. Similarly, in dogs and cats, when the main secretory product is a steroid other than cortisol, the adrenal tumour is usually a carcinoma.

Dogs and cats with sex-hormone-secreting tumours may have clinical signs consistent with hypercortisolism but they can have reference interval (or subnormal) ACTH response and low-dose dexamethasone suppression test results, and different combinations of increased production of 17-alpha-hydroxyprogesterone, progesterone, oestradiol, testosterone and androstenedione. Pre- and post-ACTH concentrations of these hormones can be measured if required.

Progesterone-secreting adrenal tumours are the most common sex-hormone-secreting adrenal tumours in cats. Progesterone may have some intrinsic glucocorticoid effects, but it is more likely that high concentrations of progesterone result in clinical signs of hypercortisolaemia by displacing cortisol from cortisol-binding proteins. This results in high concentrations of free cortisol, giving rise to clinical signs of cortisol excess (see Chapter 30). A similar presentation has been described in dogs with 17-alpha-hydroxyprogesterone excess. Pre- and/or post-ACTH concentrations of sex hormones, including progesterone, 17-alpha-hydroxyprogesterone and dehydroepiandrosterone, are also commonly increased in dogs with ACTH-dependent hypercortisolism; therefore, hypercortisolism should always be ruled out before testing for sex hormone excess.

Behavioural changes are the main clinical signs in cats with androgen- or oestrogen-secreting tumours. Adrenal neoplasia should be considered as a differential in neutered males showing 'male-type' behaviour or in neutered females with signs of oestrus. Males with androstenedione- and/or testosterone-secreting adrenal tumours can be aggressive; urine spraying and spines on the penis are also observed despite castration (Millard et al., 2009; Summer et al., 2019). Neutered females with either benign or malignant oestradiol-secreting tumours have shown cyclic oestrous behaviours (pacing, vocalizing, lordosis, head rubbing, licking the vulva) (Meler et al., 2011; Summer et al., 2019). Several sex hormones might be simultaneously increased; for example, in one neutered female cat with an adrenocortical carcinoma, the concentrations of androstenedione, oestradiol, progesterone and 17-alpha-hydroxyprogesterone were increased (Meler et al., 2011).

with phaeochromocytoma may also present with another endocrine disorder, particularly adrenocortical tumours.

Phaeochromocytomas can be malignant (presence of distant metastasis), although local invasion is more common. They commonly compress or invade the vena cava and phrenicoabdominal vein, but can also involve the aorta, renal vessels, adrenal vessels, hepatic veins or kidneys (Figure 34.6). Non-traumatic rupture can occur in dogs, resulting in life-threatening blood loss into the peritoneal cavity or retroperitoneal space.

Clinical manifestations may develop as a result of excessive secretion of catecholamines and their effect on blood pressure and cardiac function or, less commonly, as a result of the space-occupying nature of the tumour and its metastasis (Galac and Korpershoek, 2017). However, diagnosis can be challenging as dogs and cats may remain asymptomatic; in these cases, the diagnosis commonly occurs incidentally during imaging procedures.

To confirm the diagnosis, the concentrations of the plasma catecholamine metabolites normetanephrine (normetadrenaline) and metanephrine (metadrenaline) can be measured in dogs and cats with suspected phaeochromocytoma. Additionally, urine normetanephrine:creatinine and metanephrine:creatinine are useful as diagnostic tests for phaeochromocytoma in dogs. Plasma or urinary normetanephrine has superior sensitivity compared with metanephrine for detecting phaeochromocytoma in dogs. However, diagnosis of phaeochromocytoma is challenging, as dogs with hypercortisolism might also have increased concentrations of these catecholamine metabolites (Sieber-Ruckstuhl et al., 2017).

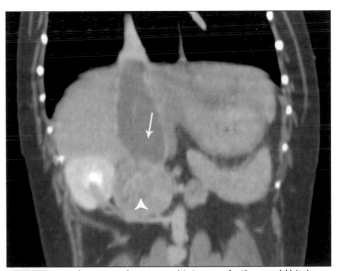

34.6 Dorsal computed tomographic image of a 12-year-old bitch with a phaeochromocytoma in the right adrenal gland (arrowhead). Cranial to the adrenal mass, the vena cava is markedly distended due to tumour invasion and thrombosis (arrowed).

Phaeochromocytoma

A phaeochromocytoma is a catecholamine-producing tumour of chromaffin cells of the adrenal medulla or sympathetic paraganglia and is the second most frequent canine adrenal neoplasm (see Chapter 33). In cats, phaeochromocytoma is considered a rare disease, with only six cases of histopathologically confirmed phaeochromocytoma reported.

Phaeochromocytomas are generally unilateral, although they can involve both adrenal glands. Furthermore, dogs

Non-functional adrenal mass

Adrenal tumours can be hormonally inactive. It is not an easy task to confirm a non-functional adrenal mass or nodule because of the difficulties in completely evaluating all hormones that could potentially be secreted by a functional tumour.

The origin of non-functional adrenal tumours varies. Tumours arising from the adrenal cortex or medulla, adrenal metastases or other masses such as myelolipoma may be non-functional (see Figure 34.1). However, dogs and cats can develop hypoadrenocorticism due to bilateral non-functional adrenal masses or adrenal metastasis (Labelle and De Cock, 2005; Kook et al., 2010; Merino-Gutierrez et al., 2020) (see Chapters 28 and 31).

A non-functional adrenal mass should be suspected in dogs and cats that remain apparently asymptomatic, normotensive and maintain reference interval routine clinicopathological results. In addition, there should be evidence of normal pituitary–adrenal function when evaluated for hypercortisolism, hyperaldosteronism and sex hormone hypersecretion, as well as reference interval plasma or urinary free metanephrine or norm-etanephrine concentrations.

The approach to non-functional adrenal incidentaloma may vary depending on the characteristics of the tumour (size, growth rate or signs of malignancy). Adrenalectomy should be considered in non-functional masses larger than 2 cm, as the likelihood of malignancy is greater. In cases with a small adrenal mass that is considered likely to be non-functional, a conservative approach is recommended. In these asymptomatic animals, clinical signs and tumour growth should be assessed monthly. If there is no change in the clinical picture and adrenal appearance after 3 months, the case should be rechecked in another 3 months. If the adrenal mass does not change in size, the time between ultrasound evaluations can be increased to every 6 months. This follow-up is important as some apparently non-functional tumours might become functional with time or increase in size. If the tumour size increases, adrenalectomy should be considered.

References and further reading

Baum JI, Boston SE and Case JB (2016) Prevalence of adrenal gland masses as incidental findings during abdominal computed tomography in dogs: 270 cases (2013–2014). Journal of the American Veterinary Medical Association **249**, 1165–1169

Bertazzolo W, Didier M, Gelain ME et al. (2014) Accuracy of cytology in distinguishing adrenocortical tumors from pheochromocytoma in companion animals. Veterinary Clinical Pathology **43**, 453–459

Briscoe K, Barrs VR, Foster DF and Beatty JA (2009) Hyperaldosteronism and hyperprogesteronism in a cat. Journal of Feline Medicine and Surgery **11**, 758–762

Cook AK, Spaulding KA and Edwards JF (2014) Clinical findings in dogs with incidental adrenal gland lesions determined by ultrasonography: 151 cases (2007–2010). Journal of the American Veterinary Medical Association **244**, 1181–1185

Fassnacht M, Arlt W, Bancos I et al. (2016) Management of adrenal incidentalomas: European Society of Endocrinology Clinical Practice Guideline in collaboration with the European Network for the Study of Adrenal Tumors. European Journal of Endocrinology **175**, G1–G34

Galac S (2019) Adrenal anatomy and physiology. In: Feline Endocrinology, ed. EC Feldman, F Fracassi and ME Peterson, pp. 357–362. Edra, Milan

Galac S and Korpershoek E (2017) Pheochromocytomas and paragangliomas in humans and dogs. Veterinary and Comparative Oncology **15**, 1158–1170

Guerios SD, Souza CHM and Bacon NJ (2015) Adrenocortical tumor in a cat secreting more than one type of corticosteroid. Journal of Feline Medicine and Surgery Open Reports **1**, 2055116915617970

Kook PH, Grest P, Raute-Kreinsen U, Leo C and Reusch CE (2010) Addison's disease due to bilateral adrenal malignancy in a dog. Journal of Small Animal Practice **51**, 333–336

Labelle P and De Cock HEV (2005) Metastatic tumors to the adrenal glands in domestic animals. Veterinary Pathology **42**, 52–58

Mayo-Smith WW, Song JH, Boland GL et al. (2017) Management of incidental adrenal masses: a white paper of the ACR Incidental Findings Committee. Journal of the American College of Radiology **14**, 1038–1044

Meler EN, Scott-Moncrieff JC, Peter AT et al. (2011) Cyclic estrous-like behavior in a spayed cat associated with excessive sex-hormone production by an adrenocortical carcinoma. Journal of Feline Medicine and Surgery **13**, 473–478

Melián C, Pérez-López L, Saavedra P et al. (2021) Ultrasound evaluation of adrenal gland size in healthy dogs and in dogs with hyperadrenocorticism. Veterinary Record **188**, e80

Millard RP, Pickens EH and Wells KL (2009) Excessive production of sex hormones in a cat with an adrenocortical tumor. Journal of the American Veterinary Medical Association **234**, 505–508

Merino-Gutierrez V, Feo-Bernabé L, Clemente-Vicario F and Puig J (2020) Addison's disease secondary to bilateral adrenal gland metastatic mammary carcinoma in a dog. Journal of the American Animal Hospital Association **56**, e56203

Pagani E, Tursi M, Lorenzi C et al. (2016) Ultrasonographic features of adrenal gland lesions in dogs can aid in diagnosis. BMC Veterinary Research **12**, 267

Pérez-López L, Wägner AM, Saavedra P, Jaber JR and Melián C (2021) Ultrasonographic evaluation of adrenal gland size in two body weight categories of healthy adult cats. Journal of Feline Medicine and Surgery **23**, 804–808

Pey P, Diana A, Rossi F et al. (2020) Safety of percutaneous ultrasound-guided fine-needle aspiration of adrenal lesions in dogs: perception of the procedure by radiologists and presentation of 50 cases. Journal of Veterinary Internal Medicine **34**, 626–635

Pey P, Specchi S, Rossi F et al. (2022) Prediction of vascular invasion using a 7-point scale computed tomography grading system in adrenal tumors in dogs. Journal of Veterinary Internal Medicine **36**, 713–725

Sanders K, Cirkel K, Grinwis GCM et al. (2019) The Utrecht Score: a novel histopathological scoring system to assess the prognosis of dogs with cortisol-secreting adrenocortical tumours. Veterinary and Comparative Oncology **17**, 329–337

Sieber-Ruckstuhl N, Salesov F, Quante S et al. (2017) Effect of trilostane on urinary catecholamines and their metabolites in dogs with hypercortisolism. BMC Veterinary Research **13**, 279

Summer JP, Hulsebosch SE, Dudley RM, Miller ML and Hayes GM (2019) Sex-hormone producing adrenal tumors causing behavioral changes as the sole clinical sign in 3 cats. Canadian Veterinary Journal **60**, 305–310

van Bokhorst KL, Kooistra HS, Boroffka SAEB and Galac S (2019) Concurrent pituitary and adrenocortical lesions on computed tomography imaging in dogs with spontaneous hypercortisolism. Journal of Veterinary Internal Medicine **33**, 72–78

Chapter 35

Concurrent endocrine neoplasia

Sara Galac

Introduction

Multiple endocrine neoplasia (MEN) in humans describes the simultaneous or sequential development of neoplasia in two or more endocrine glands and occasionally nonendocrine tissues. It has been classified into several types based on the endocrine glands affected. Human patients with MEN type 1 (MEN-1) typically have tumours of the parathyroid, enteropancreatic endocrine and anterior pituitary glands. Multiple endocrine neoplasia type 2 (MEN-2, previously MEN-2A) is characterized by medullary thyroid carcinoma, unilateral or bilateral phaeochromocytoma, and parathyroid hyperplasia or adenoma. In MEN type 3 (MEN-3, previously MEN-2B), medullary thyroid carcinoma and phaeochromocytoma occur in association with mucosal neuromas but in the absence of parathyroid disease. Recently, MEN type 4 (MEN-4), involving endocrine glands also affected in MEN-1, has been recognized (Alrezk et al., 2017). Once diagnosed, affected human patients can expect ongoing monitoring for new tumour development and may require multiple surgeries and other treatments for their management. In veterinary medicine, syndromes resembling MEN types have been described in dogs, horses, cattle, ferrets and cats, but whether they are truly reflective of the human condition is arguable (Reusch, 2015).

Aetiology

The estimated worldwide prevalence is 2–20 per 100,000 for MEN-1 and 1–10 per 100,000 for MEN-2/MEN-3 in the general human population. The vast majority of MEN syndromes in humans are familial and inherited as autosomal dominant disorders. Multiple gene mutations responsible for these syndromes have been identified (Newey and Takker, 2011). Multiple endocrine neoplasia type 1 is related to inactivating mutations of the tumour suppressor gene *MEN1*. Activating mutations of the *RET* proto-oncogene are responsible for MEN-2 and -3. Inactivating mutations of another tumour suppressor gene, *CDKN1B*, are responsible for MEN-4. In animals, there are no studies thus far determining the genetic background of MEN-like syndromes. The occurrence of more than one endocrine tumour could just be coincidental, in particular in elderly animals. Therefore, the term concurrent endocrine neoplasia (CEN) has been introduced as more appropriate for use in animals with two or more endocrine tumours and/or hyperplasia (Beatrice et al., 2018).

In dogs and cats, the description of CEN is restricted to case reports and one retrospective study (Figure 35.1). The condition is considered to be rare, but the exact prevalence is unknown. There is no apparent breed or sex

Neoplasms involved	Studies
Dogs	
Pituitary adenoma, adrenocortical tumour	Greco et al., 1999; Beatrice et al., 2018; van Bokhorst et al., 2019
Pituitary adenoma, phaeochromocytoma	Bennett and Norman, 1998; Beatrice et al., 2018
Pituitary adenoma, phaeochromocytoma, adrenocortical tumour	Thuróczy et al., 1998; Beatrice et al., 2018
Phaeochromocytoma, adrenocortical tumour	Von Dehn et al., 1995; Beatrice et al., 2018
Phaeochromocytoma, parathyroid adenoma	Wright et al., 1995
Parathyroid adenoma, pituitary adenoma	Walker et al., 2000
Insulinoma, adrenocortical carcinoma, paraganglioma	Kiupel et al., 2000
Thyroid adenoma, Leydig cell tumour	Beatrice et al., 2018
Medullary thyroid carcinoma, bilateral phaeochromocytoma, parathyroid hyperplasia	Peterson et al., 2016
Medullary thyroid carcinoma, bilateral phaeochromocytoma, parathyroid adenoma	Soler Arias et al., 2016
Medullary thyroid carcinoma, adrenocortical carcinoma, bilateral interstitial cell carcinoma	Proverbio et al., 2012
Leydig cell tumour, adrenocortical carcinoma	Beatrice et al., 2018
Leydig cell tumour, Sertoli cell tumour	Beatrice et al., 2018

35.1 Overview of published concurrent endocrine neoplasia combinations in dogs and cats. (continues) ▶

Neoplasms involved	Studies
Cats	
Thyroid hyperplasia, adenoma, carcinoma	Beatrice *et al.*, 2018
Thyroid neoplasia, adrenocortical carcinoma	Beatrice *et al.*, 2018
Thyroid and parathyroid hyperplasia and/or neoplasia	Beatrice *et al.*, 2018
Pituitary adenoma, phaeochromocytoma, unilateral thyroid hyperplasia	Beatrice *et al.*, 2018
Parathyroid adenoma, insulinoma, adrenocortical adenoma	Reimer *et al.*, 2005
Pancreatic beta cell carcinoma, pituitary adenoma, thyroid C-cell and parathyroid chief cell hyperplasia	Roccabianca *et al.*, 2006

35.1 (continued) Overview of published concurrent endocrine neoplasia combinations in dogs and cats.

predisposition. The tumours included in CEN can be functional or non-functional and associated with non-endocrine tumours or non-neoplastic abnormalities. It is possible for one tumour or its secretory product to predominate the clinical manifestation (Reusch, 2015).

Dogs

In dogs, concurrent adrenomedullary, adrenocortical and/or pituitary gland pathology is the most commonly described CEN (Figure 35.2). The diagnosis is based on the clinical presentation and endocrine testing; however, confirmation of the origin of the CEN can only be achieved by histopathology and staining with immune markers (Beatrice *et al.*, 2018). The most frequently reported forms of CEN are phaeochromocytoma with an adrenocortical tumour, and an adrenocorticotropic hormone (ACTH)-secreting pituitary tumour with an adrenocortical tumour or phaeochromocytoma (von Dehn *et al.*, 1995; Thuróczy *et al.*, 1998; Greco *et al.*, 1999; van Bokhorst *et al.*, 2019). The differentiation between spontaneous hypercortisolism and phaeochromocytoma may be difficult because they can present with similar clinical signs and because endocrine testing can give false-positive results for either disorder (Quante *et al.*, 2010; Gostelow *et al.*, 2013). Advanced diagnostic imaging with computed tomography (CT) is required to evaluate the size of the pituitary gland, and to determine the size and structure of both adrenal glands (Gregori *et al.*, 2015, Van Bokhorst *et al.*, 2019). While CT imaging is reliable in making a diagnosis of a pituitary tumour, it cannot differentiate between a cortisol-secreting adrenocortical tumour and a phaeochromocytoma. However, evaluating the size of the pituitary and adrenal glands can help in choosing the optimal treatment option. If the adrenal mass is operable, pre-treatment with phenoxybenzamine is usually recommended to reduce the risk of complications associated with catecholamine release during phaeochromocytoma surgery (Herrera *et al.*, 2008), although the added value of preoperative treatment has been questioned recently (Appelgrein *et al.*, 2020). Reaching a specific diagnosis in a dog suspected of an adrenocortical or adrenomedullary tumour can be done by measuring the plasma or urinary normetanephrine (normetadrenaline) concentration or by cytological examination of a fine-needle aspirate. Reference interval normetanephrine values in either plasma or urine exclude phaeochromocytoma, and concentrations of two to four times the upper reference limit are judged as increased in coexistence with hypercortisolism (Reusch, 2015). Cytology is reliable for establishing the origin of an adrenal tumour. However, fine-needle aspiration of adrenal masses is controversial, although recent studies in small numbers of animals report it as relatively safe (Sumner *et al.*, 2018; Pey *et al.*, 2020).

Coexistence of an ACTH-secreting pituitary adenoma with a cortisol-secreting adrenocortical tumour has been reported to occur in approximately 10% of dogs with hypercortisolism (van Bokhorst *et al.*, 2019). In such cases, medical treatment with trilostane is usually applied, although it may not represent the optimal treatment option. During trilostane therapy, the clinical signs of hypercortisolism will improve, but an ACTH-secreting pituitary tumour will continue to grow, and an adrenocortical tumour will expand in size and may also metastasize. A large pituitary tumour may lead to reduced appetite, headaches, behavioural and neurological problems, and poor quality of life. Screening for both entities is advisable to decide on the optimal treatment of hypercortisolism, in particular in relatively young dogs that will require long-term medical treatment.

A rather common CEN is the coexistence of phaeochromocytoma and paraganglioma (chemodectoma). The main difference between these two tumour types is that paragangliomas are not considered hormonally active in dogs, while phaeochromocytomas usually secrete excessive amounts of catecholamines. In humans, both types are associated with hormonal activity (Galac and Korpershoek, 2017). Phaeochromocytoma and paraganglioma originate from the same cell origin – the chromaffin cell. They also share similar genetic alterations. Succinate dehydrogenase family D and B mutations and chromosomal alterations have been demonstrated in both tumour types in dogs (Korpershoek *et al.*, 2019). A CEN involving paraganglioma, insulinoma and an adrenocortical tumour (Kiupel *et al.*, 2000), and a CEN with pituitary and parathyroid adenomas (Walker *et al.*, 2000) have been described in dogs.

Thyroid medullary carcinoma is most often concomitant with adrenal (either cortical or medullary) and testicular neoplasia (Proverbio *et al.*, 2012; Arias *et al.*, 2017).

In a retrospective study of CEN, the testicles were the second most affected endocrine organs (Beatrice *et al.*, 2018). Among histological types of testicular tumours, the concurrence of Sertoli cell tumour or Leydig cell tumour with seminoma were reported. A Leydig cell tumour combined with an adrenocortical tumour, and a Leydig cell tumour with thyroid medullary tumour, have also been described (Beatrice *et al.*, 2018). The diagnosis of testicular and thyroid neoplasia in dogs is straightforward as both organs are relatively easy to evaluate by physical examination and ultrasonography. Fine-needle aspiration can provide an initial indication of tumour type, although the final diagnosis is only possible with histopathological confirmation and immunohistochemistry staining.

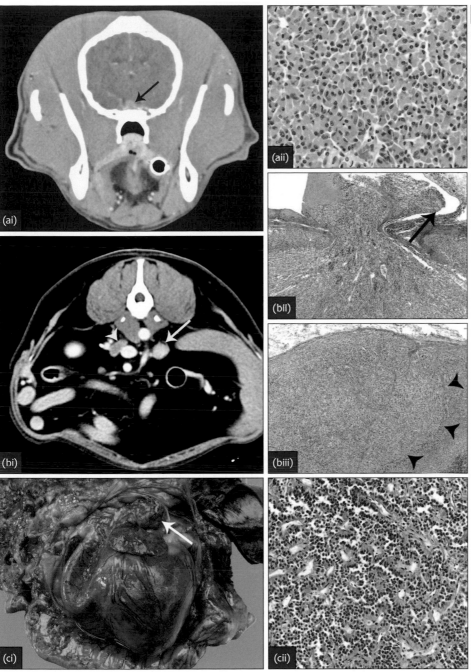

35.2 A 10-year-old neutered male Boston Terrier diagnosed with pituitary adenoma, phaeochromocytoma and paraganglioma. (ai) A computed tomographic image of the head demonstrated an enlarged pituitary gland (arrowed). (aii) An acidophil pituitary adenoma was diagnosed by histopathology. (bi) On abdominal CT, bilateral adrenomegaly was noted (arrow = left adrenal gland, arrowhead = right adrenal gland). (bii) Ingrowth of the right phaeochromocytoma into the adrenal capsule was present (arrowed) and (biii) nodular hyperplasia was detected in the left adrenal gland cortex (arrowheads). (ci) A mass was found on the heart base (arrowed). (cii) Histopathology revealed a paraganglioma.

Cats

In cats, the thyroid gland is the most frequently affected endocrine organ in CEN (Beatrice *et al.*, 2018). Hyperplasia is most commonly reported, followed by adenoma. Concurrent presence of thyroid hyperplasia, adenoma and carcinoma in the thyroid gland is possible. Hyperthyroidism is one of the most common endocrinopathies in cats (see Chapter 19). Careful monitoring for CEN in hyperthyroid cats is important, especially in cats receiving medical therapy for hyperthyroidism (Peterson *et al.*, 2016). Thyroid pathology is not arrested by management with antithyroid drugs, and malignant transformation is possible during prolonged medical therapy. Therefore, in younger cats that will require years of treatment, other treatment options are often recommended.

Concurrent thyroid and parathyroid lesions in cats involve thyroid hyperplasia and neoplasia, combined with parathyroid hyperplasia with hypertrophy of the chief cells. Neoplastic lesions in the adrenal gland in cats are predominantly detected in the cortex and not in the medulla. Concurrent adrenocortical, thyroid and parathyroid hyperplasia and neoplasia have been reported (Beatrice *et al.*, 2018). An aldosterone-secreting adrenocortical tumour and a single parathyroid adenoma in combination with thyroid lesions and an insulinoma have been described in one cat (Reimer *et al.*, 2005). In two cats with insulin-resistant diabetes mellitus and pituitary-dependent hypercortisolism, invasive pancreatic beta cell carcinoma, pituitary corticotropic adenoma, and thyroid C-cell and parathyroid chief cell hyperplasia were diagnosed by histopathology and immunohistochemistry (Roccabianca *et al.*, 2006).

This type of CEN in cats resembles MEN-1 in humans, with its known mutation of the *MEN1* gene (Newey and Thakker, 2011). Attempts to demonstrate this mutation in affected cats were not successful.

Concurrent endocrine neoplasia involving the pituitary gland in cats has only been reported in a retrospective study and was considered to be rare (Beatrice *et al.*, 2018). This might be because the pituitary gland is not routinely assessed during post-mortem examination and clinical signs may not be present with small and non-functional tumours.

Histopathology

Concurrent endocrine neoplasia includes hyperplasia and tumourous enlargement, either malignant or benign. Making a diagnosis of endocrine malignancy remains challenging. One of the general principles in histopathology is that infiltrative growth of a tumour spreading beyond the organ capsule, infiltration into adjacent blood vessels and distant metastasis are characteristics of malignancy (Grone and Rosol, 2016). However, in adrenal and thyroid tumours, these characteristics remain controversial and the significance of capsular and vascular invasion by neoplastic cells is debatable. There is no doubt that the presence of distant metastasis is the most reliable indicator of malignancy.

Maybe even more challenging is the differentiation between hyperplasia and adenoma (Derwahl and Studer, 2002). The traditional view holds that adenoma cells function autonomously. Adenomas are identified by factors such as a well defined capsule and more or less homogeneous morphology that may compress adjacent tissues and cause distortion of the organ contour. On the other hand, hyperplasia of endocrine tissue classically occurs secondary to over-secretion of the relevant tropic hormone. This leads to diffuse and uniform enlargement of the target gland due to an increased number of cells with identical morphological characteristics (Grone and Rosol, 2016). However, spontaneous proliferation of benign tissues can occur in hyperplasia. Therefore, a continuum of morphological structures has been proposed, with focal nodular hyperplasia at one end of the spectrum and adenoma at the other (van Vonderen *et al.*, 2003). As both hyperplasia and adenoma are presumably driven by intrinsic processes, hyperplasia needs to be included in CEN. In MEN syndromes, hyperplasia is regarded as a precursor to tumour formation in the adrenal and thyroid glands.

The significance of progression from benign to malignant lesions is well documented in cats with hyperthyroidism receiving long-term treatment with thyrostatic drugs (Peterson *et al.*, 2016). Although this is speculative, the feline thyroid gland may be one of the endocrine tissues in animals that can undergo a transition from hyperplasia to adenoma and even carcinoma.

Summary

The prevalence of CEN may be higher than currently realized. The ageing animal population, high level of veterinary care and increasing awareness of CEN by clinicians will very likely lead to documentation of more cases in the future. Diagnosing CEN is of clinical importance to be able to make an effective treatment plan. Therefore, thorough clinical assessment, including screening for common CEN combinations, is recommended. The prognosis for

CEN depends on the endocrine glands involved and the biological behaviour of the various tumours. Even when curative treatment of CEN is not possible, reaching a definitive diagnosis can help improve the expectations of owners concerning their animals' quality of life and duration of response to treatment.

References and further reading

Alrezk R, Hannah-Shmouni F and Stratakis CA (2017) MEN4 and *CDKN1B* mutations: the latest of the MEN syndromes. *Endocrine-Related Cancer* **24**, 195–208

Appelgrein C, Hosgood G, Drynan E and Nesbitt A (2020) Short-term outcome of adrenalectomy in dogs with adrenal gland tumours that did not receive pre-operative medical management. *Australian Veterinary Journal* **98**, 449–454

Arias EAS, Castillo VA and Trigo RH (2017) Addison disease and normocalcemic primary hyperparathyroidism in a dog with multiple endocrine neoplasia. *Open Veterinary Journal* **7**, 332–336

Beatrice L, Boretti FS, Sieber-Ruckstuhl NS *et al.* (2018) Concurrent endocrine neoplasias in dogs and cats: a retrospective study (2004–2014). *The Veterinary Record* **182**, 323–326

Bennett PF and Norman EJ (1998) Mitotane (o,p'-DDD) resistance in a dog with pituitary-dependent hyperadrenocorticism and phaeochromocytoma. *Australian Veterinary Journal* **76**, 101–103

Derwahl M and Studer H (2002) Hyperplasia versus adenoma in endocrine tissues: are they different? *Trends in Endocrinology and Metabolism* **13**, 23–28

Galac S and Korpershoek E (2017) Pheochromocytomas and paragangliomas in humans and dogs. *Veterinary and Comparative Oncology* **15**, 12–16

Gostelow R, Bridger N and Syme HM (2013) Plasma-free metanephrine and free normetanephrine measurement for the diagnosis of pheochromocytoma in dogs. *Journal of Veterinary Internal Medicine* **27**, 83–90

Greco DS, Peterson ME, Davidson AP, Feldman EC and Komurek K (1999) Concurrent pituitary and adrenal tumors in dogs with hyperadrenocorticism: 17 cases (1978–1995). *Journal of the American Animal Hospital Association* **214**, 1349–1353

Gregori T, Mantis P, Benigni L, Priestnall SL and Lamb CR (2015) Comparison of computed tomographic and pathologic findings in 17 dogs with primary adrenal neoplasia. *Veterinary Radiology and Ultrasound* **56**, 153–159

Grone A and Rosol T (2016) Endocrine tumors. In: *Pathology of Domestic Animals, 6th edn*, ed. M Maxie, pp. 269–357. Elsevier, St Louis

Herrera MA, Mehl ML, Kass PH *et al.* (2008) Predictive factors and the effect of phenoxybenzamine on outcome in dogs undergoing adrenalectomy for pheochromocytoma. *Journal of Veterinary Internal Medicine* **22**, 1333–1339

Kiupel M, Mueller PB, Ramos Vara J, Irizarry A and Lin TL (2000) Multiple endocrine neoplasia in a dog. *Journal of Comparative Pathology* **123**, 210–217

Korpershoek E, Dieduksman DAER, Grinwis GCM *et al.* (2019) Molecular alterations in dog pheochromocytomas and paragangliomas. *Cancers* **11**, 607–612

McDonnell JE, Gild ML, Clifton-Bligh RJ and Robinson BG (2019) Multiple endocrine neoplasia: an update. *Internal Medicine Journal* **49**, 954–961

Newey PJ and Thakker RV (2011) Role of multiple endocrine neoplasia type 1 mutational analysis in clinical practice. *Endocrine Practice* **17**, 8–17

Peterson ME, Broome MR and Rishniw M (2016) Prevalence and degree of thyroid pathology in hyperthyroid cats increases with disease duration: a cross-sectional analysis of 2096 cats referred for radioiodine therapy. *Journal of Feline Medicine and Surgery* **18**, 92–103

Pey P, Diana A, Rossi F *et al.* (2020) Safety of percutaneous ultrasound-guided fine-needle aspiration of adrenal lesions in dogs: perception of the procedure by radiologists and presentation of 50 cases. *Journal of Veterinary Internal Medicine* **34**, 626–635

Proverbio D, Spada E, Perego R *et al.* (2012) Potential variant of multiple endocrine neoplasia in a dog. *Journal of the American Animal Hospital Association* **48**, 132–138

Quante S, Boretti FS, Kook PH *et al.* (2010) Urinary catecholamine and metanephrine to creatinine ratios in dogs with hyperadrenocorticism or pheochromocytoma, and in healthy dogs. *Journal of Veterinary Internal Medicine* **24**, 1093–1097

Reimer SB, Pelosi A and Frank JD (2005) Multiple endocrine neoplasia type I in a cat. *Journal of the American Veterinary Medical Association* **227**, 101–104

Reusch C (2015) Pheochromocytoma and multiple endocrine neoplasia. In: *Canine and Feline Endocrinology, 3rd edn*, ed. EC Feldman, RW Nelson, CE Reusch, J Scott-Moncrieff and EN Behrend, pp. 521–544. Elsevier, Boston

Roccabianca P, Rondena M, Paltrinieri S *et al.* (2006) Multiple endocrine neoplasia type-I-like syndrome in two cats. *Veterinary Pathology* **43**, 345–352

Soler Arias EA, Castillo VA, Trigo RH and Caneda Aristarain ME (2016) Multiple endocrine neoplasia similar to human subtype 2A in a dog: medullary thyroid carcinoma, bilateral pheochromocytoma and parathyroid adenoma. *Open Veterinary Journal* **6**, 165–171

Sumner JA, Lacorcia L, Rose AM, Woodward AP and Carter JE (2018) Clinical safety of percutaneous ultrasound-guided fine-needle aspiration of adrenal gland lesions in 19 dogs. *Journal of Small Animal Practice* **59**, 357–363

Thakker RV (2001) Multiple endocrine neoplasia. *Hormone Research* **56**, 67–72

Thuróczy J, van Sluijs FJ, Kooistra HS *et al.* (1998) Multiple endocrine neoplasias in a dog: corticotrophic tumour, bilateral adrenocortical tumours, and pheochromocytoma. *The Veterinary Quarterly* **20**, 56–61

van Bokhorst KL, Kooistra HS, Boroffka SAEB and Galac S (2019) Concurrent pituitary and adrenocortical lesions on computed tomography imaging in dogs with spontaneous hypercortisolism. *Journal of Veterinary Internal Medicine* **33**, 72–77

van Vonderen IK, Kooistra HS, Peeters ME, Rijnberk A and van den Ingh TSGAM (2003) Parathyroid hormone immunohistochemistry in dogs with primary and secondary hyperparathyroidism: the question of adenoma and primary hyperplasia. *Journal of Comparative Pathology* **129**, 61–69

von Dehn BJ, Nelson RW, Feldman EC and Griffey SM (1995) Pheochromocytoma and hyperadrenocorticism in dogs: six cases (1982–1992). *Journal of the American Veterinary Medical Association* **207**, 322–324

Walker MC, Jones BR, Guildford WG, Burbidge HM and Alley MR (2000) Multiple endocrine neoplasia type 1 in a crossbred dog. *Journal of Small Animal Practice* **41**, 67–70

Wright KN, Breitschwerdt EB, Feldman JM *et al.* (1995) Diagnostic and therapeutic considerations in a hypercalcemic dog with multiple endocrine neoplasia. *Journal of the American Animal Hospital Association* **31**, 156–162

Chapter 36

Autoimmune polyendocrine syndromes

Kevin Murtagh

Introduction

In human medicine, autoimmune polyendocrine syndromes (APSs) are a well described and diverse group of clinical conditions that typically involve failure of at least two endocrine glands either concurrently or, more frequently, sequentially over many years and even decades. They are associated with defects in humoral and cellular immunity and characterized by the presence of circulating autoantibodies and lymphocytic infiltration in affected organs and tissues (Husebye *et al.*, 2018). Serological autoantibody screening is performed to predict the development of future autoimmune endocrine disease (Frommer and Kahaly, 2019). Should positive serological testing be demonstrated, functional screening is recommended for the associated endocrine deficiency. Autoimmune polyendocrine syndromes can also be associated with non-endocrine autoimmune diseases (Cutolo, 2014; Husebye *et al.*, 2018). There is a strong genetic susceptibility.

Undoubtedly, multiple endocrine disorders do occur in dogs and cats for a variety of reasons. Examples include hypercortisolism associated with the development of diabetes mellitus or hypothyroidism. Widespread neoplasia could potentially destroy more than one endocrine gland. Hypothyroidism and hypoparathyroidism or hypocortisolism could potentially occur after bilateral thyroidectomy or hypophysectomy, respectively. However, these need to be distinguished from APSs as described in humans. If similar aetiological and diagnostic criteria are extrapolated from humans, the true existence of APSs in dogs is controversial. Potentially immune-mediated diseases occurring concurrently may be purely coincidental. Immune-mediated endocrine disease is rare in cats and no study to date has described a possible APS in this species (Blois *et al.*, 2010).

Autoimmune polyendocrine syndromes in humans

In humans, APSs are divided into two major groups, the monogenic juvenile-onset type 1 disease and the polygenic adult-onset type 2 disease. Whilst the latter is more common than the former, these syndromes remain rarely described (Cutolo, 2014) – so much so that they are all recognized as orphan syndromes (Frommer and Kahaly, 2019), defined as a condition with a prevalence of 1–500 per 1,000,000. These disorders are summarized in Figure 36.1.

Characteristic	APS-1	APS-2
Inheritance	Autosomal recessive	Polygenic
Genetics	*AIRE* mutation	HLA association
Sex association	None	Female
Age at onset	Infancy	20–60 years
Main clinical features	Mucocutaneous candidiasis Hypoparathyroidism Hypoadrenocorticism	Hypoadrenocorticism Type 1 diabetes mellitus Autoimmune thyroid disease

36.1 General characteristics of autoimmune polyendocrine syndromes (APS) types 1 and 2 in humans. HLA = human leucocyte antigen.

Autoimmune polyendocrine syndrome type 1

Autoimmune polyendocrine syndrome type 1 (APS-1), also referred to as autoimmune polyendocrinopathy–candidiasis–ectodermal dystrophy (APECED), is characterized by the development during childhood of at least two of the following three diseases:

- Chronic mucocutaneous candidiasis
- Hypoparathyroidism
- Primary hypoadrenocorticism.

Other manifestations that can also occur with APS-1 include enamel hypoplasia, enteropathy with diarrhoea or constipation and pernicious anaemia. Affected women often develop early-onset primary ovarian insufficiency, and male hypogonadism has also been described. Unusual features include bilateral keratitis, periodic fever with rash and hepatitis, pneumonitis, pancreatitis, nephritis and functional asplenia. The number of disorders and the age at which they occur can vary widely. There may be one manifestation early in life and a second later on, and some affected individuals develop as many as 20 possible manifestations of the disease.

In humans, APS-1 is inherited as an autosomal recessive disease caused by mutations in the autoimmune regulator (*AIRE*) gene. This is an important transcriptional regulator that activates the expression of tissue-restricted proteins in a subset of thymic epithelial cells. The presentation of these antigens to developing T cells induces apoptosis of autoreactive clones, promoting self-tolerance. Therefore, if autoimmune regulator proteins are absent or non-functional as a result of a defective gene, T cells could initiate autoimmune disease. The variation in manifestations from one affected individual to another suggests that other genes or environmental factors may play a role. Human patients with isolated hypoadrenocorticism without APS-1 do not have *AIRE* mutations (Cutolo, 2014).

Autoimmune polyendocrine syndrome type 2

Autoimmune polyendocrine syndrome type 2 (APS-2) (also referred to as Schmidt's syndrome) originally referred to the presence of primary hypoadrenocorticism and either primary hypothyroidism or type 1 diabetes mellitus. Type 3 disease referred to autoimmune thyroid disease and type 1 diabetes mellitus without evidence of adrenal dysfunction. Type 4 disease represented autoimmune endocrinopathies that could not be classified as either type 2 or type 3 (Husebye *et al.*, 2018). In reality, the underlying genetic associations are similar for types 2–4, and it is generally accepted that APS-2 is a term that can be used to describe all these types with the development of any two or more of:

- Primary hypoadrenocorticism
- Autoimmune hypothyroidism
- Type 1 diabetes mellitus.

The initial onset is usually in young adulthood and it is more common in women. Other autoimmune conditions that can develop include coeliac disease, alopecia, vitiligo, primary ovarian insufficiency and pernicious anaemia.

Heritability is complex and polygenic. Typically, genetic associations involve the adaptive and innate immune systems, and a sex-dependent alteration of the human leucocyte antigen system has been described (Frommer and Kahaly, 2019).

Potential autoimmune polyendocrine syndromes in dogs

In one of the largest retrospective studies of multiple endocrinopathies in dogs, only 35 of 13,512 (0.3%) dogs with two or more endocrinopathies were identified over a 13-year period (Blois *et al.*, 2011). Twenty of these dogs had concurrent diabetes mellitus and hypercortisolism, in which a common immune-mediated aetiology is not implicated and, therefore, would not fit the definition of APS. Multiple hormone deficiencies within the same individuals were identified in only 18 of the 35 dogs (51%), suggesting that even if APSs accounted for some or all of these cases, the syndrome is rare in dogs. The most common combination of endocrine deficiencies was diabetes mellitus and hypothyroidism, identified in 10 dogs. Concurrent hypoadrenocorticism and hypothyroidism were identified in eight dogs. These and other combinations of endocrine deficiencies or autoimmunity have also been described in several single case reports. The different combinations are summarized in Figure 36.2. However, evidence of autoimmunity based on the existence of thyroid or adrenal autoantibodies (by indirect immunofluorescence or measurement of circulating thyroglobulin autoantibodies (TgAAs) or 21-hydroxylase autoantibodies) or supportive histopathological changes (lymphocytic infiltration) has only been demonstrated in five cases (Bowen *et al.*, 1986;

- Hypothyroidism and diabetes mellitus
- Hypoadrenocorticism and hypothyroidism
- Hypoadrenocorticism and diabetes mellitus
- Adenohypophysitis, hypoadrenocorticism and hypothyroidism

36.2 Potential combined autoimmune endocrine disorders reported in dogs, in approximate descending order of prevalence.
(Bowen *et al.*, 1986; Ford *et al.*, 1993; Kooistra *et al.*, 1995; Smallwood and Barsanti, 1995; Melendez *et al.*, 1996; Paik *et al.*, 1996; Peterson *et al.*, 1996; Hess *et al.*, 2000; Pikula *et al.*, 2007; Adissu *et al.*, 2010; Blois *et al.*, 2011; McGonigle *et al.*, 2013; Archontakis *et al.*, 2016; Cartwright *et al.*, 2016; Vanmal *et al.*, 2016; Furukawa *et al.*, 2021; Kuijlaars *et al.*, 2021)

Kooistra *et al.*, 1995; Pikula *et al.*, 2007; Adissu *et al.*, 2010; Cartwright *et al.*, 2016). It remains possible that the concurrence of these endocrine disorders is coincidental rather than reflective of a true APS.

There are also several case reports describing other immune-mediated disorders in dogs with hypothyroidism, hypoadrenocorticism or diabetes mellitus, including myasthenia gravis and immune-mediated haemolytic anaemia. More recently, a case report describing a dog with hypoadrenocorticism and hypothyroidism with concurrent keratoconjunctivitis sicca, exocrine pancreatic insufficiency and possible myositis was described but, again, evidence of autoantibody formation was not provided (Kuijlaars *et al.*, 2021).

Although the existence of true APSs in dogs remains uncertain, it is known that similar dog leucocyte antigen haplotypes confer risk for the development of hypothyroidism, hypoadrenocorticism and diabetes mellitus in some breeds (Massey *et al.*, 2013) (see Chapter 2). Nevertheless, from a clinical viewpoint, combined endocrine deficiencies can and do occur. It is estimated that between 5% and 10% of diabetic dogs and approximately 5% of dogs with hypoadrenocorticism have or develop hypothyroidism. Diabetes mellitus or hypoadrenocorticism develop in less than 2% of hypothyroid dogs, and development of diabetes mellitus in dogs with hypoadrenocorticism appears to be rare.

Clinical features

The clinical presentation of dogs with multiple endocrine deficiencies will depend on the combination of disorders present and is reviewed in the relevant chapters covering individual disorders. Careful review of the historical and clinical data is required to identify abnormalities that would not be explained by a single hormone deficiency. Some clinical signs such as lethargy are non-specific and can be features of many endocrine disorders, including hypothyroidism, diabetes mellitus and hypoadrenocorticism. Dogs with hypothyroidism usually experience some dermatological abnormalities and these are not features of either diabetes mellitus or hypoadrenocorticism. Thus, the existence or development of, for example, alopecia in diabetes mellitus or hypoadrenocorticism should prompt investigation for hypothyroidism. Polyuria and polydipsia are not features of hypothyroidism and if present diabetes mellitus or hypoadrenocorticism could be considered. Equally, polyphagia occurs with diabetes mellitus but is unexpected in both hypothyroidism and hypoadrenocorticism. Heat seeking occurs in hypothyroidism but not with other endocrine deficiencies. Signs of chronic gastrointestinal disease are much more likely with hypoadrenocorticism than with hypothyroidism or diabetes mellitus. Response to treatment may also be important. For example, markedly increased sensitivity to exogenous insulin therapy in a diabetic dog may raise concerns for hypocortisolaemia and prompt investigation for hypoadrenocorticism.

Clinicopathological abnormalities

As with clinical signs, the clinicopathological abnormalities present depend on the combination of hormone deficiencies in each individual. Unusual abnormalities may increase the index of suspicion for additional endocrine deficiencies. For example, should a dog diagnosed with hypoadrenocorticism have hypercholesterolaemia, further investigation for hypothyroidism should be considered as this disorder is more frequently associated with hypocholesterolaemia. Similarly, should hypocholesterolaemia be identified in a hypothyroid dog, hypoadrenocorticism may need consideration. The combination of hyponatraemia and hyperkalaemia supports hypoadrenocorticism. However, the absence of electrolyte abnormalities cannot be used to rule out hypoadrenocorticism. Approximately 50% of dogs diagnosed with both hypothyroidism and hypoadrenocorticism do not have any electrolyte abnormalities, reflective of atypical disease. Persistent hyponatraemia after instituting treatment for hypoadrenocorticism may prompt investigation for hypothyroidism.

Diagnosis

The diagnosis of diabetes mellitus is relatively straightforward, relying on demonstration of hyperglycaemia and glucosuria. Confirmation of hypoadrenocorticism relies on depicting minimal cortisol stimulation after administration of adrenocorticotropic hormone (ACTH). Hyperglycaemia and glucosuria are not features of hypothyroidism or hypoadrenocorticism and there will be adequate cortisol production during an ACTH response test in diabetic or hypothyroid dogs, effectively ruling out hypoadrenocorticism. The only difficulty in diagnosing hypoadrenocorticism arises because so many dogs with combined disorders do not have typical electrolyte abnormalities. Measurement of serum aldosterone pre and post ACTH administration may be required to ascertain mineralocorticoid status, as well as endogenous ACTH measurement to determine whether the disease is primary or secondary.

The diagnosis of hypothyroidism in dogs with pre-existing disorders remains challenging. For confirmation of primary hypothyroidism, the combination of decreased total thyroxine (T4) and increased canine thyrotropin (thyroid-stimulating hormone (cTSH)) concentrations is required. However, it is known that a proportion of hypothyroid dogs do not have an increased cTSH concentration. Dogs with non-thyroidal illness (NTI) such as diabetes mellitus also frequently have decreased total T4 and reference interval cTSH concentrations. In diabetic dogs, the combination of decreased total T4 and increased cTSH concentration is specific for hypothyroidism. If the cTSH concentration is not increased, further diagnostic tests such as free T4 measurement are required to distinguish the effects of hypothyroidism from NTI. Alternatively, consideration could be given to repeat testing at a later date once the diabetes mellitus has been well controlled.

Diagnosing hypothyroidism in dogs with concurrent hypoadrenocorticism is even more challenging. Increased cTSH concentrations have been demonstrated in euthyroid dogs with untreated hypoadrenocorticism, occasionally with concurrent decreased total T4 concentrations. In one study of 30 dogs with hypoadrenocorticism, 11 (37%) had increased cTSH concentrations (Reusch et al., 2017). Treatment with corticosteroids for 2–4 weeks normalized the cTSH in the majority of cases, although several months of treatment was required in a few. Care must therefore be taken to prevent a misdiagnosis of primary hypothyroidism in untreated primary hypoadrenocorticism. There should be other supportive evidence for hypothyroidism, and additional diagnostic tests for hypothyroidism should be undertken or testing delayed for several weeks after instituting treatment for hypoadrenocorticism.

By definition, the ante-mortem diagnosis of an APS requires the demonstration of autoantibodies directed against the gland in question or supportive histopathological changes. This is challenging in dogs where biopsies are invasive and not clinically indicated and where there is poor availability of autoantibody tests. In the case of primary hypothyroidism, circulating TgAAs or in some cases thyroid peroxidase autoantibodies can be measured (Skopek et al., 2006; Husebye et al., 2018). It has been shown that dogs with thyroid peroxidase autoantibodies all have TgAAs, and that their assessment over TgAAs is not particularly helpful (Graham et al., 2007). Immune-mediated destruction of the adrenal glands can be indirectly assessed by measuring 21-hydroxylase autoantibodies (Rick et al., 2014; Cartwright et al., 2016); however, this test is not yet available commercially. For diabetes mellitus, an immune-mediated aetiology can be demonstrated by measuring glutamic acid decarboxylase-65 (GAD65) and/or insulinoma antigen-2 (IA-2) autoantibodies. In one study involving 30 diabetic dogs, four had significant autoreactivity to GAD65, three were positive for IA-2 autoantibodies and two had dual autoantigen reactivity, suggesting an immune-mediated aetiology (Davison et al., 2008). However, these tests are not commercially available.

Treatment
Hormone replacement

The same principles apply for the treatment of each endocrine deficiency in dogs with multiple disorders occurring concurrently (see the relevant chapter for each disorder), with a few caveats. Initiating levothyroxine replacement therapy prior to glucocorticoid therapy in dogs with hypothyroidism and hypoadrenocorticism could theoretically precipitate an adrenal crisis due to enhanced hepatic corticosteroid metabolism. Therefore, glucocorticoid therapy should be started prior to initiating therapy with levothyroxine. For treatment of hypothyroidism in dogs with pre-existing disease a gradual introduction of supplementation (25–50% of the starting dose) is often recommended in order to minimize the effect of a sudden change in metabolic rate and its consequences. However, this is more important when using higher doses as using a moderate dose of 20 µg/kg q24h is not associated with adverse effects in such cases. Diabetic dogs that develop hypoadrenocorticism can demonstrate enhanced insulin sensitivity and, should this be noted, care must be taken to decrease the dose of insulin until the hypoadrenocorticism is controlled. Longer-term glucocorticoid supplementation may contribute to insulin resistance, and care should be taken to use the lowest dose possible to control the signs of hypocortisolaemia. Similarly, hypothyroidism can be associated with insulin resistance, and insulin dose alterations may be required after commencing thyroid hormone supplementation (Ford et al., 1993).

There is one case report of a dog with concurrent hypoadrenocorticism and hypothyroidism developing congestive heart failure (CHF) following treatment with fludrocortisone, prednisolone and levothyroxine, despite having no evidence of heart disease prior to treatment (Paik et al., 2016). The CHF resolved with treatment and clinical signs did not return despite discontinuation of cardiac medications after a 10-month follow-up, suggesting that concurrent treatment of these endocrinopathies contributed to a transient or reversible form of CHF.

Immunosuppression

There is currently little or no evidence that immunosuppression is beneficial in animals with autoimmune endocrine disease as, in most cases, irreversible damage has occurred prior to the onset of signs associated with hypofunction. There is, however, a single case report that demonstrated apparent resolution of hypoparathyroidism with immunosuppression using prednisolone and ciclosporin, both of which were prescribed for concurrent immune-mediated thrombocytopenia. A definitive link between resolution of the primary hypoparathyroidism and immunosuppression was not confirmed (Warland et al., 2015). Another dog received immunosuppressive doses of prednisolone and mycophenolate for suspected immune-mediated myositis, but this did not result in resolution of concurrent hypothyroidism or hypoadrenocorticism (Kuijlaars et al., 2021).

In humans, immunosuppression may be indicated should non-endocrine autoimmune disease such as pneumonitis, hepatitis or enteritis develop, but it is not used with the goal of regaining endocrine function.

Monitoring for future endocrine organ dysfunction

Serological testing for autoimmune endocrine disease in veterinary medicine is currently limited to assessment of TgAAs. Thus, other endocrine diseases are usually only considered if appropriate clinical signs arise or if there is an unexpected response to treatment of another known endocrine deficiency, such as enhanced response to exogenous insulin in a newly diagnosed diabetic animal with concurrent undiagnosed hypoadrenocorticism or a poor response to exogenous mineralocorticoid and glucocorticoid in a newly diagnosed hypoadrenocorticism case with undiagnosed hypothyroidism.

Prognosis

If APS exists in dogs, it should carry a relatively favourable prognosis, providing each endocrine deficiency is appropriately treated. Most dogs with combined disorders survive months to years following their initial diagnosis. Regular monitoring of the different endocrine deficiencies and their treatment is paramount for success.

References and further reading

Adissu HA, Hamel-Jolette A and Foster RA (2010) Lymphocytic adenohypophysitis and adrenalitis in a dog with adrenal and thyroid atrophy. *Veterinary Pathology* **47**, 1082–1085

Archontakis P, Kalogianni L, Tselekis D et al. (2016) Concurrent hypothyroidism and diabetes mellitus in the dog: 3 cases (2006–2015). In: *BSAVA Congress Proceedings*, 7–10 April 2016. BSAVA, Gloucester, pp. 563–564

Blois SL, Dickie EL, Kruth SA and Allen DG (2010) Multiple endocrine disease in cats: 15 cases (1997–2008). *Journal of Feline Medicine and Surgery* **12**, 637–642

Blois SL, Dickie EL, Kruth SA and Allen DG (2011) Multiple endocrine diseases in dogs: 35 cases (1996–2009). *Journal of the American Veterinary Medical Association* **238**, 1616–1621

Bowen D, Schaer M and Riley W (1986) Autoimmune polyglandular syndrome in a dog: a case report. *Journal of the American Animal Hospital Association* **22**, 649–654

Cartwright JA, Stone J, Rick M and Dunning MD (2016) Polyglandular endocrinopathy type II (Schmidt's syndrome) in a Dobermann pinscher. *Journal of Small Animal Practice* **57**, 491–494

Cutolo M (2014) Autoimmune polyendocrine syndromes. *Autoimmunity Reviews* **13**, 85–89

Davison LJ, Weenink SM, Christie MR, Herrtage ME and Catchpole B (2008) Autoantibodies to GAD65 and IA-2 in canine diabetes mellitus. *Veterinary Immunology and Immunopathology* **126**, 83–90

Ford SL, Nelson RW, Feldman EC and Niwa D (1993) Insulin resistance in three dogs with hypothyroidism and diabetes mellitus. *Journal of the American Veterinary Medical Association* **202**, 1478–1480

Frommer L and Kahaly G (2019) Autoimmune polyendocrinopathy. *Journal of Clinical Endocrinology & Metabolism* **104**, 4769–4782

Furukawa S, Meguri N, Koura K, Koura H and Matsuda A (2021) A case of canine polyglandular deficiency syndrome with diabetes mellitus and hypoadrenocorticism. *Veterinary Sciences* **8**, 43

Graham P, Refsal KR and Nachreiner RF (2007) Etiopathologic findings of canine hypothyroidism. *Veterinary Clinics of North America: Small Animal Practice* **37**, 617–631

Hess RS, Saunders HM, Van Winkle TJ and Ward CR (2000) Concurrent disorders in dogs with diabetes mellitus. *Journal of the American Veterinary Medical Association* **8**, 1166–1173

Husebye ES, Anderson MS and Kampe O (2018) Autoimmune polyendocrine syndromes. *New England Journal of Medicine* **378**, 1132–1141

Kooistra HS, Rijnberk A and van den Ingh TSGAM (1995) Polyglandular deficiency syndrome in a boxer dog: thyroid hormone and glucocorticoid deficiency. *Veterinary Quarterly* **17**, 59–63

Kuijlaars M, Yool DA and Ridyard AE (2021) Autoimmune polyendocrine syndrome in a standard poodle with concurrent non-endocrine immune-mediated diseases. *Veterinary Record Case Reports* **9**, e90

McGonigle KM, Randolph JF, Center SA and Goldstein RE (2013) Mineralocorticoid before glucocorticoid deficiency in a dog with primary hypoadrenocorticism and hypothyroidism. *Journal of the American Animal Hospital Association* **49**, 54–57

Massey J, Boag A, Scholey RA et al. (2013) MHC class II association study in eight breeds of dog with hypoadrenocorticism. *Immunogenetics* **65**, 291–297

Melendez LD, Greco DS, Turner JL, Hay DA and VanLiew CH (1996) Concurrent hypoadrenocorticism and hypothyroidism in 10 dogs (abstract). *Journal of Veterinary Internal Medicine* **10**, 182

Paik J, Kang JH, Chang D and Yang MP (2016) Cardiogenic pulmonary oedema in a dog with hypoadrenocorticism and hypothyroidism. *Journal of the American Animal Hospital Association* **52**, 378–384

Peterson ME, Kintzer PP and Kass PH (1996) Pretreatment clinical and laboratory findings in dogs with hypoadrenocorticism: 225 cases (1979–1993). *Journal of the American Veterinary Medical Association* **208**, 85–91

Pikula J, Pikulova J, Bandouchova H, Hajkova P and Faldyna M (2007) Schmidt's syndrome in a dog: a case report. *Veterinarni Medicina* **52**, 419–422

Reusch CE, Sieber-Ruckstuhl NS, Burkhardt WA et al. (2017) Altered serum thyrotropin concentrations in dogs with primary hypoadrenocorticism before and during treatment. *Journal of Veterinary Internal Medicine* **31**, 1643–1648

Rick MR, Refsal KR, Callewaert DM and Rader T (2014) The measurement of 21-hydroxylase antibodies in dogs via enzyme-linked immunosorbent assay. In: Oral Research Communications of the 23rd ECVIM-CA Congress. *Journal of Veterinary Internal Medicine* **28**, 743–744

Skopek E, Patzl M and Nachreiner RF (2006) Detection of autoantibodies against thyroid peroxidase in serum samples of hypothyroid dogs. *American Journal of Veterinary Research* **67**, 809–814

Smallwood LJ and Barsanti JA (1995) Hypoadrenocorticism in a family of Leonbergers. *Journal of the American Animal Hospital Association* **31**, 301–305

Vanmal B, Martlé V, Binst D et al. (2016) Combined atypical primary hypoadrenocorticism and primary hypothyroidism in a dog. *Vlaams Diergeneeskundig Tijdschrift* **85**, 355–364

Warland J, Skelly B, Knudsen C and Herrtage M (2015) Apparent resolution of canine primary hypoparathyroidism with immunosuppressive treatment. *Journal of Veterinary Internal Medicine* **29**, 400–404

Chapter 37

Erythropoietin excess

Eilidh Gunn

Introduction

Erythropoietin (EPO) is a polypeptide hormone synthesized in the kidneys that acts on bone marrow to stimulate red blood cell (RBC) production. The degree of tissue oxygenation is monitored by type 1 cells of the renal interstitium. During periods of hypoxia, the kidney produces EPO, leading to increased red cell production and oxygen-carrying capacity. Once normal tissue oxygenation is restored, EPO production reduces, thus completing a cycle of negative feedback. Pathologies associated with an excess production of EPO are therefore also associated with increased RBC mass.

Although the structure of canine and feline EPO is similar (approximately 95% sequence homology), both have only 80–85% sequence homology with the human peptide. This is an important consideration when using immunoassays that are designed to measure human EPO concentrations as they may not reliably measure either canine or feline EPO.

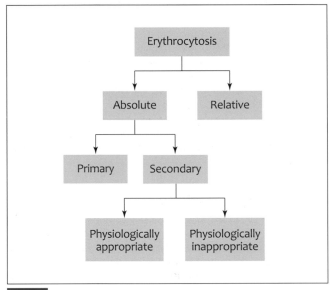

37.1 Physiological classification of erythrocytosis.

Erythrocytosis

Erythrocytosis is demonstrated by identifying an increase in haematocrit or packed cell volume (PCV), haemoglobin concentration or RBC count. Both haematocrit and PCV describe the proportion of blood made up by RBCs and are therefore affected by changes in either RBCs or plasma volume. Haematocrit is calculated by an automated haematology analyser from the RBC count and mean corpuscular volume, while PCV is a direct measurement made by visual inspection of a centrifuged microhaematocrit tube.

Erythrocytosis is generally classified as relative or absolute. Absolute erythrocytosis is further classified as primary or secondary, with the latter subcategorized as physiologically appropriate or inappropriate (Figure 37.1).

Definition of erythrocytosis

In human medicine, a diagnosis of erythrocytosis is dependent on haematocrit and haemoglobin concentrations exceeding sex-specific and well defined cut points. Such strict criteria have not been well defined for dogs or cats. However, using a guideline upper reference limit of 0.55 and 0.45 l/l for haematocrit in dogs and cats, respectively, a persistent increase above 0.65 and 0.55 l/l

warrants investigation. Extreme excitement, stress and exercise can cause a temporary increase in haematocrit through splenic contraction. Thus, the history and temperament of the animal are important considerations in interpreting erythrocytosis, as is demonstrating persistence of the abnormality.

Whilst the above guidelines apply to the general dog population, significant breed differences do occur. The Dachshund, Dogue de Bordeaux, Greyhound and other sighthound breeds naturally have higher PCV and haemoglobin concentrations compared with most other breeds. Breed-specific reference intervals should ideally be used when interpreting erythrocyte parameters and, where known, these are illustrated in Figure 37.2.

Relative erythrocytosis

Relative erythrocytosis describes an increased haematocrit without an overall increase in the animal's total red cell mass. This most commonly arises due to a decrease in plasma volume (haemoconcentration), as seen, for example, in animals with severe diarrhoea or cutaneous fluid loss arising from thermal burns. Relative erythrocytosis typically causes a mild increase in haematocrit (e.g. 0.55–0.65 l/l) and a corresponding increase in total

Breed	Reference interval (l/l)	Reference
Greyhound	0.50–0.68	Campora et al., 2011
Scottish Deerhound	0.44–0.62	Sheerer et al., 2013
Irish Wolfhound	0.46–0.62	Clark and Parry, 1997
Dachshund	0.41–0.63	Torres et al., 2014
Dogue de Bordeaux	0.35–0.56	Lavoué et al., 2014
Saluki	0.44–0.66	Uhríková et al., 2013
Whippet	0.46–0.66	
Pharaoh Hound	0.43–0.62	
Borzoi	0.43–0.65	
Italian Greyhound	0.44–0.61	

37.2 Reference intervals for haematocrit in a variety of breeds recognized to have higher haematocrit values than the general dog population. Methods of calculation of reference intervals vary and, in some cases, are estimated from a small number of dogs.

protein concentration (assuming no concurrent protein loss). However, in animals with more severe haemoconcentration (e.g. those with hypoadrenocorticism or acute haemorrhagic diarrhoea syndrome), the increase in haematocrit can be more dramatic (Peterson et al., 1996; Mortier et al., 2015). The diagnosis of relative erythrocytosis is usually based on clinical signs of hypovolaemia or dehydration, and resolution of erythrocytosis after rehydration.

Absolute erythrocytosis

Absolute erythrocytosis occurs when an increase in haematocrit is caused by a true increase in RBC mass. It is further classified as primary, where the pathology occurs at the level of the bone marrow and is independent of EPO, or secondary, where erythrocytosis is the result of EPO excess.

Primary erythrocytosis

Primary erythrocytosis is a myeloproliferative disorder caused by clonal expansion of erythroid stem cells. In such cases, the bone marrow continues to produce RBCs even in the face of low EPO concentrations. While previously referred to as polycythaemia vera in veterinary medicine, this term is now more accurately reserved for a distinct myeloproliferative disorder in humans, where an increase of several haematological cell lines (i.e. RBCs, white blood cells or platelets) is often observed. In humans, JAK2 mutations that allow dysregulated production of RBCs are identified in most affected individuals. Human and canine JAK2 share 94% sequence homology but only one analogous mutation in this gene, rarely associated with erythrocytosis in humans, has been identified in one of five dogs investigated (Beurlet et al., 2011).

Secondary erythrocytosis

Secondary erythrocytosis is driven principally by increased concentrations of EPO. This can be a physiologically appropriate response to hypoxia, or physiologically inappropriate when produced in the absence of such a stimulus, as summarized in Figure 37.3. Iatrogenic causes of erythrocytosis (i.e. overzealous administration of exogenous EPO) are possible but extremely rare.

Appropriate
- Cyanotic heart disease
  - Reverse patent ductus arteriosus
  - Tetralogy of Fallot
- Hypoxaemic respiratory disease
  - Diffuse parenchymal lung disease
  - Upper airway obstruction
- Methaemoglobinaemia
- High altitude
- Carbon monoxide poisoning

Inappropriate
- Renal neoplasia
  - Carcinoma
  - Lymphoma
  - Fibrosarcoma
  - Nephroblastoma
- Non-renal neoplasia
  - Nasal fibrosarcoma
  - Schwannoma
  - Caecal leiomyosarcoma
  - Splenic haemangiosarcoma
  - Multiple myeloma
- Non-neoplastic renal disease
  - Pyelonephritis
  - Renal replacement therapy (cats)

37.3 Differential diagnoses for erythropoietin excess.

Appropriate secondary erythrocytosis: Conditions with sustained chronic tissue hypoxia may result in a physiologically appropriate increase in EPO concentration as a compensatory effort to increase RBC mass and oxygen-carrying capacity. Chronic respiratory conditions (e.g. obstructive upper airway disease, tracheal collapse, pulmonary fibrosis) or cardiovascular conditions associated with right-to-left cardiac shunting may be associated with EPO excess. The latter tends to be due to congenital heart disorders such as reverse patent ductus arteriosus or tetralogy of Fallot (large ventricular septal defect, pulmonic stenosis, right ventricular hypertrophy and dextroposition/overriding of the aorta). These conditions allow deoxygenated blood to enter the systemic circulation; the resultant renal hypoxia increases EPO release and leads to erythrocytosis. Dogs with right-to-left shunting are more likely to suffer effects of chronic hypoxaemia and erythrocytosis, as opposed to developing congestive heart failure (Beijerink et al., 2017).

Appropriate erythrocytosis may also occur in animals living at high altitude or those with congenital methaemoglobinaemia, such as congenital methaemoglobin reductase deficiency (Giger, 2010). Obesity is a recognized cause of physiologically appropriate secondary erythrocytosis in humans, but this has not been conclusively documented in dogs or cats.

Inappropriate secondary erythrocytosis: Physiologically inappropriate secondary erythrocytosis occurs when increased concentrations of EPO are produced in the absence of hypoxaemia. There are two main theories regarding the pathophysiology of secondary inappropriate erythrocytosis:

- A tumour autonomously secretes EPO or EPO-like substances as part of a true paraneoplastic syndrome
- Associated kidney pathology induces local hypoxia and EPO is secreted by 'normal cells' in response to the hypoxia.

In some cases, it is plausible that both mechanisms occur simultaneously, and often a distinction is not made (Durno et al., 2011). Erythrocytosis has been reported most frequently with renal carcinoma/adenocarcinoma but also with lymphoma, fibrosarcoma and nephroblastoma (Bryan *et al.*, 2006; Durno *et al.*, 2011; Hergt *et al.*, 2019; Michael *et al.*, 2019).

Non-renal neoplasia causing secondary erythrocytosis has also been reported, albeit less commonly. In the dog, this has been described secondary to a nasal fibrosarcoma, caecal leiomyosarcoma, schwannoma and multiple myeloma, and in a cat secondary to splenic haemangiosarcoma (Couto *et al.*, 1989; Sato *et al.*, 2002; Yamauchi *et al.*, 2004; Seo *et al.*, 2018; Ricci *et al.*, 2021). In most cases, surgical excision or treatment of the primary neoplasm was associated with normalization of haematocrit and reduction in EPO concentration, when measured.

Non-neoplastic kidney disease has also been associated with secondary erythrocytosis. In dogs, this has been described secondary to pyelonephritis (both fungal and bacterial) and in cats secondary to renal replacement therapy (Waters and Prueter, 1988; Kessler, 2008; Giger, 2010).

Other causes of secondary erythrocytosis: There are some other causes of secondary erythrocytosis that have a variety of pathophysiological mechanisms. Thyroxine, glucocorticoids and growth hormone variably stimulate EPO production and/or directly stimulate bone marrow, likely accounting for the erythrocytosis observed in some animals with hyperthyroidism, naturally occurring hypercortisolism and hypersomatotropism. In these diseases, the erythrocytosis is typically mild and noted as an incidental finding. Occasionally, significant erythrocytosis is observed (Mansfield *et al.*, 2000) but usually these disorders are relatively easy to eliminate as a concern prior to exhaustive investigation of other causes of erythrocytosis.

Clinical features

Signalment and clinical signs may vary depending on the underlying cause (Figure 37.4). In general, clinical signs associated with absolute erythrocytosis are due to hyperviscosity or hypervolaemia. These can lead to engorgement of small blood vessels, which in turn can precipitate vessel rupture and haemorrhage. Humans with polycythaemia are predisposed to both arterial and venous thrombosis, described as a presenting feature in approximately 20% of patients. The prevalence and types of thrombosis are not well characterized in dogs or cats. Although there is the potential to affect a wide range of body systems, the brain, eye and kidney are particularly susceptible to the effects of hyperviscosity.

While engorged/red mucous membranes (Figure 37.5) are expected in animals with increased red cell mass, this can be subtle and difficult to detect clinically. Neurological signs range from lethargy and weakness to ataxia and seizures. Ocular features include retinal detachment, haemorrhage or vessel tortuosity on fundic examination. Other haemorrhagic signs, such as epistaxis, haematochezia and haematuria, can also be observed. Polyuria and polydipsia may also occur, potentially due to altered arginine vasopressin release in response to hypervolaemia and hyperviscosity (van Vonderen *et al.*, 1997).

Clinicopathological changes include increased haematocrit, haemoglobin concentration and RBC count. Biochemistry may reveal hypoglycaemia (due to increased glucose consumption from the increased number of RBCs). Urinalysis may reveal a decrease in urine specific gravity (SG) and proteinuria.

Neurological
• Lethargy
• Weakness
• Ataxia
• Seizures

Haemorrhagic
• Epistaxis
• Haematuria
• Haematochezia
• Haematemesis

Ocular
• Tortuous retinal vessels
• Retinal detachment
• Retinal haemorrhage
• Uveitis

Other
• Erythema
• Engorged mucous membranes
• Polyuria and polydipsia
• Thrombosis

37.4 Clinical signs associated with absolute erythrocytosis.

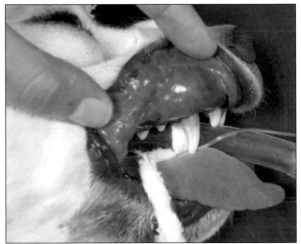

37.5 Erythematous mucous membranes in a dog with secondary erythrocytosis.
(Courtesy of Fiona Adam)

Diagnostic approach

Using a problem-oriented approach, the diagnostic work-up of erythrocytosis is relatively straightforward (Figure 37.6). The first step is to confirm an appropriate and sustained increase in haematocrit (e.g. dogs >0.65 l/l, cats >0.55 l/l), haemoglobin concentration and RBC count. While measurement of total RBC mass using labelled radioisotopes represents a definitive method for distinguishing absolute erythrocytosis from relative erythrocytosis, in practice this is rarely performed or available.

A thorough history and physical examination will help to exclude relative erythrocytosis. It may also provide clues as to other differentials for secondary erythrocytosis (e.g. a heart murmur in a young dog or a palpable abdominal mass). Assessment of total protein concentration (or total solids if using a manual refractometer) may further guide assessment of hydration status. Increased serum urea and creatinine concentrations and high urine SG may

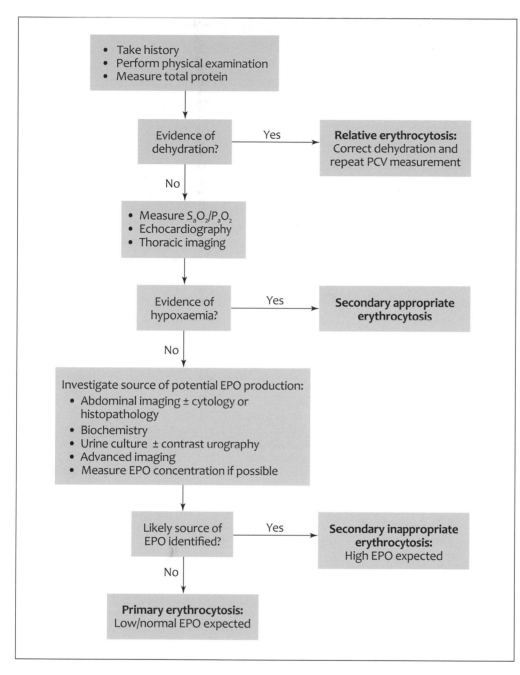

37.6 Diagnostic algorithm for investigation of erythrocytosis. EPO = erythropoietin; P_aO_2 = arterial partial pressure of oxygen; PCV = packed cell volume; S_aO_2 = arterial oxygen saturation.

Flowchart contents:

- Take history
- Perform physical examination
- Measure total protein

↓

Evidence of dehydration? — **Yes** → **Relative erythrocytosis:** Correct dehydration and repeat PCV measurement

No ↓

- Measure S_aO_2/P_aO_2
- Echocardiography
- Thoracic imaging

↓

Evidence of hypoxaemia? — **Yes** → **Secondary appropriate erythrocytosis**

No ↓

Investigate source of potential EPO production:
- Abdominal imaging ± cytology or histopathology
- Biochemistry
- Urine culture ± contrast urography
- Advanced imaging
- Measure EPO concentration if possible

↓

Likely source of EPO identified? — **Yes** → **Secondary inappropriate erythrocytosis:** High EPO expected

No ↓

Primary erythrocytosis: Low/normal EPO expected

support volume depletion. It is, however, important to note that proteinuria and a decrease in urine SG may be direct consequences of erythrocytosis itself and thus cannot be reliably used to identify kidney disease or distinguish between renal and prerenal azotaemia.

While direct measurement of EPO concentration is the next intuitive step in distinguishing primary erythrocytosis (low EPO concentration expected) from secondary erythrocytosis (high EPO concentration expected), not all commercially available EPO assays are validated for use in cats and dogs. Careful sample handling is necessary (usually frozen serum is required).

There can be an overlap between EPO concentrations found in animals with primary and secondary erythrocytosis, which can sometimes make interpretation challenging (Cook and Lothrop, 1994). As with all other endocrine disorders, interpretation of EPO concentration requires laboratory-specific reference intervals and consideration of clinical context, such as the severity of erythrocytosis. In most cases, EPO measurement forms only part of the diagnostic process, and therefore additional tests are usually performed to determine the underlying cause.

The next step is usually to rule out conditions causing appropriate secondary erythrocytosis by screening for hypoxaemia. Physical examination findings (e.g. cyanosis, cardiac murmur), thoracic imaging or echocardiography may provide evidence of an underlying disease causing hypoxaemia. Assessment of haemoglobin saturation with a pulse oximeter may be useful or ideally direct measurement of arterial blood gas if available. An arterial oxygen saturation (S_aO_2) lower than 92% or arterial partial pressure of oxygen (P_aO_2) lower than 8 kPa (60 mmHg) would be supportive of hypoxaemia. For a dog or cat breathing room air, P_aO_2 should be 10.67–13.33 kPa (80–100 mmHg). It should be noted that if hyperviscosity is marked, erythrocytosis itself can decrease tissue perfusion irrespective of the underlying aetiology and mildly reduce both S_aO_2 and P_aO_2. As a result, repeat assessment may be required following phlebotomy. For animals with reverse patent ductus arteriosus where differential cyanosis (present caudally but not cranially) is present, the pulse oximeter probe should be placed on the prepuce or vulva, or arterial blood collected from a hindlimb or the tail.

Assuming physiologically appropriate causes of secondary erythrocytosis have been excluded, the next step is to consider inappropriate causes such as neoplasia or kidney disease. Abdominal imaging, with a particular focus on evaluation of the kidneys, is important and most practically achievable with ultrasound. If structural lesions are identified, ultrasound-guided fine-needle aspirates or percutaneous core biopsies may be appropriate. If secondary erythrocytosis is suspected based upon an increased EPO concentration but neither hypoxia nor renal pathology can be identified, then careful assessment for non-renal neoplasia should be made (e.g. computed tomography of the skull, thorax and abdomen). It should be emphasized that although non-renal neoplastic causes of EPO excess have been documented, they remain rare.

Finally, if disorders causing secondary erythrocytosis have been reliably excluded, then a diagnosis of primary erythrocytosis can be made. Such a diagnosis would be supported by a low or low-normal concentration of EPO. Bone marrow sampling does not reliably distinguish between primary and secondary erythrocytosis in dogs and cats.

Treatment

In animals with secondary erythrocytosis, treatment of the underlying cause is important if possible. However, irrespective of the underlying aetiology, emergency stabilization of the erythrocytosis may be required.

Acute management

Acute management of erythrocytosis is indicated when severe clinical signs related to hypervolaemia or hyperviscosity are present, or to reduce the risk of haemorrhage or vascular thrombosis prior to surgery to address the underlying cause. Phlebotomy is the mainstay of acute treatment and can be achieved in a similar manner to blood collection from the jugular vein of a blood donor. In cats, a 60 ml syringe attached to a 19 G butterfly catheter can be used. In dogs, commercially available blood collection systems are easiest to use. Ideally, blood should be collected with anticoagulant within the line to prevent clotting. Removal of 10–15 ml/kg of blood is performed and followed by replacement of volume with a crystalloid solution. This should be repeated until a target haematocrit is reached (usually <0.60 l/l for dogs and <0.50 l/l for cats). Sedation may be necessary, particularly in cats. Phlebotomy itself can be technically challenging in severely polycythaemic animals due to the viscosity of the blood, and larger-gauge needles may be required.

As an alternative to traditional phlebotomy, the use of medical leeches (e.g. *Hirudo medicinalis*) has been documented in veterinary medicine (Nett *et al.*, 2001) (Figure 37.7). It is possible that hirudotherapy is well tolerated because leech saliva has been shown to exert local anaesthetic properties. Leeches are applied to a clipped area and typically feed for 10–20 minutes before they detach. In addition to the blood lost through feeding, blood often continues to ooze from the sites of leech attachment over the following 24 hours due to anticoagulant substances secreted by the leech. Animals are ideally hospitalized during this time for monitoring of wounds and possible

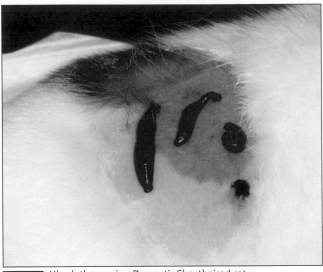

37.7 Hirudotherapy in a Domestic Shorthaired cat.
(Courtesy of Sara-Ann Dickson)

crystalloid fluid therapy. Between feeding and subsequent wound bleeding, it is possible for each leech to remove up to 20 ml of blood in a 24-hour period. The availability of hirudotherapy in an acute emergency setting may limit its use.

In an animal with physiologically appropriate secondary erythrocytosis, the benefits of phlebotomy or hirudotherapy have to be balanced against the risks associated with removing the body's 'coping mechanism' for hypoxaemia. In such cases, a gentler approach should be considered, such as removal of smaller 5 ml/kg aliquots of blood, with a higher target PCV of <0.65 l/l in dogs and <0.55 l/l in cats. Similarly, the use of fluid therapy following phlebotomy may be contraindicated in animals with some forms of cardiac disease.

Chronic management

In cases of inappropriate secondary erythrocytosis, treatment of the underlying disease usually resolves the erythrocytosis. This may involve surgical resection of a primary renal tumour or other non-renal EPO-secreting masses.

For cases of secondary erythrocytosis where the underlying disease cannot be reversed (e.g. congenital cyanotic heart disease), chronic management of erythrocytosis may be required to improve quality of life. Repeated phlebotomy may be an option if tolerated. The interval between required phlebotomies is variable and should be determined by regular monitoring of individual cases. Possible complications of chronic phlebotomy include thrombotic disease, hypoproteinaemia and iron deficiency.

Myelosuppressive agents can also be considered in animals requiring chronic therapy. In veterinary medicine, this is most commonly achieved with hydroxycarbamide (also known as hydroxyurea). In dogs, a loading dose of 30 mg/kg orally q24h for 7 days has been described, before decreasing to a maintenance dose of 15 mg/kg orally q24h. Regular monitoring is recommended to screen for neutropenic and thrombocytopenic complications as well as to assess the treatment response. Haematology should be performed every 7–14 days until the haematocrit is stable, and then the interval gradually extended to every 4–8 weeks. Other reported side effects include gastrointestinal signs such as anorexia and vomiting and dermatological signs such as alopecia and sloughing of the nails.

In cats, haemolytic crises as a result of methaemoglobinaemia have been reported. Doses of 25 mg/kg orally three times per week are recommended as an alternative in cats. If possible, the drug should be compounded to increase dosing accuracy in smaller animals.

Antithrombotic drugs are not routinely recommended in most dogs or cats. In human medicine, low-dose aspirin does not significantly decrease the risk of thrombosis, but antithrombotic drugs are often advocated due to the low risk of major bleeding associated with their use (Squizzato et al., 2013).

In a small case series of appropriate secondary erythrocytosis in dogs with cyanotic heart disease, the use of sildenafil (0.5 mg/kg q12h) was associated with an improvement in exercise tolerance as well as a more prolonged reduction in erythrocytosis (Nakamura et al., 2011). This may represent an alternative (and potentially better tolerated) strategy to myelosuppressive therapy in this subset of cases.

Prognosis

For disorders of EPO excess, the prognosis is highly variable and largely depends on the underlying cause. For dogs with underlying renal carcinoma, survival times of 7.5–32 months have been reported following nephrectomy in a small case series (Bryan et al., 2006). Thus far, the presence of erythrocytosis preoperatively has not been associated with a decrease in survival in this species (Bryan et al., 2006). In dogs with appropriate erythrocytosis secondary to reverse patent ductus arteriosus, survival of 6–22 months was reported in a small case series (Moore and Stepien, 2001).

References and further reading

Beijerink NJ, Oyama MA and Bonagura JD (2017) Congenital heart disease. In: Textbook of Veterinary Internal Medicine: Diseases of the Dog and Cat, 8th edn, ed. SJ Ettinger, EC Feldman and E Côté, pp. 1207–1248. Elsevier, St Louis

Beurlet S, Krief P, Sansonetti A et al. (2011) Identification of JAK2 mutations in canine primary polycythemia. Experimental Hematology 39, 542–545

Bryan JN, Henry CJ, Turnquist SE et al. (2006) Primary renal neoplasia of dogs. Journal of Veterinary Internal Medicine 20, 1155–1160

Campora C, Freeman KP, Lewis FI et al. (2011) Determination of haematological reference intervals in healthy adult greyhounds. Journal of Small Animal Practice 52, 301–309

Clark P and Parry BW (1997) Some haematological values of Irish Wolfhounds in Australia. Australian Veterinary Journal 75, 523–523

Cook SM and Lothrop CDJ (1994) Serum erythropoietin concentrations measured by radioimmunoassay in normal, polycythemic, and anemic dogs and cats. Journal of Veterinary Internal Medicine 8, 18–25

Couto CG, Boudrieau RJ and Zanjani ED (1989) Tumor-associated erythrocytosis in a dog with nasal fibrosarcoma. Journal of Veterinary Internal Medicine 3, 183–185

Durno AS, Webb JA, Gauthier MJ and Bienzle D (2011) Polycythemia and inappropriate erythropoietin concentrations in two dogs with renal T-cell lymphoma. Journal of the American Animal Hospital Association 47, 122–128

Giger U (2010) Polycythemia and erythrocytosis. In: Textbook of Veterinary Internal Medicine, 7th edn, ed. SJ Ettinger and EC Feldman, pp. 279–283. Saunders Elsevier, St Louis

Hergt F, Mortier F, Werres C, Flatz K and von Bomhard W (2019) Renal nephroblastoma in a 17-month-old Jack Russell Terrier. Journal of the American Animal Hospital Association 55, e55503

Kessler M (2008) Secondary polycythaemia associated with high plasma erythropoietin concentrations in a dog with a necrotising pyelonephritis. Journal of Small Animal Practice 49, 363–366

Lavoué R, Geffré A, Braun JP et al. (2014) Breed-specific hematologic reference intervals in healthy adult Dogues de Bordeaux. Veterinary Clinical Pathology 43, 352–361

Mansfield C, Mooney CT and Jones B (2000) Secondary polycythaemia, hyperviscosity syndrome and unilateral adrenocortical adenoma in a dog. Australian Veterinary Practitioner 30, 162–167

Michael AE, Grimes JA, Volstad NJ, Osekavage KE and Koenig A (2019) inappropriate secondary erythrocytosis in a dog with renal sarcoma. Topics in Companion Animal Medicine 36, 9–11

Moore KW and Stepien RL (2001) Hydroxyurea for treatment of polycythemia secondary to right-to-left shunting patent ductus arteriosus in 4 dogs. Journal of Veterinary Internal Medicine 15, 418–421

Mortier F, Strohmeyer K, Hartmann K and Unterer S (2015) Acute haemorrhagic diarrhoea syndrome in dogs: 108 cases. Veterinary Record 176, 627

Nakamura K, Yamasaki M, Ohta H et al. (2011) Effects of sildenafil citrate on five dogs with Eisenmenger's syndrome. Journal of Small Animal Practice 52, 595–598

Nett CS, Arnold P and Glaus TM (2001) Leeching as initial treatment in a cat with polycythaemia vera. Journal of Small Animal Practice 42, 554–556

Peterson ME, Kintzer PP and Kass PH (1996) Pretreatment clinical and laboratory findings in dogs with hypoadrenocorticism: 225 cases (1979–1993). Journal of the American Veterinary Medical Association 208, 85–91

Ricci M, De Feo G, Konar M et al. (2021) Multiple myeloma and primary erythrocytosis in a dog. Canadian Veterinary Journal 62, 849–853

Sato K, Hikasa Y, Morita T et al. (2002) Secondary erythrocytosis associated with high plasma erythropoietin concentrations in a dog with cecal leiomyosarcoma. Journal of the American Veterinary Medical Association 220, 486–490

Seo KW, Hong H, An SA, Lee JK and Rebhun R (2018) Secondary inappropriate polycythemia with splenic hemangiosarcoma in a young adult cat. Canadian Veterinary Journal 59, 1320–1324

Sheerer KN, Couto CG, Marin LM et al. (2013) Haematological and biochemical values in North American Scottish deerhounds. Journal of Small Animal Practice 54, 354–360

Squizzato A, Romualdi E, Passamonti F and Middeldorp S (2013) Antiplatelet drugs for polycythaemia vera and essential thrombocythaemia. Cochrane Database of Systematic Reviews 4, CD006503

Torres AR, Cassle SE, Haymore M and Hill RC (2014) Hematologic differences between Dachshunds and mixed breed dogs. Veterinary Clinical Pathology 43, 519–524

Uhríková I, Lačňáková A, Tandlerová K et al. (2013) Haematological and biochemical variations among eight sighthound breeds. Australian Veterinary Journal 91, 452–459

van Vonderen IK, Meyer HP, Kraus JS and Kooistra HS (1997) Polyuria and polydipsia and disturbed vasopressin release in 2 dogs with secondary polycythemia. Journal of Veterinary Internal Medicine 11, 300–303

Waters DJ and Prueter JC (1988) Secondary polycythemia associated with renal disease in the dog: two case reports and review of literature. Journal of the American Animal Hospital Association 24, 109–114

Yamauchi A, Ohta T, Okada T et al. (2004) Secondary erythrocytosis associated with schwannoma in a dog. Journal of Veterinary Medical Science 66, 1605–1608

Zaldívar-López S, Marín LM, Iazbik MC et al. (2011) Clinical pathology of Greyhounds and other sighthounds. Veterinary Clinical Pathology 40, 414–425

Chapter 38

Gastrointestinal tumours

Patty Lathan

Introduction

The gastrointestinal tract is considered by many to be the largest endocrine gland in the body. Cells that synthesize gastrin, glucagon, pancreatic peptide and many other peptide hormones are called amine precursor uptake and decarboxylation (APUD) cells, as they are able to produce and metabolize biogenic amines such as adrenaline (epinephrine), noradrenaline (norepinephrine), dopamine and serotonin. The central nervous system, thyroid gland (C cells that secrete calcitonin), parathyroid gland and placenta also contain APUD cells. The term 'APUDoma' refers to tumours arising from APUD cells. They are also known as neuroendocrine tumours. These tumours are typically named after the hormones they secrete, including gastrinomas, glucagonomas, somatostatinomas and pancreatic polypeptidomas. An exception to this nomenclature is carcinoid tumours, which originate from neuroendocrine cells throughout the gastrointestinal and respiratory tracts. Somatostatinoma has been reported in one dog with concurrent gastrinoma (Hoenerhoff and Kiupel, 2004); clinical signs were likely due to hypergastrinaemia.

Gastrinoma

Gastrinoma is a rare tumour in dogs and cats; the largest case series included only four dogs (Green and Gartrell, 1997). It has also been reported in a Mexican wolf (Struthers *et al.*, 2018). The clinical syndrome associated with gastrinoma was first described in humans in 1955, when Zollinger and Ellison reported two patients with pancreatic islet cell tumours and intractable peptic ulcers in the jejunum. In healthy adult humans, dogs and cats, gastrin is produced by G cells in the gastric antrum and duodenum; however, most gastrinomas in all three species arise from non-beta islet cells of the pancreas. Gastrin stimulates the release of histamine from enterochromaffin-like cells in the body of the stomach; histamine binds to H2 receptors on the parietal cells, triggering the release of hydrochloric acid. Gastrin also has a trophic effect on gastric and duodenal mucosa.

Clinical features and diagnosis

Gastrinomas and the resultant excess gastrin concentrations cause gastric mucosal hyperplasia, gastrointestinal tract ulceration, vomiting, haematemesis, diarrhoea, melaena, anorexia and weight loss. The diarrhoea may be secondary to inactivation of digestive enzymes (such as trypsin, lipase and amylase) by gastrin. Non-specific signs, small tumour size and the rarity of the condition often delay diagnosis. Older dogs and cats (>8 years old) are affected, and there is no apparent breed or sex predisposition. Physical examination is often non-specific but may reveal fever and abdominal pain; hypersalivation can also occur secondary to nausea, oesophagitis or both. Gastric or intestinal perforation may result in signs of shock.

Clinicopathological abnormalities are non-specific, and include neutrophilic leucocytosis, anaemia (likely due to blood loss from ulceration), hypoalbuminaemia, and increased alkaline phosphatase (ALP) and alanine amino transferase (ALT) activities. Hypokalaemia and hypochloraemia are occasionally present in vomiting animals.

Increased circulating gastrin concentrations are supportive of a diagnosis of gastrinoma, but histopathology is required for definitive diagnosis. Care must be taken when submitting samples for measurement of gastrin concentrations and subsequent interpretation of results. Follow specific laboratory recommendations for transporting fasted serum samples; freezing the samples is likely ideal. Dogs with gastrinoma usually have gastrin concentrations more than three times the upper limit of the reference interval, and values more than 10 times the reference interval have been reported (Altschul *et al.*, 1997; Green and Gartrell, 1997; Feldman and Nelson, 2004). Other diseases, including kidney disease and chronic enteropathies, can also result in increased gastrin concentrations. Values are less than three times the upper limit of the reference interval in approximately 95% of dogs with chronic enteropathy; however, some overlap exists (Heilmann *et al.*, 2017). Additionally, treatment with a proton pump inhibitor such as omeprazole will increase gastrin concentrations due to loss of negative feedback. The H2-blocker famotidine also causes increased gastrin concentrations, but to a lesser extent. Thus, postponing gastrin measurement for 1 week following proton pump inhibitor or H2-blocker administration is recommended (Parente *et al.*, 2014; Heilmann *et al.*, 2017).

Abdominal radiographs are usually unhelpful with diagnosis because gastrinomas tend to be very small. Ultrasound examination may identify primary lesions in the pancreas (usually single, but multiple have been reported) or metastasis to the liver or abdominal lymph nodes. Ultrasound examination may also identify non-specific thickening of the stomach and duodenum. Unfortunately, lack of identification of masses with abdominal ultrasonography does not exclude the diagnosis. The use of computed tomography (CT) for identification of gastrinoma has not been reported. Nuclear scintigraphy using a somatostatin analogue has been used to diagnose gastrinoma in a dog, but this technique has limited availability in primary care settings (Altschul et al., 1997).

In dogs or cats diagnosed with gastrinoma, gastroduodenoscopy usually reveals ulceration in the stomach and duodenum. The oesophagus may also be ulcerated. Histopathological findings from the stomach and small intestine generally reveal non-specific inflammation. Thus, although endoscopy is helpful in identifying gross masses, and ulceration may increase suspicion of gastrinoma, it does not provide a definitive diagnosis.

Histopathology is required for definitive diagnosis of gastrinoma. Unfortunately, metastases in the liver or abdominal lymph nodes, or both, are identified in most cases at surgery. The majority of gastrinomas are found in the pancreas. Masses are typically small, and may be less than 1 cm in diameter, or even microscopic. In one dog, a neuroendocrine carcinoma was identified in the regional lymph nodes when there was no gross or histopathological evidence of gastrinoma in the pancreas (Green and Gartrell, 1997). Immunohistochemical antibody staining of these neuroendocrine tumours confirms the production of gastrin.

Treatment

Surgical removal of both the primary tumour and metastases, when possible, is recommended. However, when surgery or complete resection is not possible, treatments are aimed at reducing gastric acid production. Proton pump inhibitors such as omeprazole are the mainstay of therapy. Sucralfate is often added to treat ulceration. The somatostatin analogue octreotide has also been used to inhibit gastrin production. In one dog, octreotide was administered subcutaneously, starting at 2 μg/kg twice daily, and gradually increased to 20 μg/kg three times daily over a period of 14 months (Altschul et al., 1997).

Prognosis

The prognosis for long-term survival is poor, with a median survival of 2 months. Some cases experience minimal improvement following surgery and are euthanized soon thereafter. Others respond well to surgical and/or medical management and have been reported to live for over a year. In cats that are diagnosed ante-mortem, prognosis may be better than in dogs (>1 year), but the paucity of reported feline cases makes it difficult to draw such a conclusion (Diroff et al., 2006).

Glucagonoma

Glucagon-producing tumours are rare in dogs and cats – fewer than 20 cases have been reported; only two of these cases were in cats (Asakawa et al., 2013; Sahinduran and Ozmen, 2017). Although most glucagon-producing tumours are found in the pancreas, there are reports of glucagon-staining nodules in the liver, spleen, adrenal glands and abdominal lymph nodes with no obvious pancreatic pathology (Miller et al., 1991; Allenspach et al., 2000; Mizuno et al., 2009; Asakawa et al., 2013). Glucagon is secreted from alpha cells in the pancreatic islets in healthy dogs and cats, and increases blood glucose concentration through gluconeogenesis and glycogenolysis. In healthy animals, glucagon is protective against hypoglycaemia. In animals with glucagonoma, excess glucagon may lead to hyperglycaemia and accelerated amino acid turnover. Subsequent decreased plasma amino acid concentrations result in the most recognizable clinical feature of glucagonoma – superficial necrolytic dermatitis (SND). Dogs and cats with SND have characteristic skin lesions, predominantly involving the paw pads and interdigital spaces. Even though SND is reported in most cases of glucagonoma, the majority of cases with SND do not have glucagonoma and are instead diagnosed with hepatopathy. Thus, the other, perhaps more common, name for SND is 'hepatocutaneous syndrome'. Interestingly, some dogs with characteristic liver pathology and SND, without evidence of glucagonoma, are also diabetic (Loftus et al., 2017).

Clinical features and diagnosis

Glucagonoma is most common in older dogs, with no apparent breed or sex predisposition. Most dogs eventually diagnosed with glucagonoma initially present with signs attributed to their dermatological lesions. Characteristic lesions are most common in areas exposed to mechanical trauma, including the muzzle and mucocutaneous junctions, and contact surfaces of appendages, including paw pads, elbow joints and tibiotarsal joints. Lesions are erythematous and ulcerative; crusting of the footpads is usually evident. Fissures often develop and cause severely painful paws, significantly contributing to morbidity (Figure 38.1). Lesions may also appear on the trunk. Other non-specific clinical signs include lethargy, decreased appetite and weight loss. Polyuria and polydipsia may occur, and their presence is indicative of diabetes mellitus.

Clinicopathological abnormalities include mild non-regenerative anaemia and increased ALT and ALP activities. Decreased albumin, blood urea nitrogen and cholesterol concentrations have also been noted but are non-specific. Diabetes mellitus is not uncommon in dogs with glucagonoma (present in less than 50% of cases) but can also occur in dogs with SND due to hepatic disease, so the finding of hyperglycaemia in a dog with characteristic SND lesions is not diagnostic for glucagonoma. Since the major differential diagnosis for glucagonoma is hepatic disease causing SND, liver function testing (e.g. bile acid stimulation or blood ammonia concentration) is recommended. Hepatic function should be normal in dogs with glucagonoma.

Glucagon concentrations are typically increased in dogs with glucagonoma, despite normo- or hyperglycaemia. Unfortunately, commercial availability of a glucagon assay is limited.

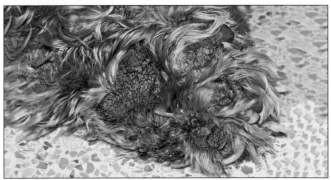

38.1 A 12-year-old intact male Cocker Spaniel presented with skin lesions characteristic of superficial necrolytic dermatitis. Note the crusting and fissures on the paw pads.
(Courtesy of Tom Thompson)

Diagnostic imaging, including thoracic radiography and abdominal ultrasonography, may help identify the primary tumour and potential metastases to the liver, spleen, adrenal glands and regional lymph nodes. Unfortunately, approximately half of the reported glucagonomas were too small to be identified with ultrasonography. Fine-needle aspirates of the primary or metastatic lesion may provide supportive evidence if findings are consistent with a neuroendocrine carcinoma. Ultrasound examination often reveals a honeycomb or Swiss-cheese appearance of the liver in dogs with SND induced by liver disease, but not in dogs with glucagonoma. Computed tomography may be helpful but is not well described.

Histopathology of skin lesions reveals marked para-keratotic hyperkeratosis, epidermal oedema and hyper-plasia, and extensive crusting (Figure 38.2). Secondary infection may also be present and should be treated. Note that these are characteristic lesions of SND, not glucago-noma. Histopathology and immunohistochemistry (staining for glucagon) of the primary or metastatic lesion is nec-essary for definitive diagnosis. Staining for other gastro-intestinal hormones may also be positive in glucagonomas; the clinical significance is unknown.

Treatment

Treatment of glucagonoma is aimed at surgical removal of the primary tumour and metastatic lesions (when possible), addressing SND and secondary infections, and treating concurrent and related disease, including diabetes mellitus and non-specific signs of tumour growth. Surgical resec-tion of the primary and metastatic lesions is the only defini-tive treatment, and metastasis is usually present at the time of diagnosis. Potential complications of surgery include pancreatitis (potentially life-threatening) and thrombo-embolic disease. There are two case reports of resolution and long-term survival in dogs following surgical excision of the primary tumours, despite lymph node metastasis in one dog (surgically excised) and hepatic metastasis in the other (not excised) (Torres et al., 1997; Langer et al., 2003).

The primary treatment for SND is amino acid infusion (8.5% amino acid solution, 28.5 ml/kg over 6–8 hours). Weekly administration is recommended initially, but

38.2 Histopathology of tissue from the paw pad of a dog with superficial necrolytic dermatitis. Note the marked hyperparakeratotic hyperkeratosis (red line), subparakeratotic oedema (black line) and basal epithelial cell hyperplasia (blue line). (Haematoxylin and eosin stain; original magnification X10)
(Courtesy of Dr Brittany Baughman)

treatments are then spaced out further as long as lesions remain significantly improved or resolved (Byrne, 1999). In a dog with SND due to hepatic disease, co-administration of intravenous lipids (Intralipid, Baxter Healthcare, 20% solution, 7 ml/kg) increased the necessary amino acid infusion interval from 1.5 weeks to 6.5 weeks (Bach and Glasser, 2013).

In a dog with metastatic glucagonoma and SND that failed to respond to amino acid therapy, the somatostatin analogue octreotide was given subcutaneously, at dosages varying from 2 µg/kg twice daily to 1 µg/kg four times daily. This improved the clinical signs for 6 weeks until the dog was euthanized due to progressive metastatic disease (Oberkirchner et al., 2010).

Prognosis

Unfortunately, the long-term prognosis for dogs with glucagonoma is poor, and cases are usually euthanized due to metastatic disease or inability to control SND. Following surgical excision of the primary lesion, two dogs that survived the immediate postoperative period lived for at least 4–6 months (Torres et al., 1997; Langer et al., 2003). Other dogs have succumbed to complications associated with pancreatitis following surgery (Gross et al., 1990). Dogs undergoing medical therapy alone tend to survive for only a few weeks. In the two reported feline cases, one survived 11 months after initial diagnosis of a hepatic glucagon-producing tumour but was euthanized following the development of SND (Asakawa et al., 2013). The other cat survived for only 2 weeks after diagnosis (Sahinduran and Ozmen, 2017).

Carcinoids

Carcinoids are uncommon tumours that originate from neuroendocrine cells and have been found throughout the gastrointestinal tract, hepatobiliary system and lungs in humans and dogs. They have been reported in the pancreas, hepatobiliary system and duodenum in cats. Carcinoids can secrete a variety of amines, including hista-mine, serotonin, bradykinin and prostaglandins. They may also produce hormones such as gastrin and glucagon out-side of the pancreas; as the clinical signs are due to the effects of the hormones, those tumours are discussed above under 'Gastrinoma' and 'Glucagonoma', respectively.

Ten percent of humans with metastatic carcinoids experience 'carcinoid syndrome', characterized by flush-ing, diarrhoea, bronchospasm and cyanosis. Not all signs are experienced by all those affected with carcinoid syndrome, and signs depend on the location of and hormones produced by the carcinoid. Most signs in dogs and cats, however, are thought to be related to the physical presence of the tumour, and include anorexia, weight loss, vomiting and diarrhoea. Vasoactive amines may contribute to clinical signs, particularly diarrhoea, but are not routinely measured. One dog with an ileocaecal mass experienced paroxysmal ventricular tachycardia and melaena that resolved following surgical excision, but vasoactive amine concentrations were not reported (Tappin et al., 2008).

Clinicopathological features depend upon the site of the carcinoid and include increased liver enzyme activities in cases with hepatobiliary tumours, and anaemia in dogs and cats with melaena due to a tumour in the gastro-intestinal tract. Abdominal ultrasonography or CT helps to identify the location and extent of the lesions, and evidence of metastasis. Fine-needle aspiration may help identify neuroendocrine cells. Laparotomy, excision and histopathology provide both treatment and definitive diagnosis.

Prognosis for carcinoids is variable. Based on single case reports, dogs and cats that had extensive disease or metastasis had a short survival time following diagnosis and either died or were euthanized within weeks. However, most dogs and cats without metastasis and with surgically resectable tumours had good long-term survival.

Pancreatic polypeptidoma

Pancreatic polypeptide is secreted by F cells in the pancreatic islets and has an inhibitory effect on gastric acid secretion, postprandial pancreatic exocrine secretion and gastric emptying. Humans with pancreatic polypeptidoma often have absent or mild signs, including abdominal pain and diarrhoea. Pancreatic polypeptidoma has been reported in two dogs, one of which had concurrent insulinoma and the other concurrent lymphoplasmacytic gastritis (Zerbe et al., 1989; Cruz Cardona et al., 2010). In these dogs, diagnosis was made based on immunohistochemical staining of the pancreatic tumours for pancreatic polypeptide; hormone concentrations were not measured. Clinical signs included chronic vomiting in both dogs, chronic diarrhoea in one dog and a gastric ulcer in the dog with concurrent insulinoma. Given the concurrent disease, it is difficult to determine which, if any, clinical signs were attributable to the pancreatic polypeptidoma, although chronic diarrhoea is consistent with signs seen in humans.

References and further reading

Allenspach K, Arnold P, Glaus T et al. (2000) Glucagon-producing neuroendocrine tumour associated with hypoaminoacidaemia and skin lesions. Journal of Small Animal Practice 41, 402–406

Altschul M, Simpson KW, Dykes NL et al. (1997) Evaluation of somatostatin analogues for the detection and treatment of gastrinoma in a dog. Journal of Small Animal Practice 38, 286–291

Asakawa MG, Cullen JM and Linder KE (2013) Necrolytic migratory erythema associated with a glucagon-producing primary hepatic neuroendocrine carcinoma in a cat. Veterinary Dermatology 24, 466–469

Bach JF and Glasser SA (2013) A case of necrolytic migratory erythema managed for 24 months with intravenous amino acid and lipid infusions. Canadian Veterinary Journal 54, 873–875

Byrne KP (1999) Metabolic epidermal necrosis-hepatocutaneous syndrome. Veterinary Clinics of North America: Small Animal Practice 29, 1337–1355

Cruz Cardona JA, Wamsley HL, Farina LL and Kiupel M (2010) Metastatic pancreatic polypeptide-secreting islet cell tumor in a dog. Veterinary Clinical Pathology 39, 371–376

Diroff JS, Sanders NA, McDonough SP and Holt DE (2006) Gastrin-secreting neoplasia in a cat. Journal of Veterinary Internal Medicine 20, 1245–1247

Feldman EC and Nelson RW (2004) Gastrinoma, glucagonoma, and other APUDomas. In: Canine and Feline Endocrinology and Reproduction, 3rd edn, ed. EC Feldman and RW Nelson, pp. 645–658. Saunders, St Louis

Green RA and Gartrell CL (1997) Gastrinoma: a retrospective study of four cases (1985–1995). Journal of the American Animal Hospital Association 33, 524–527

Gross TL, O'Brien TD, Davies AP and Long RE (1990) Glucagon-producing pancreatic endocrine tumors in two dogs with superficial necrolytic dermatitis. Journal of the American Veterinary Medical Association 197, 1619–1622

Heilmann RM, Berghoff N, Grützner N et al. (2017) Effect of gastric acid-suppressive therapy and biological variation of serum gastrin concentrations in dogs with chronic enteropathies. BMC Veterinary Research 13, 321

Hoenerhoff M and Kiupel M (2004) Concurrent gastrinoma and somatostatinoma in a 10-year-old Portuguese water dog. Journal of Comparative Pathology 130, 313–318

Langer NB, Jergens AE and Miles KG (2003) Canine glucagonoma. Compendium on Continuing Education for the Practicing Veterinarian 25, 56–63

Loftus JP, Center SA, Lucy JM et al. (2017) Characterization of aminoaciduria and hypoaminoacidemia in dogs with hepatocutaneous syndrome. American Journal of Veterinary Research 78, 735–744

Miller WH, Anderson WI and McCann JP (1991) Necrolytic migratory erythema in a dog with a glucagon-secreting endocrine tumor. Veterinary Dermatology 2, 179–182

Mizuno T, Hiraoka H, Yoshioka C et al. (2009) Superficial necrolytic dermatitis associated with extrapancreatic glucagonoma in a dog. Veterinary Dermatology 20, 72–79

Oberkirchner U, Linder KE, Zadrozny L and Olivry T (2010) Successful treatment of canine necrolytic migratory erythema (superficial necrolytic dermatitis) due to metastatic glucagonoma with octreotide. Veterinary Dermatology 21, 510–516

Parente NL, Olivier NB, Refsal KR and Johnson CA (2014) Serum concentrations of gastrin after famotidine and omeprazole administration to dogs. Journal of Veterinary Internal Medicine 28, 1465–1470

Sahinduran S and Ozmen O (2017) Necrolytic migratory erythema in a cat with glucagonoma syndrome. Acta Scientiae Veterinariae 45 (Suppl 1), 223

Struthers JD, Robl N, Wong VM and Kiupel M (2018) Gastrinoma and Zollinger–Ellison syndrome in canids: a literature review and a case in a Mexican gray wolf. Journal of Veterinary Diagnostic Investigation 30, 584–588

Tappin S, Brown P and Ferasin L (2008) An intestinal neuroendocrine tumour associated with paroxysmal ventricular tachycardia and melaena in a 10-year-old boxer. Journal of Small Animal Practice 49, 33–37

Torres SMF, Caywood DD, O'Brien TD, O'Leary TP and McKeever PJ (1997) Resolution of superficial necrolytic dermatitis following excision of a glucagon-secreting pancreatic neoplasm in a dog. Journal of the American Animal Hospital Association 33, 313–319

Zerbe CA, Boosinger TR, Grabau JH, Pletcher JM and O'Dorisio TM (1989) Pancreatic polypeptide and insulin-secreting tumor in a dog with duodenal ulcers and hypertrophic gastritis. Journal of Veterinary Internal Medicine 3, 178–182

Zollinger RM and Ellison EH (1955) Primary peptic ulcerations of the jejunum associated with islet cell tumors of the pancreas. Annals of Surgery 142, 709–723

Index

Page numbers in *italics* refer to figures.